Fundamentals of Family Medicine

Third Edition

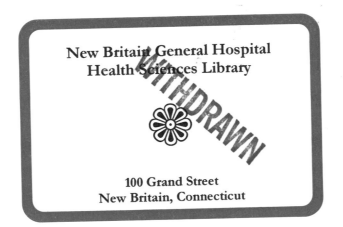

Springer
New York
Berlin
Heidelberg
Hong Kong
London
Milan
Paris
Tokyo

Fundamentals of Family Medicine

The Family Medicine Clerkship Textbook

Third Edition

ROBERT B. TAYLOR, M.D.   Editor

Professor of Family Medicine
Oregon Health & Science University
   School of Medicine
Portland, Oregon

Associate Editors

ALAN K. DAVID, M.D.
Professor and Chairman
Department of Family and
   Community Medicine
Medical College of Wisconsin
Milwaukee, Wisconsin

SCOTT A. FIELDS, M.D.
Professor and Vice Chairman
Department of Family Medicine
Oregon Health & Science University
   School of Medicine
Portland, Oregon

D. MELESSA PHILLIPS, M.D.
Professor and Chairman
Department of Family Medicine
University of Mississippi School
   of Medicine
Jackson, Mississippi

JOSEPH E. SCHERGER, M.D., M.P.H.
Dean, College of Medicine
Florida State University College
   of Medicine
Tallahassee, Florida

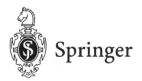

Springer

Robert B. Taylor, M.D.
Professor of Family Medicine
Department of Family Medicine
Oregon Health & Science University
  School of Medicine
Portland, OR 97201-3098, USA

Associate Editors

Alan K. David, M.D.
Professor and Chairman
Department of Family and
  Community Medicine
Medical College of Wisconsin
Milwaukee, WI 53226-0509, USA

Scott A. Fields, M.D.
Professor and Vice Chairman
Department of Family Medicine
Oregon Health & Science University
  School of Medicine
Portland, OR 97201-3098, USA

D. Melessa Phillips, M.D.
Professor and Chairman
Department of Family Medicine
University of Mississippi School
  of Medicine
Jackson, MS 39216-4500, USA

Joseph E. Scherger, M.D., M.P.H.
Dean, College of Medicine
Florida State University College
  of Medicine
Tallahassee, FL 32306-4300, USA

With 30 illustrations
Library of Congress Cataloging-in-Publication Data
Fundamentals of family medicine : the family medicine clerkship textbook /
  Robert B. Taylor, editor.—3rd ed.
    p. cm.
    "Consists of an overview of the principles of generalist healthcare followed by 27 all
  new chapters from the 6th edition of Family medicine"—Pref.
    Includes bibliographical references and index.
    ISBN 0-387-95479-1 (softcover : alk. paper)
    1. Family medicine. I. Title: Family medicine clerkship textbook. II. Taylor, Robert B.
  III. Family medicine.

RA418.5.F3 F86 2002
616—dc21   2002020938

ISBN 0-387-95479-1   Printed on acid-free paper.

Printed in the United States of America.

9 8 7 6 5 4 3 2 1   SPIN 10874621

www.springer-ny.com

Springer-Verlag   New York Berlin Heidelberg
A member of BertelsmannSpringer Science +Business Media GmbH

Preface

This third edition of *Fundamentals of Family Medicine* is designed to be the course textbook for Family Medicine/Primary Care Clerkships in medical schools and a reference source to manage the everyday health problems seen in family practice. The chapters that follow are intended to describe the process by which family physicians provide high quality, comprehensive care for their patients, and to serve as the basis for small group discussions by students and faculty.

The book consists of an overview of the Principles of Generalist Healthcare, followed by 27 all new chapters from the 6th edition of *Family Medicine: Principles and Practice*.[1] I selected the chapter topics based on the content of general and family practice as recorded in the National Ambulatory Medical Care Survey (see Chapter 1, Table 1.1) and on the patient care problems seen by the physicians in our own Family Health Center.

This third edition contains two topics not discussed in prior editions of the book. The first is Chapter 27, "The Family Physician's Role in Responding to Biological and Chemical Terrorism." Since the second edition, the possibility that the family physician may face the threat or actual event of a terrorist attack has become a grim reality. The other new chapter is "Information Mastery: Practical Evidence-Based Family Medicine," an approach that is reflected in all clinical chapters in the book.

Preparing medical students to deal with uncertainty and diverse types of clinical challenges is an important goal of medical schools.[2] One key to developing this vital competency is understanding how the family physician can identify, prioritize, and manage the multiple problems of many patients in time limited visits. The *how* is the generalist approach, described in an updated Chapter 1. This approach, which emphasizes patient- and family-centered, evidence-based concepts and focused clinical questions, is reinforced through the case presentations and discussion questions at the end of each clinical chapter. The patients in the case scenarios are all members of one extended family, affording the reader a sense of continuity of care and an awareness of the effects of illness on various family members. The Nelson family, the case presentations, and discussion questions are all explained in the section, "Notes for the Reader."

I am grateful for the contributions of the authors and the four associate editors: Alan K. David, M.D.; D. Melessa Phillips, M.D.; Scott A. Fields, M.D.;

and Joseph E. Scherger, M.D., M.P.H. I also thank Coelleda O'Neil and Lily Cha for their assistance in manuscript preparation. In preparing this third edition, I have spoken with numerous medical students and family medicine educators, and many of their thoughts are found in the pages that follow.

Robert B. Taylor, M.D.
Portland, Oregon

References

1. Taylor RB, ed., Family Medicine: Principles and Practice, 6th Edition. New York: Springer Verlag, 2003.
2. Fargason CA, Evans HH, Ashworth CS, Capper SA. The importance of preparing medical students to manage different types of uncertainty. Acad Med 1997; 72: 668–92.

Contents

Notes for the Reader

To the Student

Your time on the Family Medicine/Primary Care Clerkship may be the most important of all in medical school.[1] Here you will encounter concepts that will shape your future patient care—whether or not you choose family practice as a specialty: concepts such as personal care, longitudinal care, the meaning of illness, and the investment of self in the therapeutic relationship. The book presents these and other principles of generalist health care plus factual data regarding a broad range of common clinical problems, supplemented by case presentations that involve members of a single family.

The discussion questions are not intended to be post-tests of the factual content of each chapter and the answers to some questions may not actually be in the chapter, but rather in your ability to reason and solve problems – which, after all, are the most important skills you need as a physician. The questions are designed to stimulate thought about the issues, encourage discussion, or even inspire a quest for more information.

To the Faculty

This book, intended to be a single source text for your clerkship, has been prepared to meet the General Guidelines for a Third-Year Family Medicine Clerkship as developed by the Society of Teachers of Family Medicine (see Table 1). The 25 clinical chapters (Chapters 2 through 26) present a broad spectrum of family practice problems that are consistent with the topic categories taught in required family medicine clerkships in U.S. medical schools.[2] The case presentations and questions that follow each chapter are intended to be the basis of small group discussions. They include both traditional questions about medical history, physical examination, diagnosis, and management, as well as about psychosocial issues such as the reason for the visit, the impact of illness on the family, the patient's adaptation to illness, and the resources used in management. The case discussions have been "field-tested" with third-year medical students, and they work. Try them.

About the Case Discussions in this Book: The Nelson Family

Each chapter is followed by a case presentation with discussion questions, all involving members of a single extended family: the Nelsons. The Nelson family genogram is shown in Figure 1. During a period of 12 months, various members of the Nelson family come to the office for care, some making two or three visits during the year. The reader will find that the problems of various family members are interconnected and that they evolve over time.

Figure 1 introduces the four-generation Nelson family, some of whom have been your patients for more than a decade and who look to you as their personal physician for comprehensive health care of all family members.

Harold and Mary Nelson

The senior family members áre Harold and Mary Nelson, both in their seventies. Harold Nelson retired from his job as a welder 13 years ago at age 61. He now leads a quiet life and seldom leaves the house. He has had type 2 diabetes mellitus for 24 years and osteoarthritis of the hands for 20 years, both of which were considerations in his early retirement.

Mary Nelson, age 71, is a retired nursery school teacher. She has been hypertensive, taking medication, for 10 years. In addition, she has episodes of depression that require treatment. She wishes that she and Harold were "doing more" in their retirement, and worries about what will happen to their son, Samuel, when they die.

Harold and Mary Nelson have four children: Ruth, Samuel, Ken, and Lois— all in their 40s and 50s.

John and Ruth McCarthy

Ruth, the oldest Nelson child, is married to John McCarthy. Together they own and operate a small delicatessen-style restaurant. Their restaurant business struggles financially, and Ruth and John sometimes seek "loans" from her parents during lean times. Both work long hours in the restaurant. Ruth enjoys good health, but John has coronary artery disease with angina pectoris for which he had been treated by an internist downtown. John McCarthy's previous physician retired recently, and John has decided to transfer his care to you.

John and Ruth McCarthy have two children. Their oldest son is Mark, age 28, who dropped out of college to organize a rock group which disbanded about two years ago. Mark now works as a waiter in his parents' restaurant. John and Ruth openly disapprove of Mark's lifestyle, which includes cigarette smoking, marijuana use, and numerous sexual contacts. Recently Mark was found to be positive for human immunodeficiency virus (HIV).

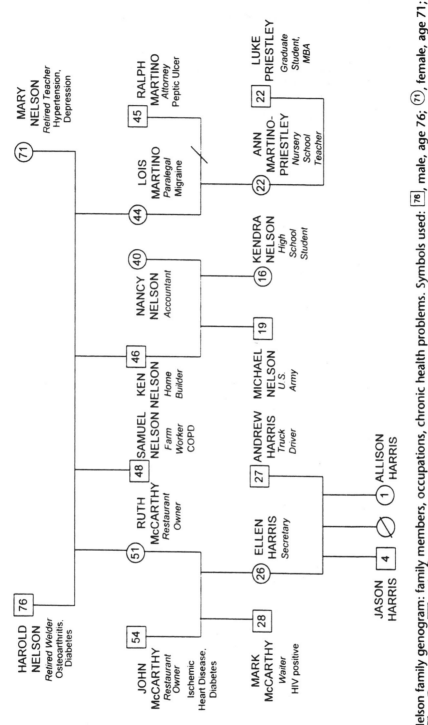

FIGURE 1. Nelson family genogram: family members, occupations, chronic health problems. Symbols used: ☐, male, age 76; ⊙, female, age 71; 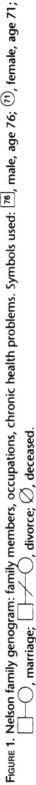, marriage; ⎯⊘⎯, divorce; ⊘, deceased.

The McCarthys' second child is Ellen, age 26, who works as a secretary in a business office. Ellen is married to Andrew Harris, a truck driver who is on the road a good deal of the time. Ellen and Andrew Harris have two children: Jason, age 4, and Allison, age 1. A third child, who would have been 3 years old this year, died in infancy of meningitis.

Samuel Nelson

Samuel Nelson, age 48, is the second child of Harold and Mary Nelson. Samuel was a high school dropout at age 16 when he began work at a nearby orchard. Today he lives with his parents and has no close friends. He has kept the same job as a farm worker for 32 years and spends his spare time watching television. Samuel has been a heavy smoker since his teens and now has chronic obstructive pulmonary disease.

Ken and Nancy Nelson

The third child is Kenneth Nelson, age 46, who works as a contractor, building new homes in middle-class neighborhoods. Ken is married to Nancy, who has an accounting degree and works part-time for a public accounting firm. Nancy has always described herself as "nervous," which has limited her ability to take a full-time job.

TABLE 1. General Guidelines for a Third-Year Family Medicine Clerkship

By the completion of a third-year family medicine clerkship, the medical student is expected to possess, at a level appropriate for a third-year student, the knowledge, attitudes, and skills needed to:
1. Provide personal care for individuals and families as the physician of first contact and continuing care in health as well as in illness.
2. Assess and manage acute and chronic medical problems frequently encountered in the community.
3. Provide anticipatory health care using education, risk reduction, and health enhancement strategies.
4. Provide continuous as well as episodic health care, not limited by a specific disease, patient characteristics, or setting of the patient encounter.
5. Provide and coordinate comprehensive care of complex and severe problems using biomedical, social, personal, economic, and community resources, including consultation and referral.
6. Establish effective physician–patient relationships by using appropriate interpersonal communication skills to provide quality health care.

Source: Working Committee to Develop Curricular Guidelines for a Third-Year Family Medicine Clerkship. Curricular Guidelines for a Third-Year Family Medicine Clerkship. Kansas City, MO: The Society of Teachers of Family Medicine, 1990. Used with permission.
Note: At the time of this printing, the Society of Teachers of Family Medicine is engaged in a federally supported project to develop a resource manual for medical educators who design and implement curricula intended to prepare students for the tomorrow's health care system. This project will delineate the goals and objectives of third-year clerkships and help provide resources to those responsible for these experiences.

Ken and Nancy Nelson have two children. The oldest is Michael Nelson, age 19, a U.S. Army paratrooper stationed at Fort Bragg, North Carolina. Still living at home is their 16-year-old daughter, Kendra, a high-school sophomore. Kendra is an above average student and a varsity athlete. Over the past year she has had her first serious relationship with a boyfriend.

Lois and Ralph Martino

The fourth child is Lois, age 44, who has training as a paralegal and works in a large law firm. Ten years ago, Lois separated from her husband, Ralph Martino, an attorney previously employed in the same law firm as Lois and now in solo practice. Although Ralph's relationship with Lois and the Nelson family is strained, he has continued to consider you his personal physician.

Lois and Ralph have one child, Ann, age 22, who works mornings as a nursery school teacher. A year ago, Ann married Luke Priestley, a graduate student now working on his Masters of Business Administration degree. Ann's parents secretly worry about Ann's marriage since Luke seems very distant and moody.

References

1. Senf JH, Campos-Outcalt D. The effect of a required third-year family medicine clerkship on medical students' attitudes; value indoctrination and value clarification. Acad Med 1995; 70:142–8.
2. Schwiebert LP, Aspy CB. Didactic content and teaching methodologies on required allopathic U.S. family medicine clerkships. Fam Med 1999; 31(2): 95–100.

Contributors

Alan M. Adelman, M.D., M.S., Professor and Associate Chair, Department of Family and Community Medicine, Penn State University College of Medicine, Hershey, Pennsylvania

Bruce Ambuel, Ph.D., Associate Professor of Family and Community Medicine, Medical College of Wisconsin, Milwaukee; Waukesha Family Practice Residency Program, Waukesha, Wisconsin

Boyd L. Bailey JR, M.D., Associate Professor of Family Medicine, University of Alabama at Birmingham, School of Medicine; Director, University of Alabama-Selma Family Medicine Residency Program, Selma, Alabama

Steven P. Bromer, M.D., Assistant Clinical Professor of Family and Community Medicine, University of California—San Francisco School of Medicine, San Francisco, California

Cora Collette Breuner, M.D., M.P.H., Department of Pediatrics, University of Washington Medical Center, Seattle, Washington

Stephen A. Brunton, M.D., Director of Faculty Development, Stamford Hospital/ Columbia University Family Practice Residency Program, Stamford, Connecticut

Walter L. Calmbach, M.D., Associate Professor of Family and Community Medicine, Director of Sports Medicine Fellowship and South Texas Ambulatory Research Network (STARNET), University of Texas Health Science Center, San Antonio, Texas

Bryan J. Campbell, M.D., Assistant Professor of Family and Preventive Medicine, University of Utah School of Medicine, Salt Lake City, Utah

Douglas J. Campbell, M.D., Community Attending Physician, Good Samaritan Regional Family Practice Center, Yavapai Regional Medical Center, Prescott, Arizona

Frank S. Celestino, M.D., Associate Professor and Director of Geriatrics, Department of Family and Community Medicine, Wake Forest University School of Medicine, Winston-Salem, North Carolina

Margaret V. Elizondo, M.D., Clinical Instructor of Family Medicine, University of California-San Diego School of Medicine, LaJolla; Grossmont Hospital, LaMesa, California

Paul Evans, D.O., Associate Dean for Curricular Affairs and Associate Professor of Family Medicine, Oklahoma State University College of Osteopathic Medicine, Tulsa, Oklahoma

Scott A. Fields, M.D., Professor of Family Medicine, Oregon Health & Science University School of Medicine, Portland, Oregon

Cheryl A. Flynn, M.D., M.S., Assistant Professor of Family Medicine, Upstate Medical University, State University of New York, Syracuse, New York

Valerie J. Gilchrist, M.D., Professor and Chair, Department of Family Medicine, Northeastern Ohio Universities College of Medicine, Rootstown; Associate Director, Aultman Family Practice Center, Aultman Hospital, Canton, Ohio

Rupert R. Goetz, M.D., Adjunct Associate Professor, Department of Psychiatry and Department of Family Medicine, Oregon Health & Science University School of Medicine, Portland, Oregon

Ronald H. Goldschmidt, M.D., Professor of Clinical Family and Community Medicine, University of California-San Francisco School of Medicine, San Francisco, California

Anthony F. Jerant, M.D., Assistant Professor of Family Medicine, University of California—Davis School of Medicine, Sacramento, California.

George L. Kirkpatrick, M.D., Emergency Department Physician, Mobile Infirmary Medical Center, Mobile, Alabama

Aubrey L. Knight, M.D., Associate Professor of Clinical Family Medicine, University of Virginia School of Medicine, Charlottesville; Director, Family Practice Education, Carilion Health System, Roanoke, Virginia

Richard B. Lewan, M.D., Associate Professor of Family and Community Medicine, Medical College of Wisconsin, Milwaukee; Director, Family Practice Residency Program, Waukesha Memorial Hospital, Waukesha, Wisconsin

Peter R. Lewis, M.D., Assistant Professor of Family and Community Medicine, Penn State University College of Medicine, Hershey, Pennsylvania

Deborah S. McPherson, M.D., Assistant Director of Medical Education, American Academy of Family Physicians, Leawood, Kansas

Alan L. Melnick, M.D., M.P.H., Assistant Professor of Family Medicine, Oregon Health & Science University School of Medicine, Portland; Health Officer, Clackamas County, Oregon

William F. Miser, M.D., Associate Professor of Family Medicine, The Ohio State University College of Medicine and Public Health; Residency Director, The Ohio State University Family Practice Residency Program, Columbus, Ohio

Alicia D. Monroe, M.D., Associate Professor of Family Medicine, Brown Medical School, Providence; Memorial Hospital of Rhode Island, Pawtucket, Rhode Island

John B. Murphy, M.D., Professor of Family Medicine, Brown Medical School, Providence, Rhode Island

Jim Nuovo, M.D., Associate Professor of Family and Community Medicine, University of California-Davis School of Medicine, Sacramento, California

James P. Richardson, M.D., M.P.H., Medical Director of Senior Care Services, St. Agnes Health Care, Baltimore, Maryland

Joseph E. Scherger, M.D., M.P.H., Dean, College of Medicine, Florida State University, Tallahassee, Florida

Allen F. Shaughnessy, Pharm.D., Clinical Associate Professor of Family Medicine, Medical College of Pennsylvania—Hahnemann School of Medicine, Philadelphia; Harrisburg Family Practice Residency Program, Harrisburg, Pennsylvania

John P. Sheehan, M.D., Associate Clinical Professor of Medicine, Case Western Reserve University School of Medicine, Cleveland, Ohio

David C. Slawson, M.D., B. Lewis Barnett, Jr. Professor of Family Medicine, University of Virginia School of Medicine, Charlottesville, Virginia

Charles Kent Smith, M.D., Dorothy Jones Weatherhead Professor of Family Medicine, Case Western Reserve University School of Medicine, Cleveland, Ohio

Robert B. Taylor, M.D., Professor of Family Medicine, Oregon Health & Science University School of Medicine, Portland, Oregon

William L. Toffler, M.D., Professor of Family Medicine, Oregon Health & Science University School of Medicine, Portland, Oregon

Michael L. Tuggy, M.D., Clinical Assistant Professor of Family Medicine, University of Washington School of Medicine; Director, Swedish Family Medicine Residency Program, Seattle, Washington

Margaret M. Ulchaker, M.S.N., R.N., C.D.E., NP-C., Clinical Instructor, Frances Payne Bolton School of Nursing, Case Western Reserve University, Cleveland, Ohio

Daniel J. Van Durme, M.D., Associate Professor and Vice-Chairman, Department of Family Medicine, University of South Florida College of Medicine, Tampa, Florida

Anne D. Walling, M.B., Ch.B., Professor of Family Medicine, University of Kansas School of Medicine, Wichita and Kansas City, Kansas

Howard N. Weinberg, M.D., Family Physician, Sentara Medical Group, Virginia Beach, Virginia

Mary Willard, M.D., Director, West Jersey-Memorial Family Practice Residency Program, Virtua Health, Voorhees, New Jersey

Christopher R. Wood, M.D., Assistant Professor, Family and Community Medicine, Medical College of Wisconsin, Milwaukee; Waukesha Family Practice Residency Program, Waukesha, Wisconsin

1
Principles of Generalist Health Care

ROBERT B. TAYLOR

This first chapter in the book is about caring for *people*—as distinct from diseases or organs—and the generalists who provide personal health care. It is about the baby with a fever, the teenager with concerns about sexually transmitted disease, the laborer with back pain, and the manager with heartburn. It is about home visits to the paraplegic young man with the flu and nursing home care of the elderly woman with a stroke—and about how these illnesses affect their lives and the lives of those close to them. Since such care is, to a great degree, a characteristic of the individual physician, I have written this chapter in the first person.

I was a general practitioner before family practice existed. In 1969, when general practice became family practice, I began to think of myself as a family physician, and then I became a *board-certified* family physician in 1971. I have practiced in the United States Public Health Service and in small town group practice. I spent 10 years in rural solo practice before entering academic medicine. Although I am currently a professor in a family medicine department in an academic medical center, I still think of myself as a rural family practitioner and what follows reflects that practice-oriented viewpoint.

In the 1980s the term "primary care" became popular, and has subsequently been redefined by the Institute of Medicine as "the provision of integrated, accessible health care services by clinicians who are accountable for addressing a large majority of personal health care needs, developing a sustained partnership with patients, and practicing in the context of family and community."[1] We—my colleagues in family practice, general internal medicine, and general pediatrics and I—are also called generalists.

What Is Generalist Health Care and Who Provides It?

Generalist health care is continuing, comprehensive, and coordinated medical care provided to a population undifferentiated by gender, disease, or organ system.[2] This type of care is also called primary care and the terms are often used interchangeably. Generalists offer first-contact and longitudinal care for persons with diverse problems such as earache, chest pain, fracture, or cancer. They provide care that is not problem or technology specific. They coordinate the patient's health care, whether provided in the generalist's own office or in the emergency department, consultant's office, or hospital. The spectrum of generalist care varies with the setting—suburban, rural, inner city, community health clinic, or academic medical center—and melds into a continuum in which some generalists include tertiary care activities as part of their practice.[3] My current practice is in an academic medical center, and my patients tend to have much more complicated problems than did my patients when I was in private practice.

The U.S. Department of Health and Human Services describes four primary care/generalist competencies[4]:

• Heath promotion and disease prevention
• Assessment and diagnosis of common symptoms and physical signs
• Management of common acute and chronic medical conditions
• Identification of and appropriate referral for other needed health services

Persons who choose careers in the generalist specialties are those who—like me—want to do it all. We worked hard to learn the full spectrum of medicine and do not want to give anything up. By offering a broad range of services, I can offer truly comprehensive care to my patients. If Mrs. Jones, for example, has migraine headaches, a skin rash, and irregular menstrual periods, I can provide care for all these complaints, often in a single office visit and without referrals. What is more, with each encounter the patient and I add to a cumulative fund of medical and personal knowledge—what Balint called the "mutual investment company"—that allows increasingly effective health care.[5] As I learn more and more about Mrs. Jones and her stress at work, her arguments with her teenage daughter, and her concern about her mother's Alzheimer's disease, she and I can better manage her various problems; but these issues are never fully elucidated in one visit or two.

Exactly what does the generalist do? Most generalist practice is office practice and the variety of problems is reflected in the top 20 principal diagnoses in office visits as recorded in the National Ambulatory Medical Care Survey (see Table 1.1)[6] This list covers family and general practice, and thus contains the broadest scope of generalist health care.

Generalists provide a wide spectrum of care: This includes *anticipatory care*, counseling the teenager on avoidance of injury or unplanned pregnancy, and *symptomatic care* to relieve the pain of a back strain. There is *therapeutic care* of acute asthma or chronic ulcerative colitis, and the *palliative care* of the person with terminal cancer or late-stage acquired immunodeficiency syndrome (AIDS). All of these types of care are provided in the setting of the clinical encounter, which has been described as "the procedure" of the family physician,[7] and which is evolving to include the digital office visit and virtual house call.

Generalist care occurs in many sites in addition to the physician's office. Most generalists provide hospital and nursing home services for their patients.[8] Home care is an important part of care in many communities, allowing the physician to visit the patient in his or her own "habitat." The practice site may be an of-

TABLE 1.1. Number and percent distribution of office visits by selected primary diagnosis groups: United States, 1999

Primary diagnosis	Number of visits in thousands	Percent Distribution
All visits	756,734	100.0
Essential hypertension	32,962	4.2
Acute upper respiratory infections, excluding pharyngitis	28,553	3.8
Arthropathies and related disorders	23,202	3.1
Routine infant or child health check	22,626	3.0
Diabetes mellitus	19,585	2.6
Dorsopathies (back problems)	17,439	2.3
Allergic rhinitis	16,662	2.2
Normal pregnancy	16,402	2.2
Rheumatism, excluding back	16,368	2.2
Malignant neoplasms	15,429	2.0
Otitis media and eustachian tube disorders	14,568	1.9
Follow-up examination	13,814	1.8
General medical examination	13,405	1.8
Cataract	11,039	1.5
Chronic sinustis	10,797	1.4
Heart disease, excluding ischemic	9,667	1.3
Ischemic heart disease	9,558	1.3
Potential health hazards related to personal and family history	9,543	1.3
Asthma	9,498	1.3
Benign and uncertain neoplasms	8,782	1.2
All other diagnosis	437,837	57.9

Source: Ref. 6.

fice in a medical building, a school, a community health clinic, or in the military on board a ship or at a base hospital.

Some generalists develop special areas of expertise such as care of the elderly, adolescent medicine, sports medicine, occupational medicine, or administrative medicine. At times, the focus may be on the community—community-oriented primary care—an expression of generalism in which the target is a community and the health problems that affect it (e.g., preventing cervical cancer by increasing the number of women screened with Pap smears) rather than concentrating exclusively on health problems at the level of the individual patient.

The U.S. medical workforce is changing, and will continue to do so throughout your professional career. One fact stands out, and will likely guide future workforce decisions: Today only about one third of U.S. physicians are in the generalist specialties, a figure that is significantly less than other "first world" countries. Many health care experts believe that this low proportion of primary care physicians contributes to the poor record of health care when U.S. health data are compared with that of other industrialized countries.[9]

The primary focus of generalist (and also subspecialty) care is the people who receive health care. Family practice arose in the 1960s as a social movement to combat the fragmentation in medicine, to put medicine back together again and to deliver it to the people. This same evangelical spirit continues today. Generalism is about the public need for personal health care, for a physician about whom one can say, "That's my doctor." It is about the physician who will make the commitment inherent in saying, "I am your personal physician. I will be there when you need me."

How to Provide Generalist Health Care: Asking the High Payoff Questions

How do we do it? How do I, as a generalist, stay current with all of medicine and see 25 patients per day? First of all, as a generalist, it is not my responsibility to know "all of medicine;" instead, I aspire to maintain current clinical knowledge and skills pertinent to the *common problems* of the patient population I serve. If knowledge could be weighed, my fund of knowledge would "weigh" about the same as that of an endocrinologist, neurologist, or any other limited specialist. It is just that my fund of knowledge and my competencies are broad based, while those of the more limited specialists are concerned with an organ, system, age group, or specific technology such as x-ray. Their in-depth knowledge of uncommon problems—the pheochromocytoma or myasthenia gravis—allows me to identify these "zebras" and refer them to the subspecialist for definitive care, while I maintain a supportive role with the patient and family.

The added value that I bring to the clinical encounter is my knowledge of the patient. Family practice is, first of all, a specialty grounded in the principles of relationship-based health care. Thus I aspire to know everything possible about the patient and family, including all the personal concerns that may influence health and illness. I have a longitudinal view of the health problems of a small group of people and offer a committed relationship. Also, on a practical basis, I already know the past medical history, family history, social history, and habits of most patients I see. Thus I can direct my attention, knowledge and compentencies toward the key issues that require attention today.

I apply the generalist fund of knowledge and competencies to help a relatively large number of patients daily by efficient application of the most commonly performed generalist procedure: *the focused clinical encounter*. Typically compressed into a 15-minute time slot, the focused clinical encounter flows seamlessly through five phases: (1) offering of the problem, (2) elucidation of key issues, (3) a targeted physical examination, (4) explanation of the diagnosis, and (5) negotiation of plans for management and follow-up. In approximately a quarter hour, I can elicit a history of epigastric distress and what makes it better and worse, explore life stresses, examine the abdomen, explain my findings, and work with the patient to plan for dietary change, stress management, and appropriate use of antacids, an H_2-receptor blocker, or protein pump inhibitor.[11]

Of necessity, the time-limited visit targets the high-probability diagnosis (e.g. gastritis or gastroesophageal reflux disease [GERD]) while considering the possibility of the "must-never-miss" diagnoses (e.g. gastric cancer). The focused clinical encounter will include exploration of psychosocial topics, such as the patient's need to take a second job to cover credit card debt or concerns about a child in trouble at school. The experienced physician knows how often these nonphysical issues hold the key to understanding the patient's illness.

High-yield questions are how the skilled generalist focuses the time-limited clinical encounter. These questions are open-ended and can often begin with, "Tell me about . . ." They can be phrased in ways that are most comfortable to each physician and in complexity appropriate to the patient's understanding. The high-yield questions are used along with standard queries about: "How long have you had chest pain?" "Does the pain radiate anywhere?" and "Have you taken any medicine for the chest pain?" The full scope of the problem may finally become clear with the response to the open- ended query: "Tell me about what's been going on lately." or "Let's talk about what's most stressful in your life right now."

The following are six areas of high-yield questions. For each I have described a rationale, with some examples. Specific questions are listed—in varying levels of specificity—for both the patient and for you or me, the physician.

What Is the True Reason for the Visit?

Patients visit physicians for many reasons, which are not always self-evident. A 65-year-old man came on a first visit, requesting a "complete physical examination." In response to a question, "Why?" I learned that the patient was planning a second marriage, that there had been a question of a prostate nodule in the past, and that he needed to know more about his health outlook in order to make some financial decisions. If I had not dug deeper, I would have failed to understand the patient's needs for the visit and perhaps would not have discussed important areas of concern with him.

The reasons for a visit may be classified under five headings (see Table 1.2). Most new-problem visits are for the diagnosis and treatment of physical problems, such as earache. The next most common category—concern about the meaning of a sign or symptom—includes many instances in which the patient

TABLE 1.2. Why patients visit physicians: problems and needs that prompt patients to initiate medical encounters

Reason	Example
Physical problem	Ankle sprain
Worry or concern	Coughed up sputum with flecks of blood
Administrative purpose	Insurance medical examination
Emotional problem	Anxiety
Social problem	Loneliness

with a problem is less bothered by the discomfort than by what the discomfort might *mean*. For example, in Chapter 17, Andrew Harris comes to the physician with back pain which began while lifting boxes at work; there is some radiation of pain to the right leg and foot. Is Mr. Harris in the office for relief of his pain so that he can sleep at night and return to work soon? Is he here because he is concerned about the possibility of a herniated disc necessitating back surgery, as happened to his brother? Or is the visit for an administrative purpose—to establish a workers' compensation claim?

Patients sometimes identify their problems as social or emotional, but more often such problems are offered as physical complaints—sometimes referred to as a "ticket of admission" (to health care). One young married woman visited my office repeatedly with lower abdominal pains. She and her husband had three small children and their income was limited. As she and I talked, I learned that her husband spent most evenings playing softball and drinking with his friends, leaving her alone at home with the children. Although the patient continued to offer a physical complaint, her "reason for the visit" was, in my opinion, a social problem.

Questions for the patient:

- What do we need to accomplish on this visit?
- Is there anything you are especially concerned (or worried) about?
- Tell me why you are here with this problem *at this time*.
- How can I help you at this visit?

Questions for the physician to consider:

- Does the patient's stated problem seem "not quite right?"
- Might the patient, for some reason, have misled the receptionist or nurse (or me) about the presenting complaint?
- Have I possibly made an incorrect assumption about the patient's goals for the encounter?
- Is the patient here today for *someone else's reason*?

Am I Listening Carefully to What the Patient Is Trying to Tell?

There is an old clinical aphorism: Listen to the patient; he (or she) is telling you the diagnosis.

This need to listen carefully extends to all phases of the clinical encounter. It begins with thinking about why the patient came (and perhaps why he or she came *today*) complaining of—for example—abdominal pain, the response to a remark by a family member in the room, a comment about some part of the physical examination, or the objection to a suggested therapeutic intervention. The phrase "listening with the third ear" is sometimes used to describe this type of active listening.

In the lexicon of decision analysis, all the above are defined as "cues." The following are some examples from my practice: One patient was a 14-year-old girl who asked if birth control pills might help her acne. What she really sought was a prescription for oral contraceptives because of an emerging sexual relationship with her boyfriend. In another instance, I watched as a patient's neck muscles tightened and he crossed his arms when I asked casually, "How are things at home?" In this instance, his response "Okay" turned out to be evasive, and on further inquiry I was able to link his chest pains and the repeated arguments with his wife about his perceived need to work long hours overtime. A four year old girl who had always been lively was noted to be withdrawn and avoiding eye contact; this turned out to be the tip-off to childhood sexual abuse.

In Chapter 25, high-school basketball player Kendra Nelson visits the physician with the second ankle sprain in 4 months. Although she cannot bear weight and must hop rather than walk, she insists that the pain in "not really bad." Is Kendra minimizing the pain so that she can get an early release to return to her basketball team? Is she under peer or parental pressure to return to sports? Is she concerned that the physician may apply a cast that would interfere with a planned social activity?

Following the path of a clinical cue is often accomplished over several visits. A 42-year-old school teacher with migraine headaches insisted on her first two visits that everything in her life "couldn't be better." The reportedly "perfect" life proved to be a cue, and on the third visit we discussed her threatened layoff at work, her husband's drinking problem, and the concerns about their 15-year-old son's suspected drug use. In such instances, a sense of when things don't sound quite right can be a useful diagnostic tool.

The ongoing attention—and revisiting—of clinical cues leads to the *continuing evolving diagnosis*. The clinician begins to generate hypotheses upon learning the chief complaint, or perhaps even before. Diagnostic possibilities are rejected, validated or set aside for future consideration. The complex origins of the patient's symptoms and their interrelatedness to life events is most often clarified over time, and only rarely as a "first-visit revelation."

The awareness of the evolutionary nature of diagnosis helps the generalist dealt with undifferentiated health care problems, such as fatigue and dizziness. It also helps the clinician tolerate the diagnostic ambiguity and complexity often found in primary care. This comfort with sometimes murky health problems actually characterizes those who choose family practice and other primary care specialties.[12] It also helps explain why generalists as a group tend to be those who can see possiblities, can recognize patterns and think in templates, and are intrigued by the process of clinical reasoning.

Questions for the patient:

- Is there some aspect of today's problem that we should discuss further?
- Events in a person's life can affect health. What is going on in your life that might be affecting your health?
- Is any part of the physical examination causing you concern?
- Are there ways that you and your family could improve your health that we should discuss?

Questions for the physician to consider:

- Has the patient seemed reluctant to discuss certain issues?
- Does there seem to be a aspect of the problem that I do not yet understand?
- Does the patient seem inappropriately sensitive to some part of the physical examination?
- Is there some apparently obvious resource—such as family support, time, or money—that the patient seems reluctant to use? If so, why?

What Is the Meaning of the Illness to the Patient?

Think back to the last time you had the flu, with high fever, achiness and fatigue. Along with the need to stay in bed for a few days to get well, what did the flu mean to you? Did it mean that you would miss class or a sports event? Might it have meant that you would be absent for an important examination or that you might perform poorly on the test? Could it be that you were not prepared for the examination, and were, in fact, happy for a delay? Perhaps the chief concern was the economic impact of the flu—the cost of care or the loss of a weekend job. Did the chills and fever remind you of the first stages of pneumonia that ended with the death of a grandparent? Or did the flu symptoms have some other special meaning for you?

Disease and illness are not synonymous. Disease refers to a biomechanical, physiologic, or psychologic dysfunction. Illness includes the patient's response to disease—with all its pain, worry, inconvenience, or loss—and places it in the context of the life, family, community, and society of the affected individual. Ellen Harris (Chapter 16) visits your office with a complaint of vaginal discharge. She is married and works as a secretary. A straightforward problem? Probably, but not necessarily. Could the symptom mean loss of sexual relations with her husband for a week or more? Does this mean he will be angry? Could she have passed an infection to him? Is it possible that the infection have been caught *from him*? Might that mean that he acquired it somewhere? That is, could this be a sexually transmitted disease?

The physician must never neglect the patient's unspoken concerns: Will I be able to return to work after my heart attack? Will my husband still love me after my breast surgery? Might I pass my chest cold (or infectious mononucleosis, or skin rash, or Chlamydia infection) to my partner?

Another example: In Chapter 5, Harold Nelson, age 76, develops urinary incontinence. What might this mean to him? "Will I have to go to the hospital?" "Will I need an operation?" "Will I need to go to a nursing home?" Although Mr. Nelson may be hesitant to ask these questions, it is likely that they have occurred to him.

Physicians need a keen understanding of the meaning of the sick role and the legitimization of illness. When you or I are sick, we are excused from our usual duties, and others offer medicine, food and support. That is, we are allowed to assume *the sick role*. Part of the contract, however, is that the patient will make every effort to get well—and no longer assume the sick role. Of course the sick role has definite advantages, not the least of which are reduced responsibility and increased service by others. Not surprisingly, some persons would prefer to prolong the sick-role, and the physician may become involved. Many office visits are concerned with legitimization of the sick role, whether explicitly by signing an excuse for work or implicitly by writing a prescription for a cough remedy or renewing a physical therapy order for a painful neck.

If you overlook the contextual meaning of the illness to patients like Mrs. Harris or Mr. Nelson, has your clinical encounter—your "procedure"—been successful?

Questions for the patient:

- What do you believe is the cause of the illness?
- Tell me how you feel about this illness.
- How does this illness affect your activities at home or at work?
- What would getting well mean to you?

Questions for the physician to consider:

- What are the implications of the patient assuming the sick role?
- How might this illness be affecting the patient's self-image?
- Might this illness remind the patient of something that happened to a family member or friend?
- Might you—the physician—have personal experience or feelings that are affecting your judgment about this patient's illness?

What Is the Impact of the Illness on the Family?

If you have any doubt that illness is a family affair, ask any child, sibling, or parent of a person with a chronic problem such as asthma, diabetes mellitus, or cerebral palsy. Resources and attention that should be equally shared are diverted to the identified "patient." The patient's illness eventually becomes a family burden, and other family members come to think of themselves as caregivers. Anger begets guilt and the illness permeates all family relationships. Eventually, the illness becomes part of the family self-image.

Describing the legacy of migraine in her own family, Anne Walling, MD (author of Chapter 7) writes, "My father's severe attacks were part of our family's normal pattern of life. Like spells of bad weather, they were unpredictable, significant events that appeared to take a perverse delight in disrupting the most intricately planned and eagerly anticipated events." And then, "My mother abhorred migraine and grimly warned us against developing even remotely migrainous symptoms."[13]

The effect of illness on a family is not predictable. Chronic, recurrent childhood illness such as renal failure or hyperactivity can be the stress that results in disruption of a young family, and many parents of leukemic children see their marriages end in divorce. On the other hand, I have cared for a family with a child whose asthma attacks seemed to occur at just the times needed to divert parental attention to the child and away from their own arguments.

In Chapter 3, you will meet Ann Martino-Priestley, age 22, and her husband Luke. Ann is pregnant with their first child. Of course, pregnancy is not an illness, but it will have an impact on the couple/family. How do each feel about the pregnancy? How will a child affect their relationship? Can they afford to have a baby at this time? Will Ann be able to continue to work? What about Luke's studies for his MBA degree? How might all of these issues affect health care decisions?

Questions for the patient:

• How is your spouse (or children, parents, partner, etc.) affected by this illness?
• What are you hearing from others about your illness?
• Tell me what has changed in your relationships since the illness began.
• How would things be different at home if you were well?

Questions for the physician to consider:

• Who, beside the patient, is affected by this illness?
• What emotions might the patient's family be experiencing: sorrow, anger, abandonment, frustration, guilt?
• Have I, as physician, spoken with key people in my patient's life?
• By engaging in the care of this patient's illness, what—if any—might be the effect on me and my family?

What Is the Appropriate Locus of Care for this Person's Illness?

The locus of care was studied by Green et al. in 2001, who found that of 1000 adults "at risk," each month:

• Eight hundred reported one of more illnesses or injuries.
• Two hundred and seventeen of these persons consulted a physician one or more times.
• Eight of these patients were admitted to a hospital.
• Fewer than one patient was referred to an academic medical center.

Some thoughts about this study and what it means to the medical student: Note that while 80% of adults reported an illness or injury during a month, only about one illness/injury in four resulted in a medical encounter; almost three quarters of care was "family" care in which the physician was not directly involved. Fewer than 1% of persons studied were hospitalized and there was less than one academic medical center referral per 1000 at risk adults, a key finding considering that research data and therapeutic guidelines tend to come from academic medical centers and thus are based on less than 0.1% of the population.

A current issue in health care centers around appropriate use of consultation and referral. The following family practice approach to locus of care was presented in the first edition of *Family Medicine: Principles and Practice*.[15]

- **Definitive Care**: The physician provides independent care, perhaps with the participation of ancillary personnel, but without subspecialist consultation or referral. Examples include depression, type 2 diabetes mellitus, and an undisplaced fracture of the fibular malleolus. The residency trained FP generalist should be competent to manage 85% to 90% of Definitive Care problems without need for consultation or referral.
- **Shared Care**: These problems generally necessitate *consultation* for some aspect of diagnosis or therapy. Care is thus shared by the generalist and subspecialist for problems such as a thyroid mass or active pulmonary tuberculosis. Some 7 to 10 percent of problems will be best managed by Shared Care.
- **Supportive Care**: These are clearly subspecialty *referral* problems such as extensive third degree burns or retinal detachment. The generalist has the responsibility to direct the patient to appropriate care and to maintain educational and emotional support for the patient and family.

The physician's decisions in locus of care options will be guided by the individual's interest, training, and competence. In our Family Practice Center, some physicians perform colposcopy (as a Definitive Care procedure); others refer patients needing colposcopy (for them, it is thereby a Shared Care procedure). Of course, physicians are only part of the decision making. Patient preferences play a role, as do practice guidelines of the health care organization or hospital.

In Chapter 21, we encounter an increasingly common locus-of-care decision: Mark McCarthy, age 28, is human immunodeficiency virus (HIV) positive and for 3 weeks has had a fever and cough productive of yellow-gray sputum. His parents ask, " Is it safe for him to stay at home, or should he be in the hospital? Should he have a consultation with a specialist? Should a specialist be in charge of his care? By having him living at home, are we—his parents—at risk?" Answers to these and related questions are often complex, and may be clouded by misinformation, fear, protection of turf, and concerns about maintaining practice volume.

Questions for the patient:

- Have you had this problem before and how was it managed?
- Tell me your view of the treatment needed today.
- What concerns do you have about our plans for management and follow-up?
- Tell me your understanding of the reason we are seeking consultation and the questions we hope to answer.

Questions for the physician to consider:

- Is the problem within my area of competence and comfort?
- Does the patient expect a consultation and, if so, is it medically appropriate?

- Is there an administrative need that would call for a consultation or referral: insurance, litigation, disability determination, or other?
- Am I making my consultation/referral recommendation for the right reasons?

What Resources Are Available to Help in Managing the Illness?

The rise in managed care in the United States was a reflection of what families have known all along: health care resources are not limitless. Individuals and families have always had to face limits on care that can be given in the home, cost of medication purchased, and nursing home care provided. Recognition of resources that are available—and what are not available—is important in ensuring optimal care for patients.

The categories of resources are listed in Table 1.3. Financial resources include the direct ability to pay and also medical insurance, emergency assistance in times of disaster, and loans or gifts from family. Care by family members, visiting nurses, community health workers, nurses, physicians, and other providers all constitute medical care resources. The time and energy resources may come from the patient, the family, medical personnel, and volunteers such as neighbors or church members. Patient and family knowledge of medicine, community contacts, and funding sources can affect the quality of care ultimately received as can the availability of medical equipment and supplies.

In Chapter 4, Allison Harris is brought to your office by her mother "for her one year old check-up and shots." There are resource implications even in this routine visit: Mrs. Harris missed several hours of work to bring Allison to the appointment. There is a cost to the Harris family for the check-up, that is not covered by their health insurance. There is a vaccine cost which, although covered by a state subsidized program, is inflated by the hidden cost of vaccine-related litigation.

Generalists work together with patients, families, community agencies, hospitals, and others to help ensure the appropriate and cost-effective deployment of resources. The higher priced prescription is not necessarily better, and not every patient with pneumonia needs hospitalization. The Medical Outcomes Study demonstrated that, even when data are controlled for patient mix, generalists use

TABLE 1.3. Resources used to manage patients' health care problems

Resource	Example
Emotional Support	Family and others comfort person with illness
Financial	Health insurance
Medical care	Office visit to physician
Time and energy	Middle-aged person stays at home caring for elderly parent
Knowledge	Information from medical reference book
Equipment and supplies	Wheelchair from community loan program

less health care resources than subspecialists. Among the generalist specialties, family physicians use the least resources of all.[16]

Questions for the patient:

- Who is your most important support person, and how is he or she involved in caring for this illness?
- Are you now a client of any community agencies that could help today?
- Tell me about family or friends that could help us at this time.
- Is there some special way you deal with problems—reading about them, meditation, pastoral counseling—and how can we put this to work now?

Questions for the physician to consider:

- What are the patient's personal and family resources that should be used?
- What community resources might be useful in management?
- Does the illness have public health or community implications?
- Have I appropriately involved the patient and family in resource use decisions?

Evidence-Based Medicine

After seeing thousands of persons with sore throat over 40 years of practice, I have empirically concluded that strep throat is more likely to be found in those with tonsillar or pharyngeal exudate or recent exposure to strep throat infection. On the other hand, a diagnosis of strep throat has always seemed less likely in those *without* tender anterior cervical adenopathy, tonsillar enlargement, or tonsillar exudate. Now there is research-based evidence that supports my intuitive beliefs.[17] It seems logical that diabetic patients who identify with a regular primary physician for their diabetes are more likely to receive more recommended elements of diabetes care and to have better glycemic control than patients who do not have such a physician. This logical conclusion was confirmed by a report published in 1998.[18] For a modest fee I can search on line at *www.clinicalevidence.org* to learn, for example, that for my patient with Alzheimer's disease donepezil is considered an effective medication, but tacrine is not. This site, supervised by the British Medical Journal Publishing Group and one of several presenting evidence-based medicine (EBM) data, is updated frequently.[19]

Evidence-based medicine was one of the chief areas of interest during the 1990s. We all sought to have our practice decisions guided by the careful and judicious use of the latest research findings. It was, and is, a way to move from experiential, anecdotal, and intuitive medical decision-making to methods that are as scientific as one can be with multiple studies employing different research methods and endowed with various methodologic flaws. Our quest for more precision in medical decision-making has brought some excellent reference sources.[20, 21]

For clinicians, EBM has been a step forward, encouraging the explicit use of research data as a foundation to our daily practice. Family physicians have been part of the current EBM movement, even though we *always* have tried to base our clinical recommendations on the best information available. POEMS (Problem-Oriented Evidence that Matters), presented monthly in the *Journal of Family Practice* is a practical application of EBM. In many cases, EBM analysis of available data has served to confirm what we thought we knew already, as shown by the strep throat and diabetes care studies mentioned above. Probably the most useful function of EBM is to pull together data from multiple studies on like topics and use meta-analysis to craft practical clinical recommendations.

For medical students, the EBM movement has brought curricular changes designed to teach young physicians how to recognize their information needs, find the data needed, evaluate the data found, and apply the results while not losing sight of current knowledge. For these reasons, we have included a chapter on EBM in this edition (see Chapter 28)

We recognize some potential problems. EBM and clinical recommendations run the risk of chiseling therapeutic options in stone, and, therefore, each clinical topic must be revisited frequently as new studies are reported. Also, EBM may tend to stifle patient choices. Finally, most of our family practice patients do not, conveniently, have one isolated illness, and they usually also have psychosocial and family issues that must be considered.

In this first decade of the 21st century, both EBM and family medicine continue to mature. At this time, we must keep in mind that, while research studies provide important data and their analysis may yield useful guidelines, clinical decisions must also include the *context* of the patient's wishes, beliefs, other health problems, available resources, family, and community.

Why Is Generalist Care More Important than Ever?

Writing on his own decision to become a general practitioner, British physician Robin Hull recalls, "I began to look at patients not as a means of locomotion of interesting pathology, but as people who were quite fascinating in their own right."[22] Dr. Hull's comment provides insight into why technological or organ-based medicine is unsatisfying to many. Patients are people, not machines with broken parts, and their illnesses have diverse origins which include the family, the community, the workplace and the tangled relationships of a lifetime.

Generalist health care is not a substitute for scientifically oriented and research based clinical activity; actually generalist care expands the dimensions of disease oriented clinical practice by adding the contextual basis through which both physician and patient come to understand the *illness*. Is there a clinical payoff to such patient-centered behavior? Certainly the diagnosis of acute myocardial infarction—documented on the electrocardiogram (ECG)—is enhanced by understanding the patient's high fat diet which began in childhood at the family dining room table, the cigarette smoking started with friends in high school, the long hours at work, and the recent concern about the company takeover that may cost him his job at age 56. Is all this reflected on the ECG tracing? No. Is the context important? Definitely!

Generalist health care calls for a committed investment of self. As a family physician I become, in a sense, a member of the family; on home visits I see my name and telephone number posted on the refrigerator door along with those of other family members and the clergy. The generalist physician is also an active member of the community; he or she is active in clubs, civic groups, and church—and enjoys social interactions with patients in these settings.

Most of all, generalist health care means *being there* for the patient and family. This has been called accessibility, but it's more. It is initiating the follow-up telephone call or e-mail to see how the patient has responded to therapy. It is asking the patient about the disabled parent at home. It is showing the patient that you care. Almost 40 years ago, just starting in a small town group practice, I cared for an elderly man dying at home of the multiple complications of a hard life and a poor genetic endowment. He and his wife lived in a trailer in the woods about 30 minutes from my office, and I visited him every Wednesday afternoon—my day for house calls for my practice group. One Monday morning the patient died at home, somewhat unexpectedly. My schedule was overbooked and the waiting room was full of patients. I did the logical thing. I sent my partner to pronounce the patient dead, sign the death certificate, and comfort the widow. After all, it was my partner's day to do the house calls. I next saw the widow at the viewing (yes, many of us make a final visit to our patients). Here she quietly let me know that she had expected *me* to come to the home when he died. I had failed to *be there* when she needed me. She taught me a lesson about being a physician that I still remember.

Family practice and today's family physicians are the current expression of the "horse and buggy" doctors of early America. We have assumed the role of maintaining patient-centered values while providing state-of-the-art health care in an increasingly technical age. We have aspired to be the standard-bearers of, as Pellegrino has described, medicine as a "moral enterprise grounded in a covenant of trust."[23] Current health care economics predict that the health care systems of the next few decades will be based on a primary care centered model. Things change, of course, and we will see new models of care including doctor–patient Internet communication, the digital office visit, and the virtual house call.[24,25] In fact, all of these exist somewhere now; in another decade, they will be state of the art. The secret of keeping our commitment to patients and yet achieving the technologically timely, universally accessible, economically affordable new care model will be to remain true to our first principles—offering our patients top-quality broad-based medical care that includes consideration of how their illness is part of the fabric of their lives, their family, and community.

References

1. Vanselow NA, Donaldson MS, Yordy KD. A new definition of primary care. JAMA 1995;273:192–4.

2. A statement on the generalist physician from the American Boards of Family Practice and Internal Medicine. JAMA 1994;271:315–6.
3. Wartman SA, Wilson M, Kahn N. The generalist health work force: issues and goals. J Gen Intern Med 1994; 9 supplement 1 (April):S7–S13.
4. Rivo ML. Division of Medicine Update. Washington DC: USPHS Health Resources and Services Administration, Bureau of Health Professions. Summer, 1992.
5. Balint M. The doctor, his patient and the illness. New York: International Universities Press, 1957.
6. National Ambulatory Medical Care Survey: U.S. Department of Health and Human Services, Public Health Service, National Center for Health Statistics, 2000 data. Available at http://www.cdc.gov/nchs/about/major/ahcd/ahcd1.htm.
7. Taylor RB. The contributions of family medicine to medical understanding: the first 50 years. J Fam Pract 1999;48:53–7.
8. Stadler DS, Zyzanski SJ, Stange KC. Family physicians and current inpatient practice. J Am Board Family Practice 1997;10:357–62.
9. Green LA, Dovey S, Fryer GE, Jr. It takes a balanced healthcare system to get it right. Jour Fam Pract 2001;50:1038–9.
10. Roberts RG. On "being there" in a virtual world. Fam Med 2001;33 (3):210.
11. Blumenthal D, Causino N, Chang YC et al. The duration of ambulatory visits to physicians. J Fam Pract 1999;48:264–71.
12. Taylor AD. How to choose a medical specialty, fourth edition, Philadelphia: Saunders, 2003.
13. Walling AD. The legacy of migraine. J Fam Pract 1994;38:629–30.
14. Green LA, Yawn BP, Lanier D, Dovey SM. The ecology of medical care revisited. N Engl J Med 2001;344:2021–25.
15. Taylor RB, ed. Family medicine: Principles and practice, 1st ed. New York: Springer Verlag, 1978.
16. Tarlov AR, Ware JE, Greenfield S. The medical outcomes study: an application of methods for monitoring the results of medical care. JAMA 1989;262:925–30.
17. Ebell MH, Smith MA, Barry HC, Ives K, Carey M. Does this patient have strep throat? JAMA 2000;284:2912–8.
18. O'Connor PJ, Desai J, Rush WA, Cherney LM, Solberg L, Bishop DB. Is having a regular provider of diabetes care related to intensity of care and glycemic control? J Fam Pract 1998;47;290–7.
19. www.clinicalevidence.org.
20. Geyman JP, Deyo RA, Ramsey SD. Evidence-based clinical practice: concepts and approaches. Woburn, Mass: Butterworth Heinemann, 2000.
21. Riegelman RK. Studying a study and testing a test, 4th edition: How to Read the medical evidence. Philadelphia: Lippincott Williams & Wilkins, 2000.
22. Hull R. Just a GP. Oxford, England: Radcliff, 1994.
23. Pellegrino ED. Dismembering the Hippocratic Oath. Boston: Boston University Alumni Report, fall, 1995:11–7.
24. Ebell MH, Frame P. What technology can do to, and for, family medicine. Fam Med 2001;33(4):311–9.

Suggestions for Small Group Discussion

The following are suggestions for class discussion. They are based on the model of a 6-week Family Medicine/Primary Care Clerkship in the clinical years of medical school. The assignments further assume that students are spending part of their time each week in the offices of practicing physicians. In discussing cases, evidence based data should be used whenever possible.

Week 1

Present a case that illustrates the significance of *The Reason for the Visit*. The case presented may, for example, show how a psychosocial problem was presented as a physical complaint or how the identification of the true reason for the visit was the key to understanding a puzzling clinical problem.

Week 2

Present a case that highlights the importance of *Listening to What the Patient is Trying to Tell*. An example might be an instance when you or your doctor used an open-ended question to clarify a complex clinical presentation. Or, perhaps tell about an instance when you overlooked a key clinical issue because you missed a cue offered by the patient.

Week 3

Describe a case that exemplifies the importance of *The Meaning of the Illness to the Patient*. Perhaps describe an instance in which the disease actually offered a special benefit to the patient, or tell about a patient whose symptom held some special significance that was revealed only later in the encounter.

Week 4

Present a case that highlights *The Impact of Illness on the Family*. This may be an instance of one person's illness having an unfavorable impact on the life of one or more family members. Another approach might be identifying an instance in which disease advantaged someone in the family and how this might influence the outcome of care.

Week 5

Describe an instance that illustrates the importance of the *Appropriate Locus of Care for a Person's Illness*. Your might tell of an instance of planned, timely consultation or referral, and how this might have been valuable in care. An alternative might be a time in which a patient or family member insisted on a consultation or referral that your physician believed inappropriate, and how the physician dealt with the request.

Week 6

Tell about a clinical case in which the *Resources Available to Help in Managing Illness* were important in the process of care. You may choose an instance in which your physician referred the patient to a social service agency, and tell how this influenced care. On the other hand, you may present an instance in which the lack of access to resources had a profound impact on the clinical outcome, and what might be done in the future to help patients gain access to needed resources.

2
Clinical Prevention

ANTHONY F. JERANT

Background

Definition and Focus

Clinical prevention involves the maintenance and promotion of health and the reduction of risk factors that result in injury and disease. The elements of clinical prevention include screening tests, counseling interventions, and immunizations, as well as chemoprophylaxis, the use of drugs or biologics taken by asymptomatic persons to reduce the risk of developing a disease. This chapter provides the tools for family physicians to meet the formidable challenge of providing clinical prevention services in an evidence-based manner. While mass screening is an important public health tool, the material in this chapter mostly concerns the individualized screening that is offered during single physician–patient encounters. Consistent with the approach of the U.S. Preventive Services Task Force (USPSTF), the focus of this chapter is primary and secondary prevention. *Primary prevention* is the reduction of risk factors for diseases before they occur, whereas *secondary prevention* is the identification and treatment of diseases or conditions at an early stage. Both primary and secondary prevention concern asymptomatic individuals. *Tertiary prevention*, which reduces the future negative health effects of diseases or conditions that have already become symptomatic, is discussed in many other chapters in this book.

The Ongoing Need for Clinical Preventive Services

Tremendous successes in clinical prevention have been realized in the last 50 years. For example, mortality due to coronary heart disease has declined by approximately 50%, and more than half of this decline can be attributed to preventive interventions such as reducing cigarette smoking and detecting and treating hyperlipidemia. The greater than 90% reductions in morbidity and mortality due to measles, mumps, rubella, smallpox, pertussis, tetanus, and *Haemophilus influenzae* type b resulting from mass vaccination programs are an even greater prevention success story.[1] Nevertheless, the most common underlying causes of death in the United States reflect an ongoing need to improve and expand the delivery of clinical preventive services (Table 2.1).[2]

The leading health indicators in *Healthy People 2010*, a blueprint for public health resulting from collaboration between hundreds of state and federal agencies and organizations, were clearly developed with this list in mind (Table 2.2).[3] Because the average life expectancy in America lags behind that of nearly 20 other nations, one of the main goals of *Healthy People 2010* is to increase life expectancy and years of healthy life. There are 467 specific objectives within 28 focus areas derived from population data, many pertinent to clinical prevention (Table 2.2). The full report is available on the World Wide Web (WWW) at *http://www.health.gov/healthypeople*. *Healthy People 2010* provides a critical link between public health and clinical practice. Approaching every patient with the focus areas in mind will help in detecting the most prevalent contributors to early morbidity and mortality. For example, in the focus area for cancer, one objective is to increase the proportion of adults who receive colorectal cancer screening from 35% to a target of 50%. A 55-year-old patient who has not undergone screening might be informed that while it can reduce the risk of death due to colorectal cancer, only one in three eligible Americans receives such screening. Subsequently, the patient's genetic and environmental history, health habits, and preferences can be used to develop a personalized colorectal cancer prevention plan.

Evidence-Based Clinical Prevention

Principles of Screening

Seven principles should be considered in evaluating a potential screening intervention:

1. The disease or condition in question must lead to substantial morbidity or mortality. Several conditions consistently account for the greatest disease bur-

TABLE 2.1. Actual Causes of Death in the United States in 1990

Cause of death	Estimated number of deaths	Percent of total deaths
Tobacco use	400,000	19
Diet / activity patterns	300,000	14
Alcohol	100,000	5
Microbial agents	90,000	4
Toxic agents	60,000	3
Firearms	35,000	2
Sexual behavior	30,000	1
Motor vehicles	25,000	1
Illicit use of drugs	20,000	<1
Total	1,060,000	50

Source: McGinnis and Foege,[2] with permission.

TABLE 2.2. Healthy People 2010 Leading Health Indicators and Focus Areas Pertinent to the Clinical Prevention Encounter

Leading indicators	Focus areas
Access to health care	Arthritis, osteoporosis, and chronic
Environmental quality	back conditions
Immunization	Cancer
Injury and violence	Chronic kidney disease
Mental health	Diabetes
Overweight and obesity	Disability and secondary conditions
Physical activity	Family planning
Responsible sexual behavior	Heart disease and stroke
Substance abuse	Human immunodeficiency virus
Tobacco use	Immunization and infectious disease
	Injury and violence prevention
	Maternal, infant, and child health
	Nutrition and overweight
	Oral health
	Physical activity and fitness
	Respiratory diseases
	Sexually transmitted diseases
	Substance abuse
	Tobacco abuse
	Vision and hearing

Source: Healthy People 2010,[3] with permission.

den in our society. This burden can be quantified using the disability-adjusted life year (DALY), the sum of the years of life lost due to premature mortality and the years of life lost due to disability in a population (Table 2.3).[4] Screening patients for these conditions and underlying risk factors should be given the highest priority.

2. The screening test employed to detect the condition should be accurate. An ideal screening test has both a high sensitivity (low false-negative rate) and high specificity (low false-positive rate). In practice, screening tests seldom meet this ideal. For example, the CAGE acronym screening tool for alcohol abuse and dependence has fair specificity (76–96%) but relatively low sensitivity (74–78%) at the most commonly used definition of abnormal (two or more affirmative responses). Lowering the abnormal cutoff to one or more affirmative responses would increase the number of problem drinkers detected (sensitivity 86–90%) but would also lead to more false positives (specificity 52–93%).[5] The trade-off between sensitivity and specificity is a characteristic of all screening tests.

3. The disease or condition should have a high incidence and/or prevalence. Screening is effective for some conditions only when individuals reach a certain age, are of a certain gender, or possess certain risk factors that place them at increased risk for developing the conditions. Stated another way, as the prevalence of a disease or condition increases, the positive predictive value (PPV) of a test increases, regardless of its sensitivity and specificity:

TABLE 2.3. Estimated Top 10 Leading Causes of Disability-Adjusted Life Years (DALYs) in the United States, 1996

Rank	Men			Women		
	Cause	DALYs	% of total DALYs	Cause	DALYs	% of total DALYs
	All conditions	18,314,401	100	All conditions	15,886,327	100
1	Ischemic heart disease	1,969,256	10.75	Ischemic heart disease	1,181,298	7.45
2	Road traffic collisions	933,953	5.10	Unipolar major depression	1,073,911	6.77
3	Lung/bronchus cancers	812,675	4.44	Cerebrovascular disease	836,345	5.27
4	HIV/AIDS	773,640	4.22	Lung/bronchus cancers	549,963	3.47
5	Alcohol abuse/ dependence	736,572	4.02	Osteoarthritis	521,443	3.24
6	Cerebrovascular disease	673,877	3.68	Breast cancer	514,729	3.21
7	Homicide and violence	567,322	3.10	COPD	510,084	3.19
8	COPD	545,350	2.98	Dementia/CNS degenerative disorder	506,858	3.16
9	Self-inflicted	541,640	2.96	Diabetes mellitus	500,932	2.90
10	Unipolar major depression	477,040	2.60	Road traffic collisions	459,489	2.61

CNS = central nervous system; COPD = chronic obstructive pulmonary disease.
Source: Michaud et al.[4] copyright 2001, American Medical Association, with permission

$$PPV = \frac{(Sensitivity \times Prevalence)}{[(Sensitivity \times Prevalence)] + [(1 - Specificity) \times (1 - Prevalence)]}.$$

Another way to estimate the overall "yield for effort" of a screening intervention is the number needed to screen (NNS),[6] which is analogous to the concept of number needed to treat (NNT) in clinical therapeutics. NNS is calculated by taking the reciprocal of the absolute risk reduction (ARR) conferred by screening:

NNS = 1/ARR
    = 1/[(*No. of outcome events/No. of screened patients*)
    − (*No. of outcome events / No. of controls*)]

For example, the NNS to prevent one death due to tuberculosis (TB) in programs involving intravenous drug abusers ranges from 103 to 4650, while in studies involving individuals with no identifiable risk factors for TB, the NNS to prevent one death due to TB ranges from 132,690 to 606,797.[7] These figures provide clinically tangible estimates of the yield of TB screening and reinforce the concept that the PPV of a screening test increases as the incidence of the condition in question increases in the screened population.

4. The disease or condition should have an asymptomatic period during which it can be detected. Diseases with long asymptomatic periods, such as cervical cancer, are easier to target with screening than diseases with a short preclinical duration, such as leukemia. However, for conditions with a long preclinical duration, *lead-time bias* can make it appear that a group of screened patients survives longer than a group that is not screened. In reality the screened patients may simply be finding out they have the disease earlier, during its asymptomatic phase. To avoid attributing benefit to a screening program that suffers from lead-time bias, screening decisions should be based on comparisons of actual mortality rates, rather than on measures that are affected by the time elapsed since diagnosis, such as 5-year survival rates. A second problem related to preclinical disease duration is called *length-time bias*. Less aggressive cases have a longer asymptomatic period and are more likely to be detected by screening than more aggressive cases. Thus, a screening program may appear to improve survival when it is actually only detecting more indolent cases that have a better prognosis. Prostate cancer screening has been criticized for many reasons, including strong concerns about lead-time and length-time bias.

5. The disease or condition should have a widely available and acceptable treatment known to improve outcomes. Many conditions that are otherwise worthy candidates for screening are not currently amenable to treatments that change their natural history. For example, dementia accounts for a substantial number of DALYs (Table 2.3) but fails to meet this criterion.

6. The screening procedure should entail reasonable health risks and financial cost. Screening cost estimates should include not only the cost of an initial

screening test but also costs related to repeat office visits, specialty referrals, additional testing, false positives, and complications. Formal cost-effectiveness analyses of preventive interventions account for all of these factors. The end point of such analyses is often the ratio of dollar cost per quality-adjusted life year (QALY), the product of the number of years of life and the quality of those years as measured from 0 (indifference between life and death) to 1 (full health) on a questionnaire. Thus, a screening test that provides an average of 12 more years of life with a quality rating or *utility* of 0.4 is said to provide 4.8 QALYs. Although there is no universal agreement on what dollar cost/QALY ratio cut-point defines a cost-effective screening program, Table 2.4 provides a comparative listing of ratios for some widely accepted preventive practices.[8] Cost-effectiveness must be considered from the societal perspective, but clinicians can greatly influence the costs of screening programs by taking an evidence-based approach.

7. The screening procedure should be acceptable to the patient and society. The yield of a screening program is decreased if many candidates are unwilling to undergo testing. For example, colorectal cancer screening via flexible sigmoidoscopy is supported by research evidence, but the rate of patient adherence to a physician's recommendation for flexible sigmoidoscopy is only 35%, partially due to test discomfort and inconvenience.

Family physicians can effectively individualize the following general clinical prevention guidelines by considering each of these seven screening principles and the way they apply to their specific practice settings and patient populations.

TABLE 2.4. Median, Minimum, and Maximum Estimated Cost-Utility Ratios for Various Preventive Interventions

Preventive service	Median $/QALY	Minimum $/QALY	Maximum $/QALY
Immunizations and vaccinations	1500	Cost-saving	140,000
Screening tests			
Cardiovascular disease	3300	950	130,000
Neoplasms	18,500	Cost-saving	140,000
Other diseases	11,500	Cost-saving	450,000
Counseling			
HIV risk behaviors	1200	Cost-saving	2400
Cardiovascular risk factors	74,000	Cost-saving	8,900,000

QALY = quality-adjusted life year.
Source: Reprinted by permission of Elsevier Science from Stone et al.[8]

Clinical Preventive Services Guidelines

The 1996 recommendations of the USPSTF, found in the *Guide to Clinical Preventive Services*, 2nd edition,[9] were chosen as the primary resource for this section for several reasons. First, the recommendations are generated using an explicit evidence-based approach, and the items listed in the age-specific recommendation tables are those for which the USPSTF concluded that there is either good or fair evidence to support the recommendation. Second, in contrast to the recommendations of organizations such as the American Cancer Society (ACS) and medical professional groups, the recommendations are not directly tied to public awareness efforts and professional or political agendas. Finally, the USPSTF makes recommendations throughout the life cycle and is thus highly relevant to family physicians. A revised third edition of the guide is scheduled to appear in 2002, and new recommendations and updates are being posted on the WWW as they are released; go to *www.ahrq.gov/clinic/uspstfix.htm*.

General Recommendations for All Age Groups

In general, new patients should undergo a comprehensive history and physical examination, have a health risk appraisal completed, and be educated regarding age-specific preventive services. Previous health records should be obtained to avoid duplication of services, and additional services may be added routinely based on the individual's risk profile. Because the evidence base is continually growing and changing, family physicians must frequently update their clinical prevention protocols as new evidence becomes available.

Birth to Ten Years (Table 2.5)

PERIOD IMMEDIATELY FOLLOWING BIRTH

Screening for congenital conditions is the first priority in prevention for newborns. All 50 states require testing for phenylketonuria and congenital hypothyroidism, but states vary regarding other mandated tests. In addition to mandated screening tests, infants born to mothers at risk for human immunodeficiency virus (HIV) infection but whose infection status is unknown should be considered for HIV testing. From the time of birth and throughout childhood, it is important to be aware of family psychosocial and socioeconomic factors such as poverty and parental substance abuse that place children at increased risk for multiple adverse health outcomes and developmental problems. For example, parents who smoke tobacco must be counseled regarding the risks to infants of passive smoke exposure, including higher rates of otitis media and lower respiratory tract infections. Counseling of smoking mothers has been shown to reduce their children's exposure to environmental tobacco smoke, regardless of the mothers' eventual cessation status.[10]

TABLE 2.5. Interventions Considered and Recommended for Prevention, Birth to 10 Years; Leading Causes of Death: Perinatal Conditions, Congenital Anomalies, Sudden Infant Death Syndrome (SIDS), Injuries

Interventions for the general population

SCREENING
Height and weight
Blood pressure
Vision screen (age 3–4 years)
Hemoglobinopathy screen (birth)[a]
Phenylalanine level (birth)[b]
T$_4$ and/or TSH (birth)[c]

COUNSELING
Injury prevention
Child safety car seats (age <5 years)
Lap shoulder belts (age ≥5 years)
Bicycle helmet; avoid bicycling near traffic
Smoke detector, flame retardant sleepwear
Hot water heater temperature <120–130°F
Window/stair guards, pool fence
Safe storage of drugs, toxic substances, firearms, and matches
Syrup of ipecac, poison control phone number
CPR training for parents/caregivers

Diet and exercise
Breast-feeding, iron-enriched formula, and foods (infants and toddlers)
Limit fat and cholesterol; maintain caloric balance; emphasize grains, fruits, and vegetables
Regular physical activity
Substance use
Effects of passive smoking*
Antitobacco message*
Dental health
Regular visits to dental care provider*
Floss, brush with fluoride toothpaste daily*
Advice about baby bottle tooth decay*

IMMUNIZATIONS
See Tables 2.6 and 2.7

CHEMOPROPHYLAXIS
Ocular prophylaxis (birth)

Interventions for high-risk populations (see detailed high-risk definitions in footnotes)

POPULATION
Preterm or low birth weight
Infants of mothers at risk for HIV
Low income; immigrants

TB contacts
Native American/Alaska Native

Travelers to developing countries
Residents of long-term care facilities

POTENTIAL INTERVENTIONS
Hemoglobin/hematocrit (high risk 1 [HR1])
HIV testing (HR2)
Hemoglobin/hematocrit (HR1); purified protein derivative (PPD (HR3)
PPD (HR3)
Hemoglobin/hematocrit (HR1); PPD (HR3); hepatitis A vaccine (HR4); pneumococcal vaccine (HR5)
Hepatitis A vaccine (HR4)
PPD (HR3); hepatitis A vaccine (HR4); influenza vaccine (HR6)

26

Certain chronic medical conditions	PPD (HR3); pneumococcal vaccine (HR5); influenza vaccine (HR6)
Increased individual or community lead exposure	Blood lead level (HR7)
Inadequate water fluoridation	Daily fluoride supplement (HR8)
Family history of skin cancer; nevi, fair skin, eyes, hair	Avoid excess/midday sun, use protective clothing* (HR9)

---

aWhether screening should be universal or targeted to high-risk individuals in the screening area, and other considerations.

bIf done during first 24 hours of life, repeat by age 2 weeks.

cOptimally between day 2 and 6, but in all cases before newborn nursery discharge.

*The ability of clinician counseling to influence this behavior is unproved.

HR1—Infants age 6–12 months who are living in poverty; black, Native American, or Alaska Native; immigrants from developing countries; preterm and low birth weight infants; infants whose principal dietary intake is unfortified cow's milk.

HR2—Infants born to high-risk mothers whose HIV status is unknown. Women at high risk include past or present injection drug use; persons who exchange sex for money or drugs, and their sex partners; injection drug–using, bisexual, or HIV-positive sex partners currently or in past; persons seeking treatment for sexually transmitted diseases (STDs); blood transfusion during 1978–1985.

HR3—Persons infected with HIV, close contacts of persons with known or suspected TB, persons with medical risk factors associated with TB, immigrants from countries with high TB prevalence, medically underserved low-income populations (including homeless), residents of long-term care facilities.

HR4—Persons >2 years old living in or traveling to areas where the disease is endemic and where periodic outbreaks occur (e.g., countries with high or intermediate endemicity; certain Alaska Native, Pacific Island, Native American, and religious communities). Consider for institutionalized children aged ≥2 years. Clinicians should also consider local epidemiology.

HR5—Immunocompetent persons >2 years old with certain medical conditions, including chronic cardiac or pulmonary disease, diabetes mellitus, and anatomic asplenia. Immunocompetent persons ≥2 years old living in high-risk environments or social settings (e.g., certain Native-American and Alaska-Native populations).

HR6—Annual vaccination of children ≥6 months old who are residents of chronic care facilities or who have chronic cardiopulmonary disorders, metabolic diseases (including diabetes mellitus), hemoglobinopathies, immunosuppression, or renal dysfunction.

HR7—Children about age 12 months who (1) live in communities in which the prevalence of lead levels requiring individual intervention, including residential lead hazard control or chelation, is high or undefined; (2) live in or frequently visit a home built before 1950 with dilapidated paint or with recent or ongoing renovation or remodeling; (3) have close contact with a person who has an elevated lead level; (4) live near lead industry or heavy traffic; (5) live with someone whose job or hobby involves lead exposure; (6) use lead-based pottery; or (7) take traditional ethnic remedies that contain lead.

HR8—Children living in areas with inadequate water fluoridation (see Table 2.8).

HR9—Persons with a family history of skin cancer, a large number of moles, atypical moles, poor tanning ability, or light skin, hair, and eye color.

T4 = thyroxine; TSH = thyroid-stimulating hormone.

Source: U.S. Preventive Services Task Force,[9] with permission.

27

Passive tobacco smoke exposure is also associated with an increased risk for sudden infant death syndrome (SIDS),[11] a leading cause of death in this age group. The USPSTF has not produced a recommendation regarding optimal infant sleep position, but substantial evidence suggests that SIDS is associated with the prone sleep position. Further, although no definite causal link has been established, populations in which physician counseling and media efforts has led to increased use of the supine sleeping position have observed decreased rates of SIDS, resulting in an American Academy of Pediatrics (AAP) recommendation that physicians counsel all parents to place infants to sleep on their backs on a firm surface.[12] A dialogue regarding breast-feeding should ideally be begun during the early prenatal period. Nevertheless, because it is associated with lower rates of otitis media and infectious diarrhea,[13] physicians should encourage all mothers to breast-feed at the time of birth. This protective effect follows a dose-response relationship so that infants who are not exclusively breast-fed still benefit. Newborns should ideally receive their first hepatitis B vaccination, using a thimerosal-free formulation, prior to discharge from the hospital.

INFANCY TO AGE TWO

Ensuring that appropriate growth is being maintained is an important preventive task in this group. Very low birth weight children, an increasing population, often have postnatal growth rates that lag behind those of term infants. Special growth curves, produced by several formula manufacturers, should be utilized until "catch up" growth is achieved, usually at about 3 years of age. Injury prevention counseling should also be emphasized. Injuries account for two of every five deaths in children aged 1 through 4, four times the number of deaths due to birth defects, the second leading cause of death in this age group. Clinicians must also remain alert to the various presentations of family violence, which may include injuries initially attributed to accidents. While the debate regarding lead screening in childhood continues, the USPSTF and Centers for Disease Control and Prevention (CDC) currently recommend a selective approach. Children should be screened if they live in areas with risk for lead exposure, belong to groups that may be at risk (such as the poor), or are found to be at risk based on a "yes" answer to any of the following three questions: (1) Does the child live in or regularly visit a house that was built before 1950? (2) Does the child live in or regularly visit a house that was built before 1978 with recent (within the last 6 months) or ongoing renovations or remodeling? (3) Does the child have a sibling or playmate who has or did have lead poisoning? Physicians must also be aware of local policies, since some states mandate screening.

Table 2.6 provides the most recent universal childhood immunization schedule.[14] Recent changes include the addition of pneumococcal conjugate vaccination and, in certain areas, hepatitis A vaccination. Unfortunately, many children receive immunizations late or not at all, placing them at risk for infectious diseases and increasing the chance of community infectious disease outbreaks in vaccinated individuals.[15] Physician failure to review immunization status at each visit and unnecessary practice policies against vaccination in certain circumstances, such as in the presence of acute minor illness with low-grade fever, are important causes of missed opportunities to vaccinate.[16] Evidence-based vaccination protocols, provider education, and immunization flow sheets may help to reduce missed opportunities. A "catch-up" schedule should be employed for children who have fallen behind to rapidly return them to full coverage (Table 2.7).[17] The Immunization Action Coalition produces excellent resources for both physicians and parents on the WWW: *http://www.immunize.org/*.

To help prevent dental caries, children who live in communities with low levels of fluoride in the water should be prescribed fluoride supplements beginning at 6 months of age. Other dental preventive efforts include counseling parents to put children to bed without a bottle and recommending periodic dentist visits beginning at around age 3.

TWO TO TEN YEARS

Early detection of cardiovascular disease risk factors should be a major focus of screening beginning in early childhood. The body mass index (BMI) is a practical indicator of the appropriateness of weight for height in children age 2 and older and can be plotted on recently updated growth curves. Although a low BMI can indicate poor nutrition or an underlying medical disorder, elevated BMI in childhood is a more common problem that is reaching epidemic proportions in the U.S. For children 6 and older, a BMI from the 85th to the 95th percentile indicates overweight, whereas a BMI above the 95th percentile indicates obesity. Childhood obesity is associated with a host of immediate and long-term health risks, including increased rates of obesity and early mortality in adulthood.[18] Early identification should be followed by frequent monitoring and parental counseling regarding appropriate diet and nutrition. Physicians should also screen children for a sedentary lifestyle, a major contributor to childhood obesity, and provide counseling regarding physical activity. All children should receive periodic blood pressure measurement throughout this period, and those with measurements that persistently exceed the 95th percentile values in tables based on gender, age, and height should receive further evaluation. Such tables are available on the WWW: *http://www.nhlbi.nih.gov/health/prof/heart/hbp/hbp_ped.htm*.[19] The USPSTF and other organizations recommend cholesterol measurement only in children at high risk for adult coronary artery disease. Risk factors include a family history of premature cardiovascular disease or family members with cholesterol levels greater than 240 mg/dL.

Injury prevention counseling should be continued throughout this period. Thirty-three percent of injuries in this age group are due to violence, and 67% are due to unintentional injuries. Simple measures that reduce injury-related mortality in children, such as the use of helmets when bicycling, should be emphasized. Firearm safety should also be reviewed. Safe sun precautions should be periodically reviewed for children at increased risk for skin cancer, including those with a family history, a large number of moles, atypical moles, poor tan-

TABLE 2.6. Recommended Childhood Immunization Schedule United States, 2002

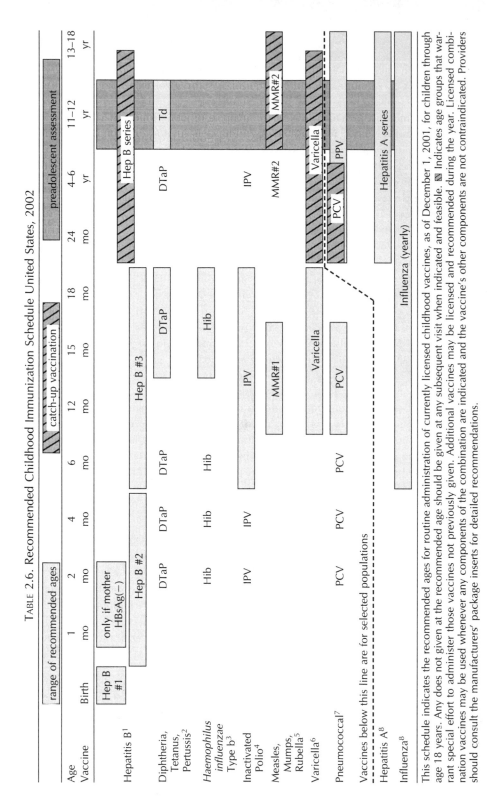

This schedule indicates the recommended ages for routine administration of currently licensed childhood vaccines, as of December 1, 2001, for children through age 18 years. Any dose not given at the recommended age should be given at any subsequent visit when indicated and feasible. ▨ Indicates age groups that warrant special effort to administer those vaccines not previously given. Additional vaccines may be licensed and recommended during the year. Licensed combination vaccines may be used whenever any components of the combination are indicated and the vaccine's other components are not contraindicated. Providers should consult the manufacturers' package inserts for detailed recommendations.

1. Hepatitis B vaccine (Hep B). All infants should receive the first dose of hepatitis B vaccine soon after birth and before hospital discharge; the first dose may also be given by age 2 months if the infant's mother is HBsAg-negative. Only monovalent hepatitis B vaccine can be used for the birth dose. Monovalent or combination vaccine containing Hep B may be used to complete the series; four doses of vaccine may be administered if combination vaccine is used. The second dose should be given at least 4 weeks after the first dose, except for Hib-containing vaccine which cannot be administered before age 6 weeks. The third dose should be given at least 16 weeks after the first dose and at least 8 weeks after the second dose. The last dose in the vaccination series (third or fourth dose) should not be administered before age 6 months.

Infants born to HBsAg-positive mothers should receive hepatitis B vaccine and 0.5 mL hepatitis B immune globulin (HBIG) within 12 hours of birth at separate sites. The second dose is recommended at age 1–2 months and the vaccination series should be completed (third or fourth dose) at age 6 months.

Infants born to mothers whose HBsAg status is unknown should receive the first dose of the hepatitis B vaccine series within 12 hours of birth. Maternal blood should be drawn at the time of delivery to determine the mother's HBsAg status; if the HBsAg test is positive, the infant should receive HBIG as soon as possible (no later than age 1 week).

2. Diphtheria and tetanus toxoids and acellular pertussis vaccine (DTaP). The fourth dose of DTaP may be administered as early as age 12 months, provided 6 months have elapsed since the third dose and the child is unlikely to return at age 15–18 months. **Tetanus and diphtheria toxoids (Td)** is recommended at age 11–12 years if at least 5 years have elapsed since the last dose of tetanus and diphtheria toxoid-containing vaccine. Subsequent routine Td boosters are recommended every 10 years.

3. Haemophilus influenzae type b (Hib) conjugate vaccine. Three Hib conjugate vaccines are licensed for infant use. If PRP-OMP (PedvaxHIB® or ComVax® [Merck]) is administered at ages 2 and 4 months, a dose at age 6 months is not required. DTaP/Hib combination products should not be used for primary immunization in infants at ages 2, 4 or 6 months, but can be used as boosters following any Hib vaccine.

4. Inactivated polio vaccine (IPV). An all-IPV schedule is recommended for routine childhood polio vaccination in the United States. All children should receive four doses of IPV at ages 2 months, 4 months, 6–18 months, and 4–6 years.

5. Measles, mumps, and rubella vaccine (MMR). The second dose of MMR is recommended routinely at age 4–6 years but may be administered during any visit, provided at least 4 weeks have elapsed since the first dose and that both doses are administered beginning at or after age 12 months. Those who have not previously received the second dose should complete the schedule by the 11–12 year old visit.

6. Varicella vaccine. Varicella vaccine is recommended at any visit at or after age 12 months for susceptible children, i.e. those who lack a reliable history of chickenpox. Susceptible persons aged ≥13 years should receive two doses, given at least 4 weeks apart.

7. Pneumococcal vaccine. The heptavalent **pneumococcal conjugate vaccine (PCV)** is recommended for all children age 2–23 months. It is also recommended for certain children age 24–59 months. **Pneumococcal polysaccharide vaccine (PPV)** is recommended in addition to PCV for certain high-risk groups. See MMWR 2000;49(RR-9);1–35.

8. Hepatitis A vaccine. Hepatitis A vaccine is recommended for use in selected states and regions, and for certain high-risk groups; consult your local public health authority. See MMWR 1999;48(RR-12);1–37.

9. Influenza vaccine. Influenza vaccine is recommended annually for children age ≥6 months with certain risk factors (including but not limited to asthma, cardiac disease, sickle cell disease, HIV, diabetes; see MMWR 2001;50(RR-4):1–44), and can be administered to all others wishing to obtain immunity. Children aged ≤12 years should receive vaccine in a dosage appropriate for their age (0.25 mL if age 6–35 months or 0.5 mL if aged ≥3 years). Children aged ≤8 years who are receiving influenza vaccine for the first time should receive two doses separated by at least 4 weeks.

For additional information about vaccines, vaccine supply, and contraindications for immunization, please visit the National Immunization Program Website at www.cdc.gov/nip or call the National Immunization Hotline at 800-232-2522 (English) or 800-232-0233 (Spanish).

Approved by the Advisory Committee on Immunization Practices (www.cdc.gov/nip/acip), the American Academy of Pediatrics (www.aap.org), and the American Academy of Family Physicians (www.aafp.org).

Reprinted from Zimmerman,[14] with permission from American Family Physician. Copyright© American Academy of Family Physicians.

Table 2.7. Minimal Age for Initial Childhood Vaccinations and Minimal Interval Between Vaccine Doses by Type of Vaccine*

Vaccine type	Minimal age for dose 1	Minimal interval between doses 1 and 2	Minimal interval between doses 2 and 3	Minimal interval between doses 3 and 4
Hepatitis B	Birth	1 month	2 months	a
DTaP (DT)[b]	6 weeks	4 weeks	4 weeks	6 months
Combined DTwP-Hib[c]	6 weeks	1 month	1 month	6 months
Hib (primary series)				
HbOC	6 weeks	1 month	1 month	c
PRP-T	6 weeks	1 month	1 month	c
PRP-OMP	6 weeks	1 month	c	
Inactivated poliovirus	6 weeks	4 weeks	4 weeks[d]	e
Pneumococcal conjugate	6 weeks	1 month	1 month	c
MMR	12 months[f]	1 month		
Varicella	12 months	4 weeks		

DTaP (DT diphtheria and tetanus toxoids and acellular pertussis vaccine (diphtheria and tetanus toxoids vaccine); DTwP-Hib = diphtheria and tetanus toxoids and whole-cell pertussis vaccine–*Haemophilus influenzae type b conjugate vaccine; HbOC* = oligosaccharides conjugated to diphtheria CRM197 toxin protein; PRP-T = polyrigosylribitol phosphate polysaccharide conjugated to tetanus toxoid; PRP-OMP = polyribosylribitol phosphate polysaccharide conjugated to a meningococcal outer membrane protein; MMR = measles-mumps-rubella.
*The minimal acceptable ages and intervals may not correspond with the optimal recommended ages and intervals for vaccination. For current recommended routine schedules, see Table 2.6.
[a]The final dose of hepatitis B vaccine is recommended at least 4 months after the first dose and no earlier than 6 months of age.
[b]The total number of doses of diphtheria and tetanus toxoids should not exceed six each before the seventh birthday.
[c]The booster doses of Hib and pneumococcal vaccines that are recommended following the primary vaccination series should be administered no earlier than 12 months of age and at least 2 months after the previous dose.
[d]For unvaccinated adults at increased risk of exposure to poliovirus with less than 3 months but more than 2 months available before protection is needed, three doses of inactivated poliovirus (IPV) should be administered at least 1 month apart.
[e]If the third dose is given after the third birthday, the fourth (booster) dose is not needed.
[f]Although the age for measles vaccination may be as young as 6 months in outbreak areas where cases are occurring in children younger than 1 year, children initially vaccinated before the first birthday should be revaccinated at 12 to 15 months of age and an additional dose of vaccine should be administered at the time of school entry or according to local policy. Doses of MMR or other measles-containing vaccines should be separated by at least one month.
Adapted from Epidemiology and Prevention of Vaccine-Preventable Diseases, 6th ed,[17] with permission.

ning ability, or light skin, hair, and eye color. The immunization series outlined in Table 2.6 should be continued as appropriate throughout childhood, so that all children will have received the full complement of vaccinations by the age of 12. Because purified protein derivative (PPD) testing of all children is exceedingly expensive and results in many false-positive tests, the USPSTF and CDC recommend a selective approach to screening based on the risk of exposure to

TB. Exposure risk factors include birth or prior residence in a region where TB is highly prevalent, such as Southeast Asia, and close exposure to persons known or suspected to have TB.[20]

Eleven to Twenty-Four Years (Table 2.8)

This period includes adolescence, a developmental period that poses unique clinical prevention challenges. Although comprehensive guidelines for preventive care in this age group have been proposed, evidence to support many of the items included is lacking. It is especially unclear whether physician counseling is capable of changing adolescent health behaviors and impacting on key adverse health outcomes. An important principle of prevention for this age group is opportunistic delivery of services. Since adolescents seldom visit a physician specifically for preventive care, every clinic visit by an adolescent should be viewed as an opportunity to provide prevention. Unfortunately, very low rates of clinical preventive services delivery have recently been observed for the typical adolescent visit.[21] Although adolescents may initially be hesitant to discuss health risk behaviors, they appear to become more willing to do so with repeated physician efforts.[22] Appointment invitation letters can increase the number of visits made by adolescents specifically to receive preventive services.[23]

Between 50% and 75% of all deaths in this age group are due to unintentional injuries, suicides, and homicides. Providing brief counseling regarding proven injury prevention measures is prudent. Important recommendations regarding motor vehicle injury reduction might include not driving at night for the first year after a driver's license is obtained, not riding in a car with an intoxicated individual, and always using a three-point seat restraint.[24] Cardiovascular risk reduction measures such as recommending tobacco avoidance and regular exercise and screening for obesity should be continued. For sexually active teens, contraception and sexually transmitted disease (STD) avoidance counseling are critical. The third USPSTF has released an advance statement regarding chlamydia, the most common STD in the United States, recommending screening all women who are sexually active and aged 25 or younger; have more than one sexual partner; have had an STD in the past; and do not use condoms consistently and correctly, regardless of age. Periodic screening for other STDs in sexually active teens and young adults should also be considered.

Because most alcohol problems begin in early adulthood, the USPSTF recommends screening for problem drinking for all adolescents and young adults using either "careful history-taking" or a standardized questionnaire such as the CAGE. Although finding insufficient evidence to recommend for or against routine screening for other drug abuse, given the increasing prevalence of amphetamine and other illicit drug use in many areas, physicians should have a low threshold for questioning young people about drug use.

In addition to ensuring that a tetanus booster is administered at about 10 years after the last childhood tetanus vaccination, physicians should inform college students about the increased risk of meningococcal infection in crowded dormi-

TABLE 2.8. Interventions Considered and Recommended for Prevention, Age 11 to 24 Years; Leading Causes of Death: Injuries, Homicide, Suicide, Malignancies, Heart Disease

Interventions for the general population

SCREENING
Height and weight
Blood pressure[a]
Papanicolaou (Pap) test (women)[b]
Chlamydia screen[c]
Rubella serology or vaccination history (females >12 years old)
Assess for problem drinking

COUNSELING
Injury prevention
Lap/shoulder belts
Bicycle/motorcycle/all-terrain vehicle (ATV) helmets*
Smoke detector*
Safe storage/removal of firearms*
Substance use
Avoid tobacco use
Avoid underage drinking and illicit drug use*
Avoid alcohol/drug use while driving, swimming, boating, etc.*

Sexual behavior
Sexually transmitted disease (STD) prevention; abstinence*; avoid high-risk behavior*; condoms/female barrier with spermicide*
Diet and exercise
Limit fat and cholesterol; maintain caloric balance; emphasize grains, fruits, and vegetables
Adequate calcium intake (females)
Regular physical activity*
Dental health
Regular visits to dental care provider*
Floss; brush with fluoride toothpaste daily*

IMMUNIZATIONS
See Tables 2.6 and 2.7
Rubella (females >12 years old)[d]

CHEMOPROPHYLAXIS
Multivitamin with folic acid (females planning/capable of pregnancy)

Interventions for high-risk populations (see detailed high-risk definitions in footnotes)

POPULATION
High-risk sexual behavior

Injection or street drug use

TB contacts; immigrants, low income
Native Americans, Alaska Natives

Travelers to developing countries
Certain chronic medical conditions

Settings where adolescents and young adults congregate
Susceptible to varicella, measles, mumps
Blood transfusion between 1975 and 1985

POTENTIAL INTERVENTIONS
RPR/VDRL (HR1); screen for gonorrhea (female) (HR2), HIV (HR3), chlamydia (female) (HR4); hepatitis A vaccine (HR5)
RPR/VDRL (HR1); HIV screen (HR3), hepatitis A vaccine (HR5); PPD (HR6); advice to reduce infection risk (HR7)
PPD (HR6)
Hepatitis A vaccine (HR5); PPD (HR6); pneumococcal vaccine (HR8)
Hepatitis A vaccine (HR5)
PPD (HR6); pneumococcal vaccine (HR8); influenza vaccine (HR9)
Second MMR (HR10)

Varicella vaccine (HR11); MMR (HR12)
HIV screen (HR3)

Institutionalized persons; health care/lab workers
Family history of skin cancer; nevi, fair skin, eyes, hair
Prior pregnancy with neural tube defect
Inadequate water fluoridation

Hepatitis A vaccine (HR5); PPD (HR6); influenza vaccine
Avoid excess/midday sun; use protective clothing* (HR13)
Folic acid 4.0 mg (HR14)
Daily fluoride supplement (HR15)

---

[a]Periodic blood pressure (BP) for persons aged ≥21 years.

[b]If sexually active at present or in the past: q ≤ 3 years. If sexual history is unreliable, begin Pap tests at age 18 years.

[c]If sexually active.

[d]Serologic testing, documented vaccination history, and routine vaccination against rubella (preferably with MMR) are equally acceptable alternatives.

*The ability of clinician counseling to influence this behavior is unproven.

HR1—Persons who exchange sex for money or drugs, and their sex partners; persons with other STDs (including HIV); and sexual contacts of persons with active syphilis. Clinicians should also consider local epidemiology.

HR2—Women who have two or more sex partners in the last year; a sex partner with multiple sexual contacts; exchanged sex for money or drugs; or a history of repeated episodes of gonorrhea. Clinicians should also consider local epidemiology.

HR3—Men who had sex with men after 1975; past or present injection drug use; persons who exchange sex for money or drugs, and their sex partners; injection drug-using, bisexual, or HIV-positive sex partner currently or in the past; blood transfusion during 1978–1985; persons seeking treatment for STDs. Clinicians should also consider local epidemiology.

HR4—Sexually active females with multiple risk factors including history of prior STD; new or multiple sex partners; age under 25; nonuse or inconsistent use of barrier contraceptives; cervical ectopy. Clinicians should also consider local epidemiology.

HR5—Persons living in, traveling in, or working in areas where the disease is endemic and where periodic outbreaks occur (e.g., countries with high or intermediate endemicity; certain Alaska-Native, Pacific Island, Native-American, and religious communities); men who have sex with men; injection or street drug users. Vaccine may be considered for institutionalized persons and workers in these institutions, military personnel, and day care, hospital, and laboratory workers. Clinicians should also consider local epidemiology.

HR6—HIV positive, close contacts of persons with known or suspected TB, health care workers, persons with medical risk factors associated with TB, immigrants from countries with high TB prevalence, medically underserved low-income populations (including homeless), alcoholics, injection drug users, and residents of long-term facilities.

HR7—Persons who continue to inject drugs.

HR8—Immunocompetent persons with certain medical conditions, including chronic cardiac or pulmonary disease, diabetes mellitus, and anatomic asplenia. Immunocompetent persons who live in high-risk environments or social settings (e.g., certain Native-American and Alaska-Native populations).

HR9—Annual vaccination of residents of chronic care facilities; persons with chronic cardiopulmonary disorders, metabolic diseases (including diabetes mellitus), hemoglobinopathies, immunosuppression, or renal dysfunction; and health care providers for high-risk patients.

HR10—Adolescents and young adults in settings where such individuals congregate (e.g., high schools and colleges), if they have not previously received a second dose.

HR11—Healthy persons aged ≥13 years without a history of chickenpox or previous immunization. Consider serologic testing for presumed susceptible persons aged ≥13 years.

HR12—Persons born after 1956 who lack evidence of immunity to measles or mumps (e.g., documented receipt of live vaccine on or after the first birthday, laboratory evidence of immunity, or a history of physician-diagnosed measles or mumps).

HR13—Persons with a family or personal history of skin cancer, a large number of moles, atypical moles, poor tanning ability, or light skin, hair, and eye color.

HR14—Women with previous pregnancy affected by neural tube defect who are planning pregnancy.

HR15—Persons aged <17 years living in areas with inadequate water fluoridation (see Table 2.8).

Source: U.S. Preventive Services Task Force,[9] with permission.

tory settings and provide them with information regarding meningococcal vaccination.[25]

Twenty-Five to Sixty-Four Years (Table 2.9)

WOMEN'S HEALTH ISSUES

Although preconception counseling is important for all young women, an opportunistic approach must be taken since few specifically request such care. Women planning pregnancy or at risk for unintended pregnancy should be advised to take folic acid, 0.4 to 0.8 mg/day, beginning at least 1 month prior to conception and continuing throughout the first trimester of pregnancy to reduce the risk of neural tube defects. This dose can be obtained by taking a prenatal vitamin daily. Physician advice about folic acid has been shown to dramatically increase patient compliance with this recommendation.[26] Screening for cervical cancer using the Papanicolaou (Pap) smear is recommended every 1 to 3 years for all women who have been sexually active and who have a cervix. Although the most cost-effective interval for repeat testing is controversial, the most important things physicians can do to reduce the incidence of cervical cancer are to ensure that as many women as possible receive at least some screening and to ensure that abnormal results are followed up appropriately. Of women who develop invasive cervical cancer, 50% have never had a Pap smear, 10% have not had a Pap smear within 5 years of diagnosis, and 10% have not received appropriate follow-up of a prior precancerous result.[27]

Breast cancer screening should be offered as women enter middle age, but the optimal time of initiation remains an emotionally charged, controversial issue. The USPSTF recommends screening with mammography alone or mammography plus clinical breast examination (CBE) for all women of ages 50 to 69. The task force found insufficient evidence to recommend for or against mammography or CBE for women of ages 40 to 49 or 70 and older, and for teaching patient breast self-examination at any age. In 1997, a National Institutes of Health (NIH) consensus panel initially issued a statement agreeing with the USPSTF position. Shortly after, following a storm of rebuttals by academicians, politicians, and professional interest and advocacy groups, the panel reversed its statement, recommending initiation of periodic mammography and CBE for all women beginning at age 40, as is advocated by the ACS. Unfortunately, these conflicting recommendations and the complexity of the medical literature in this area have greatly confused patients and physicians. It is clear that the potential mortality benefit from breast cancer screening in women of ages 40 to 49 is much smaller than that obtained by screening women of ages 50 to 75, and that beginning screening at an earlier age results in a higher lifetime incidence of false-positive tests.[28] For now, physicians must review the evidence, form their own conclusions, and then use an "informed consent" approach in negotiating a plan with patients. The National Cancer Institute's Breast Cancer Risk Assessment

TABLE 2.9. Interventions Considered and Recommended for Prevention, Age 25 to 64 Years; Leading Causes of Death: Malignancy, Heart Disease, Injuries, HIV, Suicide, and Homicide

SCREENING
Blood pressure
Height and weight
Total blood cholesterol (men beginning age 35, women beginning age 45)
Papanicolaou (Pap) test (women)[a]
Fecal occult blood test[b] and/or sigmoidoscopy (≥50 years)
Mammogram ± clinical breast exam (women 50–69 years)[c]
Assess for problem drinking
Rubella serology or vaccination history (women of childbearing age)[d]

COUNSELING
Substance use
Tobacco cessation
Avoid alcohol/drug use while driving, swimming, boating, etc.*
Diet and exercise
Limit fat and cholesterol; maintain caloric balance; emphasize grains, fruits, and vegetables
Adequate calcium intake (women)
Regular physical activity*

Injury prevention
Lap/shoulder belts
Motorcycle/bicycle/ATV helmets*
Smoke detector*
Safe storage/removal of firearms*
Sexual behavior
STD prevention: avoid high-risk behavior*; condoms/female barrier with spermicide
Unintended pregnancy: contraception
Dental health
Regular visits to dental care provider*
Floss, brush with fluoride toothpaste daily*

IMMUNIZATIONS
Tetanus-diphtheria (Td) boosters
Rubella (women of childbearing age)[d]

CHEMOPROPHYLAXIS
Multivitamin or folic acid (women planning or capable of pregnancy)
Discuss hormone prophylaxis (peri- and postmenopausal women)

Interventions for high-risk populations (see detailed high-risk definitions in footnotes)

POPULATION	POTENTIAL INTERVENTIONS
High-risk sexual behavior	RPR/VDRL (HR1); screen for gonorrhea (female) (HR2), HIV (HR3), chlamydia (female) (HR4); hepatitis B vaccine (HR5); hepatitis A vaccine (HR6)
Injection or street drug use	RPR/VDRL (HR1); HIV (HR3); hepatitis B vaccine (HR5); hepatitis A vaccine (HR6); PPD (HR7); advice to reduce infection risk (HR7)
Low income; TB contacts; immigrants; alcoholics	PPD (HR8)

37

TABLE 2.9. Interventions Considered and Recommended for Prevention, Age 25 to 64 Years; Leading Causes of Death: Malignancy, Heart Disease, Injuries, HIV, Suicide, and Homicide (*Continued*)

Native Americans/Alaska Natives	Hepatitis A vaccine (HR6); PPD (HR7); pneumococcal vaccine (HR9)
Travelers to developing countries	Hepatitis B vaccine (HR5); hepatitis A vaccine (HR6)
Certain chronic medical conditions	PPD (HR7); pneumococcal vaccine (HR9); influenza vaccine (HR10)
Blood product recipients	HIV screen (HR3); hepatitis B vaccine (HR5)
Susceptible to measles, mumps, rubella	MMR (HR11); varicella vaccine (HR12)
Institutionalized persons	Hepatitis A vaccine (HR6); PPD (HR7); pneumococcal vaccine (HR9); influenza vaccine (HR10)
Health care/lab workers	Hepatitis B vaccine (HR5); hepatitis A vaccine (HR6); PPD (HR7);
Family history of skin cancer; fair skin, eyes, hair	Avoid excess/midday sun; use protective clothing* (HR13)
Previous pregnancy with neural tube defect	Folic acid 4.0 mg (HR14)

a Women who are or have been sexually active and who have a cervix: q ≤ 3 years.
b Annually.
c Mammogram q 1–2 years, or mammogram q 1–2 years with annual clinical breast examination.
d Serologic testing, documented vaccination history, and routine vaccination (preferably with MMR) are equally acceptable.
* The ability of clinician counseling to influence this behavior is unproven.
HR1—Persons who exchange sex for money or drugs, and their sex partners; persons with other STDs (including HIV); and sexual contacts of persons with active syphilis. Clinicians should also consider local epidemiology.
HR2—Women who exchange sex for money or drugs, or who have had repeated episodes of gonorrhea. Clinicians should also consider local epidemiology.
HR3—Men who had sex with men after 1975; past or present injection drug use; persons who exchange sex for money or drugs, and their sex partners; injection drug-using, bisexual, or HIV-positive sex partner currently or in the past; blood transfusion during 1978–1985; persons seeking treatment for STDs. Clinicians should also consider local epidemiology.

HR4—Sexually active females with multiple risk factors including: history of prior STD; new or multiple sex partners; age under 25; nonuse or inconsistent use of barrier contraceptives; cervical ectopy. Clinicians should also consider local epidemiology.

HR5—Blood product recipients (including hemodialysis patients), persons with frequent occupational exposure to blood or blood products, men who have sex with men, injection drug users and their sex partners, persons with multiple recent sex partners, persons with other STDs (including HIV), travelers to countries with endemic hepatitis B.

HR6—Persons living in, traveling to, or working in areas where the disease is endemic and where periodic outbreaks occur (e.g., countries with high or intermediate endemicity; certain Alaska-Native, Pacific Island, Native-American, and religious communities); men who have sex with men; injection or street drug users. Vaccine may be considered for institutionalized persons and workers in these institutions, military personnel, and day care, hospital, and laboratory workers. Clinicians should also consider local epidemiology.

HR7—HIV positive, close contacts of persons with known or suspected TB, health care workers, persons with medical risk factors associated with TB, immigrants from countries with high TB prevalence, medically underserved low-income populations (including homeless), alcoholics, injection drug users, and residents of long-term facilities.

HR8—Persons who continue to inject drugs.

HR9—Immunocompetent persons with certain medical conditions, including chronic cardiac or pulmonary disease, diabetes mellitus, and anatomic asplenia. Immunocompetent persons who live in high-risk environments or social settings (e.g., certain Native-American and Alaska-Native populations).

HR10—Annual vaccination of residents of chronic care facilities; persons with chronic cardiopulmonary disorders, metabolic diseases (including diabetes mellitus), hemoglobinopathies, immunosuppression, or renal dysfunction; and health care providers for high-risk patients.

HR11—Persons born after 1956 who lack evidence of immunity to measles or mumps (e.g., documented receipt of live vaccine on or after the first birthday, laboratory evidence of immunity, or a history of physician-diagnosed measles or mumps).

HR12—Healthy adults without a history of chickenpox or previous immunization. Consider serologic testing for presumed susceptible adults.

HR13—Persons with a family or personal history of skin cancer, a large number of moles, atypical moles, poor tanning ability, or light skin, hair, and eye color.

HR14—Women with previous pregnancy affected by neural tube defect who are planning pregnancy.

Source: U.S. Preventive Services Task Force,[9] with permission.

Tool may help in developing individualized recommendations: *http://bcra.nci. nih.gov/brc/*.

Physicians should also provide counseling to reduce the risk of osteoporosis by encouraging women to remain physically active, consume 1000 to 1500 mg of calcium daily, and avoid tobacco use. Bone density measurement may be indicated in women with significant risk factors for osteoporosis such as Caucasian ancestry, petite body frame, low body weight, tobacco use, excessive alcohol and caffeine intake, and prolonged corticosteroid use. During the perimenopause, discussion regarding hormone replacement therapy (HRT) should be initiated. Although long-term HRT reduces the risk of osteoporosis and associated fractures, its use is associated with a slight increase in the incidence of breast cancer, and its potential benefit in the primary and secondary prevention of cardiovascular disease remains unproved. Thus, an "informed consent" approach to counseling is advised, with careful weighing of patient preferences and risk factors for osteoporosis, heart disease, and breast cancer.

MEN'S HEALTH ISSUES

Prostate cancer is the second leading cause of death for men over age 55, and African-American men have a slightly higher incidence of prostate cancer than other men. While acknowledging its clinical importance, the USPSTF found a lack of evidence to recommend for or against screening for prostate cancer with digital rectal examination (DRE), serum prostate-specific antigen (PSA), or other tests. Evidence that early diagnosis of prostate cancer improves long-term survival is lacking, and there are potential costs and psychological burdens related to the expected high number of false-positive screening tests is large.[29] Refinements in PSA testing are promising but have not yet been properly evaluated. Despite these concerns, the ACS recommends annual DRE for all men starting at age 40, annual PSA testing beginning at age 40 for African-American men and those with a history of prostate cancer, and annual PSA testing beginning at age 50 for all others. The lack of a clear evidence base for prostate cancer screening and the conflicting recommendations of various organizations have created confusion among physicians and patients alike. As with breast cancer screening in women under age 50, an "informed consent" approach to counseling and educating patients should be utilized. Because prostate neoplasms usually grow slowly, men with a life expectancy of less than 10 years should generally not be screened.

ISSUES OF IMPORTANCE TO BOTH MEN AND WOMEN

In addition to its importance as a major cardiovascular disease risk factor, tobacco use has been linked to increased risk for cervical, bladder, lung, and other cancers. Strong counseling regarding smoking cessation, adequate physical activity, and a prudent diet are part of general cancer prevention efforts. The USPSTF found insufficient evidence to recommend for or against routine screening for skin cancer by primary care providers or counseling patients to perform periodic skin self-examinations. However, because one in six Americans will develop skin cancer during their lifetime and the incidence of malignant melanoma has increased rapidly during the past decade, physicians should briefly assess skin cancer risk in all individuals. Those at increased risk should be advised to avoidance of sun exposure, particularly between 10 A.M. and 3 P.M., and to use protective clothing such as shirts and hats when outdoors. The USPSTF found insufficient evidence to recommend for or against advising sunscreen use. For patients at increased risk for malignant melanoma, such as those with familial atypical mole and melanoma syndrome, referral to a skin cancer specialist for evaluation and surveillance should be considered.

Screening for colorectal cancer should be offered to all average-risk men and women beginning at age 50. The USPSTF recommends annual fecal occult blood testing (FOBT), periodic flexible sigmoidoscopy (FS), or both, stating that there is insufficient evidence to make more specific recommendations. Colonoscopy can detect proximal adenomas and neoplasms, but it is more expensive than FS, is associated with a higher risk of complications such as perforation, and has not been shown to be superior in reducing colorectal cancer mortality. Modeling studies suggest that annual FOBT combined with FS every 5 years, beginning at age 50, is the most cost-effective approach to screening and may reduce colorectal cancer mortality by 50% to 80%.[30] As for cervical cancer screening, the major focus in colorectal cancer detection should be to ensure that as many eligible people as possible receive at least some type of screening. Less than half of eligible patients have undergone FOBT or FS within the preceding 5 years.[31] Medicare provides reimbursement for screening FOBT and FS and, beginning in July 2001, will also reimburse for screening colonoscopy once every 10 years. Even a single colonoscopy at 55 years of age may reduce colorectal cancer mortality by 30% to 50%.[30] Patients who are reluctant to undergo colorectal cancer screening may be willing to have "once in a lifetime" screening. More aggressive screening should be considered for those at increased risk for colorectal cancer, such as those with a family history of colorectal cancer or adenomatous polyps.[32]

Outside of cancer screening measures, cardiovascular disease prevention should be the major focus of preventive efforts in this age group, including periodic blood pressure screening. The third USPSTF has issued an advanced recommendation to periodically test total cholesterol levels in all men of ages 35 and older and all women of ages 45 and older. This extends the recommendations of the second USPSTF, which supported routine cholesterol screening only through age 65. High-density lipoprotein (HDL) and low-density lipoprotein (LDL) screening is recommended for individuals at high risk for cardiovascular disease. The American College of Physicians (ACP) recommends periodic total cholesterol screening in men of ages 35 to 65 and women of ages 45 to 65, with follow-up HDL testing for individuals with elevated levels.[33] Treatment decisions in the ACP recommendations are based on the ratio of total to HDL cholesterol, based on research indicating that higher ratios confer increased risk for cardiovascular disease. By contrast, the National Cholesterol Education Program's (NCEP) Adult Treatment Panel III recommends that a routine fasting lipoprotein profile (total, HDL, and LDL cholesterol and triglyceride levels) be obtained every 5 years in all adults of ages 20 or older.[34] As for the cancer screening controversies outlined above, physicians must weigh the evidence supporting each recommendation and collaborate with patients to determine the appropriate course of action.

Tobacco cessation counseling should be provided when applicable, and information on a low-fat diet that is rich in fresh fruits and vegetables and on regular physical activity should be conveyed. The incidence of obesity is increasing at an alarming rate in the United States, conferring increased risk for major cardiovascular risk factors such as hypertension and elevated cholesterol. Periodic weight and height assessment and BMI surveillance should be provided, with further evaluation and intervention offered to those individuals who are overweight (BMI 25.0–29.9) or obese (BMI ≥30.0). Although the USPSTF found insufficient evidence to recommend for or against screening for diabetes mellitus in asymptomatic adults, given its association with obesity and its role as a cardiovascular risk factor, physicians should have a low threshold for obtaining screening fasting serum glucose levels (see Chapter 20). Diabetes screening should also be considered for those with a family history of diabetes and those from high-risk ethnic groups, including Hispanics and Native Americans. Physicians often have difficulty determining the overall level of cardiovascular disease risk for individuals of varying age and either gender in the face of multiple risk factors. Coronary disease risk prediction score sheets which account for multiple variables, may be useful in this regard.[35] The score sheets are also available on the WWW: *http://www.nhlbi.nih.gov/about/framingham/riskabs.thm.* Derived from the predominantly white, middle-class Framingham Heart Study population, they may be less accurate when applied to other types of individuals.

The USPSTF found insufficient evidence to recommend for or against routine aspirin prophylaxis for the primary prevention of myocardial infarction or stroke. Because it is associated with a small increase in the risk of hemorrhagic stroke,[36] aspirin chemoprophylaxis should be employed mostly for those patients with risk factors for cardiovascular disease. Moderate alcohol consumption may reduce the risk of cardiovascular disease, but routine physician endorsement of moderate alcohol use for patients who are not already drinking is not recommended given the high prevalence of problem drinking in the U.S. Indeed, the USPSTF recommends screening for problem drinking in all adults and questioning regarding other drug abuse in those considered at increased risk.

Age 65 and Older (Table 2.10)

This group includes both the "young old" (ages 65 to 79) as well as the "oldest old" (ages 80 and beyond), which is now the fastest growing segment of the U.S. population. However, there is tremendous physiologic variability in the elderly that makes recommendations for prevention based on age alone risky. In both chronologic and physiologic terms, aging impacts on some of the criteria for preventive interventions outlined earlier in this chapter. For example, prostate cancer screening is not indicated for many individuals in this group given the long interval between detection via screening and the earliest time of expected impact on mortality. In addition, older adults may wish to focus primarily on quality of life during their remaining days. Screening interventions that are associated with inconvenience and discomfort may not be desired, regardless of their potential to reduce mortality. Finally, there is a limited evidence base to support many preventive interventions in this age. Physicians must discuss these gaps in evidence, the risks and benefits of screening, and the quality of life goals of older adults before embarking on screening interventions.

The USPSTF recommends annual influenza vaccination as well as a single immunization against *Streptococcus pneumoniae* for all adults of ages 65 and older. Periodic vision and hearing screening are also suggested because the incidence of both functional vision and hearing problems increases dramatically with aging, rising from about 10% at age 65 to approximately 40% by age 90. Injuries, particularly falls, remain an important source of morbidity and mortality in this group but are more likely to occur while performing simple daily tasks such as walking to the bathroom at night. Fall prevention measures including regular exercise, environmental hazard reduction, and avoiding sedating medications should be discussed with all older individuals. Those who are frail, have had prior falls, or are at ongoing high risk for falls may benefit from a multifactorial intervention that includes home assessment and a hip-protective undergarment.[37] End of life planning is also an important preventive care topic for older patients. The value of medical advance directives in improving primary care physicians' and lay surrogates' accuracy in predicting a patient's wishes for care is unclear. However, advance directive discussions and documentation may improve the prediction of patients' wishes by hospital-based physicians and may improve patients' sense of well-being and satisfaction with care.[38] Finally, many elders live in poverty, and many reside in assisted living and skilled nursing facilities. These older adults are often frail and may face substantial socioeconomic disadvantages. Screening these individuals for nutritional adequacy, social isolation, depression, and the ability to perform basic and instrumental activities of daily living should be considered.

The Process of Delivering Preventive Care

The Move Toward Accountability in Preventive Services Delivery

Physicians are now being held accountable for offering and delivering evidence-based preventive services. Quality of care models such as the Health Plan Employer Data and Information Set (HEDIS) seek to provide health care purchasers and consumers with a standard against which individual plans can be compared and evaluated. The HEDIS 2001 measures are heavily weighted toward clinical prevention, including items such as breast cancer screening rates, childhood im-

TABLE 2.10. Interventions Considered and Recommended for Prevention, Age 65 and Older; Leading Causes of Death: Heart Disease, Malignancies (Lung, Colorectal, Breast), Cerebrovascular Disease, Chronic Obstructive Pulmonary Disease, Pneumonia, and Influenza

SCREENING
Blood pressure
Height and weight
Total blood cholesterol
Fecal occult blood test[a] and/or sigmoidoscopy
Mammogram ± clinical breast exam[b] (women ≤69 years)
Papanicolaou (Pap) test (women)[c]
Vision screening
Assess for hearing impairment
Assess for problem drinking

COUNSELING
Substance use
Tobacco cessation
Avoid alcohol/drug use while driving, swimming, boating, etc*
Limit fat and cholesterol; maintain caloric balance; emphasize grains, fruits, vegetables
Adequate calcium intake (women)
Regular physical activity*

Injury prevention
Lap/shoulder belts
Motorcycle and bicycle helmets*
Fall prevention*
Safe storage/removal of firearms*
Smoke detector*
Set hot water heater to <120–130°F
CPR training for household members

Dental health
Regular visits to dental care provider*
Floss, brush with fluoride toothpaste daily*

Sexual behavior
STD prevention; avoid high-risk sexual behavior*; use condoms*

IMMUNIZATIONS
Pneumococcal vaccine
Influenza (a)
Tetanus–diphtheria (Td) boosters

CHEMOPROPHYLAXIS
Discuss hormone prophylaxis (peri- and postmenopausal women)

Interventions for high-risk populations (see detailed high-risk definitions in footnotes)

POPULATION	POTENTIAL INTERVENTIONS
Institutionalized persons	PPD (HR1); hepatitis A vaccine (HR2); amantadine/rimantadine (HR4)
Chronic medical conditions; TB contacts; low income; immigrants; alcoholics	PPD (HR1)
Persons ≥75 years, or ≥70 years with risk factors for falls	Fall prevention intervention (HR5)
Family history of skin cancer; nevi, fair skin, eyes hair	Avoid excess/midday sun; use protective clothing* (HR6)
Native Americans/Alaska Natives	PPD (HR1); hepatitis A vaccine (HR2)
Travelers to developing countries	Hepatitis A vaccine (HR2); hepatitis B vaccine (HR7)
Blood product recipients	HIV screen (HR3); hepatitis B vaccine (HR7)
High-risk sexual behavior	Hepatitis A vaccine (HR2); HIV screen (HR3); hepatitis B vaccine (HR7); RPR/VDRL (HR8); advice to reduce risk of infection (HR9)

Injection or street drug use	PPD (HR1); hepatitis A vaccine (HR2); HIV screen (HR3); hepatitis B vaccine (HR7); RPR/VDRL (HR8); advice to reduce risk of infection
Health care/lab workers	PPR (HR1); hepatitis A vaccine (HR2); amantadine/rimantadine (HR4); hepatitis B vaccine (HR7)
Persons susceptible to varicella	Varicella vaccine (HR10)

---

[a]Annually.

[b]Mammogram q 1–2 years, or mammogram q 1–2 years with annual clinical breast exam.

[c]All women who are or have been sexually active and who have a cervix. Consider discontinuation of testing after age 65 years if previous regular screening with consistently normal results.

*The ability of clinician counseling to influence this behavior is unproven.

HR1—HIV positive, close contacts of persons with known or suspected TB, health care workers, persons with medical risk factors associated with TB, immigrants from countries with high TB prevalence, medically underserved low-income populations (including homeless), alcoholics, injection drug users, and residents of long-term facilities.

HR2—Persons living in, traveling to, or working in areas where the disease is endemic and where periodic outbreaks occur (e.g., countries with high or intermediate endemicity; certain Alaska-Native, Pacific Island, Native-American, and religious communities); men who have sex with men; injection or street drug users. Vaccine may be considered for institutionalized persons and workers in these institutions, military personnel, and day care, hospital, and laboratory workers. Clinicians should also consider local epidemiology.

HR3—Men who had sex with men after 1975; past or present injection drug use; persons who exchange sex for money or drugs, and their sex partners; injection drug-using, bisexual, or HIV-positive sex partner currently or in the past; blood transfusion during 1978–1985; persons seeking treatment for STDs. Clinicians should also consider local epidemiology.

HR4—Consider for persons who have not received influenza vaccine or are vaccinated late; when the vaccine may be ineffective due to major antigenic changes in the virus; for unvaccinated persons who provide home care for high-risk persons; to supplement protection provided by vaccine in persons who are expected to have a poor antibody response; and for high-risk persons in whom the vaccine is contraindicated.

HR5—Persons aged 75 years and older; or aged 70–74 with one or more additional risk factors, including use of certain psychoactive and cardiac medications (e.g., benzodiazepines, antihypertensives); use of ≥4 prescription medications; impaired cognition, strength, balance, or gait. Intensive individualized home-based multifactorial fall prevention intervention is recommended in settings where adequate resources are available to deliver such services.

HR6—Persons with a family or personal history of skin cancer, a large number of moles, atypical moles, poor tanning ability, or light skin, hair, and eye color.

HR7—Blood product recipients (including hemodialysis patients), persons with frequent occupational exposure to blood or blood products, men who have sex with men, injection drug users and their sex partners, persons with multiple recent sex partners, persons with other STDs (including HIV), travelers to countries with endemic hepatitis B.

HR8—Persons who exchange sex for money or drugs, and their sex partners; persons with other STDs (including HIV); and sexual contacts of persons with active syphilis. Clinicians should also consider local epidemiology.

HR9—Persons who continue to inject drugs.

HR10—Healthy adults without a history of chickenpox or previous immunization. Consider serologic testing for presumed susceptible adults. *Source:* U.S. Preventive Services Task Force,[9] with permission.

munization status, and rates of advising smokers to quit. Health plans and clinicians that fail to meet quality thresholds for these indicators are at risk for declining patient enrollment as consumers transfer their care to "higher performers." Nevertheless, delivering individualized, evidence-based clinical preventive services remains a formidable challenge. This section provides a list of issues hindering the delivery of optimal clinical preventive services and provides potential solutions suggested by the research literature.

Organizational Issues and Potential Solutions

ISSUE 1: TIME CONSTRAINTS OF THE CLINICAL ENCOUNTER

There is a finite amount of time that can be spent with each patient, and in this time the physicians must address a range of concerns in addition to providing clinical preventive services. In the landmark Direct Observation of Primary Care (DOPC) study, one third of 4401 patient encounters included discussion of at least one preventive service, but only 3% of the all encounter time was allotted to preventive services.[39] Time pressures will increase with the aging of the population, as more patients present with multiple chronic diseases, conditions, and functional limitations.

Potential Solutions. Physicians must employ the incremental approach to clinical prevention that is endorsed by the USPSTF. The most urgent priorities for prevention can be addressed first, leaving others for future encounters. Standard "scripts" or minipresentations concerning common preventive topics may increase efficiency.

ISSUE 2: LIMITED DISSEMINATION OF NEW FINDINGS AND EVIDENCE-BASED PREVENTION GUIDELINES

The dissemination of evidence-based prevention guidelines in textbooks and journals has limited impact. Such resources, while valuable, rapidly become out of date and may not be readily available at the point of patient care.

Potential Solutions. Evidence-based summary resources that present up-to-date information in a rapid-use format include Patient-oriented evidence that matters (POEMs), *http://www.jfponline.com*; clinical evidence, *http://www.clinicalevidenceonline.com/*; the Cochrane Library, *http://www.updateusa.com/clibhome/clib.htm*; and the ACP Journal Club, *http://www.acponline.org/journals/acpjc/jcmenu.htm*. The Internet is already an established tool for the delivery of recommendations at the point of care. In the near future, palm-top computers will allow even better point of care access to recommendations.

ISSUE 3: COMPETING AND CONFLICTING RECOMMENDATIONS

Many organizations publish recommendations advocating clinical preventive services that are not evidence-based. Clinicians may become confused by conflicting guidelines and are often faced with patients requesting interventions that are promoted by these organizations but not supported by rigorous evidence.

Potential Solutions. The USPSTF recommendations should be utilized whenever possible, and patients should be informed about the levels of evidence for specific interventions. Prevention plans that account for local practice characteristics and patient risk factors, preferences, and beliefs can then be negotiated.

Issue 4: Lack of Office Systems Organized to Provide Effective Preventive Services

Office systems used by practices with successful prevention efforts include designated roles for staff at all levels, paper and computer-based health risk appraisal tools, reminder systems, patient education materials, and record systems, and a quality monitoring and improvement process.

Potential Solutions. The best-known set of materials aimed at improving clinical prevention is Put Prevention into Practice (PPIP). The PPIP kit is paper-based and includes flow sheets, patient-held prevention records, a clinician handbook, prevention prescription pads, medical record reminder stickers, patient reminder postcards, and posters for waiting and examination rooms. Implementing the PPIP office system has been shown to modestly increase the rates of delivery of multiple USPSTF-recommended preventive services. However, dissemination of PPIP has been slow and limited, the absolute increase in rates of delivery for specific services is small, and the positive effects related to its implementation diminish beyond 1 year of follow-up.[40] Both paper and computer-based reminder systems, including those linked to comprehensive electronic medical records, have been shown to improve rates of preventive services delivery, and the impact appears greatest when the reminder is provided to the physician at the time of a patient visit.[41] As for PPIP, the number of practices utilizing such resources is small and their absolute impact has been limited.

The smaller than anticipated impact of these tools has led to the recognition that the problem of low preventive service delivery rates is a complex, systems issue. The DOPC study suggests there are two major differences between practices delivering limited preventive services and those providing higher levels of these services: (1) the degree of pro-activity in dealing with competing practice demands, and (2) physician philosophy.[42] Practices with the greatest need to improve preventive care may be the least likely to implement programs like PPIP due to overwhelming competing demands, such as a practice that is heavily weighted toward acute medical care or physicians with a low "prevention orientation." Developing and testing approaches to dealing with competing demands in primary care and changing physician behavior should be given the highest priority. In the meantime, adapting generic materials to individual practice circumstances and enlisting nonphysician clinic staff in prevention efforts are useful first steps. For example, modification of PPIP flow sheets to meet local needs may result in better acceptance of the materials and higher rates of flow sheet completion,[43] and simple mailed or telephone call reminders provided by non-physician staff can increase childhood immunization "up to date" rates.[44] In the future, remote home-based health risk appraisals, conducted using the Internet and other distance communications technologies, are likely to become routine.

ISSUE 5: POOR REIMBURSEMENT FOR PREVENTIVE SERVICES

In 1988 less than 5% of health care expenditures in the United States was allocated to prevention, and only one third of those expenditures were allocated to clinical prevention.[45] Tobacco cessation counseling and hearing, vision, and blood pressure screening are all endorsed by the USPSTF for older adults, yet none are covered by Medicare. Paradoxically, many states mandate coverage for screening services not recommended by the USPSTF.

Potential Solutions.   Physicians must remain advocates for a preventive health care agenda, making sure local congressional representatives and health plans are aware of shortfalls and misplaced priorities.

Physician and Patient Issues and Potential Solutions

ISSUE 1: FAILURE TO ADOPT AND MAINTAIN A PREVENTION ORIENTATION

Despite the proven benefits of many clinical preventive efforts, some physicians have a practice style that de-emphasizes prevention. In the DOPC study, physicians with a higher volume practice had lower up-to-date rates of preventive screening and counseling services and immunizations.[46] Female physicians have consistently been shown to offer more clinical preventive services than male physicians, and the effect is not limited to gender-specific interventions.[47] In addition, some patients do not embrace the concept of clinical prevention.

Potential Solutions.   All physicians, and particularly males and those working in high-volume settings, should carefully examine their practice style to ensure it is prevention-centered. Physicians must open a dialogue with patients who do not have a prevention orientation by providing individually tailored information and collaborating to determine the areas in which the patient is most ready to accept preventive interventions.

ISSUE 2: HOLDING ON TO NON–EVIDENCE-BASED BELIEFS AND PRACTICES

Given the time constraints of the modern clinical encounter, it is critical to discard disproved and questionable preventive practices. Focusing on such services reduces the amount of time and money that can be devoted to providing evidence-based services and compounds many of the issues listed above. For example, the "complete physical" appointment accounts for as much as one third of physicians' time spent seeing patients in some practices, yet many elements of this venerable activity have no proven value.

Potential Solutions. Physicians must let go of non–evidence-based prevention ideas as part of the solution to the competing demands issue. Since many patients never make check-up visits, preventive services are best delivered over time, during acute illness and other visits. Making the shift away from the "complete physical" model will require patient education, since people have come to expect certain low-yield maneuvers and interventions. A caring, "high-touch" manner can be conveyed to patients without resorting to the misleading reassurance of a normal heart and lung examination. Patients who request non–evidence-based interventions should be congratulated for their interest in prevention and their health. The dialogue should focus on the reasons for the patient's concern about the health issue in question. The evidence to support the intervention should be summarized and placed in the context of the individual. Finally, a prevention plan is negotiated. Although some patients may still insist on non–evidence-based interventions, most will be satisfied with this approach.

ISSUE 3: FAILURE TO ACCOUNT FOR VARYING PATIENT HEALTH-BELIEF MODELS

The United States is increasingly multicultural, and culture and ethnicity impact on every aspect of preventive care, from genetics to health behavior. Some traditional cultural health belief models do not include the Western construct of the concept of prevention.

Potential Solutions. Physicians should learn about the ethnic groups, cultures, and socioeconomic strata represented in their patient population. A rapid overview can be obtained using the U.S. Census Bureau's web site at *http://www. census.gov*, which includes color maps and tables detailing the ethnic distribution of local neighborhoods, language spoken at home, and aggregate family incomes. Becoming involved in community cultural and ethnic activities is an important next step. Perhaps the most important skill in providing multicultural care is to approach each patient without relying on cultural stereotypes. Differing degrees of acculturation and interindividual variability in beliefs make such generalizations dangerous.

ISSUE 4: POOR PREVENTIVE COMMUNICATION SKILLS

Just as physicians must learn key physical examination and history-taking skills to diagnose acute medical illnesses, they must also acquire and maintain the communication skills needed to provide optimal clinical prevention. These skills include the ability to (1) translate research and statistics into lay terms, (2) determine patient readiness to modify a health risk behavior, and (3) negotiate a clinical prevention plan.

Potential Solutions. Health systems increasingly offer communication skills training to physicians, recognizing that deficiencies result in poorer health care outcomes and higher costs. Although the best method of conveying health risk information to patients remains unclear, helping patients to understand how a health problem develops (its antecedents) and to recognize what could happen to them as a result (its consequences) may be more successful than simply providing numerical risk information.[48] In determining a patient's readiness to change a risk behavior, the transtheoretical model provides a useful framework (Table 2.11).[49] The model illustrates that changes in behavior occur gradually, through a predictable series of steps. Individuals seldom skip steps, so that the physician's role is to assist them in moving to the next stage of change rather than to push them toward behavior change in one giant leap. The model also acknowledges that most individuals undergo behavior relapses after successful change. Knowledge of the model may remove the sense of fatalism many physicians feel when trying to help patients change their behaviors and reinforce the importance of providing the right input at the right stage. For example, repeatedly pressuring a smoker at the precontemplation stage to pick a quit smoking date may create an adversarial relationship, reinforcing the negative behavior and making it less likely the individual will consider cessation. Instead, acknowledging the lack of readiness to quit, spending a few moments to explore the reasons for smoking, and providing education about the harmful health effects of smoking may encourage patient contemplation, setting the stage for eventual cessation.

Issue 5: Failure to Recognize and Acknowledge the Harms of Screening

Clinical prevention saves many lives but also has potential harms, such as complications of diagnostic procedures and patient anxiety. Physicians generally underemphasize the harms of screening in a well-intentioned effort to help as many people as possible. For example, although FOBT has been shown to reduce the

TABLE 2.11. Ladder of Behavioral Change

Model stage	Patient manifestations
Precontemplation health	Not thinking about change; may be resigned to behavior; feeling of no control; denial of problem; may believe consequences are not serious
↓ ↑	
Contemplation	Weighing benefits and costs of the current behavior and the proposed change
↓ ↑	
Preparation	Experimenting with small changes in behavior
↓ ↑	
Action	Taking a definitive action to change
↓ ↑	
Maintenance	Maintaining the new behavior over time
↓ ↑	
Relapse	Experiencing normal part of the process of change; often feel demoralized, may interpret small "slips" as irrevocable slide back to prior behavior

Source: Prochaska et al,[49] with permission.

relative risk of colorectal cancer death by 33%, the absolute reduction in all-cause mortality associated with testing is only 0.3% and the false-positive rate is high. Many screened individuals must undergo potentially morbid procedures such as colonoscopy to realize the small absolute reduction in mortality. In addition, some physicians continue to offer worthless services due to misguided medicolegal concerns. Patients have also been conditioned by the health care system and the media to believe all preventive care is more beneficial than harmful. These beliefs and practices place patients at an unjustifiably increased risk of harm.

Potential Solutions.   When possible, decisions regarding whether to offer a preventive service should be based on absolute reductions in all-cause mortality rather than relative reductions in disease-specific outcomes. Harm counseling must be provided when screening also has the potential for adverse consequences. The informed consent model, developed for clinical research, should be applied. For interventions with proven benefit and minimal or no adverse consequences, such as counseling regarding infant car seat use, informed consent is not necessary.

References

1. Ten great public health achievements: United States, 1900–99. MMWR 1999;48:241–64.
2. McGinnis JM, Foege WH. Actual causes of death in the United States. JAMA 1993;270:2207–12.
3. U.S. Department of Health and Human Services. Healthy people 2010, 2nd ed.: With understanding and improving health and objectives for improving health. 2 vols. Washington, DC: U.S. Government Printing Office, November 2000.
4. Michaud CM, Murray CJL, Bloom BR. Burden of disease: implications for future research. JAMA 2001;285:535–9.
5. Schorling JB, Buchsbaum DG. Screening for alcohol and drug abuse. Med Clin North Am 1997;81:845–65.
6. Rembold CM. Number needed to screen: development of a statistic for disease screening. BMJ 1998;317:307–12.
7. Rose DN. Benefits of screening for latent *Mycobacterium tuberculosis* infection. Arch Intern Med 2000;160:1513–21.
8. Stone PW, Teutsch S, Chapman RH, Bell C, Goldie SJ, Neumann PJ. Cost-utility analyses of clinical preventive services: published ratios, 1976–97. Am J Prev Med 2000;19:15–23.
9. U.S. Preventive Services Task Force. Guide to clinical preventive services, 2nd ed. Baltimore: Lippincott Williams & Wilkins, 1996.
10. Hovell MF, Zakarian JM, Matt GE, Hofstetter CR, Bernert JT, Pirkle J. Effect of counseling mothers on their children's exposure to environmental tobacco smoke: a randomized controlled trial. BMJ 2000;321:337–42.
11. Cook DG, Strachan DP. Health effects of passive smoking—10: summary of effects of parental smoking on the respiratory health of children and implications for research. Thorax 1999;54:357–66.

12. Willinger M, Hoffman HJ, Wu K, et al. Factors associated with the transition to non-prone sleep positions of infants in the United States. JAMA 1998;280:329–35.

13. Scariati PD, Grummer-Strawn LM, Fein SB. A longitudinal analysis of infant morbidity and the extent of breast feeding in the United States. Pediatrics 1997;99:E5.

14. Zimmerman RK. The 2001 recommended childhood immunization schedule. Am Fam Physician 2000;63:151–4.

15. Feikin DR, Lezotte DC, Hamman RF, Salmon DA, Chen RT, Hoffman RE. Individual and community risks of measles and pertussis associated with personal exemptions to immunizations. JAMA 2000;284:3145–50.

16. Santoli JM, Szilagyi PG, Rodewald LE. Barriers to immunization and missed opportunities. Pediatr Ann 1998;27:366–74.

17. Epidemiology and prevention of vaccine-preventable diseases, 6th ed. Atlanta: Centers for Disease Control and Prevention, 2000.

18. Schonfeld-Warden N, Warden CH. Pediatric obesity: an overview of etiology and treatment. Pediatr Clin North Am 1997;44:339–61.

19. National High Blood Pressure Education Program. Update on the task force report (1987) on high blood pressure in children and adolescents: a working group report from the National High Blood Pressure Education Program. Bethesda, MD: National Heart, Lung, and Blood Institute, 1996.

20. American Thoracic Society/Centers for Disease Control and Prevention. Targeted tuberculin testing and treatment of latent tuberculosis infection. Am J Respir Crit Care Med 2000;161 (part 2):S221–47.

21. Merenstein D, Green L, Fryer GE, Dovey S. Shortchanging adolescents: room for improvement in preventive care by physicians. Fam Med 2001;33:120–3.

22. Steiner BD, Gest KL. Do adolescents want to hear preventive counseling messages in outpatient settings? J Fam Pract 1996;43:375–81.

23. Knishkowy B, Palti H, Schein M, Yaphe J, Edman R, Baras M. Adolescent preventive health visits: a comparison of two invitation protocols. J Am Board Fam Pract 2000;13:11–16.

24. Grossman D. Adolescent injury prevention and clinicians: time for instant messaging. West J Med 2000;172:151–2.

25. Meningococcal disease and college students: recommendations of the Advisory Committee on Immunization Practices (ACIP). MMWR 2000;49:11–20.

26. Patuszak A, Bhatia D, Okotore B, Koren G. Preconception counseling and women's compliance with folic acid supplementation. Can Fam Physician 1999;45:2053–7.

27. Cervical cancer. National Institutes of Health consensus statement. Bethesda, MD: National Institutes of Health, 1996.

28. Ernster VL. Mammography screening for women aged 40–49: a guidelines saga and a clarion call for informed decision making. Am J Public Health 1997;87:1103–6.

29. Coley CM, Barry MJ, Fleming C, Fahs MC, Mulley AG. Early detection of prostate cancer. Part II: estimating the risks, benefits, and costs. American College of Physicians. Ann Intern Med 1997;126:468–79.

30. Frazier AL, Colditz GA, Fuchs CS, Kuntz KM. Cost-effectiveness of screening for colorectal cancer in the general population. JAMA 2000;284:1954–61.

31. Screening for colorectal cancer—United States, 1997. MMWR 1999;48:116–21.

32. American Gastroenterological Association. Colorectal cancer screening: clinical guidelines and rationale. Gastroenterology 1997;112:594–42.

33. American College of Physicians. Guidelines for using serum cholesterol, high-den-

sity lipoprotein cholesterol, and triglyceride levels as screening tests for preventing coronary heart disease in adults. Part 1. Ann Intern Med 1996;124:515–7.

34. Expert Panel on Detection, Evaluation, and Treatment of High Blood Cholesterol in Adults. Executive summary of the Third Report of the National Cholesterol Education Program (NCEP) Expert Panel on Detection, Evaluation, and Treatment of High Blood Cholesterol in Adults (Adult Treatment Panel III). JAMA 2001;285:2486–97.

35. Wilson PWF, D'Agostino RB, Levy D, Belanger AM, Silbershatz H, Kannel WB. Prediction of coronary heart disease using risk factor categories. Circulation 1998;97:1837–47.

36. He J, Whelton PK, Vu B, Klag MJ. Aspirin and risk of hemorrhagic stroke: a meta-analysis of randomized controlled trials. JAMA 1998;280:1930–5.

37. Kanus P, Parkkari J, Niemi S, et al. Prevention of hip fracture in elderly people with use of a hip protector. N Engl J Med 2000;343:1506–13.

38. Ditto PH, Danks JH, Smucker WD, et al. Advance directives as acts of communication: a randomized controlled trial. Arch Intern Med 2001;161:421–30.

39. Stange KC, Zyzanski SJ, Jaen CR, et al. Illuminating the "black box": a description of 4454 patient visits to 138 family physicians. J Fam Pract 1998;46:377–89.

40. Melnikow J, Kohatsu ND, Chan BKS. Put prevention into practice: a controlled evaluation. Am J Public Health 2000;90:1622–5.

41. Jerant AF, Hill DB. Does the use of electronic medical records improve surrogate patient outcomes in outpatient settings? J Fam Pract 2000;49:349–57.

42. Stange KC. One size doesn't fit all: multimethod research yields new insights into interventions to increase prevention in family practice. J Fam Pract 1996;43:358–60.

43. Moser SE, Goering TL. Implementing preventive care flow sheets. Fam Pract Manag 2001;8:51–3.

44. Udovic SL, Lieu TA. Evidence on office-based interventions to improve childhood immunization delivery. Pediatr Ann 1998;27:355–61.

45. Estimated national spending on prevention: United States, 1988. MMWR 1988;41:529–31.

46. Zyzanski SJ, Stange KC, Langa D, Flocke SA. Trade-offs in high-volume primary care practice. J Fam Pract 1998;46:397–402.

47. Kreuter MW, Strecher VJ, Harris R, Kobrin SC, Skinner CS. Are patients of women physicians screened more aggressively? A prospective study of physician gender and screening. J Gen Intern Med 1995;10:119–25.

48. Rothman AJ, Kiviniemi MT. Treating people with information: an analysis and review of approaches to communicating health risk information. J Natl Cancer Inst Monogr 1999;25:44–51.

49. Prochaska JO, DiClemente CC, Norcross JC. In search of how people change: applications to addictive behaviors. Am Psychol 1992;47:1102–14.

CASE PRESENTATION

Subjective

PATIENT PROFILE

Ruth Nelson McCarthy is a 51-year-old married female restaurant owner.

PRESENTING PROBLEM

"Here for my pap smear."

PRESENT ILLNESS

Mrs. McCarthy has a periodic examination every 2 years. Her menses ceased 3 years ago, and she has not used estrogen replacement. She has no other medical complaints.

PAST MEDICAL HISTORY

Asthma in childhood.

SOCIAL HISTORY

She and her husband have owned and operated a small restaurant for 11 years. She works long hours 6 days per week.

HABITS

She uses no tobacco, alcohol, or drugs.

FAMILY HISTORY

Her father, aged 76, has diabetes mellitus and "arthritis." Her mother is 71 years old and has high blood pressure. She and her husband have two children. Her daughter is living and well at age 26. Their son, aged 28, has recently been diagnosed as HIV-positive.

REVIEW OF SYSTEMS

She reports an occasional mild rash on her hands that becomes red and itching but is not present at this time.

- What other historical information would be useful for this periodic health maintenance examination?
- What are common areas of concern for patients of this age group, and how would you approach these possibilities?
- What else would you like to know regarding her menopausal symptoms?
- What might be the meaning of her health status to the patient, and what unspoken reasons might be bringing her to the physician today?

Objective

VITAL SIGNS

Height, 5 ft 4 in; weight, 182 lb; blood pressure, 138/90; pulse, 72; temperature, 37.2°C.

EXAMINATION

The patient is overweight for height. The eyes, ears, nose, and throat are normal. The neck and thyroid glands are unremarkable. Examination of the chest, heart, and breasts is normal. There is no mass, tenderness, or organ enlargement in the abdomen. The vaginal introitus is mildly atrophic; the cervix, fundus, adnexa, and rectal examination are normal. The neurologic examination and peripheral pulses are normal. Examination of the skin, including the hands, reveals no abnormalities.

LABORATORY

A pap smear is performed today.

- What more—if anything—should be included in this health maintenance examination? Why?
- What might point to a physical cause for obesity?
- What—if any—laboratory tests would you order today, and why?
- What—if any—diagnostic imaging would you order today, and why?

Assessment

- What is your diagnosis regarding Mrs. McCarthy's menopausal status, and how would you describe this to the patient?
- What is the patient's ideal weight, and how would you initiate a discussion regarding weight control?

- How might decreased estrogen and increased weight influence the patient's relationship with her husband? How might you address this issue?
- What are likely to be key stressors in the patient's life, and how might these affect her future health status?

Plan

- What are the disease prevention and health promotion opportunities for this visit?
- Describe your recommendation regarding weight control.
- Describe your recommendation regarding estrogen use.
- What continuing care would you advise for Mrs. McCarthy?

3
Normal Pregnancy, Labor, and Delivery

Margaret V. Elizondo and Joseph E. Scherger

Pregnancy and birth are normal physiologic processes for most women. The cesarean delivery rate of nearly 25%, which has persisted in the United States for many years now, is a reflection of the degree of medical intervention in the birth process. Unfortunately, modern medicine has been guilty of using a disease model for the management of pregnancy and birth, resulting in higher than expected rates of complications. At least 90% of women should have a normal birth outcome without medical intervention.[1]

The disease model for pregnancy and birth took hold during the 1920s led by a Chicago obstetrician, Joseph DeLee, who questioned what is normal and pioneered efforts to improve medically on the "cruelty of nature."[2] During this period, childbirth in America went from the home to the hospital, and the legacy of hospital interventions in the birth process began. Much good has come from modern hospital obstetric care, with maternal mortality having decreased to low levels; moreover, infant mortality has steadily declined for populations having access to perinatal care. Modern prenatal care also developed during the first half of the 20th century; and with a focus on good nutrition and screening for problems during pregnancy, it has improved birth outcome.[3]

A renewed respect for normal childbirth came about as a reaction to hospital interventions, led by Dick-Read[4] during the 1930s and 1940s, Lamaze during the 1950s,[5] Kitzinger[6] during the 1960s, and eventually a social movement in America during the 1970s with the widespread development of childbirth education. Odent's[1] *Birth Reborn* represents a culmination of the effort to rediscover normal pregnancy and birth.

Technologic obstetrics, with its steady focus on improving the uncertainty of nature and sparing women the pain of childbirth, continues to march onward. Prenatal care has become preoccupied with serial ultrasound evaluations and screening for α-fetoprotein (AFP) abnormalities, gestational diabetes, genetic disorders, and every potentially infectious agent. Continuous electronic fetal monitoring, developed during the early 1970s, quickly became the standard of care in most American hospitals, despite little evidence of benefit and cumulative evidence that it causes unnecessary cesarean interventions.[7,8] Epidural anesthesia has become so commonplace in some hospitals that labor units are quiet and nurses have little experience helping women through natural labor.

Approximately 30% of U.S. family physicians provide maternity care. The current lack of access to prenatal care for many women in both rural and urban areas is a compelling reason for more family physicians to deliver these services. Knowledgeable about scientific medicine, yet with a humanistic approach to pregnancy and birth similar to that of midwives, the family physician is well suited to provide a balance between nature and technology and may be a guiding force to appropriate maternity care.[9]

This chapter focuses on normal pregnancy and delivery from a perspective of family-centered care. Family-centered maternity care has been defined by the International Childbirth Association as care that focuses on how the birth of a child affects the entire family. A woman who gives birth forms new relationships with those close to her, and all family members take on new responsibilities to each other, the baby, and the community. Family-centered maternity care is an attitude rather than a specific program. It respects the woman's individuality and need for autonomy and requires that a woman be guided, not directed, and that she be allowed to make her own decisions in accordance with her goals.[10] The family physician, as physician for the woman, the father, and the children, is well suited to provide family-centered maternity care. This chapter reviews the principles and practice of normal pregnancy, labor, and delivery.[11]

Prenatal Care

Current prenatal care begins before conception. This important early phase of preventing complications is referred to as preconception care. Prenatal care after conception should begin as early as possible, as health screening and intervention early during pregnancy may improve birth outcome. For example, taking folic acid in doses present in multivitamins during the first 6 weeks of pregnancy provides a three- to fourfold reduction in the chance of neural tube defects in the offspring.[12] Early screening and intervention is useful for control of diabetes, genetic testing, changing teratogenic drugs such as phenytoin (Dilantin), treating infections, and lifestyle modifications of such factors as smoking, alcohol use, recreational drugs, and maternal nutrition.

The traditional approach to prenatal care, developed early during the 20th century, has been modified by an expert panel convened by the U.S. Public Health Service.[13] Rather than a single comprehensive initial visit followed by monthly visits until the third trimester, this panel recommended more intensive intervention early in pregnancy if risk factors exist that can be modified. For example, women who smoke, have poor nutrition, or have a high-risk home environment may benefit from frequent visits and a multidisciplinary team approach early in pregnancy. Women at low risk may require fewer visits than are scheduled with the traditional protocol.

Health Promotion

All those who care for childbearing women should approach pregnancy as an opportunity to promote the health and well-being of the family. Counseling to reinforce healthful behaviors and education about pregnancy, childbirth, and parenting are crucial parts of perinatal care—not "extras."

Table 3.1 is an outline of topics to be covered in the education of all pregnant women and their support persons.[14] Experienced parents require only an abbreviated program, focusing on selected areas of interest to them. Preparation for natural childbirth (birth without regional or systemic analgesic drugs) and for vaginal

Table 3.1. Sample Topics for Birth and Parenting Classes

Early pregnancy

Nutrition; optimum weight gain; iron, calcium, vitamin supplements

Exercise and sex during pregnancy

Common symptoms and remedies: fatigue, nausea/vomiting, backache, round ligament pain, syncope, constipation

Danger signs: bleeding, contractions, dysuria, vaginitis, weight loss

Psychology of pregnancy: body image, libido; need for security; education for self-help; changing family roles; acceptance of pregnancy

Fevers, hot tubs, saunas

Environmental and occupational hazards and how to mitigate them; stress management

Exposure to infectious agents (e.g., toxoplasmosis, rubella, HIV, varicella)

Avoidance of tobacco, alcohol, x-rays, other drugs

Resources available for pregnant and parenting families

Late pregnancy

Common symptoms and remedies: heartburn, backache "loose joints," hemorrhoids, edema, insomnia

Nutrition/fetal growth

Avoidance of tobacco and other drugs

Potentially serious symptoms: edema, bleeding, headache, meconium-stained fluid, decreased fetal movements

Exercise (e.g., Kegel's, pelvic tilt), sex, travel (avoid prolonged sitting because of risk of deep vein thrombosis)

Occupational adjustments (avoid excessive exertion, prolonged standing, stress) and postpartum plans

Breast-feeding

Signs of labor

Stages of labor

Techniques for pain control (and practice relaxation, visualization)

Cesarean section, vaginal birth after cesarean, other potential interventions

Birth plan; importance of labor companion and early parent–infant contact

Positions for labor and birth

Seat belt use; infant car seats

Circumcision

Sibling preparation

Postpartum/parenting

Care of the perineum, Kegel's exercises

Practical support for breast-feeding

Reasons to contact provider (e.g., maternal hemorrhage, fever, increased pain; infant jaundice, respiratory distress)

Postpartum exercises

Nutrition, especially calcium and iron

Rest and sleep

Return to work

Sex, contraception

Sibling adjustment

Infant immunizations and preventive care schedule

Infant growth and development: normal expectations and parenting issues at each age birth after a previous cesarean section can reduce maternal anxiety and the rates of operative delivery and associated complications.[15] Childbirth preparation classes, often run by hospitals, clinics, or private childbirth educators, fulfill this function well. The benefits of breast-feeding for baby and mother should be discussed with women and their family members prior to or early during pregnancy and then modeled at delivery. The effectiveness of education on preventing low birth weight has not been proved.[3] However, information about smoking, alcohol and drug use, prevention of sexually transmitted infection, and mobilizing family supports and social services in the community are likely to be beneficial.

Motivation to adopt more healthy behaviors is probably stronger during pregnancy than at most other times, though a woman may curb behavior such as smoking during pregnancy only to resume it after delivery. All family members involved should be educated on the benefits of a non-smoking household, including decreased incidence of sudden infant death syndrome (SIDS) and respiratory illnesses.[16]

Abstention from alcohol and recreational drugs is also important. Alcohol exposure during gestation is a more common cause of mental retardation than Down syndrome.[17] The prevalence of cocaine use during pregnancy is reported at 17% in some populations but often is not admitted to the physician.[18] With a paucity of research on substance use by women and few treatment programs accepting pregnant women, this area is a challenge to professionals caring for them.

Women will often ask for advice on working during pregnancy. The physician should review the effects of physical exertion and prolonged standing during pregnancy, occupational and environmental hazards (e.g., heat, heavy metals, anesthetic gases, x-rays, and possibly cathode ray tubes). Day-care and health care workers need to be apprised of the risks of certain infectious disease exposures in pregnancy.[19] Physicians should also be prepared to counsel on the legal rights of pregnant workers, child care, and breast-feeding issues. In general, women may continue moderate activities, but should strive to keep their heart rate <140 and their temperature within 1 to 2 degrees of normal.[20] Attention should be given to appropriate hydration, and women at risk for preterm labor may need to curtail some activities as pregnancy progresses.

Nutrition and weight should be closely monitored during prenatal care. Physicians must be knowledgeable about nutritional requirements and offer practical suggestions for management of nausea and vomiting, gastroesophageal reflux, constipation, backache, and hemorrhoids. Anticipatory guidance about body image changes, risks of obesity, and ways of modifying the diet within various constraints (e.g., vegetarianism, lactose intolerance) are also important considerations. Optimal weight gain during pregnancy varies depending on the prepregnancy weight. An underweight woman may benefit from gaining 40 pounds, whereas an obese woman might do well gaining 10 to 15 pounds. The normal weight gain of 25 to 35 pounds is often exceeded without harm to the fetus. Nutritional advice to pregnant women should focus on a high-quality, high-protein diet with a steady, gradual weight gain profiled to the woman's size and eating habits. Pregnant women should be instructed to avoid the presence of cat feces and eating raw meat (toxoplasmosis). Caffeine intake should be limited.

Prenatal Screening

The purpose of prenatal screening is to identify problems that could affect the outcome of pregnancy and for which effective interventions are available. The number of conditions for which screening is available seems limitless. Therefore, the choice of items should be based on a rational assessment of the current literature, legislation, medicolegal climate, cost-effectiveness, and treatment effectiveness. Each screening test should be evaluated to ensure that the benefits of the test and the planned intervention outweigh the risks and complications. Prenatal screening should be discussed with each patient at the first prenatal visit.

Traditional medical teaching focuses on screening for medical conditions using blood tests, ultrasonography, amniocentesis, and physical examination. A comprehensive approach would also include screening through questioning about family and social dysfunction, such as single parent status, a history of domestic abuse, substance abuse, economic hardship, and work-related stresses. The relation between psychosocial stress and outcome of pregnancy is now well established.[21,22] Physicians should be knowledgeable about public social service programs available to support pregnant patients and their families.

Table 3.2 outlines the screening tests offered to most patients. Genetic history determines which patients are offered special testing such as hemoglobin electrophoresis (e.g., African Americans, who are at higher risk for sickle cell disease, or those of Asian or Mediterranean background, who are at higher risk for

TABLE 3.2. Common Screening Tests in Pregnancy

Initial
  Blood type/Rh factor/antibody screen (indirect Coombs' test)
  Complete blood count (CBC)
  Rubella immunoglobulin G (IgG)
  Rapid plasma reagin (RPR)
  Hepatitis B surface antigen
  Urinalysis and culture
  Papanicolaou smear
  Gonorrhea culture (GC)/chlamydia
  Consider screening for bacterial vaginosis
  Offer human immunodeficiency virus (HIV) testing
  Hemoglobin electrophoresis, if indicated
  Consider Tay-Sachs and cystic fibrosis genetic testing
  Purified protein derivative (PPD), if indicated
10–20 weeks
  Offer triple marker [expanded α-fetoprotein (AFP) screening] at 15–20 weeks
    (16–18 ideally)
  Consider chorionic villus sampling (CVS) or amniocentesis, if indicated
  Offer ultrasonography for fetal age and anatomy (generally 17–20 weeks)
24–28 weeks
  Screen for gestational diabetes (1-hour 50-g glucose load)
  Repeat CBC
  Repeat antibody screen (ABS) if Rh negative (Give RhoGAM at 28 weeks)
32–36 weeks
  Group B streptococcal screening (35–37 weeks)
  Repeat CBC, if indicated
  Repeat GC/chlamydia/RPR, if indicated

thalassemia). Testing for Tay-Sachs disease and cystic fibrosis carrier states is becoming more common, and some authorities recommend screening more than just those with a family history of these disorders.[23,24] All women who will be 35 years of age or older by their due date should be offered amniocentesis and/or chorionic villus sampling (CVS) for chromosomal analysis. CVS has the advantage of testing earlier in gestation (generally 10 to 14 weeks) and providing results rapidly (a few days). It is only available through experienced perinatologists, though, and may be associated with a slightly higher complication rate than amniocentesis. Amniocentesis has the advantage of measuring amniotic fluid AFP level as well as analyzing chromosomes, so that neural tube defects (NTDs) can be more readily detected.[23] Amniocentesis is generally performed at 14 to 20 weeks and results return in about 10 days. Other women with personal or family history of genetic problems, including Down syndrome (trisomy 21), should have the opportunity to meet with a genetics counselor, if possible, and review options for prenatal testing.

The expanded AFP screen (triple marker) uses blood levels of AFP, human chorionic gonadotropin (hCG), and unconjugated estriol (uE3) to screen for NTDs, Down syndrome, and trisomy 18; 85% of NTDs are detected by an increase in AFP level, but this result can also indicate multiple gestation, abdominal wall defects, congenital nephrotic syndrome, maternal hemorrhage, fetal demise, inaccurate dating, and even normal pregnancy. A low level of AFP may also be found with fetal demise, inaccurate dating, and normal pregnancy, or may be associated with molar gestation or Down syndrome. Down syndrome is also associated with increased hCG levels and decreased uE3 levels; 60% of Down syndrome cases are detected using these three markers. Trisomy 18 is associated with low levels of all three markers.[25] If the initial triple marker screening is abnormal, it may be necessary to repeat the test or to order a diagnostic ultrasound scan to confirm gestational age and evaluate for fetal abnormalities. Amniocentesis may be indicated to measure amniotic fluid AFP and for chromosome evaluation. Because expanded AFP screening is widely available and is considered standard by some, the test should be discussed with all patients, with a mutual agreement of patient and practitioner regarding its use. The screening is done between 15 and 20 weeks' gestation, optimally at 16 to 18 weeks.

Routine ultrasonography currently falls into a gray area. In the United States, a National Institutes of Health (NIH) consensus conference recognized 27 indications for prenatal ultrasonography that result in examinations in most pregnancies.[26] The American College of Obstetricians and Gynecologists recommended adherence to these guidelines.[27] In most of Western Europe, ultrasonography is done routinely at 16 to 18 weeks. The benefits and cost-effectiveness of universal screening are still controversial and are the subject of ongoing study.[28,29]

Screening for gestational diabetes mellitus (GDM) is generally recommended for all pregnant patients at 24 to 28 weeks' gestation. A 50-g glucose solution is given and plasma glucose measured 1 hour later. An abnormal value of 140 or more is further evaluated with a 3-hour 100-g glucose tolerance test, following measurement of fasting plasma glucose. Two or more abnormal values on this test confirm the diagnosis of GDM. One abnormal value may warrant retesting in 4 to 6 weeks.

The Expert Committee on the Diagnosis and Classification of Diabetes Mellitus allows a small subset of women to forgo routine screening: those who are under 25 years of age, of normal weight, with *no* family history of diabetes, and *not* of Hispanic, Native-American, Asian, or African-American background, are at very low risk for GDM.[30] Women with the above risk factors, however, and others including prior GDM or glucosuria, may benefit from earlier screening, in addition to routine screening at 24 to 28 weeks (see Chapter 20).

Bacterial vaginosis has been associated with preterm birth. Metronidazole (Flagyl) (500 mg po bid × 7 days) and clindamycin (300 mg po bid × 7 days) have been shown to decrease preterm birth rates in women with bacterial vaginosis.[31] It is unclear if asymptomatic women should be screened routinely. Group B streptococcal (GBS) infection can be devastating to newborns. The Centers for Disease Control and Prevention (CDC) reports that 10% to 30% of women carry these bacteria in the genital region, though fewer than 1% of infants are actually infected.[32] Despite this low rate of infection, given the mortality rate of up to 20%, screening for GBS in pregnant women is becoming standard. The outer vagina, perineum, and rectum are cultured at 35 to 37 weeks, with positive carriers treated with intravenous antibiotics intrapartum (penicillin 5 million units intravenously followed by 2.5 million units every 4 hours or clindamycin 900 mg intravenously every 8 hours until delivery). The CDC also endorses another strategy to prevent GBS disease, based on risk factors rather than universal screening. In this case, mothers are treated with intrapartum antibiotics only if they have risk factors such as previous infant with invasive GBS disease, GBS bacteriuria in this pregnancy, delivery at <37 weeks' gestation, ruptured membranes >18 hours, or intrapartum temperature of 100.4°F or greater.

Risk Assessment

The outcome of screening is identification of patients at risk for complications during pregnancy. Conventional risk assessment divides patients into low-, medium-, and high-risk categories. Because most family physicians are trained to care for low- and medium-risk patients, and to refer or share the care of high-risk patients with perinatal specialists, proper risk assessment is crucial. Table 3.3 indicates risk factors recognized by the American Board of Family Practice, the American College of Obstetricians and Gynecologists, and the American Academy of Pediatrics.[3,33] Family physicians in some areas and with appropriate training provide obstetric care for high-risk patients, but the classification of risk status remains important for guiding clinical care. The prenatal record should conveniently assist in the evaluation and indication of risk status.

High-risk categories should not be absolute contraindications to care by family physicians. For example, family physicians may be the best qualified to handle high-risk social situations and substance abuse. Because of broad medical training, family physicians may have more experience than some obstetricians in

Table 3.3. Obstetric Risk Criteria

Category I: higher risk factors	Category II: medium risk factors
Initial prenatal factors	*Initial prenatal factors*
Age ≥40 or ≤16	Ages 35–39, 16–17
Multiple gestation	Drug dependence/alcohol abuse
Preexisting or insulin-dependent diabetes	High-risk family—lack of family/ social support
Chronic hypertension	Uterine or cervical malformation or incompetence
Renal failure	
Heart disease, class II or greater	Contracted pelvis
Hyperthyroidism	Previous cesarean section
Rh isoimmunization	Multiple spontaneous abortions (>3)
Chronic active hepatitis	Grand multiparity (>8)
Convulsive disorder	History of gestational diabetes
Isoimmune thrombocytopenia	Previous fetal or neonatal demise
Severe asthma	Hypothyroidism
HIV infection	Heart disease, class I
Significant hemoglobinopathy (e.g. sickle cell disease)	Severe anemia (unresponsive to iron)
	Pelvic mass or neoplasia
Subsequent prenatal and intrapartum factors	Prior deep vein thrombosis/ pulmonary embolism
Vaginal bleeding, second or third trimester	Prior preterm delivery
	Pyelonephritis
Pregnancy-induced hypertension (or toxemia), moderate or severe	Threatened preterm labor
	Preterm rupture of membranes
Fetal malformation, by α-fetoprotein (AFP) screening, ultrasonography, or amniocentesis	*Subsequent prenatal and intrapartum factors*
	Gestational diabetes, diet-controlled
Abnormal presentation: breech, face, brow, transverse	Pregnancy-induced hypertension (toxemia), mild
Intrauterine growth retardation	Pregnancy at >41 weeks, obtain appropriate fetal/placental tests
Polyhydramnios/oligohydramnios	
Pregnancy >42 weeks or <35 weeks	Active genital herpes
Abnormal fetal/placental tests	Positive high or low AFP screen
Persistent severe variable or late decelerations	Estimated fetal weight >10 pounds (4.5 kg) or <5.5 pounds (2.5 kg)
Macrosomia	Abnormal nonstress test
Cord prolapse	Arrest of normal labor curve
Mid-forceps delivery	Persistent moderate variable decelerations or poor baseline variability
	Ruptured membranes beyond 24 hours
	Second stage beyond 2 hours
	Induction of labor

an area dealing with medical problems, such as thyroid or pulmonary disease. Consultation does not preclude shared care. Some high-risk problems may resolve during the pregnancy, and the birth may be a low-risk event.

Prenatal Visits

The schedule of prenatal visits has traditionally been every 4 weeks through the 28th week of pregnancy, every 2 weeks until the 36th week of pregnancy, and then weekly until delivery. A U.S. Public Health Service report suggested that low-risk patients require fewer visits, whereas patients with risk factors may need modified or intensive care.[13] For example, risk factors identified early in pregnancy, such as smoking, alcohol or drug use, family dysfunction, or lack of social support, should be aggressively managed with frequent visits early during pregnancy. Subsequent risk factors, such as elevated blood pressure or preterm labor, require more frequent visits beginning as soon as the condition develops.

The initial prenatal visit consists of a detailed history, physical examination, and laboratory assessment. A complete physical examination is performed as early as possible. The pelvic assessment, which includes a bimanual examination, is helpful for dating the pregnancy and evaluating the pelvic structure. Screening laboratory investigations are undertaken as stated above. Accurate dating of the pregnancy is critically important for prenatal care, including the proper performance and interpretation of screening tests, and avoidance of unnecessary testing due to a misdiagnosis of prematurity or postdates. If dating is not clear from the initial visit, an ultrasound scan should be performed promptly to establish an accurate due date. Ultrasound dating is less accurate the further pregnancy progresses. Clinical dating is based on number of weeks since the start of the last menstrual period (LMP), assuming the usual 4-week cycle, with the due date (estimated date of confinement, EDC) being 40 weeks after the start of the LMP. Uterine size grows in a predictable manner in normal pregnancies, with fundal height (measured from the symphysis pubis to the top of the uterus, in centimeters) roughly equal to estimated gestational age (EGA) between 20 and 36 weeks. Prior to an EGA of 20 weeks, the uterus, on bimanual exam, is roughly lemon size at 6 weeks, orange size at 8 weeks, grapefruit size at 10 weeks, and cantaloupe size at 12 weeks, filling the pelvis at that point.[34]

First-trimester prenatal care (up to 14 weeks) includes a determination of the patient's well-being during pregnancy, a review of family and lifestyle issues, and a reevaluation of the risk status. The clinical assessment includes measuring maternal weight gain, blood pressure, uterine growth, detecting fetal heart tones by Doppler ultrasonography, and counseling patients toward a healthy pregnancy. Common problems in the first trimester include nausea, vomiting, and gastroesophageal reflux. Patients should be counseled to eat frequent small meals and may use antacids such as calcium carbonate (e.g., Tums) or magnesium hydroxide (e.g., Maalox/Mylanta). Prenatal vitamins may help some patients, but be intolerable to others. Severe nausea and vomiting, associated with significant weight loss, ketonuria and/or electrolyte abnormalities, should be investigated with laboratory testing to rule out medical conditions associated with nausea and vomiting, and ultrasonography to rule out twin or molar gestation.[23] These cases may require intravenous hydration and antiemetics, with informed consent regarding teratogen issues with medication use.

Vaginal bleeding should be investigated carefully to rule out infection, threatened abortion, or placental abnormality, though patients may often report self-limited bleeding after sexual intercourse or vaginal exam. Rh-negative patients need to receive RhoGAM intramuscularly after episodes of vaginal bleeding, and after procedures such as amniocentesis.

Second-trimester prenatal care (14 to 28 weeks) includes confirmation of the estimated date of delivery by quickening (perception of fetal movements) at 18 to 20 weeks or earlier, uterine size at the umbilicus at 20 weeks, and fetal heart tones being heard using a fetoscope at 20 weeks. The fetus may be evaluated by ultrasonography if fetal age or size is in doubt. Health education during the second trimester includes planning for labor and delivery through childbirth education classes, initial discussion of infant feeding including encouragement of breast-feeding, and planning for parenting by recommending reading and/or classes. Mothers should be instructed to report symptoms that would indicate a pregnancy risk, such as vaginal bleeding, significant edema (especially of the face or fingers), continuous headache, blurring of vision, abdominal pain, persistent vomiting, chills, fever, dysuria, leakage of amniotic fluid, or change in frequency or intensity of fetal movements.

More frequent visits are generally made during the third trimester to evaluate for elevated blood pressure or other signs of preeclampsia, such as sudden excessive weight gain or edema, or significant proteinuria. Labor signs are taught to the patient with careful attention to the possibility of preterm labor. Fetal presentation is determined by Leopold's maneuvers, or by digital vaginal exam and/or ultrasonography when in question. Labor and delivery preferences of the mother and father should be clarified, and a completed prenatal record, including documentation of the parent's birth request, should be given to the patient or sent to the hospital. Predelivery lactation consultation should be considered in patients with nipple abnormalities that might preclude normal breast-feeding.

Other pregnancy complaints such as varicosities, hemorrhoids, and backaches are common in the latter part of pregnancy. Patients should avoid prolonged standing at this point in pregnancy, and may find relief with maternity support hose. Constipation, which aggravates hemorrhoids, can be alleviated with proper hydration and fiber laxatives. Back pains late in pregnancy should always be evaluated with the specter of preterm labor in mind. Tylenol is considered safe to use in recommended doses at any gestational age.

Fetal Assessment

Methods have been developed to assess the well-being of the fetus during pregnancy, including fetal movement records ("kick counts"), the nonstress test (NST), nipple stimulation or oxytocin contraction stress test (CST), and ultrasonography for amniotic fluid evaluation. These methods are used according to accepted protocols when risk factors are present that may jeopardize the fetus. They are routinely applied when pregnancy continues past 41 weeks, or earlier for certain conditions, such as diabetes, hypertension, decreased fetal movement, polyhydramnios/oligohydramnios, intrauterine growth retardation (IUGR), Rh sensitization, or previous unexplained stillbirth. Some authorities recommend that women monitor fetal movements regularly during the third trimester of pregnancy. Family physicians should understand these methods and be aware of their relative usefulness, including their sensitivity, specificity, and predictive values.[35]

Duration of Pregnancy

The normal duration of human pregnancy has considerable variation. The bell-shaped curve of human pregnancy is illustrated in Figure 3.1. The median is just past 280 days, or 40 weeks, from the last menstrual period. Two standard deviations from the mean would be 37 to 43 weeks. About 10% of pregnancies reach 42 weeks, confirming the normalcy of postdates pregnancy for many women. However, as pregnancies extend beyond 42 weeks, conditions such as oligohydramnios, passage of meconium into the amniotic fluid, macrosomia, and dysmaturity with potential IUGR, increase in frequency and can cause significant risk for the fetus.[23]

Labor and Delivery

Labor

Labor in the first stage is defined as progressive dilation of the cervix with uterine contractions. The early (latent) phase of labor occurs up to 4 cm dilation and is variable in duration. Progress during this phase is often slow because of the time needed for effacement of the cervix.

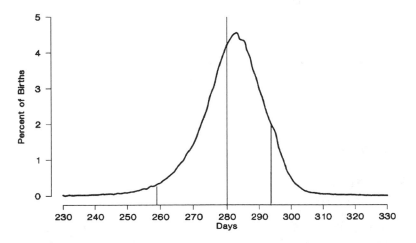

FIGURE 3.1. Distribution of duration of pregnancy, in days from last menstrual period to birth, among 383,484 singleton, noncesarean births with certain menstrual dates in Sweden, 1976–1980. Vertical lines are drawn at 259, 280, and 294 completed days. The line has been drawn between day-to-day percentage values, without any smoothing of the curve ("raw data"). (From Bergsjo et al,[43] with permission.)

The active phase of labor is more rapid and predictable, yet there is still considerable individual variation. With frequent, regular contractions, the average is 1.2 cm dilation per hour in primigravidas and 1.5 cm per hour in multigravidas, but flexibility is important. Friedman[36] attempted to describe labor, not to define parameters women must follow. Arrest of labor is present where there has been no cervical dilation for 2 hours during this active phase.

When the pregnant patient presents in labor, her prenatal record must be carefully reviewed and risk assessment done. Decisions regarding need for antibiotics (e.g., positive group B streptococcus screening or prolonged rupture of membranes) should be made early. Current or recent active genital herpes is an indication for cesarean delivery to avoid neonatal herpes infection.

Support and observation are the hallmarks of managing normal labor. Women in labor should be given as much freedom of movement as possible. During the first stage of labor the blood pressure and the frequency and duration of contractions are measured every 15 to 30 minutes. The fetal heart rate should be monitored during and immediately after a contraction every 30 minutes during the first stage by whatever method is most convenient (electronically, Doppler ultrasonography, or fetoscopic auscultation). Intermittent fetal heart rate monitoring is preferable to continuous monitoring in normal or low-risk patients, as continuous monitoring interferes with freedom of movement and has a high false-positive rate.[7,8] Continuous electronic fetal monitoring in low-risk patients has resulted in three times the diagnosis of fetal distress and twice the frequency of cesarean sections without improving birth outcome.[37]

Women succeed best during the second stage of labor (expulsion of the fetus) when they are allowed and encouraged to use their instincts about pushing. Prolonged breath-holding and Valsalva maneuvers should be avoided, as they may result in decreased oxygenation of the placenta and fetal hypoxia. Women push more effectively and are in less pain when upright: sitting, squatting, kneeling, or standing.[38] Fatigued or hypotensive women may push while lying on their side. The dorsal lithotomy position should be avoided to prevent inferior vena cava compression, with resultant maternal hypotension and fetal distress. The fetal heart rate should be monitored every 15 minutes during the second stage in low-risk patients.[39]

SUPPORT DURING LABOR

Continuous emotional support of the woman during labor enhances the birth process. It may be provided by a labor support team consisting of the nurse, the delivering physician or midwife, the father, and any other person close to the mother. A "doula" is a lay person trained to provide continuous support to the woman in labor and may be provided by the hospital to ensure that all women in labor receive optimal emotional support for labor and birth. Support during labor may reduce the need for intrapartum medication and technologic intervention.[40]

INTRAPARTUM ANALGESIA AND ANESTHESIA

Because all medications given during labor have side effects for both the mother and fetus, none is given routinely. Pain during labor may be managed by non-pharmacologic methods primarily, such as support from labor attendants, change of position, rest, physical contact, ambulation, and a warm shower or bath. Labor and birth without medication may be preferable for the woman and her partner. Some women benefit from pain medication during labor. A short-acting narcotic given parenterally during the first stage of labor may help the woman cope, and it may even facilitate dilation of the cervix.

Lumbar epidural anesthesia has become increasingly common and provides effective pain relief. It has a place in the management of dystocia and is of benefit for cesarean section. Its use during labor should be carefully considered, not elective. Studies in Europe and North America have shown that elective use of epidural anesthesia during labor increases the need for oxytocin augmentation and may increase the cesarean rate.[36,41] Documented effects of epidural anesthesia on labor include decreased uterine activity, prolongation of the first stage of labor, relaxation of the pelvic diaphragm predisposing to minor malpresentation, decreased maternal urge and ability to push, prolonged second stage of labor, and increased use of instrumental vaginal delivery.[42]

Despite these effects, epidural anesthesia has become almost routine in many hospitals, including hospitals with residency programs, and is requested by many women. If women and their birth attendants hope to avoid epidural anesthesia, prenatal education, support during labor, and management of the birthing environment must receive high priority.

Delivery

Normal delivery of the infant should occur in whatever position is comfortable for the woman, and the physician should be as flexible as possible with birth positions. The infant's head should remain flexed during delivery to lessen the diameter presenting to the perineum. An episiotomy is avoided unless the infant is large or delivery must occur quickly. Sometimes delivery of the head can be more controlled by gently pushing between contractions. After the head is delivered the physician should not rush to deliver the shoulders. The physician should assess for shoulder dystocia (Is the infant's head tightly retracted to the perineum?), check for a nuchal cord and reduce or clamp and cut it if necessary, suction the mouth and nose, and allow spontaneous delivery of the shoulders. The anterior and posterior shoulders should be delivered during a contraction with limited traction. Patience and gentleness result in fewer perineal lacerations.

The delivered infant is assessed immediately for color, tone, and respiratory effort. If no resuscitation efforts are necessary, the infant is placed against the mother for bonding, warming, and drying. Clamping and cutting the cord and assigning of Apgar scores may follow these initial steps.

Delivery of the placenta (third stage of labor) should not be attempted until separation has occurred from the uterus (up to 30 minutes). Placental separation is likely when there is a sudden gush of blood, the uterus becomes globular or firm and rises in the abdomen, and the cord protrudes farther out of the vagina. Gentle traction on the cord and suprapubic pressure to avoid uterine inversion spontaneously delivers the placenta. The placenta is examined for completeness, number of vessels, and abnormalities. The mother is examined for cervical, vaginal, or perineal lacerations. Most first-degree lacerations (skin or mucosal tears) do not require suturing. Conditions that require action immediately postpartum include hepatitis immunization of infants from mothers with positive hepatitis B surface antigen, rubella vaccine for susceptible women, and RhoGam for Rh-negative women.

Summary

The family physician can be skillful in the management of normal pregnancy, labor, and delivery. Inclusion of this joyous part of the family life cycle into the physician's practice has numerous benefits for diversifying the practice and bonding the family with the physician. The family physician may play an important role in advocating the proper support and management of normal pregnancy, labor, and delivery in an environment filled with extensive technology.

Acknowledgment

Some of the material in this chapter has been published in a paper by members of the Working Group on Teaching Family-Centered Perinatal Care of the Society of Teachers of Family Medicine (with permission).[11]

References

1. Odent M. Birth reborn. New York: Pantheon, 1984.
2. Wertz RW, Wertz DC. Lying-in: a history of childbirth in America. New Haven: Yale University Press, 1989.
3. American Academy of Pediatrics and the American College of Obstetricians and Gynecologists. Guidelines for perinatal care, 4th ed. Elk Grove Village, IL: American Academy of Pediatrics, 1997.
4. Dick-Read G. Childbirth without fear, 2nd ed. New York: Harper & Row, 1959.
5. Karmel M. Thank you, Dr. Lamaze. Philadelphia: Lippincott, 1959.
6. Kitzinger S. The experience of childbirth. New York: Pelican, 1967.
7. Freeman R. Intrapartum fetal monitoring—a disappointing story. N Engl J Med 1990;322:624–6.
8. Banta HD, Thacker SB. The case for reassessment of health care technology. JAMA 1990;264:235–40.
9. Larimore WL, Reynolds JL. Family practice maternity care in America: ruminations

on reproducing an endangered species—family physicians who deliver babies. J Am Board Fam Pract 1994;7:478–88.

10. International Childbirth Education Association. Definition of family-centered maternity care. Int J Childbirth Educ 1987;2(1):4.

11. Scherger JE, Levitt C, Acheson LS, et al. Teaching family centered perinatal care in family medicine. Parts 1 and 2. Fam Med 1992;24:288–98, 368–74.

12. Willett WC. Folic acid and neural tube defect: can't we come to closure? Am J Public Health 1992;82:666–8.

13. Expert panel on the content of prenatal care: the content of prenatal care. Washington, DC: US Public Health Service, 1989.

14. Nichols FH, Humenick SS. Childbirth education: practice, research and theory. Philadelphia: WB Saunders, 1988.

15. Scott JR, Rose NB. Effect of psychoprophylaxis (Lamaze preparation) on labor and delivery in primiparas. N Engl J Med 1976;294:1205–7.

16. Blair PS, Fleming PJ, Bensley D, et al. Smoking and sudden infant death syndrome: results from 1993–5 case-control study for confidential inquiry into stillbirths and deaths in infancy. BMJ 1996;313:195–198.

17. U.S. Preventive Services Task Force. Guide to clinical preventive services. Baltimore: Williams & Wilkins, 1989;289–95.

18. Volpe JJ. Effect of cocaine use on the fetus. N Engl J Med 1992;327:399–404.

19. Crump WJ. The pregnant day-care worker: What are the infectious risks? Fam Pract Recert 2000;22(11):21–28.

20. Copeland JA, Andolsek KM. Exercise in pregnancy. In: Andolsek KM, ed. Obstetric care: standards of prenatal, intrapartum, and post-partum management. Philadelphia: Lea & Febiger; 1990;113–16.

21. Gjerdingen DK, Froberg DG, Fontaine P. The effects of social support on women's health during pregnancy, labor and delivery, and the postpartum period. Fam Med 1991;23:370–5.

22. Williamson HA, LeFevre M, Hector M. Association between life stress and serious perinatal complications. J Fam Pract 1989;29:489–96.

23. Gabbe SG, Niebyl JR, Simpson JL, eds. Obstetrics: normal and problem pregnancies, 3rd ed. New York: Churchill Livingstone, 1996.

24. National Institutes of Health Consensus Development Conference. Genetic testing for cystic fibrosis. Arch Intern Med 1999;159:1529–39.

25. American College of Obstetricians and Gynecologists. Maternal serum screening. ACOG educational bulletin no. 228. Washington, DC: ACOG, 1996.

26. U.S. Department of Health and Human Services, Public Health Service, National Institutes of Health. Diagnostic ultrasound imaging in pregnancy. NIH publication no. 84-667. Washington, DC: Government Printing Office, 1984.

27. American College of Obstetricians and Gynecologists. Ultrasonography in pregnancy. ACOG technical bulletin no. 187. Washington, DC: ACOG, 1993.

28. Bucher H, Schmidt JG. Does routine ultrasound scanning improve outcome in pregnancy? Meta-analysis of various outcome measures. BMJ 1993;307:13–17.

29. Ewigman BG, Crane JP, Frigoletto FD, et al. Effect of prenatal ultrasound screening on perinatal outcome. N Engl J Med 1993;329:821–7.

30. The Expert Committee on the Diagnosis and Classification of Diabetes Mellitus. Report of the Expert Committee on the Diagnosis and Classification of Diabetes Mellitus. Diabetes Care 1997;20:1183–97.

31. McGregor JA, French JI, Parker R, et al. Prevention of premature birth by screening

and treatment for common genital infections: results of a prospective controlled evaluation. Am J Obstet Gynecol 1995;173(1):157–67.

32. Centers for Disease Control and Prevention. Prevention of perinatal group B streptococcal disease: a public health perspective. MMWR 1996;45(RR-7):1–24.

33. American Board of Family Practice. Normal pregnancy: reference guide 17. Lexington, KY: American Board of Family Practice, 1983.

34. Fox GN. Teaching first trimester uterine sizing. J Fam Pract 1985;21:400–1.

35. American College of Obstetricians and Gynecologists. Antepartum fetal surveillance. ACOG practice bulletin no. 9. Washington, DC: ACOG, 1999.

36. Friedman EA. Disordered labor: objective evaluation and management. J Fam Pract 1975;2:167–72.

37. Neilson JP. Electronic fetal heart rate monitoring during labor: information from randomized trials. Birth 1994;21(2):101–4.

38. Olsen R, Olsen C, Cox NS. Maternal birthing positions and perineal injury. J Fam Pract 1990;30:553–7.

39. American College of Obstetricians and Gynecologists. Fetal heart rate patterns: monitoring, interpretation, and management. ACOG technical bulletin no. 207. Washington, DC: ACOG 1995.

40. Kennell J, Klaus M, McGrath S, et al. Continuous emotional support during labor in a U.S. hospital. JAMA 1991;265:2197–201.

41. Ramin SM, Grambling DR, Lucas MJ, et al. Randomized trial of epidural versus intravenous analgesia during labor. Obstet Gynecol 1995;86:783–9.

42. Johnson S, Rosenfeld JA. The effect of epidural anesthesia on the length of labor. J Fam Pract 1995;40:244–7.

43. Bergsjo P, Denman DW III, Hoffman HY, et al. Duration of human singleton pregnancy. Acta Obstet Gynecol Scand 1990;69:197–207.

Case Presentation

Subjective

Patient Profile

Ann Martino-Priestley is a 22-year-old married female nursery school teacher.

Presenting Problem

"Possible pregnancy."

Present Illness

Mrs. Martino-Priestley, who has never been pregnant in the past, reports that her last normal period was 7 weeks ago. She has had morning nausea and urinary frequency, and an over-the-counter pregnancy test was positive. She has had a few episodes of spotting over the past week.

Past Medical History

No serious illnesses or hospitalization.

Social History

Mrs. Martino-Priestley graduated from college a few months ago and is working part-time as a nursery school teacher. She has been married for 1 year to Luke, who is a graduate student in an MBA program.

Habits

She does not smoke, she takes alcohol occasionally on weekends, and she uses no drugs.

Family History

Her parents are divorced. Her biological father, aged 45, has peptic ulcer disease. Her mother has migraine headaches. She has no siblings.

Review of Systems

Her only other symptom is occasional heartburn if she is under stress and drinks too much coffee.

- What other information about her current health status would you like to know? Why?
- What more would you like to know about her social history? Explain.
- What might be the meaning of pregnancy to Ann and Luke at this time, and how would you approach this issue?
- Is there anything in the patient's history that might concern you at this time? Why?

Objective

Vital Signs

Height, 5 ft 5 in; weight, 130 lb; blood pressure, 130/88; pulse, 70; temperature, 37.3°C.

Examination

The head, eyes, ears, nose, and throat are normal. The neck and thyroid glands are normal. The chest and heart are unremarkable. There are no breast masses. The abdomen has no tenderness or mass palpable. On pelvic examination, there is a thin vaginal discharge. The cervical isthmus is soft. The fundus is enlarged to a 6- to 8-week pregnancy size and is nontender. The adnexa and the rectal examination are normal.

Laboratory

An office pregnancy test is positive.

- What more—if anything—would you include in the physical examination, and why?
- What—if anything—would you do today to evaluate the blood pressure reading of 130/88?
- What are your concerns regarding the vaginal discharge, and what would you do to further evaluate this finding?
- What laboratory studies would you order on this first prenatal visit?

Assessment

- How would you describe your conclusions and prognosis to Mrs. Martino-Priestley?
- What are your concerns regarding this pregnancy?
- What might be the impact of this pregnancy on the patient as an individual? How might you address this topic?
- What changes are this pregnancy likely to cause in Ann and Luke's life as a couple, and how should these issues be addressed?

Plan

- What advice would you offer the patient at this time regarding diet, vitamins, medications, and activity?
- If the patient is found to have a trichomonas vaginitis, how would you explain this to the patient, and what therapy would you recommend?
- What community agencies might be helpful to Ann and Luke, and how might these agencies be contacted?
- Describe your plans for continuing care of this patient and her pregnancy.

4
Problems of the Newborn and Infant

RICHARD B. LEWAN, CHRISTOPHER R. WOOD, AND BRUCE AMBUEL

Family-centered care offers diverse opportunities for reducing risk and improving the health of newborns and infants. Premarital, preconception, and prenatal visits allow assessment for genetic disorders, ensure healthy lifestyle changes (e.g., nutrition), provide preconception vitamins, manage chronic diseases such as diabetes, and intervene when prenatal disorders such as toxemia threaten. Optimal care requires preparation for emergencies (e.g., neonatal resuscitation, sepsis), management of common problems, timely referral for complicated conditions, and prevention through early identification of feeding, growth and developmental problems, and family violence. Full family involvement prepares each member for new roles, recruits participation in healthy habits, and maintains cohesiveness when problems arise.

Newborn Care

Newborn Resuscitation

Skillful resuscitation can prevent lifelong complications of common neonatal emergencies. Proper preparation for the distressed newborn begins with a search for risk factors with each delivery. Participation in a resuscitation course or hospital-based practice sessions promotes teamwork and leadership. Then team members can develop and maintain skills using an organized plan of assessment and intervention. Figure 4.1 outlines an intervention protocol for a term newborn based on meconium, respiratory effort, heart rate, and color. This figure can be posted with a list of tested equipment in a visible location in the resuscitation area. Ready access must be provided to the equipment and medications listed. When time permits, all equipment is laid out and tested. Prior to obtaining intravenous access, epinephrine and naloxone can be given by endotracheal tube followed by 1 to 2 mL of saline. Basic resuscitation skills for a depressed newborn include (1) controlling the thermal environment with proper use of a radiant warmer and rapid, thorough drying; (2) positioning, suctioning, and gentle tactile stimulation; (3) catheter suctioning of meconium from the airway on the perineum followed by gentle bulb syringe suctioning after delivery and adding prompt tracheal suctioning of any meconium through an endotracheal tube if the newborn is not vigorous (e.g., if depressed respirations, tone or heart rate below 100 beats per minute; repeat until clear unless the heart rate is low); (4) providing immediate bag and mask ventilation for newborns with apnea, gasping, or poor respiratory effort; and (5) administration of naloxone or IV normal saline if indicated. Effective positioning and skillful assisted ventilation revive most distressed neonates. Short delays greatly prolong recovery time and increase the risk of complications.

Advanced skills for patients without immediate consultation include (1) endotracheal tube placement with ventilation for patients not responding or requiring more prolonged bag and mask ventilation; (2) chest compressions at 120 per minute for a sustained heart rate of less than 60 beats per minute (cycles of three compressions followed by one breath); (3) central circulation access through the umbilical venous catheter because peripheral intravenous access is often unsuccessful; and (4) chest puncture at the fourth intercostal space in the anterior axillary line with a 21-gauge angiocatheter or butterfly for tension pneumothorax.[1]

Stabilization for Transfer to the Nursery or Transport to Intensive Care

Postresuscitation priorities include assessment for emergent anomalies, maintenance of basic needs, effective communication with and support of the family, and deciding on the level of care required. Pulse oximetry and a cardiorespiratory monitor are used to monitor ongoing success. Oxygen saturations should be kept at 88% to 92% for preterm newborns and 92% to 94% for term newborns. Baseline tests for unstable newborns include a chest radiograph, complete blood count (CBC), glucose, and blood gases (arterial if possible, otherwise capillary). A sepsis workup and other laboratory tests may then be considered. Ventilatory support is needed for persistent respiratory distress, apnea, or deteriorating blood gases (especially PCO_2 >60 with acidosis). Feedings should then be avoided and a nasogastric tube placed. Intravenous fluids are started with 10% dextrose in water ($D_{10}W$) at 65 to 80 mL/kg/day for the first 24 hours. Timely transport of unstable or high-risk neonates for tertiary care enhances outcome (e.g., early surfactant therapy for hyaline membrane disease).

Giving Bad News to Parents After Delivery

Family physicians will confront situations where they need to discuss bad news with parents regarding their newborn. These situations can range from a stillbirth, to a neonatal death, to a multisystem serious anomaly, or to isolated problems such as cleft palate. Studies have surveyed patients and family members to determine how they believe physicians should give bad news.[2] These studies have covered a wide range of patient and family experiences including cancer, birth defects, traumatic injury and death, etc. Four common themes emerge from this

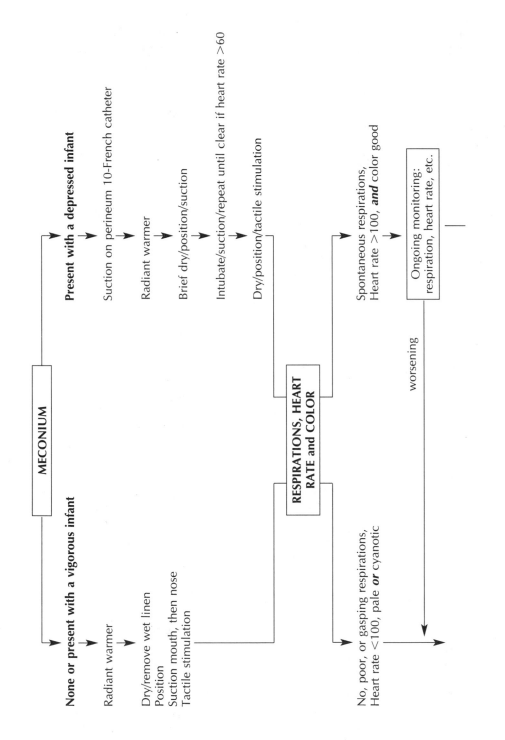

MECONIUM

None or present with a vigorous infant

Radiant warmer

Dry/remove wet linen
Position
Suction mouth, then nose
Tactile stimulation

Present with a depressed infant

Suction on perineum 10-French catheter

Radiant warmer

Brief dry/position/suction

Intubate/suction/repeat until clear if heart rate >60

Dry/position/tactile stimulation

RESPIRATIONS, HEART RATE and COLOR

Spontaneous respirations,
Heart rate >100, **and** color good

No, poor, or gasping respirations,
Heart rate <100, pale **or** cyanotic

Ongoing monitoring:
respiration, heart rate, etc.

worsening

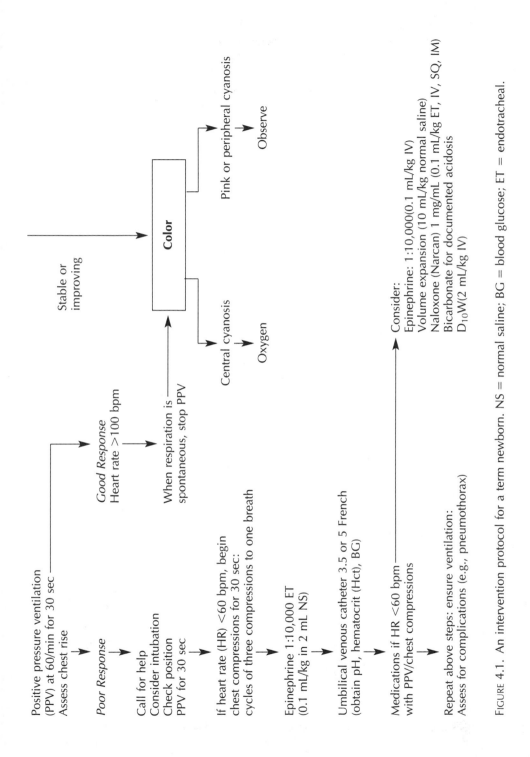

Positive pressure ventilation (PPV) at 60/min for 30 sec
Assess chest rise

Poor Response

Call for help
Consider intubation
Check position
PPV for 30 sec

If heart rate (HR) <60 bpm, begin chest compressions for 30 sec: cycles of three compressions to one breath

Epinephrine 1:10,000 ET (0.1 mL/kg in 2 mL NS)

Umbilical venous catheter 3.5 or 5 French (obtain pH, hematocrit (Hct), BG)

Medications if HR <60 bpm with PPV/chest compressions

Repeat above steps: ensure ventilation: Assess for complications (e.g., pneumothorax)

Good Response
Heart rate >100 bpm

When respiration is spontaneous, stop PPV

Stable or improving

Color

Central cyanosis
→ Oxygen

Pink or peripheral cyanosis
→ Observe

Consider:
Epinephrine: 1:10,000(0.1 mL/kg IV)
Volume expansion (10 mL/kg normal saline)
Naloxone (Narcan) 1 mg/mL (0.1 mL/kg ET, IV, SQ, IM)
Bicarbonate for documented acidosis
$D_{10}W$(2 mL/kg IV)

FIGURE 4.1. An intervention protocol for a term newborn. NS = normal saline; BG = blood glucose; ET = endotracheal.

79

work indicating that patients want (1) a clear, direct statement of the news; (2) time to talk together in private; (3) openness to emotion; and (4) ongoing involvement in decision making.[2] In addition, when physicians are discussing bad news with parents regarding a newborn, parents prefer that the physician talk to both parents together and early. Parents also prefer that the physician, when possible, discuss the news with the baby present and being held by a parent or the physician.[3,4]

Common Problems in the Nursery

Low Birth Weight Newborns

Every hospital should provide a standard graph that allows plotting of weight to gestational age (by dates and examination) to identify newborns who are premature (<37 weeks), small for gestational age (SGA) (weight <10th percentile), or both. Once classified, problems unique to each can be prevented or anticipated. For example, prematurity is associated with hyaline membrane disease, apnea, jaundice, and intracranial hemorrhage. Asymmetric SGA newborns (small trunk relative to head size, caused by uteroplacental insufficiency) are at risk for asphyxia, meconium aspiration, hypoglycemia, hypothermia, and polycythemia. Symmetric SGA [small head and body, caused by genetic or TORCH (toxoplasmosis, other agents, rubella, cytomegalovirus, herpes simplex) syndromes] adds risk for congenital malformations and poor subsequent catch-up growth. All may be at risk for sepsis.

Those newborns cared for in a level I nursery are ready for discharge when they are (1) medically stable, (2) tolerating feedings well with consistent weight gain, (3) able to maintain stable body temperature in an open crib for 24 hours, and (4) free of apneic or bradycardic spells requiring intervention for a number of days (or home monitoring is established), and when their caregivers are educated and able to cope with the infant at home, and discharge planning is complete.

Postterm Newborns

After 42 weeks' gestation, some newborns are large and at risk for birth trauma and asphyxia. Others are postmature with absent lanugo and vernix, long nails, thin and scaly skin, abundant scalp hair, increased alertness, and low birth weight (SGA due to placental insufficiency with the risks described above). Early feedings are indicated.

Neonatal Sepsis

Sepsis is often accompanied by nonspecific signs and symptoms, making early detection difficult; 2/1000 neonates have bacterial sepsis. Risk increases with preterm labor, premature rupture of membranes, or intrapartum fever. Group B streptococcus (GBS) and *Escherichia coli* are responsible for 70% of the bacterial infections, and *Listeria monocytogenes,* enterococcus, staphylococcus, and other gram-negative bacteria (e.g., *Haemophilus influenzae*) are responsible for most of the rest. Early manifestations include temperature instability, lethargy, and poor feeding. Only about 50% have a temperature higher than 37.8°C (100°F) axillary. Prompt evaluation and careful observation every few hours can clarify when a thorough workup is needed. Hepatosplenomegaly, jaundice, petechiae, seizures, stiff neck, and bulging fontanel occur late and denote a poor prognosis.

Group B streptococcal infection is associated with 20% mortality and often presents at or just after birth with rapid deterioration, unexplained apnea, tachypnea, respiratory distress, or shock. Late-onset disease (mean 24 days) usually presents as meningitis. Intrapartum chemoprophylaxis based on the 1996 Centers for Disease Control and Prevention (CDC)[5] recommendation reduces morbidity and mortality of neonatal GBS infections.

DIAGNOSIS

Helpful studies include CBC, chest radiography, and cultures of blood, cerebrospinal fluid (CSF), and urine. Catheterization or suprapubic aspiration are preferable for culture. The CSF may contain up to 32 white blood cells (WBC)/mm^3 during the first few days, so a Gram stain and protein and glucose levels in the CSF should be checked. Surface cultures are no longer recommended.

TREATMENT

Antibiotics should be initiated quickly with a combination of ampicillin (200 mg/kg/day IV or IM divided tid for infants during the first week of life, tid thereafter) plus gentamicin (2.5 mg/kg per dose bid for the first week, tid thereafter). Dosages are reduced for low birth weight infants or if meningitis is excluded. Because viruses and noninfectious disorders can produce sepsis-like illness, antibiotics can be stopped at 48 hours with sterile cultures unless the suspicion for infection continues to be high. Treatment is then continued intravenously at least 7 days while monitoring gentamicin levels. If the latter assay is not available, cefotaxime can be used instead of gentamicin. Methicillin (or vancomycin if resistance is possible) should replace ampicillin when starting antibiotics after 3 days of life. Bacteremia is treated for 7 to 10 days or 5 to 7 days after a clinical response is noted. Meningitis requires at least 14 days of therapy depending on the response and causative organism.[6]

Respiratory Distress

Tachypnea, grunting, nasal flaring, retractions, cyanosis, apnea, or stridor should be evaluated with a chest radiograph, blood gases, glucose, and hematocrit. Early-onset causes include hyaline membrane disease (HMD), meconium aspiration, transient tachypnea of the newborn (TTN), or "wet lung," and less commonly in utero acquired pneumonia or congenital defects compromising the respiratory tract. At several hours after birth sepsis, metabolic abnormalities, cardiac failure, and intraventricular hemorrhage become more likely.

Hyaline membrane disease affects preterm newborns who manifest "stiff" lungs, hypercarbia, hypoxia, and a "ground-glass" (reticulonodular) radiograph with air bronchograms. Signs are usually present within minutes after birth and progressively worsen after. Rapid stabilization and early surfactant therapy improves outcome. Meconium aspiration usually occurs after 34 weeks, causing airway obstruction and edema often within hours of birth. Radiography reveals hyperinflation and possibly pneumothorax. After resuscitation, aggressive support with ventilation and oxygen should maintain the PO$_2$ above 80 mm Hg. Sepsis workup and antibiotic coverage are indicated for HMD and meconium aspiration because the risk of pneumonia is increased.

Transient tachypnea of the newborn presents just after birth in term or preterm newborns and improves significantly within 24 hours. Tachypnea, little hypoxia or hypercarbia, and radiographic findings of perihilar streaking (not reticulonodular) and fluid in the fissures are common. Oxygen requirements gradually decrease after the first few hours. If the course is atypical or there is a risk of sepsis, neonatal pneumonia and other causes must be considered.

Apnea

A respiratory pause of 20 seconds (shorter if cyanosis or bradycardia occurs) strongly suggests pathology in the term infant. Apnea of prematurity should not occur before 1 day or after 7 days of life. The evaluation begins with a history about the event including respiratory effort, color, tone, relation to feeding, and unusual movement. Vital signs (for thermal disorders), a careful cardiorespiratory and neurologic examination, CBC, and calcium, magnesium, and electrolyte levels are assessed. Based on the suspicion, an electrocardiogram (ECG), echocardiogram, arterial blood gases, electroencephalogram (EEG), head computed tomography (CT) scan, or reflux studies may be needed. Management of the underlying problem and resolution of apnea associated with desaturations or bradycardia for several days allow discharge. Pnuemography does not predict the risk of sudden infant death syndrome. Evidence to support the use of home monitoring is lacking. It is not indicated in asymptomatic preterm patients.

Cyanosis

Blue hands and feet are sometimes normal or may be due to slowed circulation. Trunk and mucous membrane involvement (i.e., central cyanosis) after the first 20 minutes of life requires rapid evaluation. If hypothermia, hypoglycemia, narcotic respiratory depression, hypotension, and choanal atresia are not found, causes may include pulmonary, cardiac, neurologic and metabolic disorders as well as polycythemia, sepsis, and acidosis. Intermittent cyanosis with alternating "spells" of apnea and periods of normal breathing suggests a neurologic disorder. Involvement in the upper or lower part of the body or continuous cyanosis without respiratory signs strongly suggests a cardiac cause, especially if a Po_2 of 100 mm Hg is not achieved when the infant is placed in 100% oxygen for 20 minutes. Hypoxia should be reversed with oxygenation and assisted ventilation in preparation for rapid referral.

Hypotension and Shock

After quick assessment including repeated vital signs and obtaining essential laboratory tests (i.e., CBC, coagulation studies, glucose, electrolytes and pH, calcium, cultures, and if indicated the Kleihauer-Betke test), volume expansion with normal saline (10 mL/kg over 30 minutes) should be undertaken promptly for suspected hypovolemia, sepsis, or neurogenic causes. Once stabilized, the history and physical examination can direct further study. Any suggestion of sepsis requires a workup and antibiotic coverage. If cardiogenic causes are likely, inotropic agents may be indicated and should be considered when volume expansion is ineffective.

Cardiac Murmurs

Soft, benign murmurs are common during the first 24 hours of life, but early loud murmurs suggest valvular stenosis or regurgitation. Murmurs of cardiac shunts may be heard at 72 hours but more often at 2 to 3 weeks. Loud murmurs, abnormal heart sounds, or findings suggesting cardiac disease (i.e., cyanosis, poor color or feeding, tachycardia, bradycardia, abnormal blood pressure, respiratory distress, or hepatomegaly) necessitate a prompt ECG, chest radiograph, and, if pathology is suspected, cardiology consultation. All neonates require careful auscultation at the 2-week visit.

Jaundice

Jaundice is noted in at least 50% of Caucasian newborns, with 6% having total serum bilirubin (TSB) levels higher than 12.9 mg/dL. Higher levels are noted in Asian and American Indian newborns. Kernicterus leading to death or severe neurologic handicap is preventable if bilirubin levels do not exceed 25 to 30 mg/dL (lower in sick premature neonates). Two important errors are likely sources of the rising incidence of kernicterus now seen even in healthy term newborns. First, delayed recognition due to early discharge occurs if the newborn is not reassessed by day 3 of life. Second, delayed evaluation for and treatment of hemolysis makes it more likely that exchange transfusion will be needed.

DIAGNOSIS

Icterus, best detected by blanching blood from the skin, is first noted in the face and progresses to the feet as TSB levels rise. While recent studies suggest unreliability of the clinical exam in estimating TSB, if icterus does not reach the umbilicus in low-risk newborns, the TSB is unlikely to be more than 12 mg/dL.[7] Transcutaneous bilirubinometry estimates TSB but is inaccurate with rapid progression, after phototherapy, or with dark skin. TSB levels must be measured for severe or rapid-onset jaundice. Inaccuracy of ±1 mg/dL should be considered when following TSB trends.

Physiologic jaundice is common with a typical pattern of unconjugated hyperbilirubinemia, reaching an average peak of 6 mg/dL by day 3 and resolution within 1 week in term infants and within 2 weeks in preterm infants. A search for pathologic jaundice is needed with (1) icterus during the first 24 hours (assess quickly for hemolysis), (2) TSB rising more than 5 mg/dL per day, (3) TSB exceeding 15 mg/dL in term infants and 10 mg/dL in preterm infants, (4) icterus lasting longer than 10 days in term infants and 21 days in preterm infants, and (5) a direct bilirubin level exceeding 1.5 mg/dL. Review the maternal, perinatal, and family history for risk factors, reexamine, determine the infant's blood type and Rh, and perform a direct Coombs' test (on cord blood saved from the delivery, if possible). If these tests are normal, an exaggerated physiologic jaundice pattern is likely. If hemolysis is found without ABO incompatibility, hematocrit, blood smear, and red blood cell defect tests [e.g., glucose-6-phosphate dehydrogenase (G6PD)] may be indicated. A sepsis evaluation is unnecessary if the only clinical finding is unconjugated hyperbilirubinemia. The direct bilirubin level should be checked if jaundice persists or cholestasis is suspected (light stool, dark urine, jaundice with a green tinge).

TREATMENT

Despite the trend of high TSB levels before treatment, earlier treatment is needed for those at risk of kernicterus (i.e., hemolysis, asphyxia, and prematurity). Jaundice during the first 24 hours of life requires prompt evaluation and consideration for exchange transfusion if hemolysis is found.

TSB ranges are recommended for starting phototherapy in healthy term newborns as follows: TSB of 12 to 15 mg/dL at 24 to 48 hours, 15 to 18 mg/dL at 48 to 72 hours, and 17 to 20 mg/dL at more than 72 hours.[8] Increasing or high TSB levels (i.e., 20 mg/dL at 24 to 48 hours, 25 mg/dL at more than 48 hours) require intensive (double or special lights) phototherapy. If very high TSB levels do not decline 1 to 2 mg/dL within 6 hours or higher levels are encountered (i.e., 25 mg/dL at 25 to 48 hours and 30 mg/dL at any time), exchange transfusion should be added. Phototherapy precautions include increasing fluids by 15 mg/kg/day, patching eyes, and monitoring for temperature instability. A transient rash, green stools, lethargy, irritability, and abdominal distention may occur. Phototherapy can be stopped when the TSB falls by 5 mg/dL or below 14 mg/dL.[7] A rebound rise is uncommon. Home phototherapy (using a fiberoptic blanket) with uncomplicated jaundice and a reliable family allows breast-feeding and bonding to proceed with minimal interruption. If jaundice persists or bronze discoloration is noted, fractionate the bilirubin (i.e., direct) to search for cholestasis.

Breast-feeding is associated with elevated bilirubin levels beginning on the third day. More frequent feeding (i.e., 10 times in 24 hours without supplements unless milk production is low) reduces TSB levels. Breast-milk jaundice is a delayed, sometimes alarming, common form of jaundice. It begins after the third day, peaks by the end of the second week, and gradually resolves over 1 to 4 months. If the evaluation previously described reveals no pathologic cause, parental preference should strongly influence whether to breast-feed frequently (formula supplement if low output), begin phototherapy, or interrupt breast-feeding. Interruption of breast-feeding for 48 hours, while confirming the diagnosis with an abrupt decline in TSB, increases the risk of breast-feeding failure significantly and is usually unnecessary.

Hypoglycemia

Newborn blood glucose levels should be higher than 40 mg/dL. Hypoglycemia can occur without risk factors or symptoms. The most common symptoms are "jitteriness," hypothermia, poor feeding, apnea, apathy, abnormal cry, hypotonia, and seizures. A capillary glucose strip from a warmed heel allows screening of high-risk or symptomatic infants. Any value less than 45 mg/dL must be confirmed by venipuncture. Hypoglycemic injury is prevented by keeping newborns warm and initial monitoring every 30 minutes with early caloric support if high risk. Oral feeding can be attempted for levels more than 25 mg/dL. If symptomatic, a bolus of $D_{10}W$ (2 mL/kg) over 2 to 3 minutes is followed by an infusion of 8 mg/kg/min. The glucose strip is rechecked at 15 minutes and then hourly until three consecutive normal values occur.

Metabolic Disorders

Unexplained poor feeding, vomiting, lethargy, convulsion, or coma in a previously healthy newborn suggests an inborn error of metabolism even during the first few hours of life. After excluding hypoglycemia and hypocalcemia, plasma ammonia, bicarbonate, and pH should be checked. Early consultation and treatment avoids severe metabolic and neurologic disturbances.

Anemia

A central venous hematocrit less than 45% in newborns delivered after 34 weeks is often caused by blood loss and less often by hemolysis or congenital anemias. Careful review of the history, physical examination, red blood cell (RBC) indices, and peripheral smear can guide further evaluation. Coombs' test, reticulocyte count, and Kleihauer-Betke stain of maternal blood to look for fetomaternal transfusion may be needed. If the newborn is without compromise and has a hematocrit over 20%, observation is indicated. Shock requires repeated 5 mL/kg infusions over 5 minutes of crossmatched or O-negative blood until symptoms are alleviated. Severe hemolysis may require exchange transfusion.

Polycythemia

A hematocrit of more than 65% venous or 70% capillary may cause plethora, subsequent jaundice, and hyperviscosity. If the infant is symptomatic (lethargy, apnea, irritability, seizures, feeding difficulties, respiratory distress, cyanosis, hypoglycemia) and after confirming the hematocrit elevation, a partial exchange transfusion should be given to lower the hematocrit to 50%.

Birth Injuries

Head injuries include soft tissue swelling and bruising of the scalp resulting from vertex delivery (caput succedaneum), slow subperiosteal hemorrhage limited to the surface of one cranial bone that does not cross the midline or bruise (cephalohematoma), and skull fracture that requires treatment only if severely depressed. Clavicle fracture, the most common fracture, manifests as limited arm movement and crepitus over the injury. Immobilization of the affected arm and shoulder may be considered. This fracture often is undetected initially and may be found during the first outpatient visit.

Erb's palsy (neuritis of C5-C6 roots due to delivery trauma) causes arm adduction and internal rotation, elbow extension and pronation, and wrist flexion ("waiter's tip" posture). Five to nine percent have diaphragm paralysis. Early improvement or hand grasp suggests a favorable prognosis. Recovery is complete within 3 to 6 months. If no shoulder, arm, or clavicle fractures exist, the infant's sleeve can be pinned in a functional position for 1 week followed by gentle passive exercises.

Human Immunodeficiency Virus Infection in Neonates and Infants

Approximately 7000 women with HIV give birth annually in the United States. Without intervention, 1750 newly infected infants would be born every year. If currently recommended prevention practices are implemented, this number should decrease to somewhere between and 70 to 522 infants. Some have suggested that the best way to decrease this number even further is to prevent HIV transmission to fathers and mothers. The AIDS Clinical Trial Group (ACTG) protocol 076 demonstrated that if previously untreated HIV-positive pregnant women with CD4 counts >200/mm^3 are treated with zidovudine [ZDV or azidothymidine (AZT)], the risk of vertical HIV transmission drops from 25.5% to 8.3%. Multidrug regimens along with scheduled cesarean section and avoidance of breast-feeding has been suggested to decrease the rate of transmission to 1%.

However, research is still needed to assess the overall effect of multidrug regimens in pregnancy. Women should be offered counseling with an HIV expert because of the complex and varied treatment regimens, and considerations for their own health. Protocol 076 recommended that pregnant women should be started on oral ZDV (100 mg five times daily) as early as 14 weeks gestation. It is continued through delivery (loading dose of 2 mg/kg over 1 hour and then continuous infusion of 1 mg/kg/hour), and given to the newborn during the first 6 weeks of life (2 mg/kg every 6 hours, beginning 8 to 12 hours after birth).[9] All pregnant women should be screened for HIV and those positive started on ZDV.[10]

In utero infection causes 30% to 50% of the cases of vertical transmission. These infants typically have a more virulent infection with laboratory evidence of infection at birth.[11] Most of the other cases of vertical transmission occur intrapartum through exposure to infected cervical and vaginal secretions. The rate of such transmission is almost doubled when delivery follows rupture of membranes of more than 4 hours duration. A large meta-analysis of cohort studies found that scheduled cesarean section prior to labor decreased the incidence of transmission by 50%.[12,13] All factors relating to the health of the mother, the infant, and the providers must be considered when making this decision. The use of the intrapartum and neonatal portions of protocol 076 significantly decreases transmission, even in those women who have not received antepartum ZDV or cesarean section.[14] Urging HIV positive mothers to use formula instead of breast milk can further decrease the chance of vertical transmission.[15]

Newborns of HIV-positive mothers who did not receive either antepartum or intrapartum ZDV should be started on the neonatal arm of the ACTG protocol 076 within 24 hours of birth. If a woman at high risk for acquiring HIV delivers with an unknown HIV status, the CDC recommends that both the mother and infant should be screened for HIV.[10] Infants whose mothers received multidrug therapies should be monitored more closely in the antepartum period.

INFANT DIAGNOSIS

It is imperative that infants infected with HIV be quickly identified to ensure early use of antiretroviral therapies and to prevent opportunistic infections. In the majority of infected infants, physical examination at birth is normal, making early identification more difficult. Presenting symptoms are often subtle and include failure to thrive, lymphadenopathy and hepatosplenomegaly, chronic or recurrent diarrhea, interstitial pneumonia, and persistent oral thrush. The diagnosis depends on laboratory testing. Any infant exhibiting any of the above symptoms who is born to a mother at high risk for HIV, or who exhibits any other signs of immunocompromise, should be tested. Certainly all infants born to HIV-positive mothers should also be tested. The initial screen should be the DNA polymerase chain reaction (PCR) test. If this is negative, it should be repeated at 2 weeks, 1 to 2 months, and 3 to 6 months. If at any point the PCR is positive, it should be confirmed by HIV culture as soon as possible. Treatment can be started while the culture is pending.[15,16]

TREATMENT OF INFANTS

Due to the rapidly changing and complex nature of HIV treatment recommendations, management of the HIV-infected infant should be done by or in conjunction with a consultant. A detailed discussion of management will thus not be
offered; however, a few general concepts should be kept in mind. Prevention of
Pneumocystis carinii pneumonia (PCP) is one of the most important goals of
HIV management. All infants between 6 weeks and 1 year of age either born to
HIV-positive mothers or proved to be HIV infected should receive prophylaxis
with 150 mg of trimethoprim and 750 mg of sulfamethoxazole/m²/day divided
twice daily and given 3 days weekly. However, if later HIV infection can be reasonably excluded, PCP prophylaxis can be discontinued. Close attention should
be paid to nutritional status. Development should be monitored closely so that
physical or occupational therapy can be started in a timely manner if needed.
Children should be monitored for signs and symptoms of neoplastic disease, as
the effect of retroviral therapies on young children is yet unknown.[15,17] See Chapter 21 for additional information on management of the HIV-infected child.

Approaches to Common Neonatal Anomalies

Table 4.1 provides a brief overview of common anomalies encountered by those
caring for newborns.

Guidelines for Early Hospital Discharge of the Newborn

Resurgence of kernicterus demonstrates the risk of early discharge in a changing
health care environment. Careful assessment of medical risk and stability, completed education of parents on proper care and warning signs, and secured early
medical follow-up are essential components of care prior to discharge between 6
and 24 hours. Examples of eligibility criteria are adequate prenatal care, uncomplicated and low-risk pregnancy and delivery, 5-minute Apgar score over 6, weight
over 2500 g, gestational age more than 37 weeks, normal vital signs, stable medical condition including jaundice, completed physician examination, normal glucose, at least two successful feedings, voiding of urine, appropriate parent–newborn interaction, proper car seat, plans for completion of metabolic screening by 7
days of life, and ability of the parents to follow verbalized instructions. A home
visit at 2 to 3 days of life by a physician or trained nurse improves infant assessment, early identification of problems, and ongoing educational efforts.

Infant Care

Well-Child Care and Normal Development

Well-infant visits, with an emphasis on answering parents' questions and providing anticipatory guidance, are critical during this period of rapid transitions.

TABLE 4.1. Approaches to Common Neonatal Anomalies

Abnormality	Causes	Evaluation/treatment
Head		
Macrocephaly (head size >97%)	May be normal; hydrocephalus; genetic and metabolic disorders	Check for neurologic impairment; consider ultrasonography, head computed tomogram (CT)
Microcephaly (head size <3%)	Cerebral dysgenesis; prenatal insults; other syndromes; familial	Head CT or magnetic resonance imaging, maternal phenylalanine level
Large fontanels	Skeletal disorders; chromosomal anomalies; hypothyroidism; high intracranial pressure	Check for neurologic impairments
Small fontanels	Hyperthyroidism; microcephaly; craniosynostosis	Check for neurologic impairments
Craniotabes (softening of cranial bones giving a "ping-pong ball" sensation)	Prematurity; if local, benign bone demineralization; if generalized, syphilis or osteogenesis imperfecta	Should recalcify and harden over 3 months. If persists, Venereal Disease Research Laboratory (VDRL); check for blue sclera and fractures
Eyes		
Abnormal red reflex ("white pupil")	50% of patients have cataracts	Ophthalmologic evaluation
Nasolacrimal duct obstruction (6% of newborns; overflow tearing or mucopurulent drainage; erythema)	Incomplete canalization of duct with residual membrane near nasal cavity; 96% resolve spontaneously by 1 year	Nasolacrimal massage tid; topical antibiotics for mucopurulent drainage; surgery at 9–12 months, earlier if severe
Ears		
Any significant ear anomaly and preauricular pits/fistulas		Check for hearing impairment and possible renal abnormalities
Mouth/palate		
Long philtrum, thin upper lip, small jaw, large tongue		Check for genetic abnormalities
Epstein's pearls (2–3 mm white papules on the gums or palate)	Keratogenous cysts	Spontaneous resolution in weeks; reassurance
Short lingual frenulum ("tongue-tie")	Normal	Clip if feeding impaired, tip of tongue notches when extruded or cannot touch upper gums

89

TABLE 4.1. Approaches to Common Neonatal Anomalies (*Continued*)

Abnormality	Causes	Evaluation/treatment
Cleft lip or palate	Isolated variant; some genetic anomalies	Feeding assessment; lip repair usually at 3 months, palate by 1 year; revision of repair at 4–5 years; speech therapy
Neck		
Fistulas, sinuses, or cysts midline or anterior to the sterno-cleidomastoid (SCM); may retract with swallow	Branchial cleft anomalies; thyroglossal duct cysts	Nonemergent surgical referral
Neck		
Cystic hygroma (soft mass of variable size in the neck or axilla)	Dilated lymphatic spaces (failure of drainage into jugular vein)	Semiurgent surgical referral as lesion can expand rapidly
Congenital torticollis (tilting of the infant's head due to SCM spasm)	Usually an isolated muscular defect from traumatic delivery; appears at 2 weeks	Early physical therapy usually successful in 2–3 months; ortho referral if persists
Skin		
Umbilical cord granuloma	Vascular, red/pink granulation tissue after cord separation	Apply silver nitrate 1–3 times protecting surrounding skin; excise if persists
Café-au-lait spots (flat, light brown macules usually <2 cm)	Consider neurofibromatosis if more than four spots larger than 5 mm	No treatment
Hemangiomas (often raised, red, vascular nodules, deeper lesions appear blue; usually <4 cm; onset during first 3–4 weeks, increases over 6–12 months)	Multiple lesions suggest possible dissemination involving internal organs	Most involute and disappear by 7–9 years of age; observe without treatment unless involving vital structures, ulceration or infection; evaluate further if multiple.
Mongolian spots (gray-blue plaques, up to several centimeters, often lumbosacral, may appear elsewhere)	Hyperpigmentation, seen in up to 70% of nonwhite infants	Benign; most fade over first year; document location since sometimes confused with abuse during infancy
Nevi (variably sized light to dark congenital; brown macules; some others appear later during infancy)	Congenital giant (>20 cm) may undergo malignant degeneration	No treatment needed, although some advise removal of congenital nevi at puberty; refer giant nevi for evaluation

Finding	Significance	Action
Petechiae (normal only on head or upper body after vaginal births)	Infection or hematologic problem if abnormal	If abnormal, check CBC and look for signs of TORCH syndrome
Port-wine stains (permanent vascular macules)	Possible associated ocular or central nervous system (CNS) abnormalities	Cosmetic problem only, unless other abnormalities found
Subcutaneous fat necrosis (hard, purplish, defined areas on cheeks, back, buttocks, arms, or thighs, appearing during the first week)	Necrosis of fat from trauma or asphyxia	Spontaneous resolution over several weeks; rare complication of fluctuance or ulceration

Abdomen/gastrointestinal

Finding	Significance	Action
Mass	Genitourinary (GU) in 50% (either kidney or bladder)	Emergent ultrasound (US) of urinary tract
Single umbilical artery	31% have other congenital defects	Careful clinical exam for other defects
Delayed passage of meconium (99% of healthy term neonates pass meconium within 24 hours)	Small bowel obstruction with bilious vomiting (atresias, malrotations, meconium ileus) or large bowel obstruction (Hirschsprung's, anorectal atresias, meconium plug syndrome)	Anal inspection and rectal exam; if distended, abdominal x-ray and consider contrast enema, anorectal manometry and rectal biopsy; vomiting or distention requires rapid surgical evaluation
Intestinal atresia (bilious vomiting with variable degrees of distention)	If duodenal, resorption of lumen occurred. If jejunoileal, mesenteric vascular injury	Nasogastric (NG) tube, lab, chest and supine/upright abdominal x-ray; contrast enema; surgery
Meconium ileus (distended at birth, x-ray with distended loops and bubbly picture of air/stool in right lower quadrant; absent air/fluid levels)	Abnormal meconium trapping resulting in small bowel obstruction; usually caused by cystic fibrosis	Supine/upright abdominal x-ray; treat with hyperosmolar gastrografin enema (successful in two thirds), otherwise surgery; check sweat chloride test
Meconium plug syndrome (most common distal obstruction)	Inspissated colorectal meconium; diffuse gaseous distention of intestinal loops on x-ray; no air fluid levels)	Abdominal x-ray; contrast enema is diagnostic and often therapeutic; search for other causes if symptoms continue

Genitourinary tract

Finding	Significance	Action
Ambiguous genitalia (if gonads are palpable, likely to be male)	Virilization of genetic female (esp. congenital 21-hydroxylase deficiency) or undermasculinized male	Obtain karyotype and 17α-hydroxy-progesterone quickly; withhold diagnosis of sex until karyotype complete

TABLE 4.1. Approaches to Common Neonatal Anomalies *(Continued)*

Abnormality	Causes	Evaluation/treatment
Hypospadias (urethral opening proximal to tip of glans; may be associated chordee: abnormal penile curvature)	Isolated defect unless other GU anomalies present; 10–15% have first-degree relative with hypospadias	Avoid circumcision; repair 6–12 months of age by experienced surgeon; check for cryptorchidism and hernia; siblings at increased risk
Cryptorchidism (failure of testicular descent; 20% bilateral; long-term complications of infertility and cancer if left untreated)	May be normal: seen in 30% of preterm, 4% of term; if bilateral, consider ambiguous genitalia; if hypospadias and bilateral, consider urologic or endocrine problems	Observe for descent by 6 months; if not, treatment by 1 year of age; if bilateral, obtain karyotype; if also hypospadias, do full urologic and endocrine evaluation
Hydrocele (scrotal swelling that transilluminates but does not reduce during the exam)	Persistence of processus vaginalis distally without communication to the abdominal cavity	If no hernia, most spontaneously resolve in 3–12 months; prompt surgical referral if hernia or increasing size; persistence beyond 1 year makes hernia likely
Inguinal hernia (inguinal bulge that extends toward or into the scrotum; larger with crying or straining)	Processus vaginalis persists and communicates with abdominal cavity	If reducible, prompt referral for surgery to avoid incarceration; if irreducible, emergent referral
Musculoskeletal		
Syndactyly (fusion of two or more digits)	Sporadic or autosomal dominant with varying expressivity	Depending on site, surgery between 6 and 18 months of age
Polydactyly (more than five digits)	Sporadic or autosomal dominant (e.g., 5th finger in blacks)	If no cartilage/bone, remove early, otherwise surgery at 6–18 months
Metatarsus adductus (forefoot supinated and adducted; may be flexible or rigid; ankle range of motion must be normal)	Hereditary "tendency," but often due to uterine crowding; 10% association with hip dysplasia requires careful exam	If flexible and overcorrects into abduction, no treatment; if corrects only to neutral, use corrective shoe for 4–6 weeks and reassess; if rigid, needs early casting
Talipes equinovarus (clubfoot; variably rigid foot, calf atrophy, hypoplasia of tibia, fibula, and foot bones)	Multifactorial with autosomal dominant component; 3% risk in sibs and 20% to 30% for offspring of affected parent	Anteroposterior (AP) and stress dorsiflexion lateral x-ray; early serial casting; if persists, surgery by 6–12 months (90% success rate)
Nervous system		
Spina bifida occulta (spinal defect with cutaneous signs: patch of abnormal hair, dimple, lipoma, hemangioma)	Nonfusion of posterior arches of spine; may be tethering of cord or sinus to spinal space with risk of infection; clinical exam for other defects	Examine for neurologic deficits; US to document defect if cutaneous signs; nonemergent referral to neurosurgeon if dermal sinus or tethering suspected; prompt referral if deficits present

92

They facilitate the accommodation of the family to its newest member while building a relationship of trust with the physician. Cultural and socioeconomic issues, familial expectations and stresses, and an assessment of the infant's physical environment should be addressed, preferably starting prenatally. To allow early treatment of disabilities, each visit should include a systematic age-appropriate physical exam and assessment of fine and gross motor development, sensory function, language expression and comprehension, and social behavior. These visits also provide an opportunity to administer immunizations and obtain screening tests as discussed in Chapter 2. Performing this variety of tasks is simplified by the use of standardized forms.

Nutrition, Feeding, and Associated Problems

Future mothers typically decide by the second trimester of their pregnancy what nutrition, breast milk or formula, they will provide their newborns. Thus, whenever possible, discussion about the advantages and disadvantages of these two forms of nutrition should occur early in pregnancy.

BREAST MILK

It is generally recognized that breast milk is the preferred form of sustenance for newborns and young infants due to its better digestibility and enhancement of infant immunity. Breast-feeding allows the infant to share the mother's immunity to the pathogens present in the community at any given time. It also results in significant reductions in the incidence of gastrointestinal infections and otitis media as well as perhaps other respiratory infections. Although two of the principal immunologic factors have their highest concentrations in the colostrum, the immunologic protection increases with the duration of breast-feeding and is greatest for serious and persistent infections.[18,19] Considering costs of formula, visits to doctors offices, and hospital admissions, some suggest that it is much less expensive to breast-feed.[20]

Infection and Chemicals. Breast milk, unfortunately, can transmit pathogens from the mother to the infant. Thus in developed countries the presence of maternal HIV, septicemia, active tuberculosis, and typhoid fever is an absolute contraindication to breast-feeding while the presence of hepatitis B and cytomegalovirus are relative contraindications.

When seeking to explain any unexpected change in the behavior of a breast-fed infant, it is always important to examine the diet and drug history of the mother. Nicotine can cause infant irritability and reduces both the amount of milk produced and the letdown. Alcohol should be avoided for 1 to 2 hours prior to breast-feeding for each drink consumed. Marijuana is excreted for several hours after even occasional use and cocaine is excreted for 24 to 36 hours.[18]

Vitamin Supplementation. Vitamin D supplementation (400 IU) is needed in those mothers receiving little sunlight, and possibly those whose skin is darkly pigmented. Because the fluoride content of breast milk is low, the totally breast-fed baby may be supplemented with 0.25 mg of fluoride daily starting after 6 months of life. A full-term totally breast-fed infant should receive supplemental iron (2 mg/kg up to 15 mg/day) after 4 months of age and a preterm infant from birth.[18]

Supporting Breast-Feeding. Physician support is often critical to a mother's successfully breast-feeding. Prenatal visits provide an ideal opportunity for early encouragement. In addition to infant benefits, maternal health benefits should be discussed such as emotional impacts and reduced incidence of breast and ovarian cancer. Cultural and personal factors must be factored into decision making so that the patient is not pressured into a decision that may later result in failure and emotional disappointment.

After delivery, reassure mothers that it is rare not to be able to provide adequate milk for their infants and that infants often require 3 to 4 days to nurse effectively. Advise mothers that breast-fed infants often feed every 2 to 4 hours and that developing a feeding routine is often a compromise between the infant's spontaneous pattern and the mother's schedule. When problems arise the assistance of a lactation specialist can often be invaluable.

FORMULA

The vast majority of infants will thrive on cow's milk–based formula. Thus for those mothers who cannot breast-feed long-term, a good compromise may be to encourage breast-feeding for the initial few weeks after birth, and then to primarily use formula and breast-feed only a couple of times daily. In most cases such part-time breast-feeding can be accomplished as long as a nipple with a small hole is used so that the formula feeding more closely reproduces breast-feeding.

Differences between the brands of formula are generally insignificant. True infant intolerance to cow's milk–based formulas is unusual, and soy protein formulas are of value only if lactase intolerance is strongly suspected, such as after a prolonged episode of diarrhea. Even then a trial of cow's milk formula should be attempted again every 2 to 4 weeks since the intolerance is usually transient.

Because formulas do not contain fluoride, suggest the use of powdered forms mixed with fluoridated water. Low-iron formulas offer no advantages over regular iron fortification because constipation from iron is quite rare.

ADVANCING INFANT DIET

Infants should remain on either breast milk or formula until 12 months of age because the introduction of whole cow's milk before this age increases the risk of occult gastrointestinal bleeding and iron deficiency anemia. At 12 months of age, a child should generally be placed on whole or 2% milk to provide the extra calories available from the milk fat, then gradually switched to skim milk by 2 or 3 years of age in those eating well (30% of calories from fat).

Introducing nonmilk foods into the diet prior to age 4 to 6 months neither benefits the infant nor increases the likelihood of the infant sleeping through the night. On the other hand, as infants approach 12 months of age, introducing such foods can avoid making the diet too protein-dense, especially if there is a focus on whole cereals, green vegetables, legumes, and fruits. This accustoms children at a young age to nutritionally balanced high-fiber diets.

Some generally accepted guidelines for introducing nonmilk foods are the following: separate the introduction of new foods by at least 3 days to more easily determine the cause of any food intolerance; start with easily digested foods such as cereals, especially rice, and yellow vegetables; postpone such potential allergens as citric fruits, wheat, and eggs until 9 to 12 months of age; and minimize the risk of airway obstruction by avoiding spongy foods (e.g., hot dogs and grapes) and foods with kernels (e.g., corn and nuts). Once a normal child is eating a balanced diet there is no need for supplemental vitamins and iron. Fluoride, though, should be supplemented if the supply in the water system is less than 0.6 ppm.

Obesity

The significance of being overweight as an infant is unclear. Three quarters of such infants become normal-weight adults and most obese adults are not obese as infants. However, when there is a genetic predisposition to obesity, especially if associated with a strong family history of cardiovascular disease, hypercholesterolemia, and diabetes, it is reasonable to encourage primary prevention. This can include breast-feeding and delaying introduction of solids as well as avoiding overfeeding by not using the bottle as a pacifier and using a small spoon to feed solids. However, restriction of fat prior to the age of 2 years can result in a failure to consume adequate calories and other nutrients.[21]

Colic

The syndrome of colic is defined by paroxysms of irritability, fussing, or crying with the infant seeming to be in pain and difficult to console without apparent cause. Episodes typically last for a total of more than 3 hours a day but rarely occur daily. They most often occur in the afternoon or evening and between the ages of 2 weeks and 4 months. Because half of all infants can present with this picture, the other factor that seems to define these babies is that one or both parents have difficulty dealing with this facet of the infant's behavior. Parental behavior, however, does not seem to be a cause of the colic, only a response. Before infants are given the diagnosis of colic, they should have a thorough physical exam to identify an acute processes such as infection or intussusception, especially if the onset is sudden.

Treatment of Colic

A principal focus is on reassuring parents that the process is a common, self-limited one and providing them with some basic measures to try. These include providing motion as in a mechanical swing, rocker, or papoose, or exposure to a steady hum such as in a car or a vacuum cleaner; snug bundling; warmth such as a warm water bottle on the stomach; and burping well and frequently during and after feeding. Often the physician's most important roles are providing support over time and legitimizing the parents' sense of frustration, and even anger, with the situation. The physician should also encourage parents to help each other with caring for the infant, and whenever possible to enlist the help of others so that they have an opportunity to take a break. When all else fails, parents may need permission to periodically shut the door and let the infant "cry it out."[22]

Infants with more prolonged, severe bouts of crying, especially if intermittent throughout the day, may have at least a partial organic cause. If such a child seems to pass a lot of gas with relief, some physicians prescribe simethicone (Mylicon), although studies have not revealed benefit. Constipation should be treated as it would in other infants (Table 4.2). Frequent vomiting, especially if accompanied by poor feeding and failure to thrive, suggests gastroesophageal reflux. If a trial of antacids is not effective, further workup is indicated. With signs of allergy (eczema, asthma) or a strong family history of allergies, milk allergy should be considered. Finally, although anticholinergic agents have been advocated in the past, their efficacy probably has more to do with their sedating effect than any specific effect on the gastrointestinal muscles. Because they have a potential for severe side effects, their use is discouraged.

Failure to Thrive

Failure to thrive (FTT) is a failure to grow at an appropriate rate, with weight crossing two major channels on the recently updated National Center for Health Statistics (NCHS) growth curve or falling below the 5th percentile for age and sex after correcting for parents' stature, prematurity, growth retardation at birth, and race.[23,24] Because of a high prevalence of FTT in urban and rural areas (5–10%) and significant morbidity (developmental delay, permanent cognitive deficits, behavioral disorders, short stature, chronic physical problems, and medical illness), it is advisable to begin following any child whose weight declines across one NCHS channel or if a parent suspects a growth problem.[25]

Diagnosis

Although the consequences of malnutrition sometimes obscure the original causes, a thorough history and physical examination detect most organic, behavioral, family, and environmental problems that contribute to FTT. This initial assessment should include (1) prior records including growth charts and pre-

TABLE 4.2. Approaches to Common Problems of the Infant

HEENT (head, ears, eyes, nose, and throat)

Thrush (pearly white pseudomembranes on the oral mucosa). Causes: transmission from vaginal mucosa during delivery; contaminated fomites (nipples—both breast and bottle, toys, teething rings). Rx: clean fomites (boil bottle nipples, toys); oral nystatin, 200,000–500,000 U q4–6h until clear ×48 hours.

Nasolacrimal duct obstruction (see Table 4.1). Symptoms usually delayed until days to weeks after birth. Rx: nasolacrimal massage tid and cleansing of eyelids with warm water; topical antibiotics (sulfacetamide or gentamicin drops) for secondary conjunctivitis.

Strabismus (misalignment of eyes). Screen with corneal light reflex and cover test. Rx: ophthalmology referral for persistent deviation > several weeks or any deviation >4 months of age.

Hearing loss. Screening either mandatory after delivery or for those at risk: family history; congenital infection; craniofacial abnormalities; birth weight <1500 g; hyperbilirubinemia requiring exchange transfusion; severe depression at birth; bacterial meningitis. Screening: otoacoustic emissions testing or auditory brainstem response. Treatment by 6 months can greatly improve future language development.

Teething (painful gums secondary to eruption of teeth with irritability, drooling). Fever and other systemic effects not caused by teething. Rx: chewing on soft cloth, teething ring, dry toast hastens eruption; topical and systemic analgesia.

Skin problems

Circumcision. Elective procedure performed only on healthy, stable newborns using preferably a penile block. Contraindicated if any genital abnormalities. Advantages: decreased incidence of phimosis and urinary tract infection. Risks (small): hemorrhage; sepsis; amputation; urethral injury; removal of excessive foreskin with painful scarring. Risk of general anesthesia is added since it is often used after the neonatal period.

Diaper dermatitis (erythematous, scaly eruptions that may advance to papulovesicular lesions or erosions; may be patchy or confluent; genitocrural folds often spared). Due to reaction to overhydration of skin, friction, and/or prolonged contact with urine, feces, chemicals such as in diapers, and soaps. Rx: frequent changing of diapers; exposure to air; bland, protective topical ointment (petrolatum, zinc oxide) after each diaper change; advanced cases may require 1% hydrocortisone ointment.

Candidal superinfection (pronounced erythema with sharp margins, satellite lesions, involvement of genitocrural folds). Rx: topical antifungal; treat associated thrush.

Milia (superficial 1–2 mm inclusion cysts). Common on face and gingiva. Requires no Rx.

Miliaria (clear or erythematous papulovesicles in response to heat or overdressing; especially in flexural areas). Resolves with cooling.

Seborrheic dermatitis (most commonly greasy yellow scaling of scalp or dry white scaling of inguinal regions; may be more extensive). Rx: generally clears spontaneously; may require 1% hydrocortisone cream; mild antiseborrheic shampoos for scalp lesions; mineral oil with gentle brushing after 10 minutes for thick scalp crusts.

Atopic dermatitis (intensely pruritic, dry, scaly, erythematous patches). Acute lesions may weep. Typically involves face, neck hands, abdomen, and extensor surfaces of extremities. Genetic propensity with frequent subsequent development of allergic rhinitis and asthma. Consider evaluation for food and other allergens. Rx: mainstay is avoidance of irritants (temperature and humidity extremes, foods, chemicals) and drying of the skin (frequent bathing, soaps) with frequent application of lubricants (apply to damp skin after bathing); severe disease usually requires topical steroids; acute lesions may require 1:20 Burrow's solution and antihistamines (diphenhydramine, hydroxyzine).

Heart murmur

Innocent or functional (typically diminished with decreased cardiac output, i.e., standing).

Newborn murmur. Onset within first few days of life that resolves by 2–3 weeks of age. Typically soft, short, vibratory, grade I–II/VI early systolic murmur located at lower left sternal border that subsides with mild abdominal pressure.

Still's murmur. Most common murmur of early childhood. May start in infancy. Typically loudest midway between apex and left sternal border. Musical or vibratory, grade I–III early systolic murmur.

TABLE 4.2. Approaches to Common Problems of the Infant (*Continued*)

Pulmonary outflow ejection murmur. May be heard throughout childhood. Typically soft, short, systolic ejection murmur, grade I–II and localized to upper left sternal border.

Hemic murmur. Heard with increased cardiac output (fever, anemia, stress). Typically grade I–II high-pitched systolic ejection murmur heard best in aortic/pulmonic areas.

Pathologic or organic murmurs. Any diastolic murmur. Consider when a systolic murmur has one or more of the following: grade III or louder, persistent through much of systole, presence of a thrill, abnormality of second heart sound, or a gallop. Other ominous signs: congestive heart failure, cyanosis, tachycardia. Evaluation: chest x-ray (CXR), electrocardiogram (ECG), and if persistent or any distress then cardiology consult.

Gastrointestinal

Constipation (intestinal dysfunction in which the bowels are difficult or painful to evacuate). Associated failure to thrive, vomiting, moderate to tense abdominal distention, or blood without anal fissures requires ruling out organic disease (Hirschsprung's, celiac disease, hypothyroidism, structural defects, lead toxicity). Common causes are anal fissures, undernutrition, dehydration, excessive milk intake, and lack of bulk. Less common with breast-feeding. Rarely caused by iron-fortified cereals. Rx: in early infancy increase amount of fluid or add sugars (Maltsupex); later add juices (prune, apple) and other fruits, cereals, and vegetables; may add further artificial fiber (Citrocel); severe disease may require brief use of milk of magnesia (1–2 tsp), docusate sodium, and glycerin suppositories and when persistent requires ruling out of organic disease.

Gastroesophageal reflux. Vomiting noted in 95% by 6 weeks old, resolving in 60% by age 2. Associated growth delay in 60%, aspiration pneumonia in 30% of affected infants, esophagitis and hemoccult positive stool, chronic cough, wheezing. Consider cow's-milk allergy. Dx: mild cases confirmed by history and therapeutic trial. If more severe, esophageal pH probe and barium fluoroscopic esophagography. Endoscopy if esophagitis is suspected. Rx: position prone for neonates; elevate head of bed for older infants. Thickened feedings with cereal; acid suppression if esophagitis. If more severe, consider metoclopramide (side effects are common); surgery if medical therapy fails.

Pyloric stenosis (nonbilious vomiting immediately after feeding becoming progressively more projectile). 4:1 male:female preponderance. Onset 1 week to 5 months after birth (typically 3 weeks). May be intermittent. Dx: palpation of pyloric mass (typically 2 cm in length, olive shaped) that may be easier to palpate after vomiting; ultrasound preferred method to confirm difficult cases (90% sensitivity). Rx: surgery after rehydration.

Anemia

Improved nutrition has reduced incidence but infants remain at significant risk. Additional risk factors: low socioeconomic status, consumption of cow's milk prior to age 6 months, use of formula not iron fortified, low birth weight, prematurity. Effects: fatigue, apathy, impairment of growth, and decreased resistance to infection. Causes: iron deficiency most common (usually sufficient birth stores to prevent occurrence prior to age 4 months), sickle cell disease, thalassemia, lead toxicity. Screening: hemoglobin (Hgb) or hematocrit (Hct) between ages 6 and 9 months (some recommend only for infants with risk factors). Rx: if microcytic give trial of iron (elemental iron, Feosol, 3–6 mg/kg/day); if not microcytic or unresponsive to iron consider other causes (family history, environment).

Sleep disturbances (when the infant's sleeping pattern disrupts the parent's sleep). Seventy percent of infants can sleep through the night by age 3 months. Most 6-month-olds no longer require nighttime feeding. Screening: a sudden change in sleeping pattern should prompt a search for new stresses, physical (infection, esophageal reflux, etc.) or emotional (new surroundings or household members, etc.). Rx: establish realistic parental expectations (consider the natural sleeping patterns of the infant); allow the infant awakening at night to learn how to fall asleep by himself (keep bedtime rituals simple and put the infant in his bed awake; do not respond to infant's first cry; keep interactions during the night short and simple; provide a security object for older infants); slowly change undesirable sleeping patterns (move bedtime hour up and awaken infant earlier in the morning; decrease daytime napping).

natal history (prematurity, growth retardation); (2) nutrition (diet, behavior); (3) development (cognitive, motor, behavioral, emotional); (4) social context (parental knowledge, family dysfunction, drug abuse, social support, isolation); and (5) environment (poverty, shelter, toxic exposures to lead or pesticides). Diagnostic studies can follow in a stepwise manner, with step 2 studies chosen based on history, physical exam, and severity.[26]

Step 1: CBC, fasting chemistry panel, electrolytes, urinalysis, lead level
Step 2: thyroid, stool (culture, ova and parasites, fat), sweat chloride, tuberculosis, HIV, skeletal survey, renal studies

TREATMENT

Hospitalization is indicated when there is (1) severe malnutrition; (2) suspected abuse or neglect; (3) a need to observe parent–child interaction or a documented problem with interaction; (4) family dysfunction (e.g., barriers to follow-up, disorganization, depression, chemical dependence, violence); (5) need for further diagnostic workup; or (6) failure of outpatient treatment. Outpatient treatment may be appropriate when FTT is moderate (infant's weight is more than 60% the average weight for age *and* more than 85% average for height). Weekly follow-up may be lengthened after sustained weight gain. Collaborative, interdisciplinary treatment involves the parents, physician, social worker, nutritionist, and psychologist. It implements one or more of the following strategies: (1) treating organic factors first; (2) implementing a written nutritional plan for meals and snacks with caloric intake 1.5 to 2.0 times normal; (3) beginning a vitamin supplement; (4) supporting parents with mealtime observation and coaching; (5) treating specific family problems that interfere with the family's ability to care for the infant (misunderstanding, depression, drug abuse); (5) enlisting social support (family, friends, church); (6) mobilizing community and economic resources for the family; (7) establishing continuity of care and access to the treatment team; and (8) promoting parental competence.

Fever

In children under 3 years of age, if a source for the fever cannot be found, or if otitis media is found, 3% to 11% have occult bacteremia. The risk is even higher in infants under the age of 3 months who have an 8.6 % risk of having a serious bacterial infection.[27,28] Timely evaluation prevents treatment delays. Clinicians must counsel parents carefully and avoid unnecessary testing because the sepsis evaluation creates marked parental anxiety (e.g., 30% believing their infant is dying). In an attempt to provide a framework for evaluation of these children, a set of guidelines was published in *Pediatrics* in 1993 that presents a reasonable outline of how to approach this vexing problem.[27] The basic elements of the guidelines, with some variations proposed by others are as follows[28–30]:

TOXIC-APPEARING INFANTS

Children with signs of sepsis (e.g., lethargy, poor perfusion, hypoventilation, hyperventilation, cyanosis) should be hospitalized for a full septic workup with blood urine and spinal fluid cultures. If no source is initially found, a chest x-ray is indicated for infants with high fever and leukocytosis. They should then be placed on antibiotics pending culture results. In those younger than 1 to 2 months of age, antibiotic choices should follow the recommendations made earlier in this chapter for neonates. Older children are most frequently treated with either cefotaxime, 50 mg/kg, IV, q8h, or ceftriaxone, 100 mg/kg, IV, q24h.

LOW-RISK INFANTS

The clinical criteria defining this group are the following: previously healthy, nontoxic appearance, no focal bacterial infection (except otitis media), and ability to be closely monitored by caregivers. Laboratory criteria are WBC count of 5,000 to 15,000/mm^3 (<1500 bands/mm^3); normal urinalysis [<5 WBCs/high power field (hpf)]; and when diarrhea present, <5 WBCs/hpf in stool. Most would recommend obtaining the urine sample by catheterization.

YOUNGER THAN 28 DAYS OLD

The guidelines recommend admitting all such infants with rectal temperatures >38°C (100.4°F) for the septic workup described earlier in this chapter for neonates, without or without antibiotic coverage, pending culture results. Recent research confirms serious bacterial infection can be missed in nontoxic, febrile infants who meet the above low-risk laboratory criteria.[30] However, some still would recommend performing all or part of the same workup as an outpatient because the probability of a serious bacterial infection is only 0.2% among infants meeting the criteria defining low risk.[28] Automatic admission of all febrile infants has significant cost implications, and risk of iatrogenic complications.[31] If treated as an outpatient, all infants must be reevaluated within 24 hours. If blood cultures were performed and were positive, these infants should be admitted for sepsis evaluation and parenteral antibiotics. If a urine culture was obtained and was positive, and there is a persistent fever, the infant should be admitted for septic evaluation and parenteral antibiotics; however, outpatient treatment with oral antibiotics can be used if the patient is afebrile and well.

INFANTS 28 TO 90 DAYS OLD (RECTAL TEMPERATURES >38°C)

These infants can be managed as outpatients. Some recommend culturing both urine and blood, others only one of these, and some add a lumbar puncture and analysis. If there is any suspicion of bacteremia, most would recommend getting at least a blood culture and giving a dose of parenteral antibiotics, most often IM ceftriaxone, 50 mg/kg (maximum of 1 g). These infants should be reevaluated within 24 hours, and positive cultures should be treated as for outpatients <28 days old; however, blood cultures positive for *Streptococcus pneumoniae*, known to be sensitive to penicillin, can be treated with oral penicillin or amoxicillin. Otherwise treatment should be based on clinical appearance at the time of reevaluation.

INFANTS 3 TO 36 MONTHS OLD

There is no need to screen for occult bacteremia in infants with temperatures <39°C (102.2°F). However, those infants with persistent fever for more than 2 to 3 days, worsening clinical appearance, or temperatures ≥39°C without an apparent source of the fever, other than otitis media, constitute a higher risk group. They should be evaluated with a WBC count. If the count is ≥15,000/mm³, a blood culture is indicated, as well as injection of a parenteral antibiotic (most commonly IM ceftriaxone, 50 mg/kg up to a maximum of 1 g), while the culture is pending. In addition, a urine sample by catheter should be cultured from all boys <6 months of age or girls <2 years of age who are treated with antibiotics. This higher risk group should be reevaluated and treated as described above for outpatient infants 28 to 90 days old.

Sudden Infant Death Syndrome

Sudden infant death syndrome (SIDS) is the leading cause of death in infants past the neonatal period, peaking at age 2 months. Characterized by being unexpected and without apparent cause, despite thorough postmortem examination, it represents a collection of etiologies all involving an abnormality of cardiorespiratory regulation. This divergence of etiologies has so far frustrated attempts to develop reliable screening and prevention methods. Many have recommended using electronic home monitoring of apnea and bradycardia for those infants judged to be at high risk, including siblings of SIDS casualties, infants who had apparent life-threatening episodes, and those with the other risk factors cited below. However, such monitors have generally had little effect on reducing the incidence of SIDS in part because of frequent poor parent compliance with their use. When employed, they can be discontinued if there are no episodes of true apnea for 16 consecutive weeks. The use of event recorders with the monitors has made identifying apneic episodes more objective and seems to allow shorter periods of monitoring.

At this time the greatest impact on reducing the incidence of SIDS involves targeting those risk factors known to be associated with a two- to threefold increase in the risk of SIDS. These include maternal smoking or drug use, poor prenatal care, complications of delivery and prematurity, shared sleep surface, soft sleeping surface, bedding that can cover the face, and prone (stomach) sleeping position. Infants who have no medical contraindications should be placed for sleep in the supine (back) or side position. There are no controlled studies demonstrating efficacy, but retrospective studies have showed a strong correlation between sleeping position and SIDS.[32–34]

Other Common Problems of the Infant

Table 4.2 provides short summaries of other frequent problems of infancy and their management.

Family and Community Issues

Child Care

More than 50% of infants under 1 year of age have parents who work outside the home. The physician can encourage parents to use paid and unpaid leave to maximize time with their child during the first year of life and to select child care carefully. A quality child-care setting supports normal infant development, but many settings fail to protect health and safety or provide adequate developmental stimulation. Children in day care are 2 to 18 times more likely to contract certain infectious disease including enteric pathogens, respiratory pathogens, and herpesvirus infections.[26] Parents can find quality programs in both private homes and child care centers; nonprofit centers generally provide higher quality care than for-profit centers.[35] Parents can compare several programs by making scheduled and unscheduled visits to observe the emotional atmosphere and sanitation. The optimal adult/child ratio before 1 year of age is 1:3 and should not exceed 1:4. The day-care provider should have and carefully follow written policies to minimize the spread of infectious disease. Staff should (1) be trained in child development; (2) be paid sufficiently to minimize turnover; (3) enjoy their interactions with children, respond positively to children's accomplishments, and attend quickly when a child is upset; and (4) wash their hands after diapering and before food preparation, use disposable tissue for wiping runny noses, and routinely wash changing tables. After enrollment, encourage parents to continue occasional unscheduled visits and to investigate sudden changes in their child's behavior such as withdrawal, anxiety, or agitation.

Families and Infants: Risks and Resources

Normal infant development is promoted by fostering a family's strengths and resources but is threatened by individual, family, and environmental risk factors. Infant risk factors include chronic illness, physical handicap, low birth weight, growth failure, and developmental delay. Family factors include physical or sexual abuse, family violence, neglect, parental depression, chemical dependence, and chronic illness. Environmental factors include poverty and environmental toxins such as lead. Table 4.3 outlines systematic approach for identifying some common resources and risks for early family development. When possible, screening for such risk factors should start prenatally. Early intervention programs promote healthy development and prevent developmental delay even when infants and families face serious medical, psychosocial, and environmental obstacles. Effective early intervention has five elements:

TABLE 4.3. Assessing Resources and Risks for Early Family Development

Concept	Interview questions
Social support	Do you have at least one friend or relative you can turn to for support and advice? Do you work, attend school, or participate in a religious community?
Housing	Do you have any concerns about housing?
Child care	Do you have any concerns about child care?
Transportation	Do you have any concerns about transportation?
Finances	Will you have any problems paying for food and clothing? Vitamins and medications? Health care?

Safety	During the past year, has anyone you know:
	   Made you afraid for your safety?
	   Pushed, kicked, slapped, hit, or otherwise hurt you?
	   Forced sexual or physical contact?
	   Tried to control your activities, your friends, or other parts of your life?
	 Do you have any guns in your house?
	 Do you have any concerns about safety or violence in your neighborhood?
	 Do you use a seat belt when you ride in a car?
	 Do you use an infant or car seat for each infant and toddler in your family?
	 Do your children always use a seat belt?

Personal health	In general, how healthy do you consider yourself? (Excellent, good, fair, or poor)
STD and HIV Risk	Have you ever had herpes, gonorrhea, chlamydia, trichomonas, genital warts, or a pelvic infection? Have you had two or more sexual partners in the past year?
Emotions	During the last 30 days, how much of the time have you felt downhearted and blue? (Very little, sometimes, often, most of the time)
Alcohol and drugs	Have your parents had any problems with alcohol or drugs? Does your partner have any problems with alcohol or drugs? Have you had any problems in the past with alcohol or drugs? During the past 30 days, on how many days did you have at least one drink of alcohol? During the past 30 days, on how many days did you have five or more drinks of alcohol in a row, that is, within a couple of hours?
Tobacco	Does anyone in your home smoke tobacco? Do you currently smoke or use tobacco?

HIV = human immunodeficiency virus; STD = sexually transmitted disease.

1. *Crisis intervention.* Take quick action to treat immediate threats to safety (e.g., family violence, physical or sexual abuse, severe neglect).
2. *Family-centered care.* Collaborate with parents and avoid labeling a child or parent. Describe the challenge the family faces and the strengths and resources they have to assist them. Teach parents about the unique needs and abilities of their infant. Be optimistic and adapt your interventions to the family's culture.

3. *Social support.* Help families identify supportive family, friends, church, or mutual-help groups.
4. *Community resources.* Help parents mobilize community resources to treat specific needs of the infant and family (e.g., specialized day care, parenting classes).
5. *Ecologic model of intervention.* Assess the individual infant, family, and physical environment and customize your intervention to use the family's specific strengths. Continue to coordinate the involvement of multiple professionals and ensure that the overall plan remains suitable for the family. Serve as an advocate and catalyst to ensure the treatment team addresses unanswered questions.

Chaotic families disrupted by family violence, sexual abuse, or chemical dependence may be difficult to work with, as these same problems tend to disrupt the doctor–patient relationship. It is important that family-centered care be respectful, culturally sensitive, and nonstigmatizing. The physician can take a leadership role by helping the team and family focus on the developmental potential of the infant and family.

Partner Violence (Also See Chapter 6)

One in five pregnant women experience partner violence (domestic violence) during their pregnancy, with higher rates among adolescent girls.[36] Partner violence has a well-documented negative impact on both maternal and infant health. Pregnant women who are being abused are more likely to delay seeking prenatal care, and experience higher rates of depression, anxiety, suicide attempts, alcohol or other drug abuse, and tobacco smoking. Abused women are more likely to experience pregnancy that is unwanted. Intentional injury, often the result of domestic violence, is one of the leading causes of death among pregnant women. Although the health impact of partner violence on infants needs additional study, current research shows that infants born to abused women are more likely to have low birth weight and experience premature birth. Family physicians can play a valuable role by implementing standard screening for partner violence among all pregnant patients. The most effective strategy involves screening at multiple times during the pregnancy, using written questions as well as patient interview, and using questions with demonstrated reliability and validity.

Infants of Substance-Abusing Mothers

Drug abuse during pregnancy significantly increases the risk for low birth weight, growth retardation, microcephaly, and other anomalies. Fetal alcohol syndrome includes the well-described triad of growth retardation before or after birth, nervous system abnormalities, and midfacial hypoplasia. Cardiac and renal systems may also be affected. Infants are typically irritable, have difficulty feeding, and show disorganized sleep patterns. The full syndrome occurs with heavy drinking throughout pregnancy but lower levels of exposure also affect development. The specific effects of prenatal exposure to cocaine and other drugs of abuse are less well described. Exposure to one substance is often confounded by abuse of other drugs and social and environmental factors (e.g., diet and prenatal care) that correlate with chemical dependence and are known to affect infant outcome.[37]

Parents should be encouraged to seek treatment for chemical dependence at any point during pregnancy or after birth. When maternal drug abuse is suspected, infants should be evaluated and treated for acute withdrawal symptoms and then referred for developmental assessment and early intervention.

Adolescent Parents

Adolescent parents are often perceived as high risk, when in fact adolescent girls who have access to appropriate resources, including pre- and postnatal care, give birth to healthy infants and raise children who are well adjusted. True risk factors are poverty, lack of access to health care, family violence, and substance abuse. Adolescents who grow up in a family with violence, sexual abuse, or chemical dependence initiate sexual intercourse at an earlier age than the general population and experience a higher rate of pregnancy.

When working with adolescent parents, (1) expect a positive outcome while offering respect and dignity; (2) encourage family support, if appropriate, including support of the father and his family; (3) encourage use of community resources (child care, parenting classes, education, early intervention programs); (4) initiate family planning early during the pregnancy; and (5) encourage continued education and delay of the birth of another child (delay by as little as 6 months and completion of high school improves long-term social and economic outcome).

Public Policy

Federal law PL99-457 encourages states to develop programs that identify and provide services to children at risk from birth to age 3 years. By statute these early intervention programs are to be individualized, family-centered, and involve the primary care physician. Implementation varies from state to state, making it important for physicians to familiarize themselves with local programs and resources.

References

1. Zaichkin J, Kattwinkel J, eds. International guidelines for neonatal resuscitation: an excerpt from the guidelines 2000 for cardiopulmonary resuscitation and emergency cardiovascular care: international consensus on science. Pediatrics 2000;106(3):1–16.
2. Ambuel B, Mazzone M. Breaking bad news and discussing death. Prim Care 2001;28(2):249–67.

3. Krahn GL, Hallum A, Kime C. Are there good ways to give 'bad news'? Pediatrics 1993;91(3):579–82.
4. Sharp MC, Strauss RP, Lorch SC. Communicating medical bad news: parents' experiences and preferences. J Pediatr 1992;121:539–46.
5. Centers for Disease Control and Prevention. Prevention of perinatal group B streptococcal disease: a public health perspective. MMWR 1996;45(RR-7):1–24.
6. Klein JO. Bacterial sepsis and meningitis. In: Remington JS, Klein JO, eds. Infectious diseases of the fetus and newborn, 6th ed. Philadelphia: WB Saunders, 2001.
7. Moyer VA, Ahn C, Sneed S. Accuracy of clinical judgment in neonatal jaundice. Arch Pediatr Adolesc Med 2000;154:391–4.
8. Dennery PA, Seidman DS, Stevenson DK. Neonatal hyperbilirubinemia. N Engl J Med 2001;344(8):581–90.
9. Centers for Disease Control and Prevention. Zidovudine for the prevention of HIV transmission from mother to infant. MMWR 1994;43:285–8.
10. Centers for Disease Control and Prevention. U.S. Public Health Service recommendations for human immunodeficiency virus counseling and voluntary testing for pregnant women. MMWR 1995;44(RR-7):3–11.
11. Davis SF, Byers RH, Lindegren ML, et al. Prevalence and incidence of vertically acquired HIV infecton in the United States. JAMA 1995;247:952.
12. Landesman SH, Kalish LA, Burns DN, et al. Obstetrical factors and the transmission of human immunodeficiency virus type 1 from mother to child. N Engl J Med 1996;334:1617–23.
13. The International Perinatal HIV group. The mode of delivery and the risk of vertical transmission of human immunodeficiency virus type 1—a meta-analysis of 15 prospective cohort studies. N Engl J Med 1999;340(13):977–87.
14. Centers for Disease Control and Prevention. Public Health Service task force recommendations for the use of antiretroviral drugs in pregnant women infected with HIV-1 for maternal health and reducing perinatal HIV-1 transmission in the United states. MMWR 1998;47(RR-2):16–17.
15. Chadwick EG, Yogev R. Pediatric AIDS. Pediatr Clin North Am 1995;42:969–92.
16. Luzuriaga K, Sullivan JL. DNA polymerase chain reaction for the diagnosis of vertical HIV infection. JAMA1996;275:1360–1.
17. Mofenson, Lynne M. Care and counseling of HIV-infected pregnant women to reduce perinatal HIV transmission. UpToDate (http://www.uptodate.com), May 2, 2000.
18. Lawrence PR. Breast milk: best source of nutrition for term and preterm infants. Pediatr Clin North Am 1994;41:925–42.
19. Dewey KG, Heinig MJ, Nommsen-Rivers LA. Differences in morbidity between breast-fed and formula-fed infants. J Pediatr 1995;126:696–702.
20. Montgomery AM. Breastfeeding and postpartum maternal care. Prim Care 2000;27(1):237–50.
21. Hardy SC, Kleinman RE. Fat and cholesterol in the diet of infants and young children: implications for growth, development, and long-term health. J Pediatr 1994;125:S69–75.
22. Treem WR. Infant colic: a pediatric gastroenterologist's perspective. Pediatr Clin North Am 1994;41:1121–38.
23. Drotar D. Failure to thrive (growth deficiency). In: Roberts MC, ed. Handbook of pediatric psychology. New York: Guilford, 1995;516–36.
24. Leung AKC, Robson WLM, Fagan JE. Assessment of the child with failure to thrive. Am Fam Physician 1993;48:1432–8.

25. Ambuel JP, Harris B. Failure to thrive: a study of failure to grow in height or weight. Ohio State Med J 1963;59:997–1001.
26. Behrman RE, Kliegman RM, Jenson HB. Nelson textbook of pediatrics, 16th ed. Philadelphia: WB Saunders, 2000.
27. Baraff LJ, Bass JW, Fleisher GR, et al. Practice guideline for the management of infants and children 0 to 36 months of age with fever without source. Pediatrics 1993;92:1–12.
28. Grubb NS, Lyle S, Brodie JH, et al. Management of infants and children 0 to 36 months of age with fever without a source. J Am Board Fam Pract 1995;8:114–9.
29. Young PC. The management of febrile infants by primary-care pediatricians in Utah: comparison with published practice guidelines. Pediatrics 1995;95:623–7.
30. Baker D. Evaluation and management of infants with fever. Pediatr Clin North Am 1999;46(6):1061–72.
31. Slater M, Krug S. Evaluation of the infant with fever without source: an evidence based approach. Emerg Med Clin North Am 1999;17(1):97–126, viii–ix.
32. Freed GE, Steinshneider A, Glassman M, Winn K. Sudden infant death syndrome prevention and an understanding of selected clinical issues. Pediatr Clin North Am 1994;41:967–89.
33. AAP Task Force on Infant Positioning and SIDS. Positioning and SIDS. Pediatrics 1992;89(6Pt1):1120–6.
34. Kemp JS, Unger B, Wilkins D, et al. Unsafe sleep practices and an analysis of bed-sharing among infants dying suddenly and unexpectedly: results of a four-year population based, death-scene investigation study of SIDS and related deaths. Pediatrics 2000;106(3):E41.
35. Phillips DA, Howes C, Whitebook M. The social policy context of child care: effects on quality. Am J Community Psychol 1992;20(1):25–52.
36. Hamberger LK, Ambuel B. Spousal abuse in pregnancy. Prim Care Clin North Am. 2001; 3:203–24.
37. Singer L, Farkos K, Kliegman R. Childhood medical and behavioral consequences of maternal cocaine use. J Pediatr Psychol 1992;17:389–406.

CASE PRESENTATION

Subjective

PATIENT PROFILE

Allison Harris is a 1-year-old female child, here today with her mother.

PRESENTING PROBLEM

"For checkup and shots."

PRESENT ILLNESS

Over the first year of life, you have treated Allison for three episodes of otitis media. She has otherwise been well. She knows three words, walks alone, eats some table food, and drinks almost 2 quarts of milk daily.

PAST MEDICAL HISTORY

No serious illnesses or hospitalization during her first year of life.

SOCIAL HISTORY

She is the second child of her father who is a truck driver and her mother who works as a secretary in a business office.

FAMILY HISTORY

Her parents are living and well. Her grandfather has diabetes and coronary artery disease with angina, and her uncle is HIV-positive.

- What other information regarding Allison's health status would you like to know? Why?
- What are the possible implications of both parents working, and how might you address this issue?
- What more would you like to know about Allison's ear infections and her ability to hear?
- What is the possible significance of her milk consumption, and what else would you ask about her current diet?

Objective

VITAL SIGNS

Height 28 in; weight 32 lb; pulse, 82; respirations, 22; temperature, 37.2°C.

EXAMINATION

The 1-year-old child is alert and cheerful and makes good eye contact. Her left tympanic membrane is slightly dull but moves freely. Her eyes, throat, and neck are normal. The chest, heart, abdomen, and genitalia are unremarkable. Her musculoskeletal examination, including gait, is normal for her age.

- What other information derived from the physical examination might be important, and why?
- Are the patient's weight and height appropriate for her age, and how is this calculation made?
- How might you further evaluate Allison's ability to hear?
- What—if any—laboratory tests would you perform today?

Assessment

- How would you describe Allison's health status to her parents?
- What is the developmental status of this patient?
- What are your concerns regarding Allison's diet, and how would you further assess the potential problem?
- Would you do anything special in view of the family history of diabetes mellitus and coronary artery disease? Explain.

Plan

- Describe your recommendation regarding vitamins, medication, and follow-up on her ear infections.
- What immunizations would generally be appropriate at this visit?
- What diet recommendations would be appropriate? How might a problem have developed?
- Describe your recommendations for follow-up care of Allison.

5
Common Problems of the Elderly

JAMES P. RICHARDSON AND AUBREY L. KNIGHT

Older patients are a challenging but satisfying part of most family physicians' practices. Optimal care of geriatric patients occurs when the precepts of continuity of care, the team approach to the management of illness, the importance of the family, and the biopsychosocial model are followed. Because of the prevalence of chronic disease in the elderly, cure may be elusive, but appropriate care always improves the quality of the older adult's life. Some common problems of the elderly are reviewed in this chapter. More complete discussions may be found in textbooks of geriatric medicine.[1,2]

Urinary Incontinence

Urinary incontinence (UI) is defined as an involuntary loss of urine sufficient to be a problem. UI is a common clinical entity, affecting 15% to 30% of community-dwelling older adults. The prevalence is twice as high in women as in men. Institutionalized, hospitalized, and homebound elders have higher prevalence rates. It translates into a huge cost burden in both economic and human terms. UI is more common in the elderly population, but there are other identifiable risk factors, including pregnancy, urinary tract infection, medications, dementia, immobility, diabetes mellitus, estrogen deficiency, pelvic muscle weakness, and smoking.

Types of Urinary Incontinence

Most cases of UI can be divided into one of five causes: (1) involuntary loss of urine with a strong urinary urgency (urge incontinence); (2) urethral sphincter pressure insufficient to hold urine (stress incontinence); (3) too high urethral resistance or insufficient bladder contractions (overflow incontinence); (4) chronic impairment of physical or cognitive function (functional incontinence); and (5) a combination of features of more than one type (mixed incontinence) (Table 5.1).

Urge incontinence, also referred to as detrusor instability, occurs when the involuntary bladder contractions overcome the normal resistance of the urethra.

TABLE 5.1. Treatment of Urinary Incontinence

Type	Signs and symptoms	Treatment
Urge (detrusor instability)	Inability to get to toilet Large volume loss Normal postvoid residual (PVR)	Treat underlying condition Prompted voiding Bladder training Anticholinergic agents
Stress (sphincter insufficiency)	Urine loss with increased intraabdominal pressure Small volume loss Normal PVR	Pelvic muscle exercises Estrogen α-Adrenergic agents Surgical correction
Overflow (outlet obstruction or hypoactive bladder)	Constant urine loss Abdominal pain/distention High PVR	Treat underlying condition α-Adrenergic blockers Intermittent catheterization Surgical correction
Functional	Inability or unwillingness to be continent Large or small volume loss Normal PVR	Treat underlying condition Remove hindrances

This type of incontinence is likely the most common cause of problematic incontinence, affecting up to 70% of persons with incontinence. The three basic mechanisms of action for this type of incontinence are loss of brain inhibition, as might occur with a stroke or in parkinsonism; involuntary detrusor contractions, as might occur with a urinary tract infection; and loss of the normal voiding reflexes. It is characterized by a strong desire to void followed by a loss of urine, often on the way to the bathroom.

Stress incontinence, also referred to as sphincter insufficiency, is most frequently encountered in postmenopausal women and is the result of reduced intraurethral pressure. The loss of urine occurs when there is an associated increase in intraabdominal pressure, such as during coughing, sneezing, or laughing.

Overflow incontinence is the result of the bladder not emptying properly. It can be secondary to an atonic or hypotonic detrusor or an obstruction of the bladder outlet from an enlarged prostate, urethral stricture, or stone. Detrusor hypoactivity can result from diabetes mellitus, lower spinal cord injury, or drugs. Overflow incontinence is characterized by a variety of symptoms that may be confused with symptoms more frequently associated with urge or stress incontinence. The urinary stream is often weak, and there is the sensation of incomplete emptying of the bladder.

Functional incontinence occurs in persons who, despite normal urinary tract functioning, are incontinent. It results from physical, psychiatric, or cognitive dysfunction or environmental limitations. This type of incontinence is frequently seen in the hospital setting when restraints or bed rails are utilized.

Mixed incontinence is common in older persons and usually is associated with features of stress and urge incontinence.

Evaluation

The evaluation of UI has as its goal confirmation of the diagnosis, identification of any reversible causes, and identification of factors that require further diagnostic or therapeutic interventions. History focuses on the neurologic and urologic systems. Additionally, complete review of the medications, both prescribed and over the counter, is necessary. This phase should be accompanied by detailed exploration of the UI symptoms, including duration, frequency, timing, precipitants, and amount of urine lost. Associated symptoms such as nocturia, dysuria, hesitancy, urgency, hematuria, straining, and frequency should be noted. Finally, it is important to inquire about such conditions as diabetes mellitus, neurologic diseases, or urologic problems. At the conclusion of the initial visit, if the patient cannot characterize the incontinence, a bladder record should be kept for several days.[3]

The physical examination focuses on abdominal, neurologic, and genitourinary tract examinations. Specifically, during the abdominal examination the bladder is palpated. The physician assesses both cognitive function and nerve roots S2–3 during the neurologic examination. In men, the physician examines the genitalia to detect abnormalities of the foreskin, glans penis, and perineal skin and does a rectal examination, testing for perineal sensation, sphincter tone, fecal impaction, and prostatic enlargement. In women, a pelvic examination is done to assess perineal skin condition, pelvic prolapse, pelvic mass, and muscle tone. Finally, one can perform the cough stress test to observe urine loss with a full bladder.

Additional tests performed to evaluate all patients with UI include urinalysis and assessment of postvoid residual (PVR). A PVR of more than 100 mL is strongly suggestive of incomplete emptying of the bladder. The patient should be observed for leakage of urine while straining with a full bladder. Urine flow can be calculated simply by dividing the amount voided by the time it takes to void. A rate slower than 10 to 15 mL/sec is considered abnormal. Selected patients have a urine culture or blood testing that might include blood urea nitrogen (BUN), creatinine, glucose, calcium, electrolytes, and urine cytology. Further testing, including intravenous pyelography, ultrasonography, and computed tomography (CT), or referral to a specialist should be pursued when indicated by the history, physical examination, and simple testing.

Management

The first step in management is to identify and treat any reversible factors, remembering that there may be more than one cause. Seemingly small improvements may make a big difference to patients, and in many patients cure is possible. The type of UI dictates further treatment. Management can be behavioral, surgical, or pharmacologic. Many of the medications used to treat UI can, if used in the wrong circumstance, worsen the symptoms. Dosages listed below are average; both starting and maintenance doses must be individualized.

Nonpharmacologic Therapy

Clinical guidelines from the Agency for Health Care Policy and Research (AHCPR)[3] recommend behavioral therapy in the form of bladder training, prompted voiding, or pelvic muscle exercises for most forms of UI. Bladder training is most effective in the setting of urge incontinence but also may be helpful for other forms of UI. It involves behavioral education through the use of urge inhibition and scheduled voiding; it requires a cognitively intact individual. Prompted voiding, the nonpharmacologic treatment of choice in the cognitively impaired incontinent individual, involves scheduled voiding and requires prompting by the caregiver. Pelvic muscle exercises (Kegel's exercises), a regimen of planned, active exercises of the pelvic muscles to increase periurethral muscle strength, are particularly helpful in women with stress incontinence.

Other nonpharmacologic means of managing stress UI include biofeedback with or without electrical stimulation, collagen injection into the periurethral area, and vaginal pessaries. Nonpharmacologic treatments for overflow incontinence include intermittent catheterization, indwelling urethral or suprapubic catheters, external collection systems, and protective undergarments. Chronic indwelling catheters should not be viewed as a viable treatment option except when all else has failed or when there is accompanying local skin breakdown.

Pharmacologic Agents

Postmenopausal women with stress incontinence should use topical or oral estrogen in postmenopausal doses unless contraindicated. For those with an intact uterus, a progestin is added. α-Adrenergic agents such as pseudoephedrine (Sudafed, 15–30 mg PO tid) are also helpful in the setting of stress incontinence.

Anticholinergic agents such as oxybutinin (Ditropan, 2.5–5.0 mg PO tid or qid), tolterodine (Detrol, 1.0–2.0 mg PO bid), propantheline (Pro-Banthine, 7.5–30.0 mg PO tid), dicyclomide (Bentyl, 10–20 mg PO tid), and imipramine (Tofranil) or desipramine (Norpramin) (both at 25–100 mg PO a day) are often effective for urge incontinence. Anticholinergic medications should be used with caution, especially in the elderly, because of their side effects (confusion, constipation, and dizziness—see below).

In patients with overflow incontinence, bethanechol (Urecholine, 10–50 mg PO tid) can help facilitate bladder emptying. Men with prostatic hypertrophy and overflow incontinence can likely benefit from the α-adrenergic blockers prazosin (Minipress), terazosin (Hytrin), or doxazosin (Cardura) (all titrated up to 1–5 mg PO per day), or tamsulosin (Flomax), at either 0.4 or 0.8 mg PO per day.

Surgical Treatment

Surgical therapy is indicated in certain circumstances. Stress incontinence with urethrocele has an 80% to 95% 1-year success rate with suspension of the bladder neck.[3] Obstructive overflow incontinence with prostatic enlargement is often best treated with prostate surgery. Patients with urge incontinence and detrusor instability refractory to medical therapy often benefit from augmentation cystoplasty.

Falls

Falls are common, alarming, and worrisome to patients, their families, and their physicians. Most falls by the elderly do not result in serious consequences, but some cause hip fractures, other injuries, and rarely death. Unintentional injury is the sixth leading cause of death among the elderly, and most of these deaths are the result of falls.[4] Frequent falls may lead to consideration of a change in living arrangements or a severe limitation in socialization. Studies have clarified both the evaluation and management of patients who fall.[5–10]

The cause of a fall that results from loss of consciousness, a stroke or seizure, or an accidental or intentional blow to the body usually is easily discerned and managed. In most cases, however, the cause of a fall is not readily apparent. Falls may be classified as extrinsic (caused by slips or trips), intrinsic (caused by poor gait or balance, impaired sensation or proprioception, or cognitive impairment), nonbipedal (e.g., a fall out of bed), or nonclassifiable. Risk factors for falls from prospective studies include older age, white race, cognitive impairment, medication use, chronic diseases such as arthritis and Parkinson disease, foot problems, dizziness, and impaired muscle strength, gait, and balance.[5] Acute illnesses such as pneumonia, sepsis, and myocardial infarction also may present with a fall.

Most falls occur in the patient's home, and the home environment is usually a factor in these falls. Many falls occur on stairs, with injuries more likely to occur while descending rather than climbing stairs. Other hazards are electrical cords, uneven surfaces such as throw rugs or carpeting, or objects left on the floor. Poor lighting may contribute to these hazards.

Medication use is a potentially easily modifiable risk factor for falls. Long-acting benzodiazepines, barbiturates, antidepressants [including selective serotonin reuptake inhibitors (SSRIs)], and neuroleptics are associated with an increased risk of falls. Diuretics and other antihypertensive medicines also may increase the risk of falls by producing postural hypotension (see below).

Numerous trials have been completed that examine methods of fall reduction and injuries due to falls. Low-level exercise appears to reduce the frequency of falls but may not reduce the number of falls resulting in medical treatment[6] or fractures.[7] The multisite FICSIT (Frailty and Injuries: Cooperative Studies of Intervention Techniques) trial has demonstrated a modest decline in frequency of falls for the groups that underwent a variety of exercise interventions.[8] One FICSIT site used a multidisciplinary program to identify and reduce risk factors for falls. The intervention group underwent environmental hazard assessment, review of medications, treatment of postural hypotension, and physical therapy to improve strength and treat any balance or gait impairments. The rate of falls during the following year was reduced by 31%. In another FICSIT study, this time of tai chi, a low-intensity exercise derived from Chinese martial arts, falls were cut by almost half.[9] Known risk factors can be used to target the elderly for interventions, but because some elderly without risk factors experience falls as well, probably all elderly should be questioned periodically about falls. At this time, effective strategies for the practicing physician include (1) a home assessment to eliminate environmental hazards, such as throw rugs, unlit stairs, or poorly arranged furniture (by the physician during a housecall or a home care agency); (2) review of all medications, with elimination of problematic drugs when possible; (3) office evaluation of gait and balance (by the physician with a screening instrument[10] or by a physical therapist); (4) detection and treatment of postural hypotension or other chronic diseases that may cause weakness with standing (e.g., congestive heart failure, chronic obstructive pulmonary disease); (5) detection and treatment of sensory losses, including poor vision and proprioception (e.g., vitamin B_{12} deficiency); and (6) physical, medical, or surgical therapy for arthritis or other musculoskeletal disorders, especially when the feet are involved.

Postural Hypotension

Postural or orthostatic hypotension is defined as a drop in systolic blood pressure of at least 20 mm Hg 1 minute after a patient changes from a supine to a standing position. Syncope or near-syncope may be presenting symptoms, but elderly persons with postural hypotension may complain of nonspecific symptoms such as weakness, fatigue, or difficulty concentrating.

The most common causes of postural hypotension in older people are deconditioning, usually due to a long hospitalization requiring prolonged bed rest and loss of compensating autonomic reflexes, and medications, especially diuretics, tricyclic antidepressants, neuroleptics, antihypertensives, and dopaminergic drugs [e.g., levodopa (Sinemet)]. Treatment is the same for these patients. Deconditioned patients should be encouraged to gradually increase their activity, under the supervision of a physical therapist if necessary. Salt intake can be liberalized for most patients without heart failure. Raising the head of the bed on blocks 4 to 6 inches high also helps improve postural hypotension by stimulating autonomic reflexes and fluid retention. Offending drugs should be eliminated whenever possible. Patients with hypertension can be switched from a diuretic to a calcium channel blocker, angiotensin-converting enzyme inhibitor, or a beta-blocker, as these classes of antihypertensives have a low incidence of postural hypotension when used alone. Until the postural hypotension improves, patients should be reminded to change positions slowly to give compensating mechanisms some time to work. Patients also can be instructed to tighten their calf muscles while standing, thereby decreasing the pooling of blood in the legs.

Patients with rarer causes of postural hypotension (e.g., Shy-Drager syndrome) may need to be evaluated and treated by a neurologist experienced in these conditions. In severe cases, salt tablets and fludrocortisone (Florinef) may be necessary.

Polypharmacy

Elderly patients consume a disproportionate number of drugs; consequently, they suffer a disproportionate number of adverse drug reactions. Inappropriate over-prescribing, or poly-pharmacy, has been defined as taking too many drugs, using drugs for too long a time, or using drugs at too high a dose. The recent Institute of Medicine report has drawn attention to the number of adverse events that occur in hospitals, many of which are due to adverse drugs reactions.[11] Careful attention to appropriate prescribing can avoid many of these problems.

Risk Factors

Several risk factors for polypharmacy have been identified. Older adults with chronic medical problems often consult several physicians. Vague complaints may tempt physicians to prescribe, or patients or their families may pressure physicians to prescribe. Both hospitalization and nursing home placement usually result in more medications being prescribed. Medication is often added to a patient's regimen to treat the side effects of another drug. Physiologic changes of aging, including decreased body water and increased proportion of fat, can change the volume of distribution of some drugs and other pharmocokinetic characteristics and make the older person more prone to adverse drug effects.

Problematic Drug Classes

Neuroleptics, long-acting benzodiazepines, and tricyclic antidepressants have been associated with hip fractures resulting from falls[12] (see above and Chapters 22 and 23). Antihypertensive agents can also lead to falls. Benzodiazepines, especially those with long half-lives, are associated with cognitive impairment. Anticholinergic drugs, such as those given for urinary incontinence or irritable bowel syndrome, also may worsen cognition or may even lead to delirium (see below). Cardiovascular drugs and nonsteroidal antiinflammatory drugs (NSAIDs) have high rates of adverse effects. Drug–drug interactions are less frequent causes of adverse effects, but the potential for these problems increases as the number of drugs taken increases.

Principles of Prescribing

Simple changes in a patient's drug regimen can result in substantial improvements in a patient's condition. The following principles, modified from those first espoused by Vestal,[13] are helpful when prescribing for older adults.

1. Evaluate the need for drug therapy. Drug therapy is not always necessary or helpful.
2. Make a diagnosis before prescribing. The potential for adverse reactions is reduced when a specific drug is given for a specific, confirmed diagnosis.
3. A careful drug history is essential. Patients do not always immediately recall drugs prescribed by other physicians.
4. Know the pharmacology of the drugs you prescribe, especially with respect to the influence of the changes of aging. Patient reactions are more predictable when the prescriber uses few drugs in each drug class.
5. Start with small doses and titrate slowly to the desired response. Establish reasonable goals, stopping titration when the goals are achieved or side effects develop.
6. Keep the regimen simple to encourage compliance. Once- or twice-a-day dosing is ideal. Careful instruction should be given to both the patient and a relative or friend, if possible.
7. Review all medications regularly and discontinue those that are ineffective or no longer indicated. Ask the patient to throw all the drugs in their medicine cabinet into a paper bag and bring them to the office for review twice a year.
8. Remember that drugs cause illness. A new symptom may not be the result of a chronic or new medical condition. Always eliminate drug causes first.

Pain Management

Pain, acute or chronic, is one of the most common complaints of older individuals. Evaluating and treating pain syndromes in the elderly can be difficult. Many elderly patients are stoic. Cognitive impairment, especially in residents of nursing homes, may cause physicians to question the reliability of complaints of pain. Painful syndromes such as acute myocardial infarction and intraabdominal emergencies often present atypically or even silently in the elderly population. As a result, elderly patients are at risk for both over- and undertreatment of pain syndromes. Other consequences of improperly treated pain include depression, malnutrition, polypharmacy, cognitive dysfunction, and immobility. Acute pain is defined by its distinct onset and duration of less than 6 weeks; chronic pain lasts longer. Guidelines to the management of pain have been published.[14-16]

WHO Analgesic Ladder

Drug therapy is the cornerstone of treatment of acute and chronic pain due to cancer. The World Health Organization (WHO) analgesic ladder organizes drug therapy into three steps: (1) nonopioid drugs, (2) low-dose opioids, and (3) higher-dose opioids.[16] Treatment is begun with nonopioids, and opioid drugs are added as necessary. It is important to realize that when opioid–acetaminophen combinations are used [e.g., acetaminophen with codeine (Tylenol no. 3), oxycodone with acetaminophen (Percocet)], patients should receive no more than 4000 mg of acetaminophen per day. Adjuvant therapy, such as tricyclic antidepressants, caffeine, or anticonvulsants, may be added at any step.

Acute Pain

In the older patient with acute pain, physicians should determine the etiology of the pain while simultaneously making the patient comfortable. Rest, ice, compression, and elevation comprise the mainstay of treatment for acute injuries. In the elderly population, however, the period of rest should not exceed 48 to 72 hours, and early mobilization is encouraged. Physicians should start with the safest analgesics, such as acetaminophen, and add or substitute stronger analgesics as necessary. With respect to drug therapy, special considerations apply to the elderly. Older persons are more sensitive to the analgesic properties of opioids and to their side effects, such as sedation and respiratory depression. In addition, constipation and central nervous system (CNS) effects (e.g., delirium and depression) are more common in elderly patients treated with narcotics. NSAIDs should be used with care because of their gastrointestinal, renal, and hepatic effects, especially in the frail elderly. Some physicians believe that older patients have higher pain thresholds, but there is no experimental evidence to support this belief.[14]

Chronic Cancer Pain[15,16]

As in the case of patients with acute pain, the WHO analgesic ladder is followed for those with chronic pain, beginning with nonopioids such as acetaminophen and NSAIDs, adding opioids as necessary. NSAIDs may be particularly effective in cancer patients with bony metastases. Tricyclic antidepressants and the anticonvulsants carbamazepine (Tegretol) and valproic acid (Depakote) are usually helpful for neuropathic pain, although side effects (orthostatic hypotension, constipation, dry mouth) may limit the use of tricyclics.

Several principles help the physician provide optimal relief of cancer pain. Wide variation exists in the response of elderly patients to analgesics. Titration must be done carefully, with frequent follow-up to ensure that the drug is effective. Patients who have pain most of the day should receive their drugs regularly, not as needed. Side effects are treated aggressively. For example, sedation due to opioids can be particularly bothersome but can be treated by adding a stimulant such as caffeine or dextroamphetamine (Dexedrine). Long-acting morphine (MS Contin), oxycodone (OxyContin), and fentanyl patches (Duragesic) are helpful for patients with severe cancer pain, but care must be taken when calculating equianalgesic doses.[14] Other patients may require patient-controlled analgesia (PCA), continuous epidural morphine, or local radiation therapy. Lastly, nonpharmacologic adjunctive therapies including exercise, transcutaneous nerve stimulation, acupuncture, chiropractic manipulation, or prayer may aid in the treatment of pain.

Nutrition

There are few data regarding the nutritional requirements in the aged population. Similarly, the effect of nutrition on the aging process in humans is unclear. Poor nutritional status, however, does contribute to the morbidity of chronic illnesses and worsens the prognosis when an older person becomes ill. Protein–calorie malnutrition is the most common nutritional abnormality in the elderly. In one study, hospitalized elders had a 44% prevalence of protein–calorie malnutrition as defined by height/weight and serum albumin.[17] Conversely, up to 25% to 30% of older persons are overweight, defined as a body mass index (BMI) >28. Obesity increases the likelihood of developing coronary artery disease, diabetes mellitus, hypertension, and sleep apnea.

Many factors increase the risk for malnutrition in the elderly. A decrease in the acuity of taste and smell with aging lessens the enjoyment of eating. Poor dentition or poorly fitting dentures may lead to chewing difficulties. Swallowing disorders are more common in older persons, and gastrointestinal motility declines with age. Other risk factors for malnutrition include depression, poverty, social isolation, certain medications, and dementia. Such conditions as pressure ulcers, chronic infections, malabsorption, sepsis, malignancy, and alcoholism can increase the metabolic demands and result in malnutrition.

Nutritional Assessment

The key to the evaluation of malnutrition in the elderly is a high index of suspicion. Patients are asked about symptoms such as nausea, vomiting, anorexia, swallowing difficulties, and abdominal pain. They are also asked about any new medications, diagnoses, or social issues. A careful weight history is obtained and the weight loss expressed as a percentage of the patient's usual weight. Weight loss of more than 10% of the patient's usual weight usually represents severe malnutrition.

Physical signs of malnutrition may be difficult to recognize in the elderly. Anthropometric measures such as weight, height, BMI, and skinfold thickness can be helpful for the initial assessment. The total lymphocyte count, hemoglobin, serum albumin, and cholesterol levels are important screening tests. Transferrin and prealbumin levels are more sensitive measures of short-term undernutrition, but are more expensive. The farther the results are below normal values, the greater is the degree of malnutrition present. The Nutrition Screening Initiative (NSI) focused on the need for primary care physicians to consider the nutritional aspects of medical care.[18] The NSI developed a screening tool useful for evaluating risk for malnutrition.

Treatment

Treatment of malnutrition begins while efforts are made to identify the sources of nutrient losses and conditions that increase the metabolic needs. Additionally, nutritional support begins early in those individuals who are at increased risk for malnutrition. In the nonstressed elderly, approximately 22 to 25 kcal/kg body weight is required. This support increases to 30 kcal/kg in the severely stressed elderly.

Oral supplementation with food is optimal. The goal is to optimize the types of food and consistency of the diet to improve the nutritional status of the individual. The addition of liquid supplemental feedings can also improve nutritional status. When there is refusal or an inability to swallow, enteral tube feeding with a small-bore nasogastric tube or gastrostomy/jejunostomy tube is required. The decision on which of these methods to use depends on patient preference, suspected length of time the feedings will be necessary, and patient tolerance to each method. Feeding can occur in a continuous fashion or with intermittent bolus feeds. Each of these methods of feeding carries a risk of aspiration. Diarrhea is a frequent complication in the tube-fed patient.

When poor nutrition is related to depression, treatment of the depression is imperative. Buproprion (Wellbutrin) is an antidepressant that is less likely to adversely affect appetite compared to the SSRIs. Mirtazapine (Remeron) is another antidepressant that has the favorable side effect of improved appetite and weight gain in severely depressed older adults. Megestrol acetate (Megace) is a progesterone preparation that is widely studied as an appetite stimulant in cancer and acquired immunodeficiency syndrome (AIDS) patients and may be useful for older populations.

Total parenteral nutrition (TPN) is indicated in the elderly patient when there is an inability to use the gut to meet nutrient needs. Complications are more likely to occur in the elderly population, but it should not preclude the use of TPN in the appropriate clinical setting in an elderly patient. As with younger individuals, the use of TPN necessitates careful monitoring of the electrolyte and glucose levels as well as renal function.

Health Promotion and Disease Prevention

Elderly patients are living longer and longer. Average life expectancy for a 65-year-old man is at least 15 years more, and women live even longer. Thus it is important that physicians consider health promotion activities for their elderly patients, just as they do for children and younger adults.[19,20] Among the interventions that are probably helpful in the elderly are (1) immunizations for influenza, pneumococcal disease, and tetanus-diphtheria; (2) counseling for injury prevention (car safety belts, smoke detectors, hot water heater temperature (<120°F) and for smoking cessation; (3) cervical cancer screening for women who have not been previously screened; (4) guaiac stool testing, sigmoidoscopy, or colonoscopy to detect colorectal cancer; and (5) hormone replacement therapy and calcium supplementation for women at risk of osteoporosis. Currently, no evidence exists to support the use of prostate-specific antigen screening in men older than 69 years or mammography screening for breast cancer in women older than 69 years, although physicians may choose to screen some older individuals for these conditions (see Chapter 2).[20] The United States Preventive Services Task Force now recommends cholesterol screening for healthy elderly who will live long enough to realize the benefits of therapy.

Evaluating and Managing Nursing Home Patients

Every physician who takes care of older patients has some interaction with a nursing home. For some family physicians, this interaction may be limited to referring their office patients for admission when they can no longer remain in the community. Increasingly, however, family physicians will be asked to assume larger roles in nursing homes. Only about 5% of the elderly reside in nursing homes, but the lifetime chance of an older person being admitted to a nursing home is about 40%.[21]

Evaluating Elderly Patients for Nursing Home Placement

Most nursing home residents are admitted to a long-term-care facility from the hospital. Not uncommonly physicians are asked to certify that an elderly person living in the community needs nursing home care. Usually these patients and their families present at a time of crisis. Patients may have been found wandering in the neighborhood, or they may have suffered recurrent falls and are thought to be unsafe in their home. Loss of function, usually as a result of cognitive impairment, is the common denominator.[22]

Careful assessment is important because a less restrictive environment may be a better solution and because patients and families often are not aware of these possibilities. Physicians should evaluate these patients thoroughly, focusing on their functional abilities, such as activities of daily living (ADLs, such as bathing, eating, dressing) and instrumental activities of daily living (IADLs, such as using the phone or buying groceries). A mental status examination is important, as patients may appear relatively intact on casual questioning but be severely impaired. Patients and family members should be questioned closely regarding the possibility of major depression, which has a high incidence among severely medically ill elderly and nursing home residents. Medicines are reviewed to see if any can be eliminated, especially those that may impair function (see above). The social history explores personal and financial resources that could support other care options, and advance directives are reviewed. For patients found to require the services of a nursing home, a complete assessment provides an opportunity to stabilize chronic illnesses or to complete any evaluations that might be necessary prior to admission.

Integrating Nursing Home Practice into the Office Practice

Family physicians can provide continuity of care for their elderly patients who are admitted to nursing homes by continuing to follow them after their admission. To avoid disrupting an office practice, however, it is wise for the physician to limit privileges to just a few facilities. Ideally, these nursing homes are near the physician's office, home, or hospital, so visits can be incorporated into the usual workday. Another benefit of limiting privileges to a few homes is that the physician becomes more familiar with the nursing staff and capabilities of those facilities.[22]

After building up a sizable census, it is practical to set aside a half-day every 1 or 2 weeks to make rounds. Routine nursing home rounds gives the physician a chance to consult with the resident's usual nurses and observe patients during therapy or other activities. Fewer phone calls from the nursing staff usually result as well. To minimize disruptions in the office, some physicians ask nursing homes to call at previously agreed-on times for routine problems.

Physicians with an interest in the organization and administration of nursing homes may wish to work as a medical director. Most medical directors approve policies and procedures, act as liaisons with the medical staff, supervise employee health issues, address quality improvement, and help keep the facility abreast of new regulations or medical treatments. New medical directors can find resources to help them through the American Medical Directors Association (10480 Little Patuxent Parkway, Suite 760, Columbia, MD 21044; phone 1-800-876-AMDA).

Pressure Sores

Pressure sores are defined as changes in the skin and underlying tissue that result from pressure over bony prominences. If not attended to, these forces cause ulceration. The best treatment for pressure sores is prevention, but even under the best conditions it is not always possible.

Epidemiology

The incidence of pressure sores is greatest among the elderly population, especially during long hospital or nursing home confinements.[23–25] Additionally, patients with spinal cord injuries or cerebrovascular disease are at risk for the development of pressure sores. Factors that may contribute to the likelihood of developing pressure sores include nutritional deficiencies, volume depletion, increased or decreased body weight, anemia, fecal incontinence, renal failure, diabetes, malignancy, sedation, major surgery, numerous metabolic disorders, cigarette smoking, and being bed- or chair-bound. Finally, the aging skin itself, because of reduced epidermal thickness and elasticity, increases the risk for pressure changes.

Etiology

There are four primary mechanisms in the development of pressure sores: pressure, shearing forces, friction, and moisture.[26] More than 90% of pressure sores occur over the bony prominences of the lower part of the body. The amount of time and pressure necessary to cause tissue damage depends on the number of risk factors present. The second etiologic factor, shearing forces, are caused by the sliding of adjacent surfaces. This sliding results in compression of capillary flow in the subcutaneous layer. An example of shearing forces is elevation of the head of the bed, which causes the body to slide down producing a shear in the sacral and coccygeal region. Friction is the force created when two surfaces move across each other, such as would occur when maneuvering a patient on the bed. The impact of friction damages the epidermis, which is already vulnerable in the elderly. This damage accelerates the onset of ulceration. Finally, moisture increases the risk of pressure ulceration. A high correlation exists between urinary or fecal incontinence and ulceration. Because of the increased risk of skin infection, the presence of a sacral pressure sore is an indication for a chronic indwelling urethral catheter in the incontinent patient.

Clinical Evaluation

The best method for evaluating a pressure sore is to classify the sore by its severity. There are several classification schemes for pressure sores. The National Pressure Ulcer Advisory Panel has proposed a staging system[27] that divides pressure sores into four grades, depending on the depth of tissue involvement.

Grade I pressure sore (Fig. 5.1A): Acute inflammatory response in all layers of the skin. The clinical presentation of a grade I pressure sore is a well-defined area of nonblanchable erythema of the intact skin.

Grade II pressure sore (Fig. 5.1B): Presents as a break in the epidermis and dermis, with surrounding erythema, induration, or both. It is caused by an extension of the inflammatory response leading to a fibroblastic response.

Grade III pressure sore (Fig. 5.1C): Inflammatory response characterized by an irregular full-thickness ulcer extending into the subcutaneous tissue but not through underlying fascia. There is often a draining, foul-smelling, necrotic base.

Grade IV pressure sore (Fig. 5.1D): Penetrates the deep fascia, eliminating the last barrier to extensive spread. Clinically, it resembles a grade III sore except that bone, joint, or muscle can be identified.

The complications of pressure sores are associated with significant morbidity and mortality. Most of the complications occur with grade III and IV sores and include cellulitis, osteomyelitis, septic joints, pyarthrosis, and tetanus. Tetanus may complicate pressure sores, and for this reason immunoprophylaxis against tetanus is recommended in patients with pressure sores.[28]

Prevention

Because of the great morbidity and mortality associated with pressure sores and the financial burden incurred by treating this problem, their prevention is the pri-

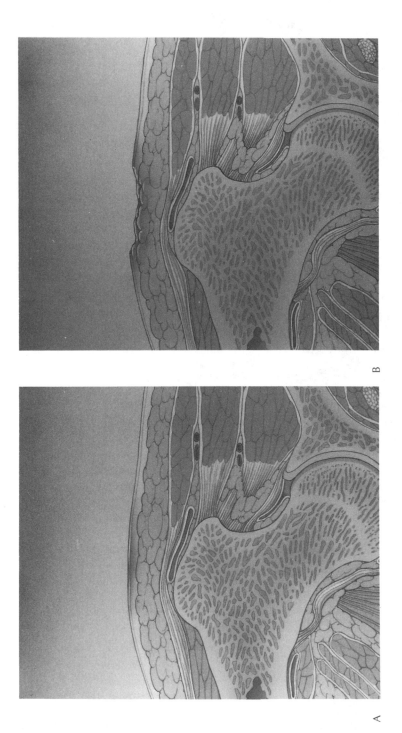

B

A

124

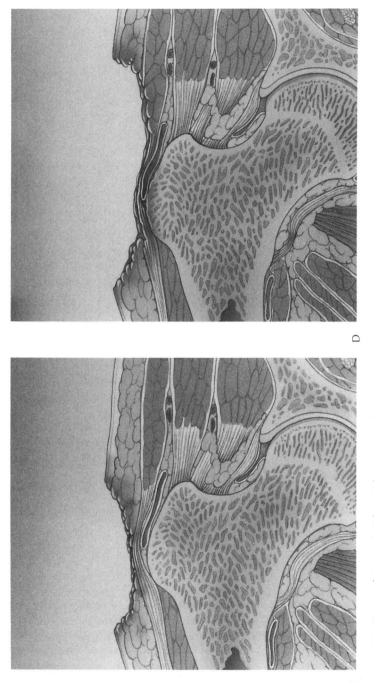

C

D

FIGURE 5.1. National Pressure Ulcer Advisory Panel staging system. (A) Grade I pressure sore, characterized by inflammatory reaction of the epidermis and dermis. It presents clinically as nonblanchable erythema over an area of pressure. (B) Grade II pressure sore, characterized by epidermal and dermal skin breakdown with surrounding erythema. (C) Grade III pressure sore, characterized by an ulcer extending into the subcutaneous tissue, frequently with necrosis. (D) Grade IV pressure sore, characterized by extension of the ulcer beyond the fascial layer and thus involving muscle, bone, or other structures. (From National Pressure Ulcer Advisory Panel,[27] with permission.)

125

mary goal of physicians and health care facilities taking care of patients at risk. Identifying persons at risk is the first step in employing intensive preventive measures.

Persons at risk should undergo frequent assessment and be placed in an environment that enhances soft tissue viability, which can be achieved through the use of proper positioning techniques and support surfaces. At the time of positioning, the patient's skin is examined for areas of redness that indicate early pressure changes. When repositioning, the patient is lifted, not dragged, from a bed or wheelchair to avoid friction and subsequent damage to the epidermis. Elevating the head of the bed to more than 30 degrees is avoided to minimize the shearing forces.

Special pads, beds, and mechanical devices are available and prevent pressure sores by altering the pressure over bony prominences. Devices such as gel pads, foam cushions, wheelchair cushions, and sheepskin pads are practical for preventing pressure sores at specific anatomic sites. No single device has yet been developed that is effective in preventing all pressure sores. Static flotation mattresses, low air loss mattresses, alternating air pressure mattresses, and air-fluidized beds help to prevent and treat pressure sores. These beds tend to relieve pressure by using air or buoyancy to keep the patient's weight evenly distributed. Such devices, however, cannot be relied on as a substitute for basic nursing care.

Preventive care of pressure sores also involves improvement of medical conditions that predispose the individual to the development of pressure changes. In particular, nutritional deficiencies, incontinence, and immobility should be minimized. Nutritional status is assessed on admission to the hospital or nursing home: Once a pressure sore has developed, nutritional status usually is already severely compromised and is difficult to correct.

Management

The first step in the management of pressure sores is assessing the extent of the sore and patients' overall status, including their nutritional state. Regardless of the grade of the sore, adherence to the principles of prevention outlined above remain important.

WOUND CLEANSING AND DEBRIDEMENT

The primary goal of therapy for pressure sores is to create an environment that promotes healthy granulation tissue. Wounds are cleansed as atraumatically as possible with normal saline-soaked gauze, wound irrigation, and whirlpool baths. Most antiseptics, such as hydrogen peroxide and povidone-iodine, are cytotoxic and should be avoided.

Necrotic tissue prevents healing and creates favorable conditions for bacterial contamination. The ideal method for debriding pressure sores is sharp dissection of the necrotic tissue. Enzymatic debridement using such agents as fibrinolysin, collagenase, and dextranomer should be used only during intervals between sur-gical debridement to help dissolve thin necrotic layers that are less accessible to excision.[29] The inability of these agents to penetrate eschar or to remove large amounts of tissue limits their usefulness. There is no proof that topical antibi-otics are superior to careful cleansing and wet-to-dry dressings. In addition, top-ical antibiotics may sensitize the tissue, promote the appearance of resistant or-ganisms, and have systemic toxicity.[26]

DRESSINGS

Once the wound is clean with granulation tissue visible, the use of dressings that promote healing is advisable. The cardinal rule is to keep the ulcer moist and the surrounding skin dry.[30] Additional factors when selecting dressings include ex-udate control and caregiver time requirements. Dressing options include saline-soaked gauze and occlusive dressings. The appeal of the occlusive dressings is that they can usually remain on the pressure sore for several days, whereas gauze dressings should be changed several times daily. This convenience is particularly useful for outpatient management of pressure sores. These dressings should be avoided in the presence of clinical infection.

MANAGING COMPLICATIONS

The two most frequently encountered complications are nonhealing and infec-tion. For clean wounds that fail to heal, reassessment of the patient's overall status and a 2-week trial of a broad-spectrum topical antibiotic are recom-mended.[30] In patients who are operative candidates, surgical repair of the non-healing wound may be considered. When these wounds are complicated by bac-teremia, soft tissue infection, or osteomyelitis, appropriate systemic antibiotics are employed.

Delirium

Delirium is a syndrome of acutely altered mental status. Delirium is frequent in older persons, especially those with dementia, typically occurring in ill inpatients and nursing home residents. Delirium may the only presenting symptom of many acute illnesses as well, including sepsis syndrome and other infections, myocar-dial infarction, surgical emergencies, adverse drug reactions, volume depletion, and electrolyte disturbances. Failure to recognize and appropriately treat delir-ium contributes to worse outcomes in these patients, regardless of etiology.

Delirium is diagnosed in the setting of a fluctuating level of consciousness, accompanied by inattentiveness and poor recent memory. Unlike dementia pa-tients (if not delirious), these patients present acutely and do not have a normal level of consciousness. Typically, speech is incoherent or disorganized. The level of consciousness may vary from hyperalert to comatose.

Evaluation and Management

As noted above, possible etiologies are numerous, and usually there is more than one cause. Treatment requires continual assessment and reassessment of causes, beginning first with a careful examination of the nervous system. Laboratory testing should include a complete blood count (CBC), chemistry panel, and liver function tests. Additional tests that may be helpful include thyroid function tests, a B_{12} level, and drug levels. Correcting electrolyte abnormalities, treating infections, and eliminating sedatives (especially benzodiazepines) and anticholinergic drugs (e.g., tricyclic antidepressants, antihistamines, drugs for urge incontinence, etc.) are the most productive strategies. Helpful environmental alterations include clear communication to delirious patients (with repeated reorientation), having a calming family member present, ensuring adequate lighting, reducing noise, and allowing uninterrupted sleep.[31] Neuroleptics are the drugs of choice, whether patients are agitated or lethargic. Low-dose oral haloperidol (Haldol) is usually sufficient in older adults. Patients may be given 0.5 to 1 mg orally or parenterally. This dose may be repeated until the patient is sedated as long as hypotension does not occur (blood pressure should be checked at least every half-hour). Benzodiazepines may worsen behavior because of disinhibition effects, but are useful for delirium that results from alcohol withdrawal or seizures.

References

1. Hazzard WR, Bierman EL, Blass JP, Ettinger WH, Halter JB, Ouslander JG, eds. Principles of geriatric medicine, 4th ed. New York: McGraw-Hill, 1999.
2. Adelman AM, Daly MP, eds. 20 common problems in geriatrics. New York: McGraw-Hill, 2001.
3. US Department of Health and Human Services. Clinical practice guideline: urinary incontinence in adults. AHCPR publ. no. 92-0038. Rockville, MD: DHHS, 1992;38–65.
4. Koogler CE, Wolf SL. Falls. In: Hazzard WR, Bierman EL, Blass JP, Ettinger WH, Halter JB, Ouslander JG, eds. Principles of geriatric medicine, 4th ed. New York: McGraw-Hill, 1999;1535–46.
5. King MB, Tinetti ME. Falls in community-dwelling older persons. J Am Geriatr Soc 1995;43:1146–54.
6. Hornbrook MC, Stevens VJ, Wingfield DJ, et al. Preventing falls among community-dwelling older persons: results from a randomized trial. Gerontologist 1994;34:16–23.
7. Vetter NJ, Lewis PA, Ford D. Can health visitors prevent fractures in elderly people? BMJ 1992;304:888–90.
8. Province MA, Hadley EC, Hornbrook MC, et al. The effects of exercise on falls in elderly patients: a pre-planned meta-analysis of the FICSIT trials. JAMA 1995;273:1341–7.
9. Wolf SL, Barnhart HX, Kutner NG, et al. Reducing frailty and falls in older persons: an investigation of Tai Chi and computerized balance training. J Am Geriatr Soc 1996;44:489–97.
10. Shumway-Cook A, Brauer S, Woollacott M. Predicting the probability of falls in com-

munity-dwelling older adults using the Timed Up and Go Test. Phys Ther 2000;80:896–903.

11. Kohn LT, Corrigan JM, Donaldson MS, eds. To err is human: building a safer health system. Washington, DC: National Academy Press, 2000.

12. Ray WA, Griffin MR, Schaffner W, et al. Psychotropic drug use and the risk of hip fracture. N Engl J Med 1987;316:363–9.

13. Vestal R. Clinical Pharmacology. In: Hazzard WR, Andres R, Bierman EL, Blass JP, eds. Principles of geriatric medicine and gerontology, 2nd ed. New York: McGraw-Hill, 1990;201–11.

14. Acute Pain Management Guideline Panel. Acute pain management: operative or medical procedures and trauma; clinical practice guideline. AHCPR publ. no. 92-0032. Rockville, MD: Agency for Health Care Policy and Research, Public Health Service, US Department of Health and Human Services, 1992.

15. American Geriatrics Society Panel on Chronic Pain in Older Persons. The management of chronic pain in older persons. J Am Geriatr Soc 1998;46:635–51.

16. World Health Organization. Cancer pain and palliative care: report of a WHO expert committee. World Health Organization Technical Report Series 804. Geneva: WHO, 1990;1–75.

17. Wilson WG, Vaswani S, Liu D, et al. Prevalence and causes of undernutrition in medical outpatients. Am J Med 1998;104:56–63.

18. White JV, Dwyer JT, Posner BM, Ham RJ, Lipschitz DA, Wellman NS. Nutrition Screening Initiative; development and implementation of the public awareness checklist and screening tools. J Am Diet Assoc 1992;92:163–7.

19. Richardson JP. Health maintenance for the elderly. In: Taylor RB, ed. The manual of family practice, 2nd ed. Philadelphia: Lippincott, Williams & Wilkins, 2002;28–32.

20. United States Preventive Services Task Force. Guide to clinical preventive services, 2nd ed. Baltimore: Williams & Wilkins, 1996.

21. Kemper P, Murtaugh CM. Lifetime use of nursing home care. N Engl J Med 1991;324:595–600.

22. Richardson JP. Outpatient evaluation for nursing home admission. In: Yoshikawa TT, Cobbs EL, Brummel-Smith K, eds. Ambulatory geriatric care, 2nd ed. St. Louis: Mosby-Year Book, 1998;113–7.

23. Brandeis GH, Morris JN, Nash DJ, Lipsitz LA. The epidemiology and natural history of pressure ulcers in elderly nursing home residents. JAMA 1990;264:2905–9.

24. Reuler JB, Cooney TG. The pressure sore: pathophysiology and principles of management. Ann Intern Med 1981;94:661–6.

25. Guralnik JM, Harris TB, White LR, Cornoni-Huntley JC. Occurrence and predictors of pressure sores in the National Health and Nutrition Examination Survey follow-up. J Am Geriatr Soc 1989;36:807–12.

26. Knight AL. Medical management of pressure sores. J Fam Pract 1988;27:95–100.

27. National Pressure Ulcer Advisory Panel. Pressure ulcers prevalence, cost and risk assessment: consensus development conference statement. Decubitus 1989;2(2):24–8.

28. Richardson JP, Knight AL. The prevention of tetanus in the elderly. Arch Intern Med 1991;151:1712–17.

29. Seiler WO, Stahelin HB. Decubitus ulcers: treatment through five therapeutic principles. Geriatrics 1985;40:30–44.

30. Pressure Ulcer Guideline Panel. Pressure ulcer treatment. Am Fam Physician 1995;51:1207–22.

31. Meagher DJ. Delirium: optimising management. BMJ 2001;322:144–9.

CASE PRESENTATION

Subjective

PATIENT PROFILE

Harold Nelson is a 76-year-old married male retired welder.

PRESENTING PROBLEM

"I can't control my urine."

PRESENT ILLNESS

There is a 2-day history of urinary incontinence, and on three occasions, the patient has lost control of his urine, wetting his clothing. This follows a several-month history of urinary hesitancy and difficulty initiating the stream. There has been no dysuria, but the patient has been out of bed several times to pass urine during each of the past few nights.

PAST MEDICAL HISTORY

Mr. Nelson has had type 2 diabetes mellitus for 24 years and is now taking glyburide. He has had osteoarthritis of multiple joints for 20 years and underwent a lumbar laminectomy at age 60.

SOCIAL HISTORY

Mr. Nelson lives with his wife, aged 71.

HABITS

He does not smoke. He takes "a few drinks" each evening and drinks 2 cups of coffee daily.

FAMILY HISTORY

Both parents died in their mid-80s of "old age."

REVIEW OF SYSTEMS

He has had a recent cold with nasal congestion and cough.

- What additional medical history might be useful, and why?
- What more might you ask about his alcohol intake? How would you address this issue?
- What might be pertinent about his "cold?"
- What might be significant about the family's reaction to his recent incontinence, and how would you inquire about this issue?

Objective

VITAL SIGNS

Height, 5 ft 7 in; weight, 156 lb; blood pressure, 150/84; pulse, 90; temperature, 37.4°C.

EXAMINATION

The abdomen has no mass or organ enlargement. There is mild suprapubic tenderness. No costovertebral angle tenderness is present. His genitalia are normal for age, and there is no hernia. The prostate is 3 plus enlarged, smooth, and symmetric.

LABORATORY

A urinalysis shows 4 to 6 white blood cells per high-powered field; no glucose is present.

- What more—if anything—would you include in the physical examination, and why?
- Are there any diagnostic maneuvers that may be helpful today?
- What—if any—additional laboratory tests might be helpful in evaluating today's problem?
- What—if any—diagnostic imaging studies should be obtained today?

Assessment

- What seems to be Mr. Nelson's problem, and how would you describe this to the patient and the family?
- What are likely causes of the problem?
- What might be the meaning of this illness to the patient and the family?

- What might be unspoken concerns of the patient regarding today's problem? How might these concerns relate to his age?

Plan

- What therapeutic recommendations would you make today?
- How would you advise the patient and his family regarding the possibility of future urinary problems?
- What is the appropriate locus of care for this patient's problem? Is a consultation with a urologist likely to be needed now or in the future?
- What follow-up would you recommend to Mr. Nelson?

6
Domestic Violence

VALERIE J. GILCHRIST

Although domestic violence may refer to all aspects of family violence, this chapter focuses on intimate partner violence (IPV). Over 95% of such abuse involves a man abusing his female partner. Although several studies have shown an almost equal number of episodes of violence perpetrated by men and by women, others show that women use violence for self-defense and escape while men use violence for control, punishment, or attention.[1] Regardless of motivation the result is both injury and fear in the female partner.[2,3]

An intimate partner's physical, emotional, or sexual abuse affects up to 50% of women in the United States at some time in their lives.[3–5] While the lifetime prevalence varies by definition of abuse, population studied, and methodology, this figure may be an underestimation because high-risk populations such as those hospitalized, homeless, institutionalized, or incarcerated are excluded. Thirty percent of female homicides in 1996 were committed by partners or expartners.[6] Battery is the single greatest cause of injury to women.[3,6]

Background

Cycle of Violence

IPV is cyclic.[7] After an abusive episode there is the *honeymoon phase*, during which the abuser is apologetic, often courting the victim with gifts and attention, promising that he will never hurt her again. This phase invariably shifts into the *tension-building phase*, during which the woman lives in an atmosphere of extreme tension and fear as her partner threatens and isolates her. The tension-building phase ultimately culminates in the *violent phase* of battery and abuse. With repetition the cycle increases in frequency and severity.

The goal of the abuse is power and control by the perpetrator. Figure 6.1 depicts tactics employed by batterers. Ongoing ego-battering erodes the victim's self-image. She is systematically stripped of the resources that would allow her to leave: her self-respect, pride, career, money, friends, and family. She often sees no options except trying to make do in her situation and hoping that somehow she can prevent further violence.[8–10]

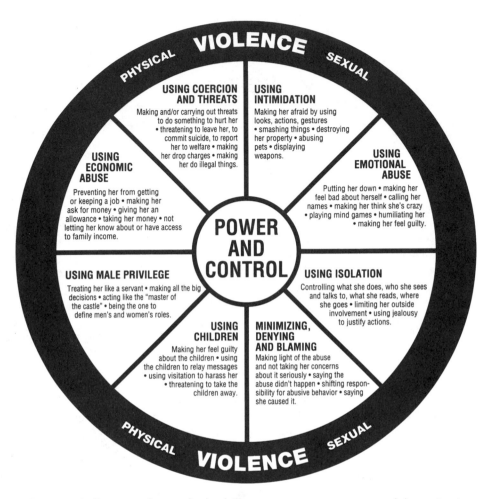

FIGURE 6.1. Power and control wheel illustrates many components of domestic violence, all of which are ultimately enforced by the threat or actuality of physical and sexual violence. (From the Domestic Abuse Intervention Project, Minnesota Program Development, 202 E. Superior, Duluth MN 55802, with permission.)

Abused Women

Women who are divorced or separated, younger, and of a lower socioeconomic status (SES) report higher prevalence rates of abuse, but there is no characteristic premorbid personality profile of the abused woman.[9] Women who have been previously traumatized will have more severe symptoms with IPV.[11]

Abusing Men

Batterers do not lose control but rather take control. Common characteristics include dependency on and jealously of their partners, a belief in traditional gender roles, a high need for control, difficulty with trust, and a refusal to accept responsibility for their violent behaviors.[12] Abusing men are not a homogeneous population. Men who batter only within their families are the least violent, and rarely have criminal records or exhibit psychopathology. Men who exhibit passive-aggressive, dependent, or borderline personality characteristics are more violent, and those who are antisocial engage in both partner and extrafamilial violence.[13,14] Ninety percent of men who batter have no criminal record.[8] The use of alcohol or drugs by the abuser is associated with increased violence.[15,16]

Abuse in Homosexual Relationships

Abuse in gay and lesbian relationships is similar in form, prevalence, and precipitants to heterosexual relationships. However, there may be pressures within the gay community not to reveal violence, there are fewer social resources, and IPV is less commonly recognized by clinicians. Batterers may use homophobic control threatening to "out" their partner. If the batterer is human immunodeficiency virus (HIV) positive, he may use this as an infective threat or a guilt-inducing control strategy. If the partner is HIV positive, the batterer may threaten to reveal this or to deny care or medication. Also, without expected gender stereotypes the batterer may use the illusion of mutual battery to maintain control.[17]

Special Populations

Up to 50% of adolescents report dating violence, and IPV for pregnant adolescents is especially high.[5,18] Many adolescent victims of IPV have also been subjected to abuse in their family of origin.[18]

Older women also experience IPV, often for many years. They are frequently financially dependent on their partner. Children may provide resources or apply pressure to keep the relationship intact. Abuse may intensify with the stress of caregiving.[19]

Immigrant women who are victims of IPV often have few resources. They may not speak English well, may fear the police and authority, especially if they are undocumented, and may live in a setting that sanctions abuse or view abuse as a "private" matter.[5]

Clinical Presentation

Battered women present with repeated, increasingly severe physical injuries, self-abuse, and psychosocial problems including depression, drug or alcohol abuse, and suicide attempts.[3,5] The battering injuries are often inconsistent with the explanation provided, bilateral, and only in areas covered by clothing. There may be contusions, lacerations, abrasions, pain without obvious tissue injury, evidence of injuries at different times, and evidence of rape. A partner, if present, may be controlling, overly solicitous, and reluctant to leave.

Twenty-five percent of battered women report receiving medical care, and 10% require hospital treatment; however, most abused women present for routine, not emergency, medical care, and most injuries do not require hospitalization.[3,10] Abused women are more likely to define their health as poor, and they have more hospitalizations, surgical procedures, pelvic pain, sexually transmitted diseases, functional gastrointestinal problems, chronic headaches, and chronic pain problems in general.[3,4,10] Poor health is just as significantly associated with psychological IPV as physical assault.[4] Abused women and their children use more health care services.[5,20] Fear of abuse has limited partner notification of HIV status.[10] IPV precipitates unemployment, homelessness, and poverty for women.[4,14]

Surveys in family practice settings revealed current abuse in 10% to 50% of women, with a lifetime prevalence of up to 40%. The diagnosis of depression was the strongest indicator of domestic violence.[5,20]

As many as 50% of women who visit emergency departments are battered, and studies in these settings reveal a lifetime prevalence of 11% to 54% depending on the definition of abuse and the method used. Victims present equally with trauma and nontraumatic complaints and more often in the evening or night.[21]

Up to one in five women are battered during pregnancy and this may become more frequent in the postpartum period.[5,20] Pregnancy may incite the initial episodes of abuse but most often there is preceding abuse.[22] Abused women have more unintended pregnancies, are twice as likely to delay seeking prenatal care, twice as likely to miscarry, and four times as likely to have a low birth weight infant, and these infants are 40% more likely to die during the first year of life.[20]

One third to one half of women presenting to mental health centers have been battered.[3,10] The diagnosis of borderline personality disorder and substance abuse are particularly common.[5,11,14,20] IPV was found in 55% of a sample of depressed women.[23] Domestic violence is a cause of posttraumatic stress disorder (PTSD). The severity of both PTSD and depression correlate directly with the intensity of the abuse.[5,20] One in 10 victims of abuse will attempt suicide[3] (also see Chapter 23).

After battery, victims have demonstrated a ninefold increased risk for drug abuse, and the use of alcohol increased 16-fold.[10,11] There is concurrent use of alcohol and drugs during 25% to 80% of the battering episodes, and this is a marker for more severe injury.[16] The presence of substance abuse should initiate questions about violence.

Children

Forty-seventy percent of children entering domestic violence shelters have been abused, and in 45% to 60% of child abuse cases there is concurrent domestic violence.[20] Children are inevitably aware of the violence and suffer from the consequences of the violence. These include direct injury while trying to intervene, decreased nuturance and social support because of maternal depression, and family dislocations with potential social and economic disadvantage.[20,24] Children's symptoms include internalizing symptoms (somatic complaints, disturbed sleep, withdrawal, anxiety, depression), externalizing behaviors (aggression, cruelty to animals, defiance of authority, destructiveness), and defects in social competence (school achievement, peer relations, self-confidence, and participation in sports and other extracurricular activities).[20,24] Children's symptoms increase with the severity, frequency, content, and resolution of parental conflict and if there is concurrent child abuse.[24,25] These children are predisposed to later enactment of abuse against, or victimization by, an intimate partner.[14]

Diagnosis

Battered women may lack money for medical care or transportation to medical facilities, or they may be prevented by their abuser from seeking medical care. Victims may withhold information from clinicians because they feel ashamed, humiliated, or that the injuries are not serious or are deserved. Victims also may lie about the source of injuries in an effort to protect the partner or children or because of fears of retribution for any disclosure or police involvement. Many women disclose abuse only after numerous inquiries.[5,26]

The single most important step medical professionals can take is to *ask every woman, confidentially,* if she is being or has been abused. Domestic violence cuts across all ages and socioeconomic, racial, ethnic, religious, and professional groups, although social and ethnic backgrounds may influence both the victim's and the perpetrator's perception of domestic violence. Domestic violence occurs at a frequency comparable to breast cancer and is more common than other conditions for which screening is routine. Questioning communicates to the patient that the problem is not trivial, shameful, or irrelevant. It opens the area to further conversation and may begin the process of the abused woman's leaving the relationship.[9]

It is important for physicians to remain nonjudgmental and relaxed because abused women are extremely sensitive to nonverbal cues. While general questions about a relationship with a partner may be a good way to open conversation ("How are things going at home? How do you resolve differences?"), explicit direct questioning is most effective.[5,6] Ask about nonviolent but psychologically abusive acts ("Are you insulted, threatened?"), and about the use of force such as grabbing or restraining, pushing, or throwing objects (be specific about the type of objects thrown). Ask about forced sex, clubbing, beating, choking, and the use of weapons. Ask about her fear: "Do you feel safe in your current relationship?" She may also fear a partner from whom she has separated but who is threatening or stalking her. Negative responses to lower levels of violence do not preclude positive responses to more severe violence.

Physician Barriers

Domestic violence is a complex social problem that requires physicians to step beyond the biomedical paradigm and confront their own personal feelings and social beliefs.[27–29] In unselected patients, physicians identified only 1.5% to 8.5% of victims.[5] Clinicians consistently underestimate the prevalence of IPV among their patients.[28] Physician education and chart reminders have been successful in increasing the identification of IPV.[30,31]

Physicians feel they have not been trained to deal with domestic violence and there is little they can do.[27,28] Physicians working with IPV recognize that it is not a problem that they can "fix" but one that requires time, as well as working with both the patient and community agencies. These physicians recognize cues, frame questions to reduce discomfort and validate concerns, and focus on establishing trust and emotional safety for women.[26]

Physicians rarely discover the abusers in their practice because they appear normal. If incidents are discovered, abusers commonly accuse their partners of exaggeration, do not define their actions as violent, or dismiss the incident as an exception. Physicians must not rationalize, minimize, or excuse the abuser's violence. Family therapy is not appropriate in a setting of violence.[3]

Management

The quality of medical care a battered woman receives often determines if she will follow through with referrals to legal, social service, and health care agencies.[9] It is critical for the physician to breach the battered woman's isolation and to validate her view of reality by telling her that spouse abuse is a crime, that she does not deserve abuse, that things can improve, and that her feelings of defeat are a result of the abuse.[9,11]

Physicians may inadvertently retraumatize the woman by blaming her, or insisting she leave, not realizing women are at the greatest risk of being brutally beaten or killed when they leave their abuser.[3,10,15,27,32] Physicians may diagnose anxiety, depression, or substance abuse without realizing these are a result of ongoing abuse. This labels the victim, delays appropriate intervention, and, if psychoactive drugs are prescribed, increases the risk of suicide.[20,27,29]

Physicians must not only diagnose domestic violence but also establish its severity and the woman's risk. Immediate danger must be assessed. The best way to ascertain the woman's risk is to ask: "Are you safe tonight? Can you go home now? Are your children safe? Where is your batterer now?" If she says she is in immediate danger, the physician should believe her and begin to explore safer options. Continued support, validation, risk assessment, documentation, and practical advice comprise the "treatment" of domestic violence. At each visit immediate danger must be assessed, features associated with increasing risk reviewed (Table 6.1), a safe plan established or reviewed (Table 6.2), and documentation provided. Scheduled follow-up visits provide the patient opportunities to acknowledge the validity of her experiences, the difficulties in her situation, and the chance to reassess her options. By facilitating rather than directing change, physicians can focus on the process of empowerment rather than on the outcome

TABLE 6.1. Features Associated with Increasing Risk of Intimate Partner Violence

Increasing frequency of violence
Increasing severity of injuries
The presence of weapons
Substance abuse
Unemployment
Threats and overt forced sexual acts
Threats of suicide or homicide
Surveillance
Abuse of children, pets, other family members, or the destruction of treasured objects
Increasing isolation
Extreme jealousy and accusations of infidelity
Failure of multiple support systems
A decrease or elimination of remorse expressed by the batterer

of leaving.[27] Physician behaviors that have been found particularly helpful or un-helpful by battered women are summarized in Table 6.3.[33,34]

Documentation

The physician's documentation provides the history and evidence of abuse. The abused woman needs to know that her records are confidential unless she decides to use them. Notes should be nonjudgmental and precise, and should document the chronology. The chief complaint and a description of abusive events should use the patient's own words. Include a complete description of any injuries with body diagrams, specifying the type, number, size, location, and age of any injuries, and the explanation offered. Photographs should be taken before medical treatment, if possible, and should include a reference object (such as a

TABLE 6.2. The Components of an Abused Woman's Safe Plan

Places to which she could flee—one primary and two backups
  Telephone numbers
  Transportation
Cash
Bag packed for her and children
Documents (or copies)
  Driver's license
  Birth certificates
  Social security card
  Welfare card
  Health and other insurance policies
  Bank statements
  Protection orders/restraining orders
  Immigration papers
An extra set of keys to home and car
Evidence of abuse such as names and addresses of witnesses, pictures of injuries, and medical reports
Something meaningful for each child (blanket, toy, book), but if the children are old enough, she should talk to them about safety—how to call for help and where to go to keep themselves safe

TABLE 6.3. The Desirability of Common Physician Behaviors Identified
by Abused Women

Desirable behaviors
Performing a careful, sensitive medical examination
Asking for concerns or questions
Listening
Expressing emotional support
Providing reassurance that the beating was not the woman's fault
Being compassionate and respectful
Noticing body language
Stating that abuse is wrong under any circumstances
Asking or offering to call the police
Undesirable behaviors
Not scheduling a follow-up visit
Insisting that the woman get away from her abuser
Calling the police without the woman's permission
Treating physical injuries without asking how they occurred
Recommending couple counseling
Going along with the patient's explanation of the injury, even if inconsistent with injuries
Acting as if the abuse was not serious because the physical injuries were not serious
Acting as if he/she did not care that an assault had occurred
Telling the woman things could be worse

ruler) to convey relative size, and the face of the woman in at least one. All photographs should be dated and kept with the consent form.[35] The physician's record should also include the results of diagnostic procedures, referrals, and recommended follow-up, and should record any contact with the abuser. The badge number of the investigating officer, if the police are notified, should be noted.[36]

The Process of Leaving

Separation from an abusive partner is an ongoing process.[14,32,37,38] Abusers respond predictably when their partner leaves, first trying to locate her, and apologizing and promising to change, but if the woman does not return, then they become threatening, embarrassing her in public or harassing her. Women are five times more likely to be murdered by their partner during the separation than before the separation or after divorce. Seventy-five percent of calls to the police and 73% of emergency room visits occur after separation.[5,32]

Most women eventually leave or change an abusive relationship, but it may involve returning repeatedly and may take years.[14,32] In one longitudinal study, after $2^{1}/_{2}$ years three fourths of the battered women were no longer in violent relationships; 43% had left, and in 32% the violence ended.[14] Women report going through stages of *reclaiming their self* as they separate from their abusive partners.[38] Initially they are shocked, fearful, and ashamed, and want to deny the abuse. After recurrent abuse, they problem solve, trying to change their behaviors or the circumstances to avoid or minimize abuse and hoping for improvement. Isolation, power imbalance, and alternating abusive and kind behaviors predispose victims to the formation of strong emotional attachments to their abusers and explain why battered women struggle to separate themselves emotionally from their abusers and often return after leaving.[9,11] Eventually, abused women realize that no matter what they do the abuse is unavoidable and they need to separate both emotionally and physically. The ability of a woman to separate depends on her resources, both material (job, housing, social supports, legal services, and child support) and psychological (self-esteem, resisting self-blame).[32,37] Subsequent violence by her partner, especially threats against the children and inadequate legal protection, are often cited by women as a reason to return to an abusive relationship. Eventual recovery from an abusive relationship is characterized by establishing a safe and separate living situation, grieving the loss, and later developing a new sense of oneself and one's abuse history.[20,32,37,38]

Legal Issues

Battered women may take civil actions, which include filing a protective order or seeking an injunction or restraining order. They may also choose to file criminal charges, including prosecution for assault and battery, aggravated assault or battery, harassment, intimidation, or attempted murder. However, the legal response to domestic violence is less than optimal. The woman is likely to know whether the batterer will adhere to court orders.[3,36] Physicians should refer batterers to an appropriate state-certified batterer treatment program, but also need to realize that the enrollment of the batterer in a program, or even a restraining order, in no way guarantees a woman's safety.[12,39]

Most states require reporting of criminal assaults; however, some states now have mandatory reporting of domestic violence. These laws have not increased reporting, and without the necessary support services this has put victims at risk and fearful of confiding in their physicians, and physicians become conflicted about their obligations to report versus their concern for their patient's safety.[36,40] The Joint Commission on Accreditation of Health Care Organizations require policies for the identification and assessment of abuse victims and the education of providers.[36]

Prevention

Primary prevention of domestic violence will be achieved only by challenging the roles of violence and patriarchy in society. This includes educating parents and teens about nonviolent problem-solving strategies and questioning gender stereotypes both in individual patient interactions and through school- or community-based programs.[8,10,18,41,42] *Secondary prevention* includes the interruption and elimination of intergenerational abuse of all kinds, challenging popular media images of gendered violence, and treating the cofactors of alcohol and substance abuse.[18,42] *Tertiary prevention* can be achieved by identifying victims and their abusers and helping each one. When available, battered women's shelters are effective, although few of the women in need can access them. Court-ordered programs for male batterers have had some success in the reduction of battery. Education, referral, outreach, and brief intervention programs by clinicians or volunteers have been shown to increase women's adoption of safe behaviors and to decrease abuse.[43,44] Comprehensive community-based programs for the identification and treatment of both victims and perpetrators are the most effective.[11,18]

Family and Community Issues

Treatment of domestic violence requires working in partnership with community agencies not only for individual patients but also as an advocate for increased and coordinated services, public education, and research.[41,45] It is hoped that the recent passage of the federal Violence Against Women Act of 2000 will increase services for families. Many communities and states operate toll-free 24-hour domestic violence hotlines. Excellent Web-based resources are available, but victims need to be warned about Internet tracking by abusers and cyber stalking.[46] Some recommended sites for victims and professionals include the following: Family Violence Prevention Fund, *http://www.fvpf.org;* Crisis Support Network, *http://crisis-support.org;* Violence Against Women Office of Department of Justice, *http://www.ojp.usdoj.gov/vamo;* Minnesota Center Against Violence and Abuse, an electronic clearing house, *http://www.mincava.umn.edu;* Centers for Disease Control and Prevention's National Center for Injury Prevention and Control and Family and Intimate Violence Prevention Program, *http://www.cdc.gov/ncipc/dvp/fivpt/fivpt.htm;* and the National Coalition Against Domestic Violence, *http://www.ncadv.org/.* The National Domestic Violence Hot Line is 1-800-799-SAFE.

Families that engage in one form of family violence are likely to engage in others.[8] Family physicians are in a unique position to interrupt the cycle of violence and to effect positive change in the lives of both the victims and the abusers, as well as the children affected by domestic violence.

References

1. Hamberger LK, Lohr J, Bonge D, Tolin D. An empirical classification of motivations for domestic violence. Violence Against Women 1997;3(4):401–23.
2. Cascardi M, Langhinrichsen VD. Marital aggression: impact, injury, and health correlates for husbands and wives. Arch Intern Med 1992;152:1178–84.
3. American Medical Association. Diagnostic and treatment guidelines on domestic violence. Chicago: AMA, 1992.
4. Coker AL, Smith PH, Bethea L, King MR, McKeown RE. Physical health consequences of physical and psychological intimate partner violence. Arch Fam Med 2000;9:451–7.
5. Nauman P, Langford D, Torres S, Campbell J, Glass N. Women battering in primary care practice. Fam Pract 1999;16(4):343–52.

6. Sisley A, Jacobs LM, Poole G, Campbell S, Esposito T. Violence in America: a public health crisis B domestic violence. J Trauma Injury Infect Crit Care 1999; 46(6):1105–13.
7. Walker LE. The battered woman syndrome. New York: Springer, 1984.
8. Gelles RJ, Cornell CP. Intimate violence in families, 2nd ed. Newbury, CA: Sage, 1990.
9. Burge SK. Violence against women as a health care issue. Fam Med 1989;21:368–73.
10. Stark E, Flitcraft A. Women at risk: domestic violence and women's health. Thousand Oaks, CA: Sage, 1996.
11. Herman JL. Trauma and recovery. New York: Basic Books, 1992.
12. Cardin AD. Wife abuse and the wife abuser: review and recommendations. Counseling Psychol 1994;22(4):539–82.
13. Holtzworth-Munroe A. A typology of men who are violent toward their female partners: making sense of the heterogeneity in husband violence. Curr Direct Psychol Sci 2000;9(4):140–3.
14. Johnson M, Ferraro K. Research on domestic violence in the 1990s: making distinctions. J Marriage Fam 2000;62:948–63.
15. Kyriacou DN, Anglin D, Taliaferro E, et al. Risk factors for injury to women from domestic violence. N Engl J Med 1999;341(25):1892–8.
16. Brookoff D, O'Brien KK, Cook CS, Thompson TD, Williams C. Characteristics of participants in domestic violence: assessment at the scene of domestic assault. JAMA 1997;277(17):1369–73.
17. West CM. Leaving a second closed: outing partner violence in same-sex couples. In: Jasinski JL, Williams LJ, eds. Partner violence: a comprehensive review of 20 years of research. Thousand Oaks, CA: Sage 1998;163–83.
18. Stringham P. Domestic violence. Prim Care 1999;26(2):373–84.
19. Phillips LR. Domestic violence and aging women. Geriatr Nurs 2000;21(4):188–93.
20. Campbell J, Lewandowski L. Mental and physical health effects of intimate partner violence on women and children. Psychiatr Clin North Am 1997;20(2):353–74.
21. Olson L, Anctil C, Fullerton L, et al. Increasing emergency physician recognition of domestic violence. Ann Emerg Med 1996;27(6):741–6.
22. Martin SL, Mackie L, Kupper LL, Buescher PA, Moracco KE. Physical abuse of women before, during and after pregnancy. JAMA 2001;285(12):1581–4.
23. Scholle SH, Rost KM, Golding JM. Physical abuse among depressed women. J Gen Intern Med 1998;13:607–13.
24. Anderson SA, Cramer-Benjamin DB. The impact of couple violence on parenting and children: an overview and clinical implications. Am J Fam Ther 1999;27:1–19.
25. Dubowitz H, Black MM, Kerr MA, et al. Type and timing of mothers' victimization: effects on mothers and children. Pediatrics 2001;107(4):728–35.
26. Gerbert B, Caspers N, Bronstone A, Moe J, Abercrombie P. A qualitative analysis of how physicians with expertise in domestic violence approach the identification of victims. Ann Intern Med 1999;131:578–84.
27. Warshaw C. Domestic violence: changing theory, changing practice. J Am Med Wom Assoc 1996;51(3):87–91.
28. Snugg NK, Thompson RS, Thompson DC, Maiuro R, Rivara FP. Domestic violence and primary care: attitudes, practices and beliefs. Arch Fam Med 1999;8:301–6.
29. Gremillion DH, Kanof EP. Overcoming barriers to physician involvement in identifying and referring victims of domestic violence. Ann Emerg Med 1996;27(6):769–73.

30. Wiist WH, McFarlane J. The effectiveness of an abuse assessment protocol in public health prenatal clinics. Am J Public Health 1999;89:1217–21.
31. Thompson RS, Rivara FP, Thompson DC, et al. Identification and management of domestic violence: a randomized trial. Am J Prev Med 2000;19(4):253–63.
32. Landenburger KM. The dynamics of leaving and recovering from an abusive relationship. J Obstet Gynecol Neonatal Nurs 1998;27(6):700–6.
33. Hamberger LK, Ambuel B, Marbella A, Donze J. Physician interaction with battered women: the women's perspective. Arch Fam Med 1998;7:575–82.
34. Rodriguez MA, Szkupinski Quiroga S, Bauer HM. Breaking the silence: battered women's perspectives on medical care. Arch Fam Med 1996;5(3):153–8.
35. Bryant W, Panico S. Physician's legal responsibilities to victims of domestic violence. NC Med J 1994;55(9):418–21.
36. Hyman A. Domestic violence: legal issues for health care practitioners and institutions. J Am Med Wom Assoc 1996;51(3):101–5.
37. Rothery M, Tutty L, Weaver G. Tough choices: women, abusive partners and the ecology of decision-making. Can J Community Mental Health 1999;18(1):5–18.
38. Merritt-Gray M, Wuest J. Counteracting abuse and breaking free: the process of leaving revealed through women's voices. Health Care Wom Int 1995;16:399–412.
39. Capshew T, McNeece CA. Empirical studies of civil protection orders in intimate violence: a review of the literature. Crisis Intervent 2000;6(2):151–67.
40. Mills L. Mandatory arrest and prosecution policies for domestic violence: a critical literature review and the case for more research to test victim empowerment approaches. Criminal Justice Behav 1998;25(3):306–18.
41. Candib LM. Primary violence prevention: taking a deeper look. J Fam Pract 2000;49(10):904–6.
42. Foshee VA, Bauman KE, Arriaga XB, et al. An evaluation of safe dates, an adolescent dating violence prevention program. Am J Public Health 1998;88(1):45–50.
43. McFarlane J, Parker B, Soeken K, Silva C, Reel R. Safety behaviors of abused women after an intervention during pregnancy. J Obstet Gynecol Neonatal Nurs 1998;27:64–9.
44. Sullivan CM, Bybee DI. Reducing violence using community-based advocacy for women with abusive partners. J Consult Clin Psychol 1999;67:43–53.
45. Chalk R, King P. Assessing family violence interventions. Am J Prevent Med 1998;14(4):289–92.
46. Finn J. Domestic violence organizations on the Web: a new arena for domestic violence services. Violence Against Women 2000;6(1):80–102.

CASE PRESENTATION

Subjective

PATIENT PROFILE

Ann Martino-Priestley is a 22-year-old married female nursery school teacher found to be pregnant on her last visit 6 weeks ago.

PRESENTING PROBLEM

"Routine prenatal visit."

PRESENT ILLNESS

The patient is now 13 weeks pregnant and no longer has nausea and urinary frequency. There is no vaginal spotting. She feels well and is "excited about this first pregnancy." Her appetite is good, and she is taking prenatal vitamins.

PAST MEDICAL HISTORY, SOCIAL HISTORY, HABITS, AND FAMILY HISTORY

These are unchanged since her first prenatal visit (see Chapter 3).

REVIEW OF SYSTEMS

While taking the history, you noticed a bruise below her left eye, although this was not mentioned by the patient. When questioned, the patient reports that she walked into a partially opened bathroom door while going to the toilet at night.

- The husband insists on being present throughout the examination and the following consultation. How do you respond to this request?
- What additional information about the progress of the pregnancy would be important today?
- What might be the patient's goals for today's visit?
- What more would you like to know about the bruise below the left eye? How would you frame the question(s)?

Objective

VITAL SIGNS

Weight, 131 lb; blood pressure, 120/72; pulse, 74; temperature, 37.2°C.

EXAMINATION

There is no abdominal tenderness. The uterus is palpable at a 3- months' size. In addition to the fading ecchymosis below the left eye, there is a recent-appearing ecchymosis 2 by 4 cm in size of the left lower abdomen and another bruise 2 by 3 cm of the lateral right breast. The patient was apparently unaware of these bruises and reports that she does not know the cause.

LABORATORY

On laboratory examination, the urine is negative for protein and glucose.

- What additional information derived from the physical examination would be useful in regard to the pregnancy?
- What additional physical examination data might help clarify the cause of the bruising?
- What laboratory specimens—if any—should you obtain today?
- What diagnostic imaging—if any—would you obtain today?

Assessment

- What are the diagnostic possibilities, and how will you share these with the patient?
- What might be the significance of the pregnancy to the patient and her husband?
- What may be the patient's concerns, and how would you elicit these?
- What physical diseases could explain the bruising? What drugs might contribute to the bruising? How readily will you accept these possible explanations?

Plan

- What is your recommendation to the patient and her husband?
- What community agencies might become involved, and how should they be contacted?

- The patient expresses concern about the cost of prenatal care, hospital confinement, and delivery. How would you respond?
- As you are concluding the visit, the patient begins to cry and says, "I'm afraid." What would you do next?

7
Headache

ANNE D. WALLING

Headache is an almost universal experience, afflicting patients of any age or characteristic, although it is reported to be particularly frequent in young adults. Nearly 60% of men and 76% of women aged 12 to 29 years report at least one headache within any 4-week period.[1] The societal costs of headache are enormous but can be estimated only indirectly in terms of days lost from work or school, expenditures on medical services, and consumption of nonprescription medications. The total burden of suffering due to this symptom, including disruption of relationships and loss of normal activities, is incalculable. Although headache is the principal reason for more than 50 million physician office visits and 2.5 million emergency room visits per year, it is important to realize that most headache episodes are not brought to medical attention. Over 20% of those headache patients who do seek medical attention are dissatisfied with the care provided, making headache the leading diagnosis associated with patient dissatisfaction.[2]

Headache is a symptom, not a diagnosis. Numerous conditions can produce cephalic pain (see Classification of Headaches, below) as part of a localized or systemic process; thus headache may be a prominent symptom in the child with fever, the adult with sinusitis, or the elderly patient with temporal arteritis. The pathophysiology of "primary" headaches, such as migraine and cluster headaches, is a controversial, rapidly developing area with the principal developments focused on the role of neurotransmitters, endothelial cells, and whether neuronal tissue can itself generate pain.[3,4]

Whatever the etiology, each headache episode is interpreted by the individual patient in terms of experience, culture, and belief systems. Thus a relatively minor degree of pain may prompt one patient to seek emergency care and comprehensive neurologic assessment, whereas a patient with extensive personal or family experience of recurrent headache may cope with several days of incapacitating symptoms without seeking medical assistance. Patients and physicians tend to be uncomfortable with the diagnosis and management of headache. In addition to extensive patient dissatisfaction,[5] headache is frequently identified as a "heart-sink" condition by physicians (i.e., the patient evokes "an overwhelming mixture of exasperation, defeat, and sometimes plain dislike"[6]). The reasons for this situation include the recurrent nature of most headache syndromes, the potential for secondary gain and iatrogenic complications (particularly overuse of narcotic analgesics), and fear of missing a potentially serious but rare intracranial lesion. The effective management of headaches requires the development of a therapeutic alliance between the physician and patient based on objectivity and mutual respect.[7] Most chronic headaches are recurrent and cannot be completely cured. Physicians can, however, greatly help patients to understand their condition, develop effective strategies to reduce the number and severity of attacks, and follow healthy lifestyles not skewed by the presence or fear of headache.

Clinical Approach to the Headache Patient

With so many potential causes and complicating circumstances, a systematic approach to the headache patient is essential for objective, effective, efficient management. It can be achieved in four stages:

1. Clarification of the reasons for the consultation
2. Diagnosis (classification) of the headache
3. Negotiation of management
4. Follow-up

Not infrequently, a significant headache history is discovered on systematic inquiry of a patient presenting for other reasons. The clinical approach to these patients reverses "clarification" to identify why the patient has avoided seeking medical help for headache symptoms.

Clarification of the Reasons for Consultation

Those headaches that lead to medical consultation have particular significance. It is important to have patients articulate their beliefs about the symptoms and expectations of treatment.[7] Reasons for consultation range from fear of cancer to seeking validation that current use of nonprescription medication is appropriate. Headache is frequently used as a "ticket of admission" symptom by the patient who wishes to discuss other medical or social problems. In practice, a change in the coping ability of the patient, family, or coworkers is as frequent a cause of consultation as any change in the severity or type of headache. Patients may also consult when they learn new information, particularly concerning situations in which a severe illness in a friend or relative presented as headache. Recent public advertising campaigns by drug companies have led to patients consulting physicians specifically to request the newer medications.

All headache patients should be asked directly what type of headache they believe they have and what causes it. These issues must be addressed during the management even if they are inaccurate. Patients should also be asked about expectations of management. Successful management avoids dependence by emphasizing the patients' role in reducing the frequency and severity of headaches and increasing their ability to cope with a recurrent condition.

Background information from relatives and friends may give useful insights. Disruptive headaches lead to highly charged situations, and the physician must remain objective and avoid becoming triangulated between the patient and others. With good listening and a few directed questions, the background to the consultation can be clarified and the groundwork laid for accurate diagnosis and successful management. This short time is well invested. In headache patients presenting to family physicians, "listening" time makes a significantly greater contribution to the diagnosis and management than time spent on the physical examination or other investigation,[8] although all are appropriate.

Classification of Headaches

The 1988 International Classification of Headaches[9] established diagnostic criteria for 13 major types of headache with approximately 70 subtypes (Table 7.1). A useful grouping for family practice uses five categories.

1. Migraine (all types)
2. Cluster headaches
3. Tension/stress (or muscle contraction) headaches
4. Headaches secondary to other pathology
5. Specific headache syndromes (e.g., cough headache)

These categories are broad with considerable overlap. "Mixed headaches," where the clinical picture contains elements of more than one headache category, are

TABLE 7.1. Headache Types

Primary headaches	Miscellaneous
Migraine	"Ice-pick"
Without aura	External compression
With aura (several types)	Cold stimulus (including ice cream)
Ophthalmoplegic	Cough
Retinal	Exertional
Childhood syndromes	Coital
Complicated migraine	
Other	**Secondary headaches**
Tension type	*Associated with*
Episodic	Head trauma
Chronic	Vascular disorders
Other	Intracranial disorders
Cluster	Substance use or withdrawal (including
Episodic	medication side effects)
Chronic	Systemic infections
Chronic paroxysmal hemicrania	Metabolic disorders
Other	Structural disorder of head or neck
	Neuralgia syndromes
	Unclassifiable headaches

TABLE 7.2. Diagnostic Criteria for Common Primary Headaches

Headache	Duration	Characteristics	Associated symptoms	Other
Migraine	4–72 hours	At least two: Unilateral Pulsating Moderate to severe Aggravated by activity	At least one: Nausea/vomiting Photophobia and phonophobia	No neurologic source for symptoms Multiple types (Table 7.1) At least five attacks for diagnosis
Cluster	Individual attacks: 15–180 minutes Cluster episodes: 1–8 attacks/day for 7 days to 1 year or longer	Unilateral orbital/temporal stabbing Severe to very severe	At least one: Conjunctival injection Lacrimation Nasal congestion Rhinorrhea Sweating Miosis Ptosis Eyelid edema	No neurologic source for symptoms At least five attacks for diagnosis
Tension/stress	Individual headaches: 30 minutes to 7 days Headaches <15 days/month or <180/year	At least two: Pressure/tightness Bilateral Mild to moderate Not aggravated by activity	No nausea Photophobia and phonophobia: absent or only one present, not both	No neurologic source for symptoms At least 10 episodes for diagnosis

common. Individual patients may also describe more than one type of headache; for example, migraineurs experience tension headaches on occasion.

Diagnosis

The diagnosis of headache syndromes (Table 7.2) requires systematic clinical reasoning based on the history augmented by physical examination and judicious use of investigations or consultation to establish the most probable etiology for the pain. A particular feature is the potential to use the diagnostic process to increase patients' understanding and prepare them to take responsibility for long-term management in cooperation with the physician.

Tension headaches are by far the most prevalent type of cephalic pain encountered in family practice,[8,10] probably followed by headaches secondary to other causes. The medical literature, research efforts, and therapeutic innovations focus on migraine and other interesting primary headache syndromes, but all headache patients deserve a competent assessment and appropriate, individualized treatment for their symptoms.

History

Headache diagnoses depend on the medical history. An open-ended approach, such as "Tell me about your headaches," followed by specific questions to elucidate essential features usually indicates which of the diagnostic categories is most probable. The history should address the criteria shown in Table 7.2 and clarify the following:

1. *Characteristics:* nature of pain, location, radiation in head, intensity, exacerbating and relieving factors or techniques, associated symptoms and signs.
2. *Pattern:* usual duration and frequency of episodes, precipitating factors, description of a typical episode, change in pattern over time, prodromes and precipitating factors, postheadache symptoms.
3. *Personal history:* age at onset, medical history (including medication, alcohol, and substance use) with special emphasis on secondary causes of headache, such as depression or trauma; environmental and occupational exposure history (see Chapter 23).
4. *Investigations and treatments:* previous diagnoses and supporting evidence, patient's degree of confidence in these diagnoses, patient's beliefs and concerns about diagnosis and potential treatments; previous treatments and degree of success; side effects of any investigations and treatments; patient preferences for treatment; current use of prescription and nonprescription medications.
5. *Family history:* headache, other conditions, family attitudes to headache.

The headache profile that emerges from the history has a high probability of correctly classifying the headache[7,8,10,11] without further investigation. It is important, however, to complete the usual review of systems to uncover additional data. Throughout the history-taking process, the physician forms a general impression of the patient. Although subjective, this should correlate with the headache profile and is particularly useful for assessing psychological components of the situation, including which management strategies are most likely to be successfully implemented and followed by the patient. By the end of the history taking, the physician should have the answer to two questions: Which of the five headache groups best fits the story? and Is this diagnosis likely in this particular patient?

Physical Examination

The physical examination continues the dual processes of confirming a specific diagnosis and laying the groundwork for successful management. Unless the consultation coincides with an attack, many migraine, cluster, and other headache patients can be expected to have no abnormal findings on physical examination. Some authors recommend that only a targeted examination be performed, focusing on the most probable cause of the secondary headache elicited from the history,[8] whereas others emphasize the importance of complete physical and neurologic examination of every headache patient.[11] The time devoted to a complete examination may be a wise investment, as it documents both positive and negative physical findings, contributes to the therapeutic alliance, and in many instances is therapeutic. Any physical examination targets the most probable diagnoses based on the symptoms presented by the patient and the physician's knowledge of conditions relevant to the individual.

Other Investigations

A logical test strategy is guided by the most probable diagnosis (or diagnoses) suggested by the history and physical examination. Targeted laboratory and radiologic investigations are most useful for confirming the underlying cause of secondary headaches. Tests are often performed to relieve either physician or patient distress and uncertainty. If the patient or family insists on tests the physician does not believe appropriate, the contributions and limitations of the test in question should be reviewed. Similarly, the physician experiencing the WHIMS (what have I missed syndrome) must review the data and attempt to make a rational decision as to the potential contribution of additional testing.

Most of the debate over the appropriate role of testing currently involves radiologic investigation, specifically computed tomography (CT) and magnetic resonance imaging (MRI). The role of these modalities is limited by the rarity in family practice of headaches caused by intracranial lesions. Serious intracranial pathology was the cause of only 0.4% of new headaches presented to primary care physicians in two studies.[8,12] When deciding to refer a patient for advanced radiologic investigation, the family physician must seriously consider the potential benefits versus the potential radiation exposure (for CT), patient distress

(MRI), and cost. As the investigations have different and often complementary abilities, one must also have a clear concept of what type of intracranial lesion is being sought and its likely location. CT is very sensitive to acute hemorrhage and certain enhancing solid lesions; MRI provides better resolution in the posterior fossa and superior detection of gliosis, infection, posttraumatic changes, and certain tumors.[13] Discussions with a neurologist or radiologist may be useful in this difficult area.

Recent guidelines developed by a consortium including the American Academy of Family physicians (available at *www.aafp.org*) recommend neuroimaging in migraine only if the result is likely to change clinical management and the patient has a significant risk of a relevant abnormality.[14] An exception may be made if patients are excessively worried about the potential etiology of headaches. This is in general agreement with the National Institutes of Health (NIH) Consensus Development Panel which recommended CT investigation of patients whose headaches were "severe, constant, unusual, or associated with neurological symptoms."[15] This recommendation can be problematic in practice, however, as more than half of the patients describe their headaches as severe.[8] The other elements of the NIH recommendations, particularly the presence of neurologic signs, are more useful. The final decision to refer for CT or MRI remains a clinical judgment based on the characteristics of the patient, the symptom complex, and risk factors for intracranial pathology.

Negotiation of Management

Migraine, cluster, tension/stress, and many secondary headaches are recurrent; hence the emphasis is on enabling the patient to successfully manage a lifestyle that includes headaches. The physician who sets a goal of abolishing headaches is being unrealistic in almost all cases.[7,8] More appropriate goals are effective treatment of individual headache episodes and minimizing the number and severity of these episodes. Most headache patients are open to the concept that they carry a vulnerability to headaches and are willing to learn how to manage this tendency. Patients who strongly resist this management approach are often highly dependent personalities who may have drug-seeking behavior or may change to another chronic pain symptom complex when offered aggressive treatment of headaches. The complete management plan includes patient education, treatment plans for both prophylaxis and acute management, and follow-up.

Patient education is essential for the patient and family to manage headaches. They must understand the type of headache and its treatment and natural history. In addition to providing information, the physician must address hidden concerns. Many myths and beliefs are associated with headaches, and patients are empowered to deal with their headaches once these beliefs are addressed. Patients may be embarrassed by their fears; for example, almost all migraine patients have feared cerebral hemorrhage during a severe attack.

Patient education and treatment overlap as the patient and family become responsible for identifying and managing situations that precipitate or exacerbate headache. These situations range from avoiding foods that trigger migraine attacks to practicing conflict resolution. Stress is implicated in almost all headaches; even the pain of secondary headaches is less easy to manage in stressful situations.

There are few "absolutes" in the pharmacologic treatment of headaches, and the large number of choices can be bewildering to both physicians and patients. In general, first-line analgesics and symptomatic treatment are effective, and narcotic use should be avoided. A common mistake is to appear tentative about therapy. The exasperated physician who uses phrases such as, "We'll try this," may convey the message that the medication is not expected to work. Conversely, implying to patients that one has selected a medication specific to their situation, and based on an understanding of the headache literature, recruits the placebo effect and is much more likely to succeed. Patients gather information about headaches and their treatment from a wide variety of sources, including news media and the experience of friends. Patient knowledge and opinions of specific treatments should be established before issuing a prescription.

Nonpharmacologic advice is a powerful factor in building the placebo effect and therapeutic alliance. Physicians gather experiences from many patients and can pass on tips for headache management, such as Lamaze-type breathing exercises for tension headaches, cold washcloth over the eyes during a migraine attack, and vigorous exercise at the start of migraine, cluster, or tension headaches. Including such information in the overall treatment plan enhances the physician's credibility and reinforces the message that headache management is not solely dependent on medications. Formal therapies such as relaxation therapy, thermal biofeedback, and cognitive-behavior therapy can be effective in individual migraine patients.[16]

Follow-Up

With the exception of headaches secondary to acute self-limiting conditions, headaches tend to be a recurrent problem. Unless follow-up is well managed, the patient returns only at times of severe symptoms or exasperation at the failure of treatment. This pattern implies the risk of emergency visits at difficult times and consultation complicated by hostility or disappointment. In practice, patients manage well if given scheduled appointments, particularly if they are combined with the expectation that the patient will come to the consultation well prepared (i.e., with information on the number, pattern, response to treatment, and any other relevant information about headaches since the last visit). Some authors recommend that patients keep a formal headache diary.[8]

Clinical Types of Headache

Migraine

Migraine-type headaches are estimated to affect more than 23 million Americans, approximately 17% of women and 6% of men.[17] Although all epidemiologic studies are complicated by differences in definitions and design, migraine is more common in women at all ages and has a peak prevalence during young adulthood. Up to 30% of women aged 21 to 34 report at least one migraine-type headache per year.[18]

Up to 90% of migraine patients have a first-degree relative, usually a parent, also affected by migraine.[18] Perhaps because of familiarity with the condition, significant numbers of migraine sufferers (approximately 50%) do not seek medical assistance. Several classifications of migraine have been suggested. As shown in Table 7.2, the current international classification[9] is based on clinical features, particularly the presence of aura. In practice, it is seldom useful to subclassify migraine.

Patients in the "classic" subgroup (approximately 20% of all migraineurs) experience a characteristic aura before the onset of migraine head pain. This aura may take several forms, but visual effects such as scotomas, zigzag lines, photopsia, or visual distortions are the most common. A much larger proportion of patients describe prodromal symptoms, which may be visceral, such as diarrhea or nausea, but are more commonly alterations in mood or behavior. Food cravings, mild euphoria (conversely, yawning), and heightened sensory perception, particularly of smell, are surprisingly common.

The headache of migraine is severe, usually unilateral, described as "throbbing" or "pulsating," and aggravated by movement. The pain usually takes 30 minutes to 3 hours to reach maximum intensity, and it may last several hours. The eye and temple are the most frequent centers of pain, but occipital involvement is common. Each patient describes a characteristic group of associated symptoms among which nausea predominates. Either nausea or both photophobia and phonophobia are required for diagnosis along with the characteristic headache. During attacks, migraine patients avoid movement and sensory stimuli, especially light. They may use pressure and either heat or cold over the areas of maximal pain. The attack usually terminates with sleep. Vomiting appears to shorten attacks, and some patients admit to self-induced vomiting, although this phenomenon is not widely described in the literature. Many patients report a "hangover" on waking after a migraine, but others report complete freedom from symptoms and a sense of euphoria. The cause of migraine remains unknown; research indicates that migraine begins in neurons as a biochemical process, and that vascular phenomena are secondary effects.[19,20]

The treatment of migraine typifies the approach of enabling patients to manage their own condition. A bewildering variety of therapies is available, and management should be individualized. The treatment plan has three aspects: avoidance of precipitants, aggressive treatment of attacks, and prophylactic therapy if indicated. Patients and their families can usually identify triggers of migraine attacks. The role of specific foods has probably been exaggerated,[21] although red wine and cheese continue to have a significant reputation as migraine triggers. Disturbance in daily routine, particularly missed meals, excessive sleeping, and relaxation after periods of stress, are notorious precipitants of migraine attacks. Certain women correlate migraines with the onset of menstruation each month, but the effect of oral contraception and postmenopausal hormone replacement are unpredictable. Migraines commonly disappear during pregnancy.

Patients should be encouraged to recognize their own aura or prodrome, as early treatment is most efficacious. Whatever treatment strategy is followed, early use of metoclopramide helps reduce nausea and counteract delayed gastric emptying. The multiple medications used for migraine may be categorized into four groups:

1. Symptom control: principally analgesics, with or without adjunctive antiemetics or sedatives
2. Ergotamines: based on the theory that migraine pain is due to cerebral vasodilation
3. Serotonin (5-hydroxytryptamine, 5-HT) receptor agonists: new class of agents (prototype is sumatriptan) based on etiology
4. Prophylactic agents: large, diverse group of medications reported to reduce the frequency of attacks (Table 7.3).

A common problem in migraine treatment is subtherapeutic dosage of medication or failure to absorb medication because of vomiting and gastric stasis.

The choice of specific medications and route of delivery must be individualized. Factors contributing to the decision include the migraine characteristics (particularly the likelihood of vomiting), patient factors such as associated medical problems, and medication issues including efficacy, speed of onset, side effects, cost, and acceptability.[17] The headache consortium guidelines stress the balance between adequate, effective treatment and the avoidance of iatrogenic effects from inappropriate medication use.[22] Patients frequently appreciate having more than one agent or combination of agents (e.g., ergotamine, analgesic, or a triptan drug) when they need to "keep going" and a combination analgesic and sedative for "backup" or situations when they can "crash." Many patients also report that a particular agent appears to work well for several months, but then they need to change it.

Narcotics have almost no place in migraine therapy. Even in the emergency room situation, controlled studies have shown that adequate analgesia, use of injections of antiemetics, or injectable ergotamines are superior to narcotics.[18] The migraine patient who demands narcotics or claims allergies to alternative treatments may be a drug abuser. Rarely, patients develop dehydration and "status migrainosus" when the attack lasts several days. These patients may require hospitalization and steroids in addition to fluids and aggressive therapy based on antiemetics plus a triptan drug or ergotamine preparation.

The introduction of the triptans has dramatically changed migraine management,[23] but the experience for individual patients may be unpredictable. Whereas

TABLE 7.3. Pharmacologic Treatment of Primary Headaches

Headache type	Acute attack[a]		Prophylactic therapy	
	Dose	Comment	Dose (per day)	Comment
Migraine	Ergotamines Inhalation (0.36 mg/dose) Oral, sublingual (1–2 mg) Rectal IM or IV (0.5–1 mg)	Many formulations and combination drugs available Side effects: nausea, vasoconstriction	Beta-blockers Propranolol (40–240 mg) Nadolol (80–240 mg) Timolol (20–30 mg) Atenolol (50–100 mg) Metoprolol (50–300 mg)	Dosage individualized; side effects are fatigue, GI upset; contraindicated with asthma, heart failure
	Analgesics Aspirin (650–1000 mg) Acetaminophen (<1000 mg) Ibuprofen (<600 mg) Naproxen (<550 mg) Ketorolac (30–60 mg IM)	Many analgesics and NSAIDs effective Dosage individualized Combinations available with sedatives and antiemetics Side effects: mainly gastric upset	Amitriptyline (25–150 mg hs) Sodium valproate (800–1500 mg) Phenelzine (Nardil) (30–75 mg)	Sedation, weight gain, dry mouth; synergistic with beta-blockers Not in liver disease Insomnia, hypotension; interacts with tyramine in food

5-HT agonists
  Sumatriptan 6 mg SC,
    25–100 mg oral,
    5–20 mg nasal
  Zolmitriptan 2.5–5 mg
  Naratriptan 1–2.5 mg
  Rizatriptan 5–10 mg

Not given if
  cerebrovascular,
  cardiovascular disease
  risk or hypertensive
Headache may recur
Expensive

Verapamil (240 mg) — Constipation; not in conduction block

Serotonin-receptor antagonists
  Methysergide (2–10 mg) — Pending FDA approval; sedation, weight gain; Vasoconstriction, fibrosis

Cluster
  Oxygen 100% 8–10 mL/min for 10 minutes
  Ergotamine 1–2 mg orally
  Ergotamine 0.36 mg/puff × 1–3
  Lidocaine 4% 1 mL into nostril
  Methoxyflurane inhale 10 drops
  Prednisone 10–80 mg daily
  Lithium 300–900 mg daily
  Indomethacin 120 mg daily
  Nifedipine 40–120 mg daily

Tension-stress
  Analgesics and NSAIDs (as for migraine but at lower dosages)
  Amitriptyline (50–100 mg hs)
  Imipramine (25–75 mg)

[a]Treatment must be of rapid onset. (1) All therapy should be started at first sign of attack but triptans are not advised during aura. (2) Other symptomatic relief may be added, especially antiemetics and sedative. (3) Encourage patients to find abortive therapy (e.g., caffeine, exercise, cold ± pressure over the site of pain) to use in addition to above. (4) Narcotics are rarely necessary for migraine.
5-HT = 5-hydroxytryptamine (serotonin); NSAID = nonsteroidal antiinflammatory drug.
AAFP treatment guidelines are available at *http://www.aafp.org/afp/20001115/practice.html.*

159

many patients experience dramatic relief, others find triptan use limited by nausea, return of headache 3 to 6 hours after initial clearing, and an unpleasant autonomic reaction of flushing, nausea, hyperventilation, and panic attack as the medication is absorbed. A European study found comparable pain relief but fewer side effects when a combination of aspirin and antiemetic was compared to sumatriptan.[24] As with all migraine treatment, the importance of working with the patient to achieve optimal results from the many options cannot be overstressed. For some patients the triptans are wonder drugs, but for others an expensive disappointment. The headache consortium concluded there was good clinical evidence of effectiveness for several drugs[25] (Table 7.3).

If patients find normal life disrupted by the frequency and severity of migraine attacks, prophylactic treatment should be considered.[16] Beta-blockers are the most widely studied agents. Those without intrinsic sympathomimetic activity (e.g., propranolol, nadolol, atenolol, metoprolol) are effective, but the dosage at which individual patients benefit must be established by clinical trial. Amitriptyline appears to prevent migraine at lower dosages than that used for treatment of depression. Beta-blockers and amitriptyline are synergistic if used together. Many other drugs have been recommended, but the studies are often small and difficult to interpret because of the placebo effect and patient selection. Verapamil appears to have some prophylactic effect, but there is little evidence to support the use of other calcium channel blocking agents. Studies indicate that the anticonvulsant medication valproic acid can be prophylactic for migraine, and interest is growing in the use of fluoxetine and other selective serotonin reuptake inhibitors for this indication.[26] A serotonin agonist, pizotifen, and a calcium-channel blocker, flunarizine, are widely used in other countries[20] but are not yet approved for use in the United States. Conversely, methysergide, which has largely fallen out of use in the United States because of the fear of retroperitoneal fibrosis, is returning to use in other countries at low dosages plus monitoring for side effects and scheduled "drug holidays."[21]

The choice of any prophylactic agent must balance potential benefit against issues of compliance, side effects, and cost.[16,26] Migraine patients can usually be assisted to find regimens that enable them to minimize attacks and deal effectively with those that do occur. They may be comforted by knowing that the condition tends to wane with age, has been associated with lower rates of cerebrovascular and ischemic heart disease than expected,[19] and has afflicted a galaxy of famous people.[18]

Cluster Headaches

The cluster headache, a rare but dramatic form, occurs predominantly in middle-aged men. The estimated prevalence is 69 per 100,000 adults with a 6:1 male preponderance.[18]

The headache is severe, unilateral, centered around the eye or temple, and accompanied by lacrimation, rhinorrhea, red eye, and other autonomic signs on the same side as the headache. Symptoms develop rapidly, reach peak intensity within

10 to 15 minutes, and last up to 2 hours. During the attack the patient is frantic with pain and may be suspected of intoxication, drug-induced behavior, or hysteria.[8] This behavior, including talk of suicide because of the severity of the pain, is characteristic, but patients may be too embarrassed to volunteer this information. The diagnosis is based on the description of attacks, especially their severity, and is confirmed by the unique time pattern described by the patient. During a cluster period, which typically lasts 4 to 8 weeks, the patient experiences attacks at the same time or times of day with bizarre regularity. Approximately half of these attacks awaken the patient and are particularly frequent around 1 A.M. Most patients experience one or two cluster periods per year and are completely free from symptoms at other times. About 10% of patients develop chronic symptoms, with daily attacks over several years. During a cluster period, drinking alcohol or taking vasodilators almost inevitably precipitates an attack. It is speculated that the cluster headache is due to a disorder of serotonin metabolism or circadian rhythm (or both), but the cause remains unknown.[18]

Management strategies aim to provide relief from individual attacks and prophylactically to suppress cluster episodes (Table 7.3). Acute treatment must be of rapid onset and able to be administered by the patient or family. Conventional analgesics do not act quickly enough to provide relief, and all the current treatments of acute cluster headaches are difficult to administer to a patient who is restless and distracted with pain. Inhalation of oxygen is the traditional treatment, and inhalation or instillation of local anesthetics into the nostril on the affected side may also be effective. The only ergotamines likely to be effective during the acute attack are those delivered by inhaler or injection. European studies indicate that self-administered injections of sumatriptan are effective.[27]

The mainstay of cluster headache management is to suppress headaches during a cluster period. As shown in Table 7.3, several drugs are effective. Drugs may also be used in combination (e.g., verapamil 80 mg qid with ergotamine 2 mg hs).[28] Treatment should be initiated as soon as a cluster period begins and continued for a few days beyond the expected duration of the cluster. Only the previous experience of each patient can be used to judge the duration of therapy. Each patient has a set length for the cluster period as well as a tendency to repeat the same time and symptom pattern of individual headaches. It is particularly important in the age group usually affected by cluster headaches to monitor prophylactic drugs such as lithium, prednisone, ergotamine, indomethacin, calcium channel blockers, and methysergide for side effects.

Tension-Stress (Muscle Contraction) Headaches

Tension-stress headaches are the most frequent of all headaches encountered in clinical practice.[10,18] In one study of family practice consultations, they accounted for 70% of all new headache patients.[8] These patients represent a select sample of all tension headache patients, as most sufferers are believed to manage their symptoms using simple analgesics or other strategies. Although physicians are familiar with the condition, it is difficult to define it because it presents in myriad forms and is known by several names. The formal definition (Table 7.2) contains both positive and negative criteria, but a common problem is to diagnose tension headaches only after searching for more interesting etiologies for the symptoms.

The etiology and pathophysiology of tension headaches are poorly understood. Stress, psychological abnormalities, muscle contraction, and abnormalities of neurotransmitters have been implicated.[29,30] The clinical syndrome may represent more than one entry, and in many cases there is considerable overlap with migraine.[19]

As with migraine, more than 70% of tension headaches occur in women, and a substantial proportion of patients (40%) give a family history of similar symptoms. Tension headaches, however, tend to have their onset at an older age (70% after 20 years) and to produce symptoms daily or on several days per week, rather than occur as episodic attacks.

The clinical picture is characterized by long periods (up to several years) of almost daily headaches that vary in intensity throughout the day. Most patients keep going with daily activities, but going to bed early is characteristic. The pain is described in many ways, among which "pressure," "tight band," and "aching" predominate. Patients usually express exhaustion, and the patient's affect and body language convey weariness and frustration. Sleep disturbances are common.

Physical examination may be negative or may reveal tightness and tenderness of the muscles of the occipital area, posterior neck, and shoulders. Physical examination is important to rule out secondary headache and to assist in establishing the therapeutic relationship. Attempts to treat the headaches with analgesics before establishing patient confidence in the diagnosis risk failure despite escalating use of analgesics including narcotics.

The treatment of tension headaches is frequently unsatisfactory. Success depends on treatment of any underlying condition (particularly depression), patient education about the nature of the condition, and the control of symptoms without creating dependence or other adverse effects (see Chapters 22 and 23). Tension headache patients frequently take large quantities of analgesics, leading to gastrointestinal and other complications, or they use combination medicines containing sedatives. A wise investment during the history is to clarify all medication use, including nonprescription medication, and to explore previous encounters with physicians. Patients may have already been investigated extensively, and prior medical experiences color expectations and evaluation of management approaches.

Acute episodes of headache are best managed by first-line analgesics, such as acetaminophen, aspirin, or ibuprofen. Narcotics and combination drugs, especially those that contain barbiturates or caffeine, should be avoided. Nonsteroidal antiinflammatory drugs (NSAIDs) may be more effective than other analgesics,[10] especially if prescribed on a regular schedule for several days rather than on an as-needed basis. It is useful to teach the patient and family simple massage and relaxation techniques and to explore methods to resolve conflicts and enhance self-esteem. Not all patients require extensive counseling or biofeedback. The most significant predictor of symptom resolution after 1 year has been shown to be patient confidence that the problem had been fully discussed with a physician.[8] In addition to treating underlying depression, amitriptyline and other antidepressants raise pain thresholds and play a significant role in enabling patients to manage symptoms. The effective dosage may be lower than that required for depressive illnesses.

Secondary Headaches

Headache is part of the clinical picture of many conditions. Particularly in children, frontal headache is a common accompaniment of fever. In all age groups, almost any condition of the head and neck and several systemic conditions can present as headache. A careful history combined with physical examination and other investigations where appropriate can almost always differentiate secondary from primary headache.[3]

There is particular concern in family practice not to miss the rare but serious intracranial condition, especially brain tumor. The symptoms of an intracranial lesion depend on its size, location, and displacement effect on other tissues. No single characteristic headache picture can therefore be given. Suspicion should be raised about headaches of recent onset that appear to become steadily more severe, do not fit any of the primary classifications, and do not respond to first-line treatment. Close follow-up and repeated physical examinations may detect the earliest neurologic abnormalities, but if there is a high degree of suspicion, early radiologic investigation or specialist consultation should be obtained. With intracranial vascular lesions, the first symptom may be a catastrophic hemorrhage.

A growing area of concern for family physicians is "rebound" headache, sometimes called chronic daily headache, which may represent up to 30% of headache consultations.[30] These patients have headaches at least 15 days per month. These patients initially have tension, migraine, or secondary headaches but inappropriate and/or excessive use of medications sets up a vicious cycle in which the treatment itself exacerbates and perpetuates headache. Drug-rebound headaches occur with analgesics, ergotamines, and triptans. In addition, headache may be an adverse effect of several drugs, including NSAIDs.[31]

Specific Headache Syndromes

The literature describes several specific primary headache syndromes that are uncommon but may be encountered in practice (e.g., cough headache) (Table 7.1). These syndromes are more common in men and are characterized by the severity of the pain and the potential for confusion with serious intracranial conditions. Despite the dramatic history, the conditions are generally benign and many respond to indomethacin.[18] Neuroimaging may be necessary to confirm the diagnosis. Explanation, reassurance, and symptom control are usually effective.

References

1. Diamond S, Feinberg DT. The classification, diagnosis and treatment of headaches. Med Times 1990;118:15–27.
2. Lake AE. Psychological impact: the personal burden of migraine. Am J Manag Care 1999;5:S111–21.
3. Olesen J. Understanding the biologic basis of migraine. N Engl J Med 1994; 331:1713–4.
4. Thomsen LL, Olesen J. Human models of headache. In: Olsen J, Tfelt-Hansen P, Welch KMA, eds. The headaches, 2nd ed. Philadelphia: Lippincott Williams & Wilkins, 1999;203–9.
5. Silberstein SD. Office management of benign headache. Postgrad Med 1996; 93:223–40.
6. O'Dowd TC. Five years of heartsink patients in general practice. BMJ 1988; 297:528–30.
7. Graham JR. Headaches. In: Noble J, ed. Textbook of primary care medicine, 2nd ed. St. Louis: Mosby, 1996;1283–319.
8. McWhinney IR. A textbook of family medicine. New York: Oxford University Press, 1989.
9. Headache Classification Committee of the International Headache Society. Classification and diagnostic criteria for all headache disorders, cranial neuralgias and facial pain. Cephalgia 1988;8(S7):1–96.
10. Clough C. Non-migrainous headaches [editorial]. BMJ 1989;299:70–2.
11. Diamond S, Dalessio DJ, eds. The practicing physician's approach to headache, 5th ed. Baltimore: Williams & Wilkins, 1992.
12. Becker L, Iverson DC, Reed FM, et al. Patients with new headache in primary care: a report from ASPN. J Fam Pract 1988;27:41–7.
13. Prager JM, Mikulis DJ. The radiology of headache. Med Clin North Am 1991; 75:525–44.
14. Morey SS. Practice guidelines. Headache consortium releases guidelines for use of CT or MRI in migraine work-up. Am Fam Physician 2000;62:1699–702.
15. NIH Consensus Development Panel. Computer tomographic scanning of the brain. In: Proceedings from NIH Consensus Development Conference, NIH, Bethesda. Washington DC: Government Printing Office, 1982;4:2.
16. Morey SS. Guidelines on migraine: part 4. General principles of preventive therapy Am Fam Physician 2000;62:2359–60, 2363.
17. Silberstein SD, Lipton RB. Overview of diagnosis and treatment of migraine. Neurology 1994;44(suppl 7):S6–16.
18. Raskin NH. Headache, 2nd ed. New York: Churchill Livingstone, 1988.
19. Blau J. Migraine: theories of pathogenesis. Lancet 1992;339:1202–7.
20. Smith R. Chronic headaches in family practice. J Am Board Fam Pract 1992;5:589–99.
21. Lance JW. Treatment of migraine. Lancet 1992;393:1207–9.
22. Morey SS. Practice guidelines. Guidelines on migraine: part 2. General principles of drug therapy. Am Fam Physician 2000;62:1915–7.
23. Cady RK, Shealy CN. Recent advances in migraine management. J Fam Pract 1993;36:85–91.
24. Tfelt-Hansen P, Henry P, Mulder LJ, et al. The effectiveness of combined oral lysine acetylsalicylate and metoclopramide compared with oral sumatriptan for migraine. Lancet 1995;346:923–6.

25. Morey SS. Practice guidelines. Guidelines on migraine: part 3. Recommendations for individual drugs. Am Fam Physician 2000;62:2145–51.
26. Morey SS. Practice guidelines. Guidelines on migraine: part 5. Recommendations for specific prophylactic drugs. Am Fam Physician 2000;62:2535–9.
27. Walling AD. Cluster headaches. Am Fam Physician 1993;47:1457–63.
28. Kudrow L. Diagnosis and treatment of cluster headache. Med Clin North Am 1991;75:579–94.
29. Olesen J, Schoenen. Synthesis of tension-type headache mechanisms. In: Olesen J, Tfelt-Hansen P, Welch KMA, eds. The headaches, 2nd ed. Philadelphia: Lippincott Williams & Wilkins, 1999;615–8.
30. Rapoport A, Strang P, Gutterman DL, et al. Analgesic rebound headache in clinical practice: data from a physician survey. Headache 1996;36:1419.
31. Walling AD. Headache. Monograph, Edition No 265, Home Study Self-Assessment Program. Leawood, KS. AAFP June 2001.

CASE PRESENTATION

Subjective

PATIENT PROFILE

Lois Nelson Martino is a 44-year-old divorced woman who works as a paralegal.

PRESENTING PROBLEM

Headaches.

PRESENT ILLNESS

For 6 months, Lois has had headaches that occur two or three times a month. The headaches are sometimes preceded by a sense of feeling a little "mentally fuzzy," and there may be slightly blurred vision. The headache pain, which begins about 20 to 30 minutes after the onset of the initial symptoms, is severe, throbbing, and generally right-sided, although it sometimes is on the left or spreads to involve the whole head. Lois reports that nausea often accompanies the pain but that she has never vomited during a headache. When the headache is present, she is especially sensitive to noise or bright lights, and she generally retreats to a dark room for the duration of the pain, which is usually some 3 to 6 hours. The patient has used aspirin and ibuprofen (Advil) for pain, but these afford little relief. She is concerned because the headaches sometimes occur during the day and are interfering with her work.

PAST MEDICAL HISTORY

She had an appendectomy at age 16 and is the mother of one child, aged 22.

SOCIAL HISTORY

Mrs. Martino has been employed with the same law firm for 8 years. She left her previous job at the time of her divorce 10 years ago; her ex-husband, Ralph Martino, is an attorney. She lives alone in an apartment not far from the home of her daughter Ann and son-in-law Luke Priestley.

Habits

She has never smoked and uses alcohol only rarely. She takes no daily medications. Her meals are often at irregular times, and she drinks approximately six cans of diet cola each day.

Family History

Her father, aged 76, has osteoarthritis and type 2 diabetes mellitus. Her mother, aged 71, has hypertension and sometimes takes medication for depression. She has three siblings.

Review of Systems

The patient believes that she sometimes feels excessively tired at the end of the day and sometimes awakes in the middle of the night and has trouble getting back to sleep.

- What more do you wish to know about the patient's headaches?
- How would you inquire to learn more about events in her personal life and at work?
- What else would you ask about the family history? Why?
- Are you listening carefully to what the patient is trying to tell you?

Objective

General

Mrs. Martino seems slightly anxious. She uses notes and a calendar while describing her symptoms.

Vital Signs

Height, 5 ft 6 in; weight, 133 lb; blood pressure, 126/82; pulse, 74; temperature, 37.1°C.

Examination

The eyes, ears, nose, and throat are normal, including an unremarkable funduscopic examination. There are no abnormalities of the neck and thyroid. Cranial nerves II to XII are normal. The finger-to-nose test, deep tendon reflexes, and Romberg test are all normal.

LABORATORY

No office laboratory tests are performed at this visit.

- What more—if anything—would you include in the physical examination, and why?
- What additional neurologic tests might be useful?
- What laboratory tests—if any—might be helpful?
- What diagnostic imaging—if any—might be important and cost-effective?

Assessment

- What appears to be Mrs. Martino's problem, and how would you explain it to her?
- What do you think is the patient's chief concern about her headaches? Explain.
- How are her headaches likely to be affecting her life at home and at work?
- What is the possible significance of her tiredness and sleep disturbance?

Plan

- What medical therapy would you recommend today? Why did you choose this regimen?
- What diet and life-style changes would you advise?
- How might you help Mrs. Martino deal with the impact of the headaches on her work?
- If the headaches become more severe or more frequent over the next few months, what would you do then?

8
Hypertension

STEPHEN A. BRUNTON

Despite widespread efforts to improve education and enhance public awareness, up to 33% of persons with hypertension remain undiagnosed, and only about 50% of those known to have hypertension are adequately controlled. The percentages of patients who are aware that they have hypertension, who are treated, and who are controlled have increased since the 1970s (Table 8.1). Most have stage 1 hypertension, and controversy still exists concerning the appropriate approach to these patients. Nonpharmacologic therapy is often the first choice, and this approach continues to evolve.[1] Of the 20 to 30 million hypertensives who receive pharmacologic therapy, fewer than 50% adhere to their therapeutic regimen for more than 1 year, and 60% of these patients reduce the dosage of their drug owing to adverse effects. A negative impact on the patient's quality-of-life may occur as a result of just making the diagnosis. Effects such as increased absenteeism, sickness behavior, hypochondria, and decreased self-esteem have been noted in cohorts of previously well individuals who have been told they were hypertensive.[2] A 1987 survey of physicians revealed that they regarded quality-of-life changes to be the primary impediment to effective pharmacologic treatment of hypertension.

The challenge to the clinician is to provide patient education and develop a hypertension regimen that effectively lowers blood pressure or reduces cardiac risk factors, minimizes changes in concomitant disease states, and maintains or improves quality of life. Putting the patient first necessitates integrating the individual patient's lifestyle and current disease states with a thorough understanding of the effect of drug and nondrug therapy on quality of life. This chapter reviews nonpharmacologic and pharmacologic therapy, with special emphasis on individualizing patient regimens to improve adherence.

Detection

The diagnosis of hypertension should not be based on any single measurement but should be established on the basis of at least three readings with an average systolic blood pressure of 140 mm Hg and a diastolic pressure of 90 mm Hg. Mechanisms should be established to standardize the measurement process: (1)

TABLE 8.1. Trends in the Awareness, Treatment, and Control of High
Blood Pressure in Adults: United States, 1976–94[a]

	NHANES II (1976–80)	NHANES III (Phase 1) 1988–91	NHANES III (Phase 2) 1991–94
Awareness	51%	73%	68.4%
Treatment	31%	55%	53.6%
Control[b]	10%	29%	27.4%

[a]Data are for adults age 18 to 74 years with SBP of 140 mm Hg or greater, DBP of 90 mm
Hg or greater, or taking antihypertensive medication.
[b]SBP below 140 mm Hg and DBP below 90 mm Hg.
Source: National Institutes of Health.[1]

The patient should be seated comfortably with the arm positioned at heart level.
(2) Caffeine or nicotine should not have been ingested within 30 minutes before
measurement. (3) The patient should be seated in a quiet environment for at least
5 minutes. (4) An appropriate sphygmomanometer cuff should be used (i.e., the
rubber bladder should encircle at least two-thirds of the arm). (5) Measurement
of the diastolic blood pressure should be based on the disappearance of sound
(phase V Korotkoff sound). Table 8.2 describes the classification of blood pressure for adults.

TABLE 8.2. Classification of Blood Pressure for Adults Aged 18 Years and Older[a]

Category	Systolic (mm Hg)	Diastolic (mm Hg)
Optimal[b]	<120	<80
Normal	<130	<85
High normal	130–139	85–89
Hypertension[c]		
Stage 1	140–159	90–99
Stage 2	160–179	100–109
Stage 3	>180	>110

Source: National Institutes of Health.[1]
Note: In addition to classifying stages of hypertension based on average blood pressure levels, the clinician should specify the presence or absence of target organ disease and additional
risk factors. For example, a patient with diabetes, a blood pressure of 142/94 mm Hg, and left
ventricular hypertrophy should be classified as "stage 1 hypertension with target organ disease (left ventricular hypertrophy) and with another major risk factor (diabetes)." This specificity is important for risk classification and management.
[a]Not taking antihypertensive drugs and not acutely ill. When systolic and diastolic pressures
fall into different categories, the higher category should be selected to classify the individual's
blood pressure status. For instance, 160/92 mm Hg should be classified as stage 2 and 174/120
mm Hg as stage 3. Isolated systolic hypertension is defined as systolic pressure of 140 mm
Hg or more and diastolic pressure of less than 90 mm Hg and staged appropriately (e.g.,
170/82 mm Hg is defined as stage 2 isolated systolic hypertension).
[b]Optimal blood pressure with respect to cardiovascular risk is systolic pressure <120 mm Hg
and diastolic pressure <80 mm Hg. However, unusually low readings should be evaluated
for clinical significance.
[c]Based on the average of two or more readings taken at each of two or more visits after an
initial screening.

Evaluation

Evaluation is directed toward establishing the etiology of hypertension, identifying other cardiovascular risk factors, and evaluating the possibility of target organ damage. Although most hypertension is considered "essential," primary, or idiopathic, it is necessary to eliminate secondary causes of hypertension, including renovascular disease, polycystic renal disease, aortic coarctation, Cushing syndrome, and pheochromocytoma. It is important to ensure that the patient is not on medications that may result in increased blood pressure, such as oral contraceptives, nasal decongestants, appetite suppressants, nonsteroidal antiinflammatory drugs (NSAIDs), steroids, and tricyclic antidepressants.

Medical History

The medical history should include a review of the family history for hypertension and cardiovascular disease, previous measurements of blood pressure, symptoms suggestive of secondary causes of hypertension, and other cardiovascular risk factors including smoking, hyperlipidemia, obesity, and diabetes. Environmental and psychosocial factors that may influence blood pressure control or the ability of the individual to comply with therapy should also be considered.

Physical Examination and Laboratory Tests

The physical examination should include more than one blood pressure measurement in both standing and seated positions with verification in the contralateral arm. (If a discrepancy exists, the higher value is used.) The rest of the physical examination includes (1) an evaluation of the optic fundi with gradation of hypertensive changes; (2) examination of the neck for bruits and thyromegaly; (3) a heart examination to evaluate for hypertrophy, arrhythmias, or additional sounds; (4) abdominal examination to search for evidence of aneur-ysms or kidney abnormalities; (5) examination of the extremities to check the pulses; and (6) a careful neurologic evaluation.

Some baseline laboratory tests may be helpful for the initial evaluation. They might include urinalysis and serum potassium, blood urea nitrogen, and creatinine levels. A lipid panel may help evaluate cardiovascular risk.

Treatment

The goal of therapy is not just to bring the blood pressure lower than 140 mm Hg systolic and 90 mm Hg diastolic, but rather to prevent the morbidity and mortality associated with hypertension. As such, the decision to treat hypertension is based on documentation that the blood pressure has remained elevated and on assessment of the risk for that particular patient.

In general, individuals with blood pressure ranges considered borderline high (i.e., systolic of 130 to 139 mm Hg or diastolic of 85 to 89 mm Hg) should have their blood pressures rechecked within 1 year. Blood pressures in the stage 1 range should be confirmed within 2 months by repeated measurements; however, certain lifestyle approaches are appropriate even at this level. Blood pressures that are markedly elevated (e.g., systolic >180 mm Hg or diastolic >110 mm Hg) or those associated with evidence of existing end-organ damage may require immediate pharmacologic intervention. In general, whether pharmacologic intervention is initiated, a nonpharmacologic approach is the foundation of any management strategy.[1]

Nonpharmacologic Therapeutic Approaches

Information concerning dietary modifications, exercise, weight reduction, the role of cations, and the possible role of relaxation and stress management techniques for reducing blood pressure have opened the door for greater acceptance of multiple nonpharmacologic approaches to the treatment of hypertension. The 1988 report of the Joint National Committee (JNC) on the Detection, Evaluation, and Treatment of High Blood Pressure recommended that "nonpharmacological approaches be used both as definitive intervention and as an adjunct for pharmacological therapy and should be considered for all antihypertensive therapy."

Several studies have shown positive correlation of increased blood pressure with alcohol consumption of more than 2 ounces/day.[3] Although smoking has not been shown to cause sustained hypertension, it is associated with increased cardiovascular, pulmonary, and hypertension risks, and therefore should be eliminated.[4]

Weight reduction has a strong correlation with decreased blood pressure in obese individuals. Stamler et al[5] reported that a 10-pound weight loss maintained over a 4-year period allowed 50% of participants previously on pharmacologic management to remain normotensive and free of medication.

Sodium restriction has been a mainstay of hypertension control, as a 100 mEq drop in daily intake can result in a 2- to 9-mm Hg decline in systolic blood pressure in salt-sensitive individuals. This goal is one of the easiest for a patient to accomplish, as moderate restriction can be accomplished by eliminating table salt for cooking, avoiding salty foods, and using a salt substitute.[6]

Regular aerobic exercise not only assists with weight reduction but also appears to lower diastolic blood pressure. Cade and associates[7] reported a decline from 117 to 97 mm Hg diastolic blood pressure after 3 months of daily walking or running for 2 miles. This effect appeared to be independent of weight loss, and some benefit persisted even if the patient became sedentary.

Vegetarian diets high in polyunsaturated fats, potassium, and fiber result in lower blood pressures than diets high in saturated fats. Dietary fat control also contributes to the reduction of cholesterol and coronary artery disease risk.[8] The role of cations such as potassium, magnesium, and calcium in lowering blood pressure has now been investigated. High potassium intake (>80 mEq/day) may result in a modest decline in blood pressure while offering a natriuretic and cardioprotective effect. These effects are more pronounced in hypokalemic individuals.[9] Magnesium and calcium supplementation of more than 300 mg/day and 800 mg/day, respectively, have been shown to lower the relative risk of developing hypertension in a large cohort of women. The impact of individual supplementation is less clear, and the role of these substances is still controversial.[10]

Stress management and relaxation techniques over a 4-year period have been shown to reduce systolic blood pressure 10 to 15 mm Hg and diastolic blood pressure 5 to 10 mm Hg. However, these results are variable and are largely dependent on the instructor–patient relationship.[11]

The effects of nonpharmacologic approaches can be additive and certainly are beneficial even if the patient requires drug therapy. Stamler and associates[12] documented that reducing weight and lowering salt and alcohol intake allowed 39% of patients previously on therapy to remain normotensive without medication over a 4-year period. In the mildly hypertensive individual, these lifestyle modifications should be tried for at least 6 months before initiating pharmacologic therapy.

Pharmacologic Therapy

The decision to initiate drug therapy requires consideration of individual patient characteristics, such as age, race, sex, family history, cardiovascular risk factors, concomitant disease states, compliance, and ability to purchase the prescribed therapeutic agent. Pharmacologic therapy is recommended when the systolic blood pressure is higher than 160 mm Hg and the diastolic blood pressure remains higher than 100 mm Hg. Treatment of stage 2 and 3 hypertension (systolic pressure >160 and diastolic pressure >100 mm Hg) has reduced cardiovascular morbidity and mortality dramatically since the 1960s. The incidence of stroke, congestive heart failure, and left ventricular hypertrophy has also decreased among treated stage 1 hypertensives, and therapy is recommended if patients have one or more cardiovascular risk factors and have not controlled their blood pressure after 6 months of lifestyle modification.

The ideal antihypertensive agent would improve quality of life, reduce coronary heart disease risk factors, maintain normal hemodynamic profiles, reduce left ventricular hypertrophy, have a positive impact on concomitant disease states, and reduce end-organ damage while effectively lowering blood pressure on a convenient dosing regimen at minimal cost to the patient. This "magic bullet" has yet to be synthesized, although several of the newer antihypertensive classes offer the possibility of many of these positive outcomes.

The selection of an appropriate antihypertensive agent may be based on the current recommendations of the JNC on the Detection, Evaluation, and Treatment of High Blood Pressure or individualized to the specific medical, social, psychological, and economic situation of each patient.[1] The previous stepped-care approach has been modified by the JNC into an algorithm that permits an individualized approach to the patient (Fig. 8.1). Many clinicians have moved

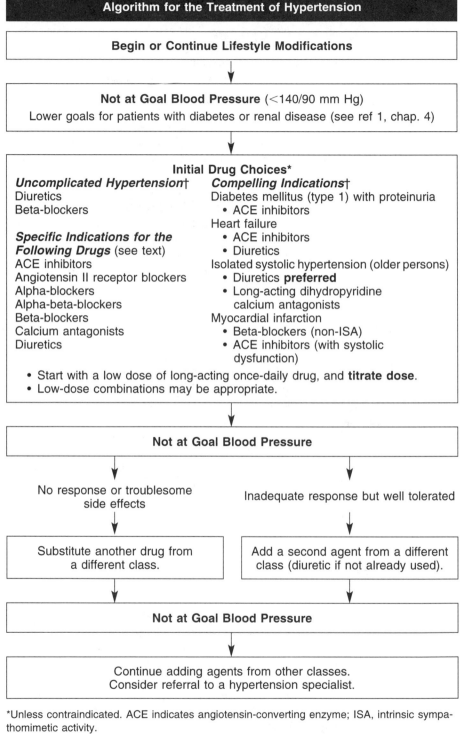

Algorithm for the Treatment of Hypertension

Begin or Continue Lifestyle Modifications

↓

Not at Goal Blood Pressure (<140/90 mm Hg)
Lower goals for patients with diabetes or renal disease (see ref 1, chap. 4)

↓

Initial Drug Choices*

Uncomplicated Hypertension†
Diuretics
Beta-blockers

**Specific Indications for the
Following Drugs** (see text)
ACE inhibitors
Angiotensin II receptor blockers
Alpha-blockers
Alpha-beta-blockers
Beta-blockers
Calcium antagonists
Diuretics

Compelling Indications†
Diabetes mellitus (type 1) with proteinuria
• ACE inhibitors
Heart failure
• ACE inhibitors
• Diuretics
Isolated systolic hypertension (older persons)
• Diuretics **preferred**
• Long-acting dihydropyridine
  calcium antagonists
Myocardial infarction
• Beta-blockers (non-ISA)
• ACE inhibitors (with systolic
  dysfunction)

• Start with a low dose of long-acting once-daily drug, and **titrate dose**.
• Low-dose combinations may be appropriate.

↓

Not at Goal Blood Pressure

↓   ↓

No response or troublesome
side effects

Inadequate response but well tolerated

↓   ↓

Substitute another drug from
a different class.

Add a second agent from a different
class (diuretic if not already used).

↓   ↓

Not at Goal Blood Pressure

↓

Continue adding agents from other classes.
Consider referral to a hypertension specialist.

*Unless contraindicated. ACE indicates angiotensin-converting enzyme; ISA, intrinsic sympathomimetic activity.
†Based on randomized controlled trials (see ref. 1, chaps. 3 and 4).

away from the stepped-care philosophy toward a monotherapy approach, which maximizes the dose of one drug before substituting or adding another. Combination therapy with lower doses of several agents may also be utilized to minimize adverse effects. Therapeutic choices must be based on a sound understanding of the mechanism of action, pharmacokinetics, adverse effect profile, and cost of available agents.

Major Antihypertensive Classes

ACE Inhibitors

Angiotensin-converting enzyme (ACE) inhibitors (Table 8.3) block the conversion of angiotensin I to angiotensin II, resulting in decreased aldosterone production with subsequent increased sodium and water excretion. Renin and potassium levels are usually increased as a result of this medication. The hemodynamic response includes decreased peripheral resistance, increased renal blood flow, and minimal changes in cardiac output and glomerular filtration rate. There is little change in insulin and glucose levels or in the lipid fractions. The adverse effects of ACE inhibitors include cough (1–30%), headache, dizziness, first-dose syncope in salt- or volume-depleted patients, acute renal failure in patients with renal artery stenosis, angioedema (0.1–0.2%), and teratogenic effects in the human fetus. Thus, ACE inhibitors should not be used during the second and third trimesters of pregnancy. Captopril (Capoten) has a higher incidence of rash, dysgeusia, neutropenia, and proteinuria than the others due to a sulfhydryl group in the ring structure.[13]

The ACE inhibitors are good first-line agents for patients with diabetes, congestive heart failure, peripheral vascular disease, elevated lipids, and renal insufficiency. This class is effective in all races and ages, although black patients respond better with the addition of a diuretic.[14,15]

Angiotensin Receptor Antagonists

Angiotensin receptor antagonists, a newer class of antihypertensive agents, binds to the angiotensin II receptors, resulting in blockade of the vasoconstrictor and aldosterone-secreting effects of angiotensin II. In addition, bradykinin production is not stimulated. The first agent available in the United States was losartan (Cozaar). The physiologic effects of losartan include a rise in plasma renin and angiotensin II levels and a decrease in aldosterone production. There is no significant change in plasma potassium levels and no effect on glomerular filtration rate, renal plasma flow, heart rate, triglycerides, total cholesterol, high-density

FIGURE 8.1. Algorithm for the treatment of hypertension. (From National Institutes of Health.[1])

TABLE 8.3. Antihypertensive Drugs

Drug class	Available doses (mg)	Usual dose/schedule (mg/day)	Half-life (hours)	Peak (hours)	Pregnancy class
ACE inhibitors					
Benazepril (Lotensin)	5, 10, 20, 40	10–40 qd	10	2–4	C (1st trimester) D (2nd and 3rd trimester)
Captopril (Capoten)	12.5, 25, 50, 100	25–50 bid–tid	2	1–2	C (1st trimester) D (2nd and 3rd trimester)
Enalapril (Vasotec)	2.5, 5, 10, 20	5–40 qd	11	4	C (1st trimester) D (2nd and 3rd trimester)
Fosinopril (Monopril)	10, 20	10–40 qd	12	2–6	C (1st trimester) D (2nd and 3rd trimester)
Lisinopril (Prinivil, Zestril)	2.5, 5, 10, 20, 40	10–40 qd	12	6	C (1st trimester) D (2nd and 3rd trimester)
Moexipril (Univasc)	7.5, 15	7.5–30 qd	2–10	1.5	C (1st trimester) D (2nd and 3rd trimester)
Quinapril (Accupril)	5, 10, 20, 40	10–80 qd	2	2–4	C (1st trimester) D (2nd and 3rd trimester)
Perindopril (Aceon)	2, 4, 8,	4–8qd	3–10	3–7	C (1st trimester) D (2nd and 3rd trimester)
Ramipril (Altace)	1.25, 2.5, 5, 10	2.5–20 qd	2	3–6	C (1st trimester) D (2nd and 3rd trimester)
Trandolapril (Mavik)	1, 2, 4	2–4 mg qd	10	4–10	C (1st trimester) D (2nd and 3rd trimester)
				Selectivity	
Beta-Blockers					
Atenolol (Tenormin)	25, 50, 100	50–100 qd	9	B_1	C
Acebutolol (Sectral)	200, 400	400–800 qd	4	B_1, ISA	B
Betaxolol (Kerlone)	10, 20	10–20 qd	22	B_1	C
Bisoprolol (Zebeta)	5, 10	5–20 qd	11	B_1	C
Carteolol (Cartrol)	2.5, 5	2.5–10 qd	6	B_1, B_2, ISA	C
Labetalol (Normodyne)	100, 200, 300	100–400 bid	6	B_1, B_2, α	C
Nadolol (Corgard)	20, 40, 80, 120, 160	40–80 qd	24	B_1, B_2	C
Metoprolol (Lopressor)	50, 100	100–450 qd	3	B_1	C

Penbutolol (Levatol)	20	20–80 qd	5	B_1, B_2, ISA	C
Pindolol (Visken)	5, 10	10–30 qd	4	B_1, B_2, ISA	B
Propranolol (Inderal)	60, 80, 120, 160, SR;	80–160 SR qd	10	B_1, B_2	C
	10, 20, 40, 60, 80, 90	20–120 bid	4		C
Timolol (Blocadren)	5, 10, 20	10–30 bid	4	B_1, B_2	C
Calcium entry antagonists					
Amlodipine (Norvasc)	2.5, 5, 10	2.5–10		6–12	C
Diltiazem (Cardizem)	SR 60, 90, 120	SR 60–120 bid	6	6–11	C
	CD 120, 180, 240, 300	CD 180–360 qd		12	
	30, 60, 90, 120,	30–90 qid		2–3	
(Dilacor XR)	120, 180, 240	120–360 qd	4	4–6	C
Felodipine (Plendil)	SR 2.5, 5, 10	5–20 qd	16	2–5	C
Isradipine (DynaCirc)	2.5, 5	2.5–5 bid	8	1.5	C
Nicardipine	SR 30, 45, 60	SR 30–60 bid	4	0.5–2	C
(Cardene)	20, 30	20–40 tid	5	0.5–6	
Nifedipine	SR 10, 20, 30, 60, 90	30–120 qd		6–12	C
(Adalat Procardia)					
Nisoldipine (Sular)	10, 20, 30, 40	20–40 qd	10	1–2	C
Verapamil (Calan,	SR 120, 180, 240	240–480 qd	7		C
Covera, Isoptin,	40, 80, 120				
Verelan)					
α_1-blockers					
Doxazosin (Cardura)	1, 2, 4, 8	1–16 mg qd	22	2–3	B
Prazosin (Minipress)	1, 2, 5	1–5 bid–tid	3	3	C
Terazosin (Hytrin)	1, 2, 5, 10	1–10 qd	12	1–2	C
Central α_2-agonists					
Clonidine (Catapres)	0.1, 0.2, 0.3;	0.2–1.2 qd	16	3–5	C
	TTS 1, 2, 3	1 patch weekly	19	2–3 days	
Guanabenz (Wytensin)	4, 8	4–8 bid	6	2–4	C
Guanfacine (Tenex)	1, 2	1–3 qd	17	3	B
Methyldopa (Aldomet)	125, 250, 500	250–500 tid–qid	2	2–4	B

TABLE 8.3. Antihypertensive Drugs (*Continued*)

Drug class	Available doses (mg)	Usual dose/ schedule (mg/day)	Half-life (hours)	Peak (hours)	Pregnancy class
Vasodilators					
Hydralazine (Apresoline)	10, 25, 50, 100	10–50 qid	7	0.5–2	C
Minoxidil (Loniten)	2.5, 10	10–40 qd	4	2–3	C
αβ-Blockers					
Carvedilol (Coreg)	6.25, 12.5, 25	6.25–12.5 bid	7	3–4	C
Labetalol (Normodyne)	100, 200, 300	100 mg–400 bid	6	2–4	C
Selected thiazide diuretics					
Chlorothiazide (Diuril)	250–500	500–2000 qd	6–12	4	
Hydrochlorothiazide (HydroDIURIL)	25, 50, 100	25–50 qd	6–12	4–6	
Chlorthalidone (Hygroton)	25, 50, 100	25–100 qd	24–72	2–6	
Indapamide (Lozol)	1.25, 2.5	2.5–5 qd	36	2	B
Metolazone (Zaroxolyn)	0.5, 2.5, 5, 10	2.5–5 qd	12–24	2.6	B
Loop diuretics					
Bumetanide (Bumex)	0.5, 1, 2	0.5–2 qd	4–6	1–2	C
Furosemide (Lasix)	20, 40, 80	20–40 qd–bid	6–8	1–2	C

Potassium-sparing diuretics

Amiloride (Midamor)	5	5–20 qd	24	6–10	B
Spironolactone (Aldactone)	25, 50, 100	25–100 qd	48–72	48–72	D
Triamterene (Dyrenium)	50, 100	100 bid	12–16	6–8	B
Angiotensin receptor antagonists					
Eprosartan (Teveten)	400, 600	400–800 qd	5–9	3–6	C (1st trimester) D (2nd and 3rd trimester)
Irbesartan (Avapro)	75, 150, 300	150–300 qd	11–15	3–6	C (1st trimester) D (2nd and 3rd trimester)
Losartan (Cozaar)	25, 50	25–100 qd	2–9	1–4	C (1st trimester) D (2nd and 3rd trimester)
Telmisartan (Micardis)	20, 40, 80	20–80 qd	24	0.5–1	C (1st trimester) D (2nd and 3rd trimester)
Valsartan (Diovan)	80, 160	80–320 qd	6	2–4	C (1st trimester) D (2nd and 3rd trimester)

ISA = Intrinsic sympathomimetic activity; D = positive evidence of human fetal risk; C = fetal risk documented in animals; B = low fetal risk; SR = slow release; CD = controlled delivery.

lipoprotein (HDL) cholesterol, or glucose. Losartan use does produce a small uricosuric effect with lowering of plasma uric acid levels.

These agents are effective antihypertensives in adults and the elderly. Blood pressure–lowering effects are not as significant in black patients. Adverse effects include muscle pain, dizziness, cough, insomnia, and nasal congestion. As with ACE inhibitors, angiotensin receptor antagonists should not be used during the second and third trimesters of pregnancy.

At this time the role of angiotensin receptor antagonists is not completely defined. Further study of the hemodynamic effects in large populations is needed to determine the role in cardiac patients. These agents are an alternative antihypertensive agent for patients experiencing adverse effects from ACE inhibitors.

Calcium Entry Antagonists

Calcium entry antagonists (CEAs) inhibit the movement of calcium across cell membranes in myocardial and smooth muscles. This action dilates coronary arteries, and additional peripheral arteriole dilation reduces total peripheral resistance, resulting in decreased blood pressure. Although the mechanism of action for lowering blood pressure is similar for these agents, structural differences result in varying effects on cardiac conduction and adverse effect profiles. Verapamil (Calan, Covera, Isoptin, Verelan) and diltiazem (Cardizem, Dilacor, Tiazac) slow atrioventricular (AV) node conduction and prolong the effective refractory period in the AV node. Cardiac output is increased by nifedipine (Procardia), nicardipine (Cardene), isradipine (DynaCirc), and felodipine (Plendil).

The calcium entry antagonists are contraindicated in patients with heart block, cardiogenic shock, or acute myocardial infarction. Common adverse effects include peripheral edema, dizziness, headache, asthenia, nausea, constipation, flushing, and tachycardia. Calcium entry antagonists have no significant impact on lipid profiles or glucose metabolism.[1]

These agents are effective at all ages and in all races. They are good choices for patients with diabetes, angina, migraine, chronic obstructive pulmonary disease (COPD)/asthma, peripheral vascular disease, renal insufficiency, and supraventricular arrhythmias.[14,15]

Diuretics

Thiazide, loop, and potassium-sparing diuretics have been the mainstay of antihypertensive therapy since the 1960s. They remain as first-line agents in the JNC VI approach, although the ACE inhibitors and calcium entry antagonists are rapidly replacing diuretics as monotherapy for hypertension.

Thiazide diuretics increase renal excretion of sodium and chloride at the distal segment of the renal tubule, resulting in decreased plasma volume, cardiac output, and renal blood flow and increased renin activity. Potassium excretion is increased, and calcium and uric acid elimination is decreased.[13] Thiazides adversely affect lipid metabolism by increasing the total cholesterol level 6% to

10% and the low-density lipoprotein (LDL) cholesterol 6% to 20%, and by causing a possible 15% to 20% rise in triglycerides.[15] Plasma glucose levels increase
secondary to a decrease in insulin secretion. Clinical adverse effects include nausea, vomiting, diarrhea, dizziness, headache, fatigue, muscle cramps, gout attacks, and impotence. Thiazides are inexpensive choices for initial therapy, but
caution must be exercised in patients with preexisting cardiac dysfunction, lipid
abnormalities, diabetes mellitus, and gout. The lowest effective dose is recommended to minimize these potential adverse effects. Suggested daily doses are
hydrochlorothiazide (HydroDIURIL) 25 mg, chlorthalidone (Hygroton) 25 mg,
and indapamide (Lozol) 2.5 mg daily. Indapamide is unique among thiazides in
that it has minimal effects on glucose, lipids, and uric acid. Thiazides are good
choices for volume/salt-dependent, low-renin hypertensives. Thiazides improve
blood pressure control when added to ACE inhibitors, beta-blockers, vasodilators, and alpha-blockers.

The loop diuretics—furosemide (Lasix), torsemide (Demadex), and
bumetanide (Bumex)—inhibit sodium and chloride reabsorption in the proximal
and distal tubules and the loop of Henle. These diuretics are effective in patients
with decreased renal function. The primary adverse effects include ototoxicity
with high doses in patients with severe renal disease and in combination with an
aminoglycoside, photosensitivity, excess potassium loss, increased serum uric
acid, decreased calcium levels, and impaired glucose metabolism. Patients may
experience nausea, vomiting, diarrhea, headache, blurred vision, tinnitus, muscle cramps, fatigue, or weakness. Furosemide and bumetanide are utilized in patients with compromised renal function or congestive heart failure (CHF) and as
adjuncts to volume-retaining agents such as hydralazine (Apresoline) and minoxidil (Loniten).

The potassium-sparing diuretics spironolactone (Aldactone), triamterene
(Dyrenium), and amiloride (Midamor) are useful for preventing potassium
wastage from thiazide and loop diuretics. Spironolactone competitively inhibits
the uptake of aldosterone at the receptor site in the distal tubule, thereby reducing aldosterone effects. It is used for treatment of primary aldosteronism, CHF,
cirrhosis with ascites, hypertension, and hirsutism. Triamterene is used in combination with hydrochlorothiazide as Dyazide or Maxzide and effectively prevents potassium loss. Amiloride inhibits potassium excretion at the collecting
duct. Adverse reactions associated with spironolactone include gynecomastia,
nausea, vomiting, diarrhea, muscle cramps, lethargy, and hyperkalemia. Triamterene and amiloride have adverse effects similar to those seen with the thiazide diuretics.[13–15]

Antiadrenergic Agents

BETA-BLOCKERS

β-adrenergic blocking agents compete with β-agonists for B_1 receptors in cardiac muscles and B_2 receptors in the bronchial and vascular musculature, in-

hibiting the dilator, inotropic, and chronotropic effects of β-adrenergic stimulation. Clinical responses to β-adrenergic blockade include decreased heart rate, cardiac output, blood pressure, renin production, and bronchiolar constriction; there is also an initial increase in total peripheral resistance, which returns to normal with chronic use.

Beta-blockers are contraindicated for sinus bradycardia, second- or third-degree heart block, cardiogenic shock, cardiac failure, and severe COPD/asthma. The adverse effect profile of beta-blocking agents is partially dependent on their receptor selectivity (Table 8.3). Acebutolol (Sectral), penbutolol (Levatol), carteolol (Cartrol), and pindolol (Visken) have intrinsic sympathomimetic activity (ISA), resulting in less effect on cardiac output and lipid profiles. Beta-blockers without ISA slow the heart rate, decrease cardiac output, increase peripheral vascular resistance, and cause bronchospasm. Common adverse effects include fatigue, impotence, depression, shortness of breath, cold extremities, cough, drowsiness, and dizziness. The more lipid-soluble agents, such as propranolol and metoprolol, have a higher incidence of central nervous system (CNS) effects. In diabetic patients beta-blockers may mask the usual symptoms of hypoglycemia, such as tremor, tachycardia, and hunger.[13] Increased triglycerides (30%) and decreased HDL cholesterol (1–20%) occur with non-ISA agents.[15] Beta-blockers are effective agents in the young and white populations. Black patients may not respond as well to monotherapy because of their lower renin levels. Beta-blockers are good choices for patients with supraventricular tachycardia, high cardiac output, angina, recent myocardial infarction, migraine, and glaucoma. Caution should be exercised in those with diabetes, CHF, peripheral vascular disease, COPD/asthma, and an elevated lipid profile.[14]

CENTRAL ACTING DRUGS

Methyldopa (Aldomet), clonidine (Catapres), guanfacine (Tenex), and guanabenz (Wytensin) are central α_2-agonists. These agents decrease dopamine and norepinephrine production in the brain, resulting in a decrease in sympathetic nervous activity throughout the body. Blood pressure declines with the decrease in peripheral resistance. Methyldopa exhibits a unique adverse effect profile as it induces autoimmune disorders, such as those with positive Coombs' and antinuclear antibody (ANA) tests, hemolytic anemia, and hepatic necrosis. The other agents produce sedation, dry mouth, and dizziness. Abrupt clonidine withdrawal may result in rebound hypertension. These drugs are good choices for patients with asthma, diabetes, high cholesterol, and peripheral vascular disease.

PERIPHERAL ACTING DRUGS

Guanadrel (Hylorel), reserpine (Serpasil), and guanethidine (Ismelin) are peripheral antiadrenergic agents. Their mechanism of action is at the storage granule level of norepinephrine release. They are infrequently chosen because of their significant side effects, which include profound hypotension, sedation, depression, and impotence.

α_1-Blockers

α_1-Receptor blockers have an affinity for the α_1-receptor on vascular smooth muscles, thereby blocking the uptake of catecholamines by smooth muscle cells. This action results in peripheral vasodilation. The currently available agents are prazosin (Minipress), terazosin (Hytrin), and doxazosin (Cardura). There is a marked reduction in blood pressure with the first dose of these drugs. It is recommended that they be started with 1 mg at bedtime and titrate slowly upward over 2 to 4 weeks. When adding a second antihypertensive the α-blocker dose should be decreased and titrated upward again. Often a diuretic is added to α_1-blocker therapy to reduce sodium and water retention. The primary adverse effects of these three drugs are dizziness, sedation, nasal congestion, headache, and postural effects. They do not significantly affect lipids, glucose, electrolytes, or exercise tolerance. α_1-Blockers are good choices for young active adults and patients with diabetes, renal insufficiency, CHF, peripheral vascular disease, COPD/asthma, or elevated lipids.

The Antihypertensive and Lipid Lowering Treatment to Prevent Heart Attack Trial (ALLHAT) was initiated in 1994 to evaluate the impact of various classes of antihypertensives on outcomes. In early 2000 the doxazosin treatment arm was discontinued because a twofold higher incidence of CHF was noted compared to those on chlorthalidone.[16]

Vasodilators

The two direct vasodilators, hydralazine (Apresoline) and minoxidil (Loniten), dilate peripheral arterioles, resulting in a significant fall in blood pressure. A sympathetic reflex increase in heart rate, renin and catecholamine release, and venous constriction occur. The renal response includes sodium and water retention. The patient often experiences tachycardia, flushing, and headache. Addition of a diuretic and a beta-blocker relieves the major adverse effects of the vasodilators. Hydralazine may cause a lupus-like reaction with fever, rash, and joint pain. Chronic use of minoxidil often results in hirsutism with increased facial and arm hair. These drugs are third- or fourth-line agents because of their adverse side-effect profile.[13–15]

Quality-of-Life Issues

The need for lifestyle changes and probable drug therapy increases the possibility that the patient's quality of life will be altered. The adverse physical, mental, and metabolic effects of antihypertensive therapy results in significant nonadherence to prescribed regimens. In 1982 Jachuck and associates[17] investigated the effect of medications on their patients by asking them, their closest relatives, and their physicians a series of questions concerning their quality of life since starting the blood pressure medications. The physicians and patients thought there was either no change or improvement, whereas 99% of the relatives thought the patients were worse. They cited side effects such as memory loss, irritability, decreased libido, hypochondria, and decreased energy as major problems.[17] Other studies during the 1980s confirm that nonselective beta-blockers, diuretics, and methyldopa compromised quality of life to a far greater extent than ACE inhibitors or calcium entry antagonists.[17–19] Further research in this area is necessary to assist the physician in determining the optimum strategy for blood pressure control to improve adherence and quality of life.

Antihypertensive Selection

It is important to consider the patient's lifestyle, economic status, belief systems, and concerns about treatment when selecting an antihypertensive agent. Therapy should be initiated with one drug in small doses to minimize adverse effects. It is important to educate the patient about the long-term benefits of therapy, including the decreased incidence of stroke and renal and cardiac disease. Adequate follow-up visits are scheduled to assess adherence and adverse effects. During these visits the patient is asked to describe the mental, physical, and emotional changes that have occurred as a result of therapy. If adverse effects are bothersome, consider an alternative selection from a different drug class and attempt to maintain monotherapy. If a second drug is needed, agents can be combined that improve efficacy without significantly altering the adverse-effect profile (e.g., adding a diuretic to an ACE inhibitor).

There are some special considerations when prescribing medications. Concomitant disease states must be considered and drugs selected that either improve or at least maintain the current clinical condition. Hypertension is a major risk factor for thrombotic and hemorrhagic strokes; smoking, CHF, diabetes, and coronary artery disease increase the risk. Patients with coronary artery disease may benefit from a calcium entry antagonist or beta-blocker with ISA to decrease anginal pain while resulting in minimal changes in lipid profiles. CHF and hypertension respond well to ACE inhibitors and diuretic therapy. Diabetes may be adversely affected by thiazide diuretics and beta-blockers. ACE inhibitors, calcium entry antagonists, and central α_2-agonists are appropriate choices.

Patients with severe renal disease are most effectively treated with loop diuretics, whereas ACE inhibitors and CEAs may decrease proteinuria and slow the progress of renal failure. As renal function declines, ACE inhibitors must be used with some caution as increased potassium and decreased renal perfusion may occur. A few agents such as methyldopa, clonidine, atenolol, nadolol, and captopril need dosage reduction in the presence of renal failure.

Asthma and COPD patients may be effectively treated with calcium entry antagonists, central α_2-agonists, and α_1-blockers. Beta-blockers and possibly diuretics should be avoided because they might exacerbate bronchospasm.

The elderly are of special concern when selecting an antihypertensive. They have decreased receptor sensitivity, changing baroreceptor response, atherosclerosis, decreased myocardial function, declining total body water, decreased renal function, and memory loss. Blood pressure should be lowered cautiously using smaller than normal doses that are slowly titrated upward. Calcium entry antagonists, ACE inhibitors, and diuretics are possible choices for the elderly. Beta-blockers are effective in the elderly especially in conjunction with diuretics. Larger doses may result in declining mental function, depression, fatigue, and impotence. α_1-Blockers and central α_2-agonists may be used with caution. First-dose syncope and sedation are the major concerns (see Chapter 5).

Black patients may not respond as well to ACE inhibitors or beta-blockers as other races, perhaps due in part to low renin, salt/volume-dependent hypertension. Thiazide diuretics may adversely affect diabetes, gout, and lipids. Calcium entry antagonists, α_1-blockers, central α_2-agonists, and ACE inhibitors are possible choices.

Young women with hyperdynamic hypertension may respond best to a beta-blocker to slow the heart rate and relieve symptoms of stress. An active young man would be better served with an ACE inhibitor, calcium entry antagonist, or alpha-blocker, as beta-blockers and diuretics may cause impotence and exercise intolerance.[14]

Severe Hypertension and Emergencies

Patients with a diastolic blood pressure (DBP) over 115 mm Hg must be treated upon diagnosis. The blood pressure should be lowered in 5- to 10-mm Hg increments with a goal of lowering it to less than 100 mm Hg after several weeks of therapy. Often more than one drug must be used initially to control the blood pressure. A hypertensive emergency exists if the DBP is over 130 mm Hg and evidence of end-organ damage exists, such as retinal hemorrhage, encephalopathy, pulmonary edema, myocardial infarction, or unstable angina. Drugs available for treatment in this situation include sodium nitroprusside, nitroglycerin, hydralazine, phentolamine, labetalol, and methyldopa. Patients must be hospitalized for appropriate monitoring. Hypertensive urgency exists when the DBP is over 115 mm Hg without evidence of end-organ damage. Oral agents such as clonidine, captopril, and minoxidil may be used to lower the DBP 10 to 15 mm Hg over several hours.[1] Nifedipine should not be used in this situation as many serious adverse events have been reported including severe hypotension, acute myocardial infarction, and death.[20]

Conclusion

Pharmacologic management of hypertension challenges the physician to understand the patient's social, psychological, and economic status in order to select an antihypertensive regimen that effectively lowers the blood pressure, alleviates concomitant disease states, and allows easy adherence to the regimen. Continual assessment of therapy is necessary to determine the effectiveness of the regimen, adverse side effects, and the patient's quality-of-life issues.

Acknowledgment

The assistance of Janet Pick-Whitsitt, Pharm. D., with Table 8.3 is gratefully acknowledged.

References

1. National Institutes of Health. Sixth Report of the Joint National Committee on Detection, Evaluation, and Treatment of High Blood Pressure. National High Blood Pressure Education. NIH publication no. 98-4080. Bethesda: National Heart, Lung and Blood Institute, 1997.
2. Haynes RB, Sackett DL, Taylor DW, et al. Increased absenteeism from work after detection and labeling of hypertensive patients. N Engl J Med 1978;297:741–4.
3. Gordon T, Doyle JT. Alcohol consumption and its relationship to smoking, weight, blood pressure, and blood lipids. Arch Intern Med 1986;146:262–5.
4. Pooling Project Research Group. Relationship of blood pressure, serum cholesterol, smoking habit, relative weight and ECG abnormalities to incidence of major coronary events. J Chronic Dis 1978;31:201–6.
5. Stamler J, Farinaro E, Majonnier LM, et al. Prevention and control of hypertension by nutritional-hygienic means. JAMA 1980;243:1819–23.
6. Rose G, Stamler J. The Intersalt Study: background, methods and main results: Intersalt Cooperative Research Group. J Hum Hypertens 1989;3:283–8.
7. Cade R, Mars D, Wagemaker H, et al. Effect of aerobic exercise training on patients with systemic arterial hypertension. Am J Med 1984;77:785–90.
8. Margetts BM, Beilin LJ, Armstrong BK. A randomized control trial of a vegetarian diet in the treatment of mild hypertension. Clin Exp Pharmacol Physiol 1985;12:263–6.
9. Kaplan NM. Non-drug treatment of hypertension. Ann Intern Med 1985;102:359–73.
10. Witteman JC, Willett WC, Stampfer MJ, et al. A prospective study of nutritional factors and hypertension among US women. Circulation 1989;80:1320–7.
11. Patel C, Marmot MG. Stress management, blood pressure and quality of life. J Hypertens 1987;5(suppl 1):521–8.
12. Stamler R, Stamler J, Grimm R, et al. Nutritional therapy for high blood pressure. JAMA 1987;257:1484–91.
13. American Hospital Formulary Service Drug Information. Bethesda: American Society of Hospital Pharmacists, 2001.
14. Kaplan NM. Clinical hypertension, 7th ed. Baltimore: Williams & Wilkins, 1998.
15. Houston MC. New insights and new approaches for the treatment of essential hypertension: selection of therapy based on coronary heart disease, risk factor analysis, hemodynamic profiles, quality of life and subsets of hypertension. Am Heart J 1989;117:911–51.
16. ALLHAT Collaborative Research Group. Major cardiovascular events in hypertensive patients randomized to doxazosin vs. chlorthalidone: the antihypertensive and

lipid-lowering treatment to prevent heart attack trial (ALLHAT) JAMA 1999;283(15):1967–75.

17. Jachuck SJ, Brierly H, Jachuck S, et al. The effect of hypotensive drugs on quality of life. J R Coll Gen Pract 1982;32:103–5.

18. Croog SH, Levine S, Testa MA, et al. The effects of antihypertensive therapy on the quality of life. N Engl J Med 1986;314:1657–64.

19. Steiner SS, Friedhoff AJ, Wilson BL, et al. Antihypertensive therapy and quality of life: a comparison of atenolol, captopril, enalapril and propranolol. J Hum Hypertens 1990;4:217–25.

20. Grossman E, Messerli FH, Grodzicki T. Should a moratorium be placed on sublingual nifedipine capsules given for hypertensive emergencies and pseudoemergencies? JAMA 1996;276(16):1328–31.

CASE PRESENTATION

Subjective

PATIENT PROFILE

Mary Nelson is a 71-year-old married female retired teacher.

PRESENTING PROBLEM

High blood pressure.

PRESENT ILLNESS

Mrs. Nelson is here for continuing care of hypertension, which has been present since age 61. She currently takes 25 mg hydrochlorothiazide daily and feels well. Her last periodic health examination with laboratory tests and x-ray was 2 years ago.

PAST MEDICAL HISTORY

She had an abdominal hysterectomy for fibroids at age 50 and is currently taking no estrogen replacement. She has been treated for depression at times but is taking no medication now.

SOCIAL HISTORY

She retired as a middle school history teacher at age 62. She lives with her husband, Harold, aged 76, whom you recently treated for urinary incontinence (see Chapter 5), and son Samuel, aged 48.

HABITS

She does not use alcohol or tobacco. She drinks one cup of coffee daily.

FAMILY HISTORY

She is an orphan, adopted in infancy, and her biological parents are unknown. She and her husband, Harold, had four children. Three are living and have no serious illnesses; their son Samuel, aged 48, has COPD.

REVIEW OF SYSTEMS

She sleeps poorly and wakes early in the morning, unable to fall asleep again. She feels tired throughout the day and occasionally is inappropriately sad.

- What additional medical history might be helpful, and why?
- What questions might help elucidate target organ damage related to hypertension or problems with medication?
- What are possible reasons why the patient is not taking antidepressant medication, and how would you address this issue?
- Have you listened carefully to everything Mrs. Nelson would like to tell you today?

Objective

VITAL SIGNS

Height, 5 ft 3 in; weight, 122 lb; blood pressure, 162/84; pulse, 72.

EXAMINATION

The patient's affect seems somewhat dull and flat compared with previous visits. The head, eyes, ears, nose, and throat are normal. The neck and thyroid gland are normal. Her chest is clear to percussion and auscultation. The heart has a regular sinus rhythm with no murmurs.

- Is there any additional information regarding the physical examination that might be helpful, and why?
- What other areas of the body—if any—should be examined today?
- What—if any—laboratory tests should be obtained today?
- What—if any—diagnostic imaging should be obtained today?

Assessment

- What is the current status of Mrs. Nelson's hypertension? How would you explain this to the patient?
- Describe the pathophysiology of hypertension in the elderly patient. How might this influence your choice of therapy?
- What is the apparent status of her recurrent depression, and how would you explain this to the patient?
- What are some possible adaptations of this patient to her illnesses, and how might these be important in care?

Plan

- What would be your therapeutic recommendations today regarding diet and medication?
- What are possible interrelationships of Mrs. Nelson's problems and the medications that might be used to treat them?
- If Mrs. Nelson is your patient in a capitated plan for which you are a case manager, how might this influence your thinking and actions?
- What continuing care would you recommend for this patient?

9

Sinusitis and Pharyngitis

PAUL EVANS AND WILLIAM F. MISER

Sinusitis

Sinusitis, or rhinosinusitis, is a common problem, with 25 million office visits per year in the United States and over $7 billion in direct costs.[1] It is primarily caused by ostial obstruction of the anterior ethmoid and middle meatal complex due to retained secretions, edema, or polyps. Barotrauma, nasal cannulation, or ciliary transport defects can also precipitate infection.[2] Most sinusitis is handled well at the primary care level; there appear to be few discernible differences in technical efficiency between generalists and specialists in its treatment.[3]

Classification and Diagnosis

There are four classification categories, all of which have similar signs and symptoms but varying durations and recurrence rates. Signs and symptoms associated with sinusitis include major and minor types. Two or more major, or one major and two or more minor, or nasal purulence typify all rhinosinusitis classifications. Major symptoms include facial pain and pressure, nasal obstruction, nasal or postnasal discharge, hyposmia, and fever (in acute sinusitis). Minor signs and symptoms include headache, fever (other than acute sinusitis), halitosis, fatigue, dental pain, cough, and ear fullness or pain.[4,5] *Acute sinusitis* lasts up to 4 weeks. *Subacute sinusitis* lasts 4 to <12 weeks and resolves completely after treatment. *Recurrent acute sinusitis* has four or more episodes per year, each lasting a week or longer, with clearing between episodes. *Chronic sinusitis* lasts 12 weeks or longer.

Clinical Presentation

Pain is localized by sinus involvement: frontal sinus pain in the lower forehead, maxillary sinus in the cheek and upper teeth, ethmoidal sinus in the retro-orbital and lateral aspect of the nose, sphenoid sinus in the skull vertex.[6] Maxillary sinuses are most commonly infected, followed by ethmoidal, sphenoidal, and frontal sinuses.[7] Sneezing, watery rhinorrhea, and conjunctivitis may be seen in sinusitis associated with an allergy.

Physical Findings

Examination reveals nasal mucosal erythema and edema with purulent nasal discharge. Palpatory or percussive tenderness over the involved sinuses, particularly the frontal and maxillary sinuses, is common. Drainage from the maxillary and frontal sinuses may be seen at the middle meatus. The ethmoids drain from either the middle meatus (anterior ethmoid) or superior meatus (posterior ethmoid). The sphenoid drains into the superior meatus.[8]

Diagnostic Imaging and Laboratory Studies

Definitive diagnosis is based on clinical presentation. No imaging studies or laboratory studies are recommended for the routine diagnosis of uncomplicated sinusitis.[1] In unusual or recurrent cases, plain sinus radiographs may show air-fluid levels, mucosal thickening, and anatomic abnormalities that predispose to the condition. Views specific to each sinus are the Caldwell (frontal), Waters (maxillary), lateral (sphenoid), and submentovertical (ethmoid).[9] Computed tomography (CT) is more sensitive and may better reveal pathology, with focused sinus CT now a cost-competitive alternative to plain films.[10,11] The severity of symptoms does not correlate with severity of CT findings.[12]

Microbiology

Bacterial pathogens responsible for acute sinusitis commonly include *Streptococcus pneumoniae, Haemophilus influenzae,* group A streptococci, and *Moraxella catarrhalis.* Less commonly *Staphylococcus aureus, Streptococcus pyogenes, Mycoplasma pneumoniae,* and *Chlamydia pneumoniae* are seen. Anaerobic organisms include *Peptostreptococcus, Corynebacterium, Bacteroides,* and *Veillonella.*[13,14] Adenovirus, parainfluenza, rhinovirus, and influenza virus may cause or exacerbate sinusitis. *Aspergillus fumigatus* and *Mucormycosis* can cause sinusitis, especially in those who are immunocompromised.[9] The immunocompromised patient also has a higher susceptibility to common pathogens.[15]

Nonmicrobiologic Causes

Sinusitis may be a complication of allergic rhinitis, foreign bodies, deviated nasal septum, nasal packing, dental procedures, facial fractures, tumors, barotraumas, and nasal polyps. The cause appears to be stasis of normal physiologic sinus drainage.[16] Prolonged nasal intubation may also be associated with sinusitis (presumably by the same mechanism) with subsequent infection by *S. aureus, Enter-*

obacter, Pseudomonas aeruginosa, Bacteroides fragilis, Bacteroides melanino-genicus, and *Candida* sp.[2]

Treatment

Initial treatment of acute sinusitis is controversial. Almost two thirds of primary care patients with an upper respiratory infection (URI) expect antibiotics.[17] Since viruses frequently cause acute sinusitis, some authors advocate no antibiotic treatment if the condition is not severe, wanes in 5 to 7 days, and resolves in 10 days ("watchful waiting").[18] If symptoms persist, antibiotics, decongestants, and non-pharmacologic measures should be used to maintain adequate sinus drainage.

ANTIBIOTICS (TABLE 9.1)[19]

For patients with no antibiotics use in the prior 30 days and in areas where drug-resistant *Streptococcus pneumoniae* (DRSP) is $\leq$ 30%, use either amoxicillin, amoxicillin-clavulanate, cefdinir, cefpodoxime, or cefuroximine axetil. If DSRP is $\geq$ 30%, use either amoxicillin-clavulanate or a fluoroquinolone. If the first regimen fails, use amoxicillin-clavulanate plus extra amoxicillin, or cefpodoxime in mild to moderate disease; and use gatifloxacin, levofloxacin, or moxifloxacin in severe disease. The duration of treatment is 10 days. In hospitalized patients with nasotracheal and or nasogastric tubes, remove tubes if possible and use imipenem 0.5 g q6h or meropenem 1.0 g q8h. Alternately, use an antipseudomonal penicillin (e.g., piperacillin) or ceftazidime plus vancomycin or cefepime 2.0 g q12h. Antibiotics are usually ineffective for chronic sinusitis, but if an acute exacerbation occurs, use one of the acute regimens above. Otorhinolaryngology consultation is appropriate.[20]

DECONGESTANTS

Normal saline nasal sprays and steam may increase sinus drainage.[21] Oxymeta zoline 0.05% topical nasal spray inhibits nitric oxide synthetase with resulting decrease in inflammation; it should be used for no more than 3 to 4 days. Guaifenesin preparations maintain sinus drainage by thinning secretions and thus decreasing stasis.[22]

NASAL STEROIDS

The addition of intranasal corticosteroids to antibiotics reduces symptoms of acute sinusitis vs. antibiotics alone. With allergic sinusitis, nasal steroids shrink edematous mucosa and allow ostial openings to increase. A two or three times per day dosage is commonly used.[23]

NONPHARMACOLOGIC

Increasing oral fluids, local steam inhalation, and application of heat or cold have had some success in reducing discomfort.[11]

TABLE 9.1. Antibiotics for Rhinosinusitis[20] and for GABHS Pharyngitis[51]

Antibiotic	Dosage		Dosing frequency[b]	Cost[c]
	Adults (mg)	Children (mg/kg/day)		
Rhinosinusitis				
Oral administration				
Suggested primary regimen				
Trimethoprim-sulfamethoxazole	160/300	8/40	bid	$
Amoxicillin-clavulanate	875/125	45/6.4	bid	$$$$–$$$$$
Cefaclor	500	40	tid	$$$$
Second-line treatment				
Clarithromycin extended release	1000	15	qd	$$$$
Amoxicillin	500	40	tid	$–$$
Cefuroxime axetil	250	30	bid	$$–$$$
Cefpodoxime-proxetil	200	10	bid	$$$$
Cefdinir	600	14	qd	$$$$$
Levofloxacin	500	*	qd	$$$$$
Moxifloxacin	400	*	qd	$$$$$
Gatifloxacin	400	*	qd	$$$$$
Parenteral administration				
Imipenem	500	15–25	q6h	$$$$$
Meropenem	1000	60–120	q8h	$$$$$
Ceftazidime	1000–2000	50	q8h	$$$$$
Vancomycin	15 mg/kg	40–60	q12q/q6h	$$$$$
Gatifloxacin	400	*	qd	$$$$$
Cefepime	2000	150	q12h/q8h	$$$$$

GABHS pharyngitis

Suggested primary regimen				
Benzathine penicillin G				
<60 pounds, 27 kg	600,000 U IM	Same	Once	$
≥60 pounds, 27 kg	1,200,000 U IM	Same	Once	$-$$
Benzathine/procaine PCN	900,000/300,000 U IM	Same	Once	$
Penicillin VK	500 mg total	250 mg total	bid	$
Penicillin-allergic				
Erythromycin estolate	Not advised	20-40	bid-qid	$$
Erythromycin ethylsuccinate	400	40	bid-qid	$
Second-line treatment				
Amoxicillin	500	40	tid	$-$$
Amoxicillin-clavulanate	500-875	40	bid-tid	$$$$-$$$$$
Cephalexin	500	25-50	bid	$-$$
Cefadroxil	1000	30	qd	$$-$$$$$
Cefaclor	250	20-30	tid	$$$$
Cefuroxime axetil	125	15	bid	$$-$$$
Cefixime	200	8	qd	$$$-$$$$$
Clarithromycin	250	—	bid	$$$$$
Azithromycin (5 days)	500 mg day 1 250 mg days 2-5	12	qd	$$-$$$

[a]Unless otherwise indicated, antibiotic is given orally for 10 days.

[b]qd = once a day; bid = twice a day; tid = three times a day; qid = four times daily.

[c]Cost for therapeutic course based on average wholesale price from 2000 Drugs Topics Red Book; prices for generic drugs were used when available; $ = 0-15 dollars; $$ = 16-30 dollars; $$$ = 31-45 dollars, $$$$ = 46-60 dollars, $$$$$ = greater than 60 dollars.

*Fluoroquinolones not recommended under 18 years of age except in cystic fibrosis.

Complications

Mucocele and osteomyelitis are rare complications of sinusitis. Mucoceles, treated surgically, may be identified by radiography or sinus CT. Osteomyelitis, a serious infection of the surrounding bone, requires prolonged parenteral antibiotics and debridement of necrotic osseous structures with later cosmetic reconstruction.[9] Meningitis, cavernous sinus thrombosis, brain abscess, or hematogenous spread may also occur. Orbital infections occur more commonly in children.[24]

Chronic Recurrent Sinusitis

More than 32 million cases of chronic sinusitis occur annually in the United States.[25] Predisposing factors include anatomic abnormalities, polyps, allergic rhinitis, ciliary dysmotility, foreign bodies, chronic irritants, adenoidal hypertrophy, nasal decongestant spray abuse (rhinitis medica-mentosa), smoking, swimming, chronic viral URIs, and immunocompromised states. Pathogens are those above with an increase in *Bacteroides* sp., *Peptostreptococcus,* and *Fusobacterium.* Parasitic sinusitis by microsporidium, cryptosporidium acanthamoeba species has been reported in acquired immunodeficiency syndrome (AIDS) patients.[26] Treatment is aimed at resolving predisposing factors, but acute sinusitis is treated with organism specific antibiotics.[20] Endoscopically guided microswab cultures from the middle meatus correlate 80% to 85% with results of more painful antral puncture in antibiotic failures.[27]

Surgical Management

When antibiotic management fails, surgical management is indicated. Chronic sinusitis patients have significant decrements in bodily pain and social functioning. Surgery reduces symptoms and medication use.[28] Functional endoscopic sinus surgery is a minimally invasive technique used to restore sinus ventilation and normal function. Improvement in symptoms have been reported in up to 90%.[29]

Sinusitis in Children

Sinusitis affects 10% of school-age children, and 21% to 30% of adolescents.[30] Chronic rhinosinusitis may affect quality of life more severely than juvenile rheumatoid arthritis, asthma, or other chronic childhood illnesses.[31] The differential diagnosis includes allergy, immunodeficiency [immunoglobulin A (IgA) is most common], cystic fibrosis, ciliary disorders (e.g., primary ciliary dyskinesia), and gastroesophageal reflux.[32] Maxillary and ethmoidal sinuses are the primary sites of infection in infants. The sphenoid sinus develops later during the third to fifth year of life and the frontal sinus during the sixth to tenth year.

Childhood sinusitis may be a challenge to diagnose. Common symptoms include fever over 39°C, periorbital edema, facial pain, and daytime cough.[24] Periorbital cellulitis is seen in infants with ethmoidal sinus disease. If a URI is severe or persists beyond 10 days in a child, suspect sinusitis. In young children, sinusitis may present only with cough and persistent rhinorrhea. Low-dose, high-resolution CT is recommended when available.[33] The radiographic diagnosis of sinusitis is based on air-fluid levels, mucosal thickening of 4 mm or more, or sinus opacification. Organisms in antral cultures include *S. pneumoniae, M. catarrhalis,* and *H. influenzae.*[34] In July 1998, the Food and Drug Administration (FDA) approved amoxicillin-clavulanate, cefprozil, cefuroxime, clarithromycin, loracarbef, levofloxacin, and trovafloxin for childhood sinusitis treatment. Quinolones are not established as safe for those younger than 18 years old. Amoxicillin is the initial antibiotic of choice. Trimethoprim-sulfamethoxazole, amoxicillin-clavulanate, cefaclor, and cefuroxime axetil are useful alternatives if β-lactamase–producing organisms are suspected. All antibiotics are given for 10 days. Antihistamines may impair ciliary clearing mechanisms and thicken secretions. If oral antibiotics are unsuccessful, parenteral antibiotics such as imipenem, ceftazadime, and cefepime have been recommended (Table 9.1).[24]

Pharyngitis

Sore throat is the third most common presenting complaint in family practice, with an annual cost of $37.5 million for antibiotics.[35] The challenge for family physicians is to determine, in a cost-effective manner, which patients need antibiotics.[35,36]

Epidemiology

The infectious causes of a sore throat are listed in Table 9.2. Although viruses are the most common infectious agents, Group A β-hemolytic *Streptococcus* (GABHS) is most important because of potential sequelae. GABHS can be isolated by throat culture in 30% to 40% of children and 5% to 10% of adults with sore throat, with the highest prevalence found in children age 5 to 15 years.[37,38] Groups C and G streptococci, *Mycoplasma pneumoniae,* and *Chlamydia pneumoniae* (TWAR agent) occur most commonly in adolescent and young adults, and usually have no serious sequelae.[38] Rare bacterial causes include *Corynebacterium diphtheriae, Neisseria gonorrhoeae* (especially in those who practice fellatio), *N. meningitidis, Treponema pallidum,* and tuberculosis. In 20% to 65% of patients, no infectious pathogen can be found. Noninfectious causes to consider are postnasal drip, low-humidity in the environment, irritant exposure to cigarette smoke or smog, and malignant disease (e.g., leukemia, lymphoma, or squamous cell carcinoma). GABHS pharyngitis is seen most frequently in late winter and early spring, while other infectious agents occur year round. All are spread

TABLE 9.2. Infectious Causes of Pharyngitis*[35,36]

Primary bacterial pathogens (30% in children age 5–11 years old, 15% in adolescents, 5% in adults)	Group A β-hemolytic streptococci (GABHS) Group B, C, and G streptococci Neisseria gonorrhoeae (uncommon) Corynebacterium diphtheriae (rare) Treponema pallidum (unusual) Tuberculosis (unusual)
Possible bacterial pathogens (5–10%, primarily in young adults)	Arcanobacterium haemolyticum Chlamydia pneumoniae (TWAR) Chlamydia trachomatis Mycoplasma pneumoniae
Probable bacterial co-pathogens (all age groups)	Staphylococcus aureus Haemophilus influenzae Klebsiella pneumoniae rhinoscleromatis Moraxella (Branhamella) catarrhalis Bacteroides melaninogenicus Bacteroides oralis Bacteroides fragilis Fusobacterium species Peptostreptococci
Viruses (15–40% in children, 30–80% in adults)	Rhinovirus (100 types)—most common Coronavirus (three or more types) Adenovirus—types 3, 4, 7, 14, and 21 Herpes simplex virus—types 1 and 2 Parainfluenza virus—types 1–4 Influenzavirus—types A and B Coxsackievirus A—types 2, 4–6, 8, 10 Epstein-Barr virus Cytomegalovirus Human immunodeficiency virus type 1
Fungal (uncommon in immunocompetent patient)	Candida albicans

*No pathogen is isolated in 20–65% (avg. 30%) of cases of sore throat.

by close contact or by droplets. A higher incidence of disease occurs in schools, day-care centers, and dormitories.

Clinical Presentation

The classic features of GABHS pharyngitis are sudden onset of severe sore throat, moderate fever (39°–40.5°C), headache, anorexia, nausea, vomiting, abdominal pain, malaise, tonsillopharyngeal erythema, patchy and discrete tonsillar or pharyngeal exudate, soft palate petechiae, and tender cervical adenopathy.[35] The majority of patients have mild disease, with overlap of these features and those of viral pharyngitis. Scarlet fever produces a fine, blanching, sandpaper-texture rash, circumoral pallor, and hyperpigmentation in the skin creases. Although highly suggestive of GABHS, it also may be caused by *Arcanobacterium haemolyticum*.

Exudative pharyngitis/tonsillitis, anterior cervical adenopathy, fever, and lack of other URI symptoms such as cough and rhinorrhea are most predictive of a positive GABHS culture, with a probability of occurrence of 56% when all four are present.[35]

Groups C and G streptococcus and *A. haemolyticum* produce tonsillopharyngitis indistinguishable from GABHS, but rarely have sequelae.[36] The tonsillopharyngitis of *M. pneumoniae* and *C. pneumoniae* is similar to GABHS infection, but is usually accompanied by a cough.[38] Membranous pharyngitis with a gangrenous exudative appearance is found in Vincent's angina or diphtheria. Herpangina (caused by the Coxsackie A virus) is characterized by a severe sore throat, fever, and 1- to 2-mm pharyngeal vesicles that subsequently ulcerate and resolve within 5 days. Hand-foot-and-mouth disease (caused by Coxsackie A-16 virus) presents as pharyngitis accompanied by vesicles on the palmar and plantar surfaces. Patients with aphthous stomatitis have a sore throat and round, painful oral lesions that resolve within 2 weeks. Herpes simplex virus causes fever, oral fetor, submaxillary adenopathy, and gingivostomatitis. Symptoms of infectious mononucleosis include sore throat, anterior and posterior adenopathy, a gray pseudomembranous pharyngitis, and palatine petechiae. Acute retroviral syndrome due to primary infection of human immunodeficiency virus (HIV) presents as fever, nonexudative pharyngitis, lymphadenopathy, and systemic symptoms such as fatigue, myalgias, and arthralgias.[36]

Diagnosis

Since no single element of the history or physical exam is diagnostic for GABHS, the standard for diagnosis is a properly processed and interpreted throat culture on sheep blood agar.[36] For best results, use a Dacron swab and thoroughly swab both tonsils and posterior pharyngeal wall, avoiding the tongue. Since it takes 24 to 48 hours to obtain definitive results from a throat culture, streptococcal rapid antigen-detection tests were developed that can provide answers within minutes. Most are highly specific (90–96%), but not as sensitive (80–90%) as throat cultures.[36,38] If a rapid antigen test is positive, one can almost be certain that GABHS is present. If the test is negative in clinically suspicious situations, national advisory committees recommend obtaining a confirmatory throat culture.[36] Recently, newer tests using optical immunoassay and chemiluminescent DNA probes have sensitivities similar to that of throat cultures, and may one day become the standard method for diagnosis.[1,36]

Complications of GABHS Tonsillopharyngitis

Suppurative complications include peritonsillar abscess (PTA), retropharyngeal abscess, and cervical lymphadenitis. Peritonsillar abscess occurs in fewer than 1% of patients treated with appropriate antibiotics.[39] It is seen most frequently in teenagers and young adults, and is rare in children. Symptoms include a severe unilateral sore throat, dysphagia, rancid breath, trismus, drooling from a partially opened mouth, and a muffled "hot potato" voice. There is generalized erythema of the pharynx and tonsils, with a deeper dusky redness overlying the involved area, swelling of the anterior pillar and soft palate above the tonsil, and uvular deviation to the opposite side.[40] Diagnostic ultrasound [41] or CT scan [42] helps distinguish between peritonsillar cellulitis and abscess. Treatment includes intravenous penicillin and needle aspiration.[40] Tonsillectomy is indicated when needle aspiration fails and in those with recurrent PTA.[43]

Once the leading cause of death in children and adolescents in the United States, acute rheumatic fever (ARF) now occurs infrequently, with a reported annual incidence of 1 case per 1,000,000 untreated patients with GABHS pharyngitis.[35] Symptoms begin 2 weeks after the pharyngitis with polyarthritis and cardiac valvulitis. Acute glomerulonephritis may occur 10 days after GABHS pharyngitis, and presents as anasarca, hypertension, hematuria, and proteinuria. It generally is a self-limited condition and almost never has permanent sequelae, and antibiotics do not prevent its occurrence.[37]

Treatment

Since a small but significant portion of patients with GABHS pharyngitis will develop complications, many physicians treat all patients who have a sore throat with antibiotics. However, treating all patients as if they had GABHS infection means overtreating at least 70% of children and 90% of adult patients. Treating GABHS pharyngitis accomplishes four goals[36]: (1) patients clinically improve quicker; (2) they become noninfectious sooner, thus preventing transmission of infection; (3) suppurative complications such as PTA are avoided; and (4) ARF is prevented. Children who complete 24 hours of antibiotics can be considered noninfectious, and if they feel better, may return to school. Although patients clinically respond within 1 to 2 days of antibiotics, treatment for 10 days remains the optimal duration to prevent ARF. Patient compliance issues should be addressed; up to 80% do not complete a 10-day course.[39]

Penicillin remains the drug of choice for treating GABHS pharyngitis because it is effective in preventing ARF, inexpensive, and relatively safe (Table 9.1).[36] Penicillin-resistant GABHS has yet to be identified. Even when started as late as 9 days after the onset of pharyngitis, penicillin effectively prevents primary attacks of ARF. Intramuscular benzathine penicillin is the definitive treatment but is infrequently used because injections are painful. Amoxicillin offers a low-cost, better-tasting alternative to penicillin, and one recent study suggested that a single daily dose for 10 days had similar efficacy.[44]

For those allergic to penicillin, erythromycin is the antibiotic of choice. Clarithromycin and azithromycin have a susceptibility pattern similar to that of erythromycin, but with less gastrointestinal distress, and may be administered once or twice a day. Azithromycin as a 5-day treatment regimen for GABHS pharyngitis is attractive, but its cost and the potential rapid development of streptococcal resistance of macrolides make this a second-line antibiotic.[36] Cephalosporins are more expensive, may hasten the development of resistant bacteria, and should not be used in patients with a history of immediate (anaphylactic) hypersensitivity to penicillin.[38] Recent evidence suggests that a 5-day course of nonpenicillin antibiotics is just as effective as a 10-day course of oral penicillin, but further studies are needed before this is accepted as the standard of care.[45]

The same antibiotic treatment choices exist for groups C and G streptococci and *A. haemolyticum*.[36] Both *M. pneumoniae* and *C. pneumoniae* are sensitive to tetracycline and erythromycin. Treatment for diphtheria includes antitoxin and erythromycin 20 to 25 mg/kg every 12 hours intravenously for 7 to 14 days. Vincent's angina is treated with penicillin, tetracycline, and oral oxidizing agents such as hydrogen peroxide to improve oral hygiene. Treatment of viral pharyngitis with antivirals is not indicated. An oral rinse consisting of corticosteroids (Kenalog suspension) and topical tetracycline (250 mg/50 cc water) may hasten recovery in those patients with aphthous stomatitis. Therapy for infectious mononucleosis is supportive and may include penicillin (avoid amoxicillin and ampicillin) for simultaneous GABHS infection, and steroids for respiratory obstruction.

Ibuprofen 400 mg every 6 hours is superior to acetaminophen in alleviating throat pain.[39] Available suspension analgesics include ibuprofen 100 mg/5 cc, naproxen 125 mg/5 cc, acetaminophen with codeine elixir, and acetaminophen with hydrocodone elixir.[39] Avoid aspirin in children and teenagers because of the risk of Reye's syndrome. Warm liquids are an effective adjuvant treatment. Patients with severe inflammatory symptoms may benefit from corticosteroids, given as a short course of oral prednisone or a single 10-mg injection of dexamethasone.[39]

Cost-Benefit Treatment Strategy

The most important task when evaluating a sore throat is to determine whether or not the patient has GABHS. Although national guidelines exist,[46] consensus on the most cost-effective approach remains elusive. A rational policy should be based on the incidence of GABHS in the population, cost containment, avoidance of adverse outcomes, reducing unnecessary use of antibiotics, and patient priorities. When the probability of GABHS is greater than 20%, treating all patients with pharyngitis without testing may be rational.[47] Otherwise, those individuals who may have GABHS based on clinical findings should have a rapid antigen test or throat culture performed.[46] In those cases where rapid antigen tests are negative and a confirmatory throat culture is pending, presumptive antibiotic use should be based on severity of illness, risk of transmission to others, need to return to school or work, and the patient's willingness to accept risks of unnecessary use of antibiotics should the culture return negative.

Treatment Failures and Chronic Carriers

Posttreatment throat cultures are indicated only in those who remain symptomatic after completion of antibiotics, who develop recurrent symptoms within 6 weeks, or who have had rheumatic fever and are at high risk for recurrence.[46] Reasons for treatment failures include poor compliance, β-lactamase–producing bacteria, and recurrent exposure to a family member who harbors GABHS ("ping-pong" infections).[48] The family pet is an unlikely reservoir for GABHS.[49] A chronic GABHS carrier is asymptomatic with a positive throat culture. As many as 50% of school-age children are GABHS carriers, are rarely contagious, and are at little risk for developing GABHS complications.[50] Indications to eradicate GABHS from the chronic carrier include a personal or family history of ARF and "ping-pong" spread occurring within a family.[50] The treatment for those who fail an adequate course of oral penicillin is a single injection of benzathine penicillin (Table 9.1). If this fails, clindamycin 20 to 30 mg/kg/day (up to 450 mg per day) may be given in three divided doses for 10 days.[46]

Tonsillectomy

Tonsillectomy is indicated in those who have recurrent peritonsillar abscesses or respiratory obstruction.[43] The American Academy of Otolaryngology and Head and Neck Surgery considers four or more infections of the tonsils per year, despite adequate medical therapy, to be sufficient indication for tonsillectomy, although the benefit of decreased frequency of GABHS tonsillitis may only last for 2 years.

References

1. Stewart M, Siff J, Cydulka R. Evaluation of the patient with sore throat, earache, and sinusitis: an evidence-based approach. Em Med Clin North Am 1999;17(1):153–87.
2. Linden B, Aguilar E, Allen S. Sinusitis in the nasotracheally intubated patient. Arch Otolaryngol Head Neck Surg 1988;114:860–1.
3. Ozcan Y, Jiang H, Pai C. Do primary care physicians or specialists provide more efficient care? Health Serv Manag Res 2000;13(2):90–6.
4. Lanza D, Kennedy D. Adult rhinosinusitis defined. Otolaryngol Head Neck Surg 1997;117:S1–7.
5. Hadley J, Schafer S. Clinical evaluation of rhinosinusitis: history and physical examination. Otolaryngol Head Neck Surg 1997;117:S8–11.
6. Kormos WA. Approach to the patient with sinusitis. In Goroll AH, May LA, Mulley AG, eds. Primary care medicine 4th ed. Philadelphia: JB Lippincott; 2000:1127–8.
7. Way L. Current surgical diagnosis and treatment, 10th ed. East Norwalk, CT: Appleton & Lange, 1994.
8. Ferguson B. Acute and chronic sinusitis—how to ease symptoms and locate the cause. Postgrad Med 1995;97(5):45–57.
9. Tierney L, McPhee S, Papadakis M. Current medical diagnosis and treatment, 34th ed. East Norwalk, CT: Appleton & Lange, 1995.
10. Burke T, Guertler A, Timmons J. Comparisons of sinus x-rays with CT scans in acute sinusitis. Acad Emerg Med 1994;1(3):235–9.
11. Hopp R, Cooperstock M. Evaluation and treatment of sinusitis: aspects for the managed care environment. JAOA 1996;96(4 suppl):S6–10.

12. Bhattacharyya T, Piccinillo J, Wippold F. Relationship between patient-based description of sinusitis and paranasal sinus CT findings. Arch Otolaryngol Head Neck Surg 1997;123:1189–92.
13. Sanford J, Gilbert D, Sande M. Sanford's guide to antimicrobial therapy, 26th ed. Dallas: Antimicrobial Therapy, 1996.
14. Nord C. The role of anaerobic bacteria in recurrent episodes of sinusitis and tonsillitis. Clin Infect Dis 1995;20:1512–24.
15. Decker C. Sinusitis in the immunocompromised host. Curr Infect Dis Rep 1999;1(1):27–32.
16. Kormos WA. Approach to the patient with sinusitis. In Goroll AH, May LA, Mulley AG, eds. Primary care medicine 4th ed. Philadelphia: JB Lippincott; 2000:1127.
17. Ray N. Healthcare expenditures for sinusitis in 1996: contributions of asthma, rhinitis, and other airway disorders. J Allergy Clin Immunol 1999;103(3 pt 1):408–14.
18. Snow V, Mottur-Pilson C JMJH. Principles of appropriate antibiotic use for acute sinusitis in adults. Ann Intern Med 2001;134:495–7.
19. Holten K, Onusko E. Appropriate prescribing of oral beta-lactam antibiotics. Am Fam Physician 2000;62:611–20.
20. Gilbert D, Moelleering R, Sande M. The Sanford's guide to antimicrobial therapy, 31st ed. Dallas,TX: Antimicrobial Therapy, 2001.
21. Taccariello M, Parikh A, Darby Y, Scadding G. Nasal douching as a valuable adjunct in the management of chronic rhinosinusitis. Rhinology 1999;37(1):29–32.
22. Malm L. Pharmacological background to decongesting and anti-inflammatory treatment of rhinitis and sinusitis. Acta Otolaryngol Suppl (Stockh) 1994;515:53–5.
23. Naclerio R. Allergic rhinitis. N Engl J Med 1991;325:860–9.
24. Parsons DS, Wilder BE. Rhinitis and sinusitis (acute and chronic). In: Burg TD, Ingelfinger JR, Wald ER, Polin RA, eds. Current pediatric therapy 16th ed. Philadelphia: WB Saunders, 1999:506–7.
25. Mellen I. Chronic sinusitis: clinical and pathophysiological aspects. Acta Otolaryngol Suppl (Stockh) 1994;515:45–8.
26. Dunand V, Hammer S, Rossi R, et al. Parasitic sinusitis and otitis in patients infected with human immunodeficiency virus: report of five cases and review. Clin Infect Dis 1997;25(2):267–72.
27. Osguthorp J. Adult rhinosinusitis: diagnosis and management. Am Fam Physician 2001;63:69–76.
28. Metson R, Gliklich R. Clinical outcomes in patients with chronic sinusitis. Laryngoscope 2000;110(3 pt 3):24–8.
29. Slack R, Bates G. Functional endoscopic sinus surgery. Am Fam Physician 1998;58:707–18.
30. Deda G, Caksen H, Ocal A. Headache etiology in children: a retrospective study of 125 cases. Pediatr Int 2000;42:668–73.
31. Cunningham J, Chiu E, Landgraf J, Gliklich R. The health impact of chronic recurrent rhinosinusitis in children. Arch Otolaryngol Head Neck Surg 2000;126(11):1363–8.
32. Lasley M, Shapiro G. Rhinitis and sinusitis in children. Immunol Allerg Clin North Am 1999;19:437–52.
33. Konen E, Faibel M, Kleinbaum Y, et al. The value of the occipitomental (Waters') view in diagnosis of sinusitis: a comparative study with computed tomography. Clin Radiol 2000;55:856–60.
34. Diaz I, Bamberger D. Acute sinusitis. Semin Respir Infect 1995;10:14–20.

35. Ebell M, Smith M, Barry H, Ives K, Carey M. Does this patient have strep throat? JAMA 2000;284:2912–8.
36. Bisno A. Acute pharyngitis. N Engl J Med 2001;344:205–11.
37. Kiselica D. Group A beta-hemolytic streptococcal pharyngitis: current clinical concepts. Am Fam Physician 1994;49(5):1147–54.
38. Pichichero M. Group A streptococcal tonsillopharyngitis: cost-effective diagnosis and treatment. Ann Emerg Med 1995;25(3):390–403.
39. Kline J, Runge J. Streptococcal pharyngitis: a review of pathophysiology, diagnosis, and management. J Emerg Med 1994;12(5):665–80.
40. Epperly T, Wood T. New trends in the management of peritonsillar abscess. Am Fam Physician 1990;42:102–12.
41. Ahmed K, Jones A, Shah K, Smethurst A. The role of ultrasound in the management of peritonsillar abscess. J Laryngol Otol 1994;108:610–2.
42. Patel K, Ahmad S, O'Leary G, Michel M. The role of computed tomography in the management of peritonsillar abscess. Otolaryngol Head Neck Surg 1992;107:727–32.
43. Richardson M. Sore throat, tonsillitis, and adenoiditis. Med Clin North Am 1999;83(1):75–83.
44. Gerber M, Tanz R. New approaches to the treatment of group A streptococcal pharyngitis. Curr Opin Pediatr 2001;13(1):51–5.
45. Adam D, Scholz H, Helmerking M. Short-course antibiotic treatment of 4782 culture-proven cases of group A streptococcal tonsillopharyngitis and incidence of post-streptococcal sequelae. Clin Infect Dis 2000;182:509–16.
46. Bisno A, Gerber M, Gwaltney J, Kaplan E, Schwartz R. Diagnosis and management of group A streptococcal pharyngitis: a practice guideline. Clin Infect Dis 1997;25:574–83.
47. Green S. Acute pharyngitis: the case for empiric antimicrobial therapy. Ann Emerg Med 1995;25(3):404–6.
48. Pinchichero M, Casey J, Mayes T, et al. Penicillin failure in streptococcal tonsillopharyngitis: causes and remedies. Pediatr Infect Dis J 2000;19:917–23.
49. Wilson K, Maroney S, Gander R. The family pet as an unlikely source of group A beta-hemolytic streptococcal infection in humans. Pediatr Infect Dis J 1995;14:372–5.
50. Gerber M. Treatment failures and carriers: perception or problems? Pediatr Infect Dis J 1994;13:576–9.
51. Hayes C, Williamson H. Management of group A beta-hemolytic streptococcal pharyngitis. Am Fam Physician 2001;63:1557–64.

CASE PRESENTATION

Subjective

PATIENT PROFILE

Luke Priestley is a 22-year-old married male graduate student.

PRESENTING PROBLEM

Sore throat.

PRESENT ILLNESS

For 2 days, Mr. Priestley has had a sore throat and fever. There has been slight pain in both ears and a mild cough. He is taking aspirin for the symptoms and has continued to attend classes.

PAST MEDICAL HISTORY

He had a positive tuberculin skin test on entering college 5 years ago. This finding followed a year as an exchange student in Korea.

SOCIAL HISTORY

Mr. Priestley is in his first year as a graduate student in an MBA program. He and his wife, Ann, are expecting their first child in 5 months.

HABITS

He uses no tobacco, alcohol, or recreational drugs.

FAMILY HISTORY

His father died of heart failure at age 55. His mother is living and well at age 57. His sister, aged 26, has mitral valve prolapse.

- What more would you like to know about the history of the present illness, and why?
- What further information would you like to know about Mr. Priestley's school work? Why?
- What family history might be pertinent, and why?

- What additional information might be pertinent about his positive tuberculin skin test?

Objective

VITAL SIGNS

Blood pressure, 120/78; pulse, 88; respirations, 26; temperature, 38.8°C.

EXAMINATION

The patient's face appears flushed, and the pitch of his voice seems altered by throat swelling. The tympanic membranes are both mildly injected but not retracted. The throat and tonsils are swollen bilaterally and erythematous. There is bilateral, tender cervical adenopathy. The thyroid is not enlarged. The chest examination reveals a few rhonchi at the bases bilaterally, but no wheezes are heard. The heart has a regular sinus rhythm without murmurs.

LABORATORY

A rapid screening test for β-hemolytic streptococcus is positive.

- What more—if anything—would you include in the physical examination, and why?
- Are there other areas of the body that should be examined, and why?
- What might cause you to be concerned about airway obstruction, and how would you address this concern?
- What—if any—laboratory or diagnostic imaging studies would you obtain today? Why?

Assessment

- What is your diagnostic impression, and how would you explain this to Mr. Priestley?
- What might be the meaning of this illness to the patient? To his wife?
- Mr. Priestley asks if he might develop complications of this illness. How would you respond?
- What are the risks that Mr. Priestley's wife or classmates might develop streptococcal pharyngitis, and what—if anything—should be done regarding this risk?

Plan

- Describe your therapeutic recommendations for the patient.
- If the patient were worse in 48 hours, what would you suspect? What would you do?
- Mrs. Priestley asks if her husband's illness presents any risk to the pregnancy. How would you respond?
- What follow-up would you advise?

10

Viral Infections of the Respiratory Tract

GEORGE L. KIRKPATRICK

Viral infections of the respiratory tract are responsible for large amounts of time lost from the workplace and significant morbidity and mortality in the very young and the very old. The worldwide pandemic of influenza in 1918 was alone responsible for nearly 30 million deaths in excess of those expected for influenza. Viral respiratory infections are the most frequent illnesses in human beings. The most frequent causes of respiratory infections are adenoviruses, influenza viruses, parainfluenza viruses, respiratory syncytial viruses, and rhinoviruses. Frequency and severity of infection are increased in the very young and the elderly, worsened by crowding and inhaling pollutants, and influenced by anatomic, metabolic, genetic, and immunologic disorders. Respiratory infections are the leading cause of death in children under age 5 living in underdeveloped countries.[1]

Viruses Involved with Upper Respiratory Tract Infections

Table 10.1 compares the results of studies over the past 15 years detailing the prevalence rates of the common respiratory viruses. These prevalence rates include data from various parts of the world, and all age groups. Prevalence rates as high as 35% reflect the reason why these viruses are such common causes of disease.[2–13]

Viral Identification and Specimen Collection

Three techniques are commonly utilized to obtain specimens for viral identification. Nasopharyngeal swabs are sterile swabs inserted 3 to 4 cm into one nostril, left in place about 5 seconds, then removed and placed in a culturette containing modified Stuart's medium for transport to the lab. (One such system is the Becton Dickinson Microbiology Systems Mini-Tip Culturette, San Diego, CA.) Nasopharyngeal wash specimens are collected according to the method described by Hall and Douglas.[14] A 1-ounce rubber ear syringe (Davol, Inc., Cranston, RI) is loaded with 3 to 5 mL of sterile phosphate-buffered saline. With

TABLE 10.1. Prevalence Rates of the Common Respiratory Viruses

	Flu A	Flu B	Para	Adeno	RSV	Rhino	Corona	Flu A & B
Croatia study[2]			2.3		7.6	33.6		0.6
Indian hospital study[3]			5	3	5			6
Nursing home study[4]			2		12	9.4		
COPD study[5]			8	0.7	3.1	6	5	4.2
Hospitalized colds[6]	5.9					12.5	4.7	
Cost-effective study[7]	1.8	1.2		0.35	18			
Early detection study[8]	5.5	2.6	2.7	4.5	12.8	35.8		
Pediatric inpatients, Taiwan[9]	7.2	0.1	2.0	4.0	1.7	12.7		
Chronically ill patients[10]	4.8	1.3	7.5	1.1	10.3	4.2	2.5	
Hospitalized Korean children[11]	7.0		6.5	3.9	11.8			
Hospitalized German children[12]		1.3	2.8	7.7	12.6			
Children in Jordan[13]		4.0	2.0	14.0				

COPD = chronic obstructive pulmonary disease; RSV = respiratory syncytial virus.

the patient's head tipped back about 70 degrees, the bulb tip is inserted until it occludes the nostril. With one complete squeeze and release, the nasal wash is collected in the bulb. The bulb contents are then emptied into a sterile screw-top tube for transport to the lab. Nasopharyngeal aspirate specimens are collected using a pediatric suction catherer (Safe-T-Vac, Kendall Healthcare Products, Mansfield, MA). Normal saline, 2 to 3 mL, is instilled into a nostril and the specimen is aspirated moments later into a sterile specimen trap.

Laboratory Testing

The standard to which laboratory tests for viral identification are compared is viral culture on monkey kidney, human lung laryngeal epidermoid carcinoma (Hep-2), and human embryonal diploid lung cell tissue culture. These cultures are studied daily for evidence of cytopathic effect. Cultures may become positive in several days to several weeks. Sensitivity of viral culture ranges from 7% to 94%. Specificity is very high. The Bartels viral respiratory screening and identification kit is an indirect fluorescence antibody procedure that contains monoclonal antibodies for seven respiratory viruses. This type of test has sensitivity of 84% to 88% and results are available in less than 24 hours after specimen collection.[15] Several laboratories are developing rapid reverse-transcription polymerase chain reaction (RT-PCR) tests (Prodesse, Inc., Milwaukee, WI) that improve sensitivity and shorten reporting time for respiratory virus identification. Sensitivities for rhinoviruses improved from 8% for tissue culture methods to 56% for the RT-PCR method.[8,16] Tests based on the reaction between viral neuraminidase from influenza viruses and a chromogenic substrate (Z Statflu Test, Zymetx, Oklahoma City, OK, USA) are available to detect influenza types A and B. Sensitivity approaches 78% and specificity nears 91% for this method with turnaround times of a few hours using throat swab specimens.[17]

Respiratory Syncytial Virus

Respiratory syncytial virus (RSV), a single-stranded RNA paramyxovirus, is the leading cause of pneumonia and bronchiolitis in infants and children. Virtually 100% of young children are infected with RSV by age 3. Two antigenically distinct groups of RSV (A and B) are recognized. Community outbreaks of RSV usually appear during the winter and spring in temperate climates. The diagnosis of RSV in the acute setting is usually made by viral culture of nasopharyngeal secretions. A rapid diagnostic test (Abbott test pack RSV; Directigen RSV by Becton Dickinson) employing antigen detection in nasal secretions is 95% sensitive and 99% specific. Results are available in an hour.

The spectrum of illness associated with RSV is broad, ranging from mild nasal congestion to high fever and respiratory distress. What seems to begin as a simple cold may suddenly become a life-threatening illness. Modes of spread are primarily via large-droplet inoculation (requiring close contact) and self-inoculation via contaminated fomites or skin. RSV is recoverable from countertops for up to 6 hours from the time of contamination, from rubber gloves for up to 90 minutes, and from skin for up to 20 minutes. Viral shedding of RSV in infants is a prolonged process averaging 7 days. Strategies for controlling spread of RSV should be aimed at interrupting hand carriage of the virus and self-inoculation of the eyes and nose. Masks commonly employed for respiratory viruses have not been shown to be an effective measure for curtailing RSV outbreaks on pediatric wards. Hand washing is probably the single most important infection control measure for RSV.

Influenza Viruses

Influenza, considered a benign disease today, has ravaged human populations recently enough that there are still those living who can recall the 1918 worldwide pandemic, called the "Spanish flu." This particular influenza began as an ordinary attack of influenza and rapidly developed into severe pneumonia. Within hours, the patients had mahogany-colored spots over the cheekbones and cyanosis began to spread over the face. Death shortly overcame them as they struggled for air and suffocated. It is important to realize that although worldwide 30 million deaths were attributed to influenza, 97% of people who were infected had a 3-day course of fever and malaise and recovered. Of the 3% who died, most died of pneumonia. A small subset died very rapidly of massive pulmonary edema and hemorrhage. Influenza pandemics occur about every 7 to 11 years. They are always associated with extensive morbidity and a marked increase in mortality.

Type A influenza is an RNA virus with a negative-sense segmented genome. It undergoes continuous antigenic drift because it has no proofreading mechanism, and is prone to mutate during replication. Influenza virus is chimeric, existing in wild bird and swine reservoirs, with minor antigenic drifts making the same virus infectious among birds, humans, or swine.[18]

In addition to the predominant influenza virus that invades an area each season, many types, subtypes, or variants are identified during each epidemic period. During the early stage of an epidemic, a disproportionate number of cases involve school-age children, 10 to 19 years old. Later in the epidemic, more cases are diagnosed in younger children and adults. The age shift suggests that the early spread of influenza viruses in a community is concentrated among schoolchildren.

Parainfluenza Viruses

Parainfluenza is a single-stranded RNA virus of which four serotypes and two subtypes are recognized (parainfluenza types 1, 2, 3, 4A, and 4B). Bronchiolitis, croup, and pneumonia occur with all parainfluenza types. In children under 1 year of age, bronchiolitis is associated mostly with type 2. In older children, croup is most commonly associated with types 1 and 2. Immunosuppression, chronic cardiac, or pulmonary diseases are associated with increased risk of parainfluenza infection.[19] Most persons have been infected with parainfluenza virus by age 5.

Immunity to parainfluenza is incomplete, and, as with RSV, reinfection occurs throughout life and probably plays a major role in the spread of virus to the young infant.

Parainfluenza types 1 and 2 tend to peak during the autumn of the year, whereas parainfluenza type 3 shows an increased prevalence during late spring. Adult infection results in mild upper respiratory tract symptoms, although pneumonia occasionally occurs. Outbreaks of parainfluenza types 1 and 3 have been reported from long-term-care facilities.[20] Illness is characterized by fever, sore throat, rhinorrhea, and cough. The rate of pneumonia is relatively high.

Most studies suggest direct person-to-person transmission. Parainfluenza is stable in small-particle aerosols at the low humidity found in hospitals. Outbreaks tend to proceed more slowly than influenza or other aerosol-spread infections.[21] Infection control policies should emphasize hand washing and isolation of patients.

Rhinoviruses

Rhinovirus is a non-enveloped, 30-nm, RNA virus with over 100 serotypes. It only replicates in primates. It is characterized by a single positive stranded genome not only acting as a template for RNA synthesis, but also encoding for a single polypeptide necessary for viral replication. It belongs to the picornavirus family, a diverse group of viral pathogens that together are the most common causes of infection in human beings. Within the picornavirus family are found the rhinoviruses, the enteroviruses, and the hepatoviruses (including hepatitis A). Rhinovirus infection is transmitted by direct contact with the eye or nasal mucous membrane. The most efficient modes of spread are hand-to-hand contact or contact with a contaminated surface followed by inoculation of the nose or conjunctiva. Rhinoviruses remain infectious for as long as 3 hours on nonporous surfaces. Transmission can be decreased by hand washing and disinfecting environmental surfaces. After deposition on nasal mucosa, the virus binds to intercellular adhesion molecule type 1 (ICAM-1) receptors on epithelial cells, initiating a cascade of inflammatory responses. Viral replication occurs in the nose, and viral shedding continues for up to 3 weeks. The cascade of interleukin-6, -8, and -16, histamine, bradykinin, and cytokines recruit neutrophils and produce the rhinorrhea, vascongestion, sinus congestion, sore throat, cough, wheezing, and middle ear inflammation.[22,23]

There is now evidence that direct invasion of the lower respiratory tract does occur, causing bronchitis and possibly triggering asthma attacks and exacerbation of chronic obstructive pulmonary disease (COPD). New antirhinoviral treatments are being tested. Intranasal interferon prevents infection, but provides no therapeutic benefit. Oral pleconaril shows therapeutic promise. Intranasal tremacamra and AG7088 are under investigation.[24,25] For the time being, treatment is mostly symptomatic, with antibiotics and steroids showing no benefit.

Coronaviruses

Coronaviruses, members of the Coronaviridae family, are single-stranded RNA viruses first identified in 1962. They do not appear to replicate in any animal models and are almost impossible to isolate in standard tissue cultures. Acute and convalescent sera for enzyme immunoassay will identify the two common subtypes, 229E and OC43. The enzyme-linked immunosorbent assay (ELISA) has been used to identify coronaviruses in nasal secretions.[26] A 1997 study of frail older persons by Falsey and McCann[27] found 37 (8%) of 451 serologies positive for coronavirus 229E over 44 months. It was noted that illnesses were indistinguishable from RSV and influenza virus infections. Lower respiratory complications, such as pneumonia, occurred in one fourth of the infected residents.

Epidemics occur during late fall through early spring. Clinical symptoms usually include nasal congestion, headache, cough, sore throat, malaise, and low-grade fever similar to rhinoviral infections. Coronavirus infections have been associated with lower respiratory tract illnesses, including pneumonia and bronchiolitis in young children. Coronavirus is the second most frequent virus associated with asthma exacerbations; rhinovirus is the most frequent. Interferon-α, tremacamra, and pleconaril have shown promise in prevention and treatment of these infections.

Adenoviruses

Adenoviruses are double-stranded DNA viruses. There are 51 serotypes divided into six subgenera (A–F) that exhibit distinctly different organ tropisms. Adenoviruses cause a broad spectrum of diseases, including conjunctivitis, kerato-conjunctivitis, pharyngoconjunctival fever, pharyngitis, tonsillitis, coryza, pneumonia, heart disease, hepatitis, nephritis, and gastroenteritis. All ages are affected, but the majority of illness occurs in children younger than 6 years old. Military recruits in the United States from 1971 to 1995 received adenovirus vaccine to types 4 and 7. Since vaccine production ceased in 1995, an average of 4555 cases of adenoviral respiratory disease occur annually on military bases, costing about $2.6 million per year.[28] Adenovirus is ubiquitous, found everywhere during all seasons of the year, with annual peaks of activity in midsummer and midwinter. Transmission can occur by aerosolized droplets, fomites, hand carriage, fecal-oral, and by contact with contaminated lake water while swimming. The virus can be isolated for prolonged periods from respiratory secretions, conjunctival secretions, and stools of infected patients. Adenoviruses are identified by cytopathic effect in tissue cultures from nasopharyngeal specimens. They are also detected by indirect fluorescence antibody procedures (e.g., Bartels, Issaquah, WA, Viral Respiratory Screening and Identification Kit) using monoclonal antibodies. Newer RT-PCR testing (Taqman PCR, Glaxo Wellcome, Research Triangle Park, NC) can provide very accurate results in 6 to 12 hours, and primers are available for all adenovirus serotypes.[18]

Disease Presentations

Common Cold

The common cold, a disease of antiquity, is characterized by objective signs and subjective symptoms that are usually self-limited. Symptoms that occur with common colds include sneezing, watering of the eyes, nasal stuffiness, nasal obstruction, postnasal discharge, sore throat, hoarseness, cough, and sputum production. The common cold is a clinical diagnosis and lacks specificity because other ailments such as allergies and early symptoms of more serious illnesses mimic common cold symptoms. In the United States colds account for 23 million lost days of work and 26 million lost school days per year.

DIAGNOSIS

Rhinoviruses and coronaviruses are the most common causes of the common cold, with RSV and adenoviruses producing a similar set of signs and symptoms especially in adults. Mild cases of influenza and parainfluenza infection can be mistaken for the common cold. Because there are now a number of specific (as well as nonspecific and symptomatic) treatments for these viruses, it has become prudent medicine to undertake identification of the infecting virus, especially in more severe cases. Direct and indirect immunofluorescent staining techniques with virus-specific monoclonal antibodies (e.g., Chemicon International, Inc., Temecula, CA) or RT-PCR tests (e.g., Taqman PCR, Glaxo Wellcome) are well tested throughout the world and provide virus identification in a matter of hours almost anywhere.

MANAGEMENT

There are as many ways to manage the common cold as there are physicians. Gwaltney and Park[29] tested the therapeutic efficacy of clemastine fumarate, a second-generation antihistamine, and found reduction in total volume of rhinorrhea and number of sneezes in their patients challenged with rhinovirus. First-generation antihistamines reduce rhinorrhea and sneezing, and nonsteroidal antiinflammatory drugs reduce coughing, headache, malaise, and myalgias.

Intranasal steroid sprays reduce symptoms, but have little effect on duration of illness. Steroids may lengthen the period of viral shedding. Renewed interest in herbal and homeopathic remedies has produced clinical trials designed as randomized double-blind, placebo-controlled, multicenter studies mostly focused on symptom relief.[30] Jackson and Lesho[31] conducted a meta-analysis of 10 clinical trials on the use of zinc gluconate lozenges for treatment of the common cold. They concluded that evidence for effectiveness of zinc lozenges in reducing the duration of common colds is still lacking. Similar negative results have been reported from studies using heated, humidified air (steam) for cold treatment. Recent improved understanding of the pathophysiology of rhinoviral colds has focused attention on the neutrophilic inflammatory reaction, chemotaxis regulation, cytokinesis, and upregulation of immunocompetent cells. Pleconaril 200 mg twice a day for 7 days decreases signs and symptoms as well as reducing viral shedding.[32] Tremacamra, a synthetic ICAM-1 glycoprotein acts as an antiadhesion molecule when sprayed into the nostrils. Tremacamra produces a significant decrease in symptoms.[33] Rest, adequate hydration, and time to recover should be stressed during management of the common cold. In the future, antirhinovirus drugs and interferon may reach development levels where alleviation of symptoms or prevention of infection exceeds side effects.

COMPLICATIONS AND SEQUELAE

When the diagnosis of the common cold is accurate, complications and sequelae are minimal. Complications generally result from assuming the cold symptoms are caused by rhinovirus or coronavirus, when in fact influenza, RSV, adenovirus, or a bacterial pathogen are responsible. Complications also occur in immunocompromised patients where rhinovirus can cause fatal pneumonia. Sequelae include asthma triggered by the rhinoviral-induced airway inflammation, and otitis media precipitated by viral-induced eustachian tube dysfunction with altered middle ear pressure.

Hand washing is the most important way to prevent transmission of these viruses. With rhinoviruses and RSV, direct contact with a contaminated surface followed by inoculation of the nose or conjunctiva can result in infection. Use of masks and gloves and isolation of infected persons is the most effective way to limit the spread of cold viruses.

Influenza

Influenza has one of the more characteristic sets of clinical findings. The onset is usually sudden, with shivering, sweating, headache, aching in the orbits, and general malaise and misery. Cough is often found early in the course, aggravating headaches and causing generalized aching. The onset is generally explosive, with fever in adults ranging up to 102°F. In children the fever may be higher than 102°F, and sore throat may be an early sign. The most consistent signs are the presence of polymyalgias, weakness, and malaise.

DIAGNOSIS

Not surprisingly, the diagnosis of influenza is more accurate during epidemics and less accurate during nonepidemic periods. Influenza in the United States usually occurs during December, January, and February. Successful presumptive diagnosis requires appropriate clinical symptomatology at the right time of the year and a knowledge of the pattern of influenza illness around the world. Virologic studies, including cultures from throat swabs and nasopharyngeal washings, cells from nasopharyngeal washings stained with monoclonal antibody fluorescence stains, and complement fixation studies on paired serum samples can confirm the diagnosis. The Zstatflu test (Zymetx, Oklahoma City, OK, USA) is a rapid detection kit for both type A and type B influenza. It is based on the reaction between influenza neuraminidase and a chromogenic substrate. Throat swab or nasopharyngeal swab specimens will generate results in a few hours. There are several rapid flu A and flu B tests available currently that report results in less than an hour.

Management

Because several new effective medications are now readily available for treatment of influenza, virologic testing to confirm the diagnosis and type the virus is important. Amantadine (Symmetrel) 100 mg twice a day, is effective treatment for influenza type A, but not type B. Patients with compromised renal function should reduce the dose to 100 mg once a day. The dose in children up to age 10 is 3 mg/pound/day as a single dose. More recently, rimantadine (Flumadine) in the same doses offers the same good results with fewer side effects. Within the past 2 years, two neuraminidase inhibitors, zanamivir (Relenza) and oseltamivir (Tamiflu), have been approved for use and are widely available to treat both types of influenza. Zanamivir is inhaled as 10 mg twice a day. Oseltamivir is taken orally as 75 mg twice a day for adults and 2 mg/kg twice a day for children, used daily for 5 days. Because of the severity of the myalgias and headache associated with influenza, aspirin and nonsteroidal antiinflammatory drugs (NSAIDs) may not suffice and a narcotic-containing product is frequently indicated.

Complications and Sequelae

Most statistical methods for assessing excess morbidity and mortality are based on an index of influenza complicated by pneumonia, which may produce an underestimation of the serious morbidity and mortality. During an influenza outbreak, there is usually an increased death rate among the elderly mostly due to pneumonia and cardiovascular disease. Influenza itself can cause severe and rapidly evolving viral pneumonia with multiorgan failure. Children under 5 years of age have the highest rates of hospitalization for acute upper and lower respiratory tract disease when infected with influenza. Pandemic strains of extreme virulence such as the 1918 influenza can cause far-reaching complications. The 1918 Spanish flu caused 5 million cases of encephalitis lethargica (of von Economo) with symptoms of acute encephalitis with or without death and postencephalitic Parkinson's disease. The 1957 pandemic produced a small number of people with massive pulmonary edema and hemorrhage with rapid death as was seen commonly in 1918. Even in the years where the circulating influenza strains are mild, there is a rise in the number of cases of otitis media, bronchitis, asthma, and exacerbation of COPD.

Control and Prevention

Influenza vaccine is produced on the recommendation of the Food and Drug Administration (FDA) Vaccines and Related Biologicals Advisory Committee. Antigenic choices are based on (1) the viruses that have been seen during the previous year, (2) the viruses that are being seen in other parts of the world during the current year, and (3) the estimated antibody response in persons previously infected or vaccinated to these viruses. The current strategy is to immunize high-risk groups (the elderly and children with underlying conditions including heart, pulmonary, malignant, and some metabolic diseases). Unfortunately, the level of acceptance by patients and the overall delivery of vaccines to high-risk children has been consistently poor. This approach leaves most of the population unvaccinated, which produces a large "at-risk" population to be infected. Another approach to the control of influenza is to immunize all schoolchildren, children in day care, college students, military personnel, and employees of large companies. These groups have the highest susceptibility and, because of the nature of their activities, are the principal vectors of influenza virus in the community. They are also an accessible population with a structured environment that permits effective distribution of influenza vaccine. Efforts should also be directed toward immunizing as many high-risk patients as possible or to start them on chemotherapy at the first evidence of an epidemic.

Bronchitis

DIAGNOSIS

Bronchitis is an inflammation of the major and minor bronchial branches. It is characterized by a cough that is frequently productive of sputum, depending on the inflammatory cause. Bacterial causes of bronchitis generally produce purulent-looking sputum. Viral causes of bronchitis more commonly produce either clear sputum or a nonproductive cough. On physical examination, a patient with bronchitis has a noticeable cough, but the lungs are usually normal to auscultation. Rales, dullness to percussion, egophony, and other lower respiratory findings are usually absent. Cigarette smoking, other air pollutants, and chemical exposures that cause bronchial irritation may prolong an episode of bronchitis. Systemic lupus erythematosus is a cause of persistent bronchitis in a small number of affected patients.[34]

SPECTRUM OF INFECTION

Acute lower respiratory tract illness in previously well adults is usually labeled acute bronchitis and treated with antibiotics before establishing the etiology. An English study of 638 patients over 1 year identified pathogens in 55% of cases; viruses were identified as 28% of the pathogens. Outcome did not relate to pathogens. Most patients improved without antibiotics in spite of the pathogen identified.[35] Viral causes of acute bronchitis tend to be more common with influenza (types A and B), parainfluenza of all four serotypes, and RSV. RSV and parainfluenza viruses are found more commonly in the young population, and coronaviruses and adenoviruses occur in older patients. Influenza causes bronchitis at all ages. Increases in frequency of bronchitis as a reason for adult hospital admissions usually occur during influenza epidemics. RSV is a significant problem in elderly populations in nursing homes. Falsey and Walsh[36] found attack rates of up to 10% per year in nursing home patients, with up to 20% going on to pneumonia, and 5% dying.

Spasmodic Croup and Laryngotracheobronchitis

Though croup is a frightening family experience, especially for parents of very young children, it is a self-limited illness. There are two variations of croup presentation, episodic (spasmodic) croup and laryngotracheobronchitis (LTB). Episodic croup presents as the sudden onset without warning of inspiratory stridor, cough, and hoarseness. The young child has not been overtly ill, but is suddenly crouping. There is minimal or no fever and no other respiratory symptoms. LTB has early warning signs of respiratory infection for several days that gradually lead to cough and inspiratory stridor. Cool night air or a steamed bathroom will usually break episodic croup, and it does not tend to recur in the same time period. At most, one treatment of aerosolized racemic epinephrine (0.25–0.5 mL of a 2.25% solution in 3 mL of normal saline) will break the attack. On the other hand, LTB may break with one epinephrine treatment, improve, and then worsen again.

On occasion, LTB will become severe enough to warrant admission for repeated aerosol treatments or a croup tent with mist and oxygen. Steroids are effective in improving the outcome of croup when given within 6 hours of symptom onset. Prednisolone (Pediapred or Prelone) 5 to 60 mg po divided bid can be continued for several days. Steroids given prior to a racemic epinephrine treatment may reduce the likelihood of rebound return of crouping as the epinephrine wears off. Physicians should look for the coexistence of underlying illnesses and reassure the family that croup is a manageable illness. Munoz and Glasso[37] reported that 70% of croup cases were caused by parainfluenza viruses. Children under 15 years of age are more likely to croup with parainfluenza types 1 and 2. Croup has peak incidence at age 2 years, and is more common in the fall and winter months. Croup is not commonly associated with rhinovirus infections, but is associated with coronavirus infections. Adenovirus is a common cause of croup in children and occurs sporadically throughout the year, being most common during the winter and spring.

Bronchiolitis

Bronchiolitis is an acute viral respiratory disease generally found in children younger than 2 years old. The typical clinical presentation is an upper respiratory infection with cough that progresses to a more severe cough and tachypnea. Respirations become rapid and shallow with a prolonged expiratory phase. Because the infants are not able to breathe well, they are also unable to suck or drink and can become dehydrated.

DIAGNOSIS

Physical findings include intercostal retractions and nasal flaring, which suggest pneumonia. A chest roentgenogram shows only hyperinflation with no infiltrates. Tight expiratory sounds (not entirely typical of wheezes found with asthma) are usually present, as are some rhonchi. Rales and dullness to percussion suggest the coexistence of pneumonia. Bronchiolitis is most commonly caused by RSV, occurring predominantly during the winter and spring. Parainfluenza viruses, particularly types 1 and 2, can cause bronchiolitis during early winter. The most severe cases of bronchiolitis are usually caused by influenza viruses, especially type A. The virus involved can be identified by culture of nasopharyngeal secretions or by RT-PCR or immunofluorescent assay.

MANAGEMENT

Management of bronchiolitis depends on the progression of signs and symptoms. Hospitalization may be necessary to correct hypoxemia or dehydration. If fever is significant, pneumonia must be ruled out. Cases that appear to be recurrent bronchiolitis may be asthma, even if the child is younger than 1 year old.

Outpatient treatment is generally supportive, with careful attention to hydration. If hospitalization becomes necessary to correct hypoxemia or dehydration, treatment is focused on oxygenation, mist, and mechanically clearing the upper airway. There is no effective antiviral agent to treat RSV and parainfluenza viruses. Ribavirin (Virazole) has shown variable effectiveness in the most severe cases of bronchiolitis, especially respirator-dependent infants. Steroids are of no proven value; however, the tight airway that reminds one of asthma may respond to both steroids and bronchodilators such as albuterol.

Infants who are at highest risk of developing severe bronchiolitis (preterm birth, bronchopulmonary dysplasia, immunocompromise and other underlying chronic diseases) can be protected during the winter season by prophylaxis with human RSV immunoglobulin or monoclonal antibodies (Palivizumab).

COMPLICATIONS AND SEQUELAE

The most serious complication of bronchiolitis is respiratory failure requiring ventilatory assistance. It is best managed with continuous positive airway pressure and oxygen. RSV accounts for an estimated 90,000 hospitalizations and 4500 deaths per year in children under 16 years of age in the United States. Mortality rates in institutionalized elderly can reach 20%.

Bronchiolitis caused by RSV is strongly associated with postinfection wheezing for as long as 10 years. Careful studies have shown rates of asthma from 23% to 30% several years after hospitalization as an infant for RSV bronchiolitis.

Pharyngoconjunctival Fever

Pharyngoconjunctival fever is an upper respiratory illness that affects teenagers and adults. It manifests as pharyngitis, cough, fever, headache, myalgias, malaise, and particularly conjunctivitis. This syndrome is caused by adenovirus, particularly serotypes 3 and 7, which are frequently found in natural bodies of water and reservoirs. Symptoms may be similar to those of influenza. Conjunctivitis is generally not present with influenza but is always found with pharyngoconjunctival fever and usually at an early stage. There is a spring and summer seasonal prevalence. It can be diagnosed by viral cultures of nasopharyngeal and throat swabs and the recently developed immunofluorescent and RT-PCR tests. Management of pharyngoconjunctival fever is symptomatic. There is no indication for systemic antibiotic treatment or ophthalmic antibiotics. There are no long-term complications or sequelae. Recovery is generally within 1 week.

Laryngitis

There are six distinct causes of laryngitis, the most common being viral infections of the upper respiratory tract. Vocal cord tumors can cause laryngitis; allergies are a frequent cause, and strain of the vocal cords caused by long periods of loud talking produces laryngitis. A fairly frequent cause of laryngitis is hard coughing associated with an upper or lower respiratory tract infection. The least frequent cause is a bacterial infection of the throat. Most of the causes of laryngitis are obvious. Viral laryngitis is difficult to distinguish from the less frequent bacterial laryngitis, which might require antibiotic treatment. Children over age 2 and adults rarely have significant swelling of the throat that would put them at risk of airway obstruction. Children under age 2 are more likely to develop airway obstruction. Viral causes of laryngitis include the parainfluenza viruses, rhinoviruses, adenoviruses, and the influenza viruses. Voice rest has the greatest impact on recovery. Patients who are able to gargle with warm, weak salt-water solution sometimes find it soothing. Patients should be told that laryngitis is not a serious disease and that adequate time to recover is the only therapy in most cases.

Viral Respiratory Tract Infections in Very Young and Very Old Patients

Patients younger than age 2 present some special problems. Perhaps as many as two thirds of pediatric emergency room visits for respiratory infections are inappropriate. Parents frequently need only reassurance that their child is not seriously ill. Although most viral respiratory infections in children appear to be self-limited and without complications, they are among the leading causes of death in the youngest children. Table 10.2 details the patterns of viral illness found in young children, adults, and elderly patients. The institutionalized elderly represent a subgroup of older people who are prone to excess morbidity and mortality from respiratory tract infections. Each year many elderly persons living in long-term-care facilities become ill with respiratory illnesses that are mistakenly

TABLE 10.2. Patterns of Viral Illness in Children and Elderly Patients

Virus	Signs and Symptoms		
	Young children	Adults	Elderly
Respiratory syncytial virus	Wheezing, bronchiolitis, pneumonia, bronchitis	Nasal congestion and cough	Nasal congestion, cough, fever, pneumonia, wheezing, bronchitis
Influenza	Sore throat, high fever, myalgias, bronchitis, croup, bronchiolitis, rhinorrhea, otitis media	Fever, headache, myalgias, malaise, cough, weakness, bronchitis, laryngitis	Bronchitis, low-grade fever, sore throat, pneumonia
Parainfluenza	Croup, bronchitis, pneumonia, sore throat, bronchiolitis	Common cold, laryngitis	Rhinorrhea, sore throat, cough, pneumonia, fever
Rhinoviruses	Sore throat, rhinorrhea	Rhinorrhea, sneezing, cough, sore throat, laryngitis	Rhinorrhea, cough, sneezing
Coronaviruses	Croup, sore throat	Common cold, malaise, headache, sore throat, low-grade fever	Exacerbation of chronic pulmonary disease, pneumonia, bronchitis
Adenoviruses	Croup, sore throat	Coryza, sore throat, pneumonia, pharyngoconjunctival fever, keratoconjunctivitis, laryngitis	Bronchitis rarely

attributed to bacterial pneumonia or influenza. The respiratory tract viruses listed in Table 10.2 (particularly RSV, parainfluenza virus, and influenza virus) are a significant cause of disease in this high-risk population. RSV ranks second to influenza as the most common cause of serious viral respiratory infections in long-term-care facility patients. The pattern of reported outbreaks of RSV in a long-term-care facility is usually a steady trickle of cases over several months—distinctly different from outbreaks of influenza, which tend to be explosive. Parainfluenza virus is a common cause of croup and bronchitis in young children; however, because full immunity does not develop, reinfection is common in the older population. In the institutionalized elderly, parainfluenza presents as rhinorrhea, pharyngitis, cough, and pneumonia.

References

1. Denny FW. The clinical impact of human respiratory virus infections. Am J Respir Crit Care Med 1995;Oct. 152(4PT2):54–12.
2. Milinaric G. Epidemiological picture of respiratory viral infections in Croatia. Acta Med Iugosl 1991;45:203–11.
3. Jain A. An Indian hospital study of viral causes of acute respiratory infection in children. J Med Microbiol 1991;35:219–23.
4. Falsey AR, Treanor JJ. Viral respiratory infections in the institutionalized elderly; clinical and epidemiology findings. J Am Geriatr Soc 1992;40:115–19.
5. Greenberg SB, Allen M. Respiratory viral infections in adults with and without chronic obstructive pulmonary disease. Am J Respir Crit Care Med 2000;162:167–73.
6. El-Sahly HM, Atmar RL. Spectrum of clinical illness in hospitalized patients with "common cold" virus infections. Clin Infect Dis 2000;31:96–100.
7. Barenfanger J, Drake C. Clinical and financial benefits of rapid detection of respiratory viruses: an outcomes study. J Clin Microbiol 2000;38:2824–8.
8. Steininger C, Aberle SW. Early detection of acute rhinovirus infections by a rapid reverse transcription–PCR assay. J Clin Microbiol 2001;39:129–33.
9. Tsai HP, Kuo PH. Respiratory viral infections among pediatric inpatients and outpatients in Taiwan from 1997 to 1999. J Clin Microbiol 2001;39:111–18.
10. Glezen WP, Greenberg SB. Impact of respiratory virus infections on persons with chronic underlying conditions. JAMA 2000;283:499–505.
11. Kim MR, Lee HR. Epidemiology of acute viral respiratory tract infections in Korean children. J Infect 2000;41:152–8.
12. Weigl JA, Puppe W. Epidemiological investigation of nine respiratory pathogens in hospitalized children in Germany using multiplex reverse-transcriptase polymerase chain reaction. Eur J Clin Microbiol Infect Dis 2000;19:336–43.
13. Nasrallah GK, Meqdam MM. Prevalence of parainfluenza and influenza viruses amongst children with upper respiratory tract infection. Saudi Med J 2000;21:1024–9.
14. Hall CB, Douglas RG. Clinically useful method for the isolation of respiratory syncytial virus. J Infect Dis 1975;131:1–5.
15. Irmen KE, Kelleher JJ. Use of monoclonal antibodies for rapid diagnosis of respiratory viruses in a community hospital. Clin Diagn Lab Immunol 2000;7:396–403.
16. Kehl SC, Henrickson KJ. Evaluation of the hexaplex assay for detection of respiratory viruses in children. J Clin Microbiol 2001;39:1696–701.

17. Shimizu H. The rapid detection kit based on neuraminidase activity of influenza virus. Nippon Rinsho 2000;58:2234–7.
18. Munoz FM, Glasso GJ. Current research on influenza and other respiratory viruses. Antiviral Res 2000;46:91–124.
19. Laurichesse H, Dedman D. Epidemiological features of parainfluenza virus infections: laboratory surveillance in England and Wales, 1975–1997. Eur J Epidemiol 1999;15:475–84.
20. Todd FJ, Drinka PJ. A serious outbreak of parainfluenza type 3 on a nursing unit. J Am Geriatr Soc 2000;48:1216–8.
21. Graman PS, Hall CB. Epidemiology and control of nosocomial viral infections. Infect Dis Clin North Am 1989;3:815–41.
22. Mygina N. The common cold as a trigger of asthma. Monaldi Arch Chest Dis 2000;55:478–83.
23. Van Kempen MJ, Bachert C. An update on the pathophysiology of rhinovirus upper respiratory tract infection. Rhinology 1999;37:97–103.
24. Hayden FG. Influenza virus and rhinovirus-related otitis media: potential for antiviral intervention. Vaccine 2000;19(suppl):566–70.
25. Rotbart HA. Antiviral therapy for enteroviruses and rhinoviruses. Antivir Chem Chemother 2000;11:261–71.
26. Isaacs D, Flowers D. Epidemiology of coronavirus respiratory infections. Arch Dis Child 1983;58:500–3.
27. Falsey AR, McCann RM. The "common cold" in frail older persons: impact of rhinovirus and coronavirus in a senior day care center. J Am Geriatr Soc 1997;45:706–11.
28. Hyer RN, Howell MR. Cost-effectiveness analysis of reacquiring and using adenovirus types 4 and 7 vaccines in naval recruits. Am J Trop Med Hyg 2000;62:613–8.
29. Gwaltney JM Jr, Park J. Randomized controlled trial of clemastine fumarate for treatment of experimental rhinovirus colds. Clin Infect Dis 1996;22:656–62.
30. Henneicke-Von Zepelin H. Efficacy and safety of a fixed combination phytomedicine in the treatment of the common cold: results of a randomized, double blind, placebo controlled, multicentre study. Curr Med Res Opin 1999;15:214–27.
31. Jackson JL, Lesho E. Zinc and the common cold: a meta-analysis revisited. J Nutr 2000;130(55 suppl):15125–55.
32. Schiff GM, Sherwood JR. Clinical activity of pleconaril in an experimentally induced coxsackievirus A21 respiratory infection. J Infect Dis 2000;181:2000–26.
33. Meddiratta PK, Sharma KK. A review on recent development of common cold therapeutic agents. Indian J Med Sci 2000;54:485–90.
34. Raz E, Bursztyn M. Severe recurrent lupus laryngitis. Am J Med 1992;92:109–10.
35. Macfarlane J, Holmes W. Prospective study of the incidence, aetiology and outcome of adult lower respiratory tract illness in the community. Thorax 2001;56:109–14.
36. Falsey AR, Walsh EE. Respiratory syncytial virus infection in adults. Clin Microbiol Rev 2000;13:371–84.
37. Munoz FM, Glasso GJ. Current research on influenza and other respiratory viruses Antiviral Res 2000;46(2):91–124.

CASE PRESENTATION

Subjective

PATIENT PROFILE

Kendra Nelson is a 16-year-old single female high school sophomore.

PRESENTING PROBLEM

Fever and weakness.

PRESENT ILLNESS

For the past day-and-a-half, Kendra has felt weak and achy. She has had a temperature of 103°F at home. There is a generalized headache, a mild cough, and a decreased appetite. A few of her schoolmates have had similar symptoms.

PAST MEDICAL HISTORY

No prior hospitalization or serious injury.

SOCIAL HISTORY

Kendra lives with her parents. She is a "good student" and has had a steady boyfriend for the past year.

HABITS

She uses no tobacco, alcohol, or coffee.

FAMILY HISTORY

Her parents are living and well. She has one sibling, aged 19, who is away from home in the Army.

- What additional historical information might be useful, and why?
- What might be the meaning of this illness to the patient?
- Would further information regarding her classmates or boyfriend be helpful? Why?

- What are likely adaptations of this teenager to her illness? Why might this be pertinent?

Objective

VITAL SIGNS

Blood pressure, 104/60; pulse, 86; respirations, 22; temperature, 38.6°C.

EXAMINATION

The patient is alert and ambulatory but looks "ill." The tympanic membranes are normal. The pharynx is mildly injected. The neck is supple without adenopathy, and the thyroid gland is normal. Her chest is clear. The heart has a normal sinus rhythm with no murmurs present.

- What further information about the physical examination might be useful, and why?
- What other areas of the body—if any—should be examined? Why?
- What—if any—laboratory tests should be obtained today? Why?
- What—if any—diagnostic imaging studies should be obtained today?

Assessment

- What is the likely diagnosis, and how would you explain this to the patient and her parents?
- Kendra's mother asks if Kendra is likely to be even worse during the next few days and what to do if this occurs. How would you reply?
- If the patient also had a rash, what diagnoses would you consider?
- What are the family/community implications of this illness?

Plan

- What would be your therapeutic recommendation to Kendra regarding medication, diet, pain relief, and return to school?
- Kendra asks about the possibility of others catching her illness. How would you reply?
- Kendra's mother asks about preventing such an illness in the future. How would you respond?
- What continuing care would you recommend?

11

Otitis Media and Externa

William F. Miser

Otitis Media

Otitis media is the most common reason for medical office visits (over 20 million a year) and for surgery in children in the United States.[1-3] The peak incidence occurs between the ages of 6 and 15 months, with a second peak at age 5 years.[4] Nearly two thirds of children have at least one episode of otitis media by their first birthday, and more than 90% have one by age 2 years.[2,3] The diagnosis of otitis media is the most common reason for antibiotic prescriptions in children.[5] Nearly $5 billion is spent each year in the United States in managing otitis media.[6,7] This cost does not take into account the disruption of child-care arrangements and work schedules, and the generation of parental anxiety and stress.[8] Despite its frequency and associated costs, controversy exists about its proper management.

Definitions

Otitis media refers to inflammation of the middle ear, which is often associated with a middle-ear effusion.[9] *Acute otitis media* (AOM) is an infection of the middle ear with rapid appearance of symptoms and signs such as fever, pain, irritability, and abnormal appearance (erythematous, bulging) of and decreased mobility of the tympanic membrane. *Otitis media with effusion* (OME), also known as "serous otitis media" and/or "glue ear," is a middle-ear effusion without the obvious signs of an acute infection. If this effusion persists for longer than 4 months, it is known as *chronic otitis media with effusion* (COME). *Persistent acute otitis media* is the persistence of symptoms and signs of AOM following at least two courses of antibiotic therapy, whereas *recurrent acute otitis media* is three or more separate episodes of AOM in a 6-month time span, or four or more episodes in a year.[10] *Chronic suppurative otitis media* is an infection of the middle ear resulting in a perforated tympanic membrane with purulent discharge (otorrhea).

226

Pathophysiology

Dysfunction of the eustachian tube, which allows reflux of bacteria and fluid from the nasopharynx into the middle ear space, contributes to the development of AOM.[3] Children are more prone to AOM because their eustachian tubes are shorter, more flexible, and inefficient at clearing secretions. Over 70% of painful ear episodes develop during a viral upper respiratory infection, which magnifies eustachian tube dysfunction.[3,11] Other major risk factors for AOM include craniofacial abnormalities (e.g., cleft palate), cigarette smoking in the home, exposure to large numbers of children (e.g., day care), and family history of frequent AOM.[12,13] It also appears that prolonged use of a pacifier, especially past age 2 years, increases the risk.[14] Breast-feeding for at least 6 months appears to be protective.[15]

In a recent study of children with AOM, middle ear fluid obtained by tympanocentesis revealed that 41% had a viral cause.[16] The most common virus was respiratory syncytial virus. The most common bacterial causes for AOM were *Streptococcus pneumoniae* (25%), *Haemophilus influenzae* (23%), and *Branhamella catarrhalis* (15%). Both bacteria and viruses were isolated in 65% of children.

Diagnosis

It is commonly accepted that AOM is overdiagnosed in the United States.[8,17] A squirming, uncooperative toddler with an ear canal occluded with cerumen seen by a busy clinician who wants to please anxious parents, often will err on the side of making a diagnosis of AOM based on history alone. Diagnostic uncertainty is as high as 33% to 42%.[18,19]

The diagnosis of AOM is based on a combination of symptoms and physical findings. Typically, symptoms are nonspecific and include fever, earache, tugging or rubbing of the ear, irritability, muffled or diminished hearing, lethargy, anorexia, vomiting, and/or diarrhea.[3] However, these symptoms need not always be present.[20]

An accurate diagnosis of AOM requires a clear and well-illuminated view of the tympanic membrane. Any cerumen obstructing the view should be gently removed with a curette. The use of a cerumenolytic with warm irrigation may be necessary to remove excessive cerumen. The light of the otoscope should work well; bulbs for most otoscopes should be changed every 2 years.[17]

Four characteristics of the tympanic membrane should be evaluated—position, mobility, degree of translucency, and color. The "normal" tympanic membrane is in a neutral position (not retracted or bulging), responds well to positive and negative pressure, and is translucent and pearly gray.[17] Pneumatic otoscopy allows for the evaluation of mobility of the tympanic membrane. If used, the ear speculum should create an air seal against the external auditory canal. A soft rubber sleeve over the speculum usually reduces the discomfort of this exam.[17]

Tympanometry and acoustic reflectometry are tools useful in confirming the presence of a middle ear effusion. Tympanometry is portable and useful in the office by providing information about the actual pressures within the middle ear space.[17] An abnormal, "flat" (type B) tympanogram in infants with acute symptoms strongly suggests AOM, although a normal test is not helpful in ruling out the diagnosis.[3]

Each of the physical findings of the tympanic membrane alone is inadequate to confirm the diagnosis of AOM. In one study, only two thirds of patients with a red tympanic membrane and 16% with a slightly red tympanic membrane had AOM.[3] Erythema of the tympanic membrane can be due to fever, crying, or cerumen removal. However, combining the findings on exam is useful. Typically, a bulging or cloudy tympanic membrane with or without erythema, middle ear effusion, and marked decrease or absence of tympanic membrane mobility is nearly 100% predictive of AOM.[3] Perforation of the tympanic membrane with purulent drainage is also diagnostic of AOM.

To avoid unnecessary antibiotic treatment, it is important to distinguish between AOM and OME, which is sometimes difficult to do. Middle-ear effusion and a decrease in, or absence of, tympanic-membrane mobility characterize both. Both will have a flat (type B) tympanogram and a "plugged ear" feeling with conductive hearing loss. The position of the tympanic membrane in AOM is usually bulging, while it is slightly retracted or in a neutral position in OME. Unlike OME, AOM is often associated with acute symptoms (e.g., ear pain and fever) and signs (erythematous or yellow, bulging tympanic membrane). Visualization of the tympanic membrane in OME often demonstrates "bubbles" or an air-fluid level. Occasionally tympanocentesis is required to determine whether the middle effusion is infected, but there are no consensus guidelines for its routine use in the management of AOM or OME.[17]

Treatment

The management of otitis media is controversial. Results from recent studies have questioned the use of antibiotics and the length of treatment if prescribed, and the role of surgical interventions such as tympanostomy (ventilating) tubes.

ACUTE OTITIS MEDIA

The growing worldwide occurrence of multidrug-resistant bacteria, the uncertainty of diagnosis, and the fact that up to a third of cases of AOM are viral in origin have made popular a "wait and see" approach to the initial prescription of antibiotics, especially in many European countries. In several randomized clinical trials, antibiotics provide only a small benefit.[21–23] The natural course of uncomplicated, untreated AOM is quite favorable. In a recent meta-analysis of over 2000 children with AOM, ear pain resolved spontaneously in two thirds by 24 hours, and in 80% by day 7.[22] This study estimated that 17 children would need to be treated with antibiotics to prevent one child from having some pain after 2 days. Children treated with antibiotics are almost twice as likely to have adverse reactions such as skin rash, vomiting, or diarrhea. Minimizing the use of antibiotics in patients with AOM does not increase the risks of perforation of the tympanic membrane, hearing loss, or contralateral or recurrent AOM.[3]

Most studies do not include children younger than 2 years of age. This group appears to have a higher risk of treatment failure, persistent symptoms, and recurrent AOM.[3] However, a recent trial in this age group found that seven to eight children with AOM need to be treated with antibiotics to improve symptomatic outcome at day 4 in one child.[24] The major benefit of antibiotics was 1 day less of fever, but adverse effects were almost twice as likely compared to placebo, and there were no differences in clinical failure rates at day 11 or in the likelihood of recurrence. The authors conclude that a watchful waiting approach is also justified in this age group.

Some will argue that untreated AOM will increase the risk of mastoiditis or meningitis, although there are insufficient data to suggest that routine antibiotic use makes a difference.[3] Mastoiditis is quite rare; in one study there was only one case among 2202 children with untreated AOM.[22] It is uncertain whether the current rarity is due to widespread antibiotic use or to a change in host defenses or in virulence of the organisms.[3] Further studies will need to be done as the wait and see approach becomes more popular.

In summary, the immediate prescription of antibiotics offers some benefits, but these are balanced by the disadvantages of increased cost, drug resistance, and adverse reactions. A practical approach is to counsel parents about the options, provide pain relief to the child, and write a prescription for antibiotics, to be filled only if the child is no better in 2 to 3 days, sooner if it appears that symptoms are worsening. This watchful waiting has been shown to be feasible and acceptable to most parents, with a 76% reduction in the use of antibiotics.[23]

Antibiotics. If antibiotics are used, amoxicillin is the drug of choice for most children.[13,25] It achieves high levels in the middle ear fluid, is effective against most bacterial pathogens known to cause AOM, is inexpensive, and has a low incidence of side effects (skin rash, nausea, diarrhea). Although there are over a dozen other clinically effective antibiotics approved by the Food and Drug Administration for treating AOM (Table 11.1), none of these more expensive options has been shown to be more effective for empiric therapy of uncomplicated AOM.[25] Rather, these other antibiotics are good alternatives for those known to be allergic to amoxicillin, to have a more severe clinical course, or to have a treatment failure, defined as no clinical improvement after 2 to 3 days or recurrence of AOM within 2 weeks of therapy.[13] Oral antihistamine-decongestant preparations offer no additional advantage when given with antibiotics, and are no more effective than placebo in decreasing the middle ear effusion.[2]

Amoxicillin is normally given at 40 to 45 mg/kg/day divided into two or three doses daily. There is recent in vitro evidence, and some clinical experience, of increasing penicillin-resistant *Streptococcus pneumoniae*. This resistance is more common in children younger than 2 years of age, especially those in a day-care

TABLE 11.1. Antibiotics for Acute Otitis Media[2,13]

Antibiotic	Dosage[a] Adults (mg)	Dosage[a] Children (mg/kg/day)	Dosing frequency[b]	Cost[c]
Suggested primary regimen				
Amoxicillin	500	80–90	bid–tid	$–$$
Second-line treatment[d]				
Amoxicillin-clavulanate (Augmentin)	875/125	90/6.4	bid	$$$$–$$$$$
Sulfonamides				
Trimethoprim-sulfamethoxazole (Bactrim, Septra)	160/800	8 (trimethoprim)	bid	$
Erythromycin-sulfisoxazole (Pediazole)	400/1200	50 (erythromycin)	qid	$$
Cephalosporins				
1st generation				
Cefaclor (Ceclor)	500	40	tid	$$$$
2nd generation				
Cefprozil (Cefzil)	250–500	30	bid	$$$$
Cefuroxime axeti (Ceftin)	250	30	bid	$$–$$$
Loracarbef (Lorabid)	200–400	30	bid	$$$–$$$$
3rd generation				
Cefdinir (Omnicef)	600	14	qd–bid	$$$$$
Cefixime (Suprax)	400	8	qd	$$$–$$$$$
Cefpodoxime (Vantin)	200	10	qd–bid	$$$$
Ceftibuten (Cedax)	400	9	qd	$$$$$
Ceftriaxone (IM)[d] (Rocephin)	—	50	qd	$$$$$
Macrolides				
Clarithromycin (Biaxin)	250	15	qd	$$$$$
Azithromycin (Zithromax)	500 mg day 1 250 mg days 2–5	10 mg day 1 5 mg day 2–5	qd qd	$$–$$$ $$–$$$

[a]Do not exceed adult doses in children weighing more than 40 kg. Initial therapy is for 5 days; duration is 10–14 days for treatment failures or recurrence.
[b]qd = once a day; bid = twice a day; tid = three times a day; qid = four times a day.
[c]Cost for therapeutic course based on average wholesale price from 2000 *Drugs Topics Red Book*; prices for generic drugs were used when available; $ = $0–$15; $$ = $16–$30; $$$ = $31–$45; $$$$ = $46–$60; $$$$$ = greater than $60.
[d]See text for further information.

setting, and in those with recurrent bouts of AOM or who have recently been treated for AOM.[10] As such, a working group of the Centers for Disease Control and Prevention advised a doubling of the amoxicillin dose to 80 to 90 mg/kg/day.[26] For those children who show no improvement with this increased dose in 3 to 5 days, alternatives such as amoxicillin-clavulanate (Augmentin), cefuroxime axetil (Ceftin), or intramuscular ceftriaxone (Rocephin) should be tried. Unfortunately, the two former antibiotics rate lowest on palatability and compliance,[27] and the latter requires two to three injections over 2 to 3 days. Although more expensive, third-generation cephalosporins are better tolerated and offer good options for amoxicillin treatment failures. Children with amoxicillin failure who develop a new episode of AOM more than 90 days later may still be treated with amoxicillin as the first choice.[28]

Duration of Therapy. There is strong evidence that 5 days of antibiotic therapy is just as effective as the traditional 10- to 14-day regimen for uncomplicated AOM in children.[29–31] Although the 5-day regimen has a slightly higher risk of treatment failure at a 1-month follow-up compared to the longer course, there appears to be no difference in long-term (2 to 3 months) outcome.[30] A minimum of 17 children would need to be treated with the longer course of antibiotics to avoid one treatment failure.[31] These studies exclude children with underlying disease, a recent bout of AOM, recurrent or chronic OM, craniofacial abnormalities (e.g., cleft palate), or a perforated tympanic membrane. It is recommended that these children be treated with the longer regimen. Most studies also exclude children younger than 2 years of age, although one recent trial demonstrated that the 10-day regimen has a slightly better success rate initially than the 5-day course (92% vs. 84%), with no difference in clinical success 4 to 6 weeks later.[32] In summary, the duration of therapy should be individualized, and most children with uncomplicated AOM can be treated with a shortened 5-day course.

Pain Relief. Analgesia is an important adjunct to therapy. Acetaminophen 10 to 15 mg/kg every 4 to 6 hours or ibuprofen 5 to 10 mg/kg every 6 to 8 hours is effective in relieving pain.[33] Occasionally, codeine is needed for severe pain. Topical analgesia with antipyrine, benzocaine and glycerin (e.g., Auralgan Otic) every 1 to 2 hours effectively relieves pain and congestion within 30 minutes of administration, but should be avoided if the tympanic membrane has ruptured.[33] Occasionally, pain is so severe that referral is needed to an otolaryngologist for relief of pressure with tympanocentesis or myringotomy.

Surgery. As initial therapy, tympanocentesis offers no advantage to antibiotics alone in treating AOM.[34] It should be reserved for those who appear septic, who have persistent AOM unresponsive to multiple courses of antibiotics, or who have a complex anatomic or immunologic abnormality.

RECURRENT AOM

About one in five children have recurrent AOM.[8] Antibiotic prophylaxis has been shown to be at least as effective as, if not more effective than, tympanostomy tubes in preventing new episodes.[35] Prophylactic doses are normally half of that required for treatment of AOM. In a large meta-analysis, antibiotic prophylaxis reduced the frequency of new episodes of AOM by 44%.[36] Amoxicillin (20 mg/kg/day in one or two doses) or sulfisoxazole (75 mg/kg/day in one or two doses) is an effective prophylactic antibiotic. In the past, 3 to 6 months of therapy was suggested for prophylaxis. However, because of increasing antimicrobial resistance, it is now recommended that therapy should begin at the first sign of an upper respiratory infection, and should continue for 10 days.[37] In addition to prophylactic antibiotics, it is important to modify known risk factors (e.g., encourage and help parents to quit smoking).

Since *S. pneumoniae* is the leading bacterial cause of otitis media, it is thought that the recent approval of the pneumococcal vaccine Prevnar (Wyeth-Ayerst Labs, Philadelphia, PA) will decrease the occurrence of otitis media. This vaccine is associated with a 6% reduction in the number of episodes of AOM, and a 9% reduction in the frequency of recurrent AOM.[7] Although not as dramatic a decline as hoped, routine vaccination of all children will prevent up to 1.2 million episodes of AOM in the United States each year. Influenza virus vaccination is also recommended for those prone to frequent AOM during the respiratory season.[25]

For those children who have severe and recurrent disease, consider referral to an otolaryngologist for placement of tympanostomy tubes. Concomitant adenoidectomy is commonly performed in the United States, but recent evidence questions its effectiveness, and suggests that it should not be considered as a first surgical intervention in children whose only indication is recurrent AOM.[38]

CHRONIC SUPPURATIVE OTITIS MEDIA

Purulent material should be removed by suctioning under direct visualization, or by gently using a cotton swab. Since the tympanic membrane is often ruptured, avoid flushing the ear canal, which may damage the inner ear with resultant hearing loss. Topical treatment with ofloxacin otic solution, 3 mg/mL, five drops twice daily for 10 days, has a similar cure rate to systemic amoxicillin-clavulanate and is better tolerated.[2,39,40]

CHRONIC OTITIS MEDIA WITH EFFUSION (COME)

Children who recover from AOM often have a residual middle ear effusion for up to 6 weeks after treatment. In 20% of these children, this effusion persists and there is concern that over time it will result in mild-to-moderate conductive hearing loss with subsequent impairment in language development and academic functioning.[8,41,42]

Initial management for COME is observation. A meta-analysis found that antibiotics offer only a marginal short-term benefit, and no long-term benefit.[36] The use of corticosteroids (prednisone or prenisolone, 1 mg/kg/day in two divided doses for 7 days) has been advised in the past,[8] but a recent study found only marginal short-term benefit in resolution of the effusion, and no long-term benefit in preventing hearing loss.[42]

If the effusion persists for longer than 4 months, the clinical practice guideline developed by the Agency for Health Care Policy and Research recommends a hearing test; if there is evidence of documented bilateral hearing impairment of 20 dB or more, tympanostomy tubes should be considered in children younger than 3 years of age.[43] Myringotomy with insertion of tympanostomy tubes is the most common operation among children beyond the newborn period in the United States.[44] It is thought that surgical resolution of the effusion will restore normal hearing and thereby prevent language and behavioral problems.

However, recent studies have suggested that the benefit from immediate insertion of tympanostomy tubes may not be as great as once thought.[44,45] Compared to watchful waiting, the insertion of tympanostomy tubes improves hearing at 6 months, but this difference disappears by 1 year.[46] In addition, there is relatively little difference in expressive or comprehensive language,[45] developmental behavior,[44] or in quality of life[47] between watchful waiting and insertion of tubes.

Children who undergo placement of tympanostomy tubes require ongoing surveillance. Showering, rinsing the hair, or submersion of the head in plain tap water or in a pool does not promote the entry of water into the middle ear.[48] As such, earplugs are not indicated for routine bathing or swimming, but are needed for deeper swimming or diving. Sequelae of tympanostomy tubes are common but generally transient.[49] Otorrhea occurs in up to 16% in the postoperative period, with 4% experiencing chronic drainage.[50] Cosmetic complications include tympanosclerosis (32%), focal atrophy (25%), and chronic perforation (17%) with long-term use.[50] The clinical implications of these changes are unknown, but this information is useful when counseling parents prior to referral to an otolaryngologist. Clearly, further long-term studies need to be conducted before abandoning the role of tympanostomy tubes in treating COME.

Some children who undergo tympanostomy tube placement for COME also benefit from concomitant adenoidectomy.[41] In one recent study, adenoidectomy or adenotonsillectomy at the time of initial insertion of tympanostomy tubes substantially reduced the likelihood of additional hospitalizations or further surgeries.[1] Eight adjuvant adenoidectomies need to be performed to avoid a single instance of rehospitalization over a 2-year period. For now these surgeries should be reserved for special cases not responding to tympanostomy tube insertion.

Otitis Externa

Otitis externa is an inflammatory process involving the external auditory canal. Cerumen normally acts as a defense against infection by creating an acidic environment that inhibits bacterial and fungal growth, and by preventing water from penetrating to the skin and causing maceration.[51] The most common precipitants for otitis externa are trauma to the ear canal (e.g., mechanical removal of cerumen by cotton swabs or other instruments, insertion of foreign objects such as fingernails or hearing aids), excessive moisture that raises the pH and removes the cerumen (e.g., swimming, diving, high humidity, perspiration), and chronic dermatologic conditions (e.g., eczema, seborrheic dermatitis).[51,52] Because otitis externa is most commonly found in persons involved in water sports, it is also known as "swimmer's ear."

The infectious agents of otitis externa are usually polymicrobial,[53] with *Pseudomonas aeruginosa* (40–60%) and *Staphylococcus aureus* (15–30%) being most common.[40,51,52,54] In about 10% of cases, fungi are involved (*Aspergillus* 80–90%, and *Candida*). Noninfectious causes of external otitis involve skin conditions such as psoriasis, seborrheic dermatitis, atopic dermatitis, lupus erythematosus, acne, and contact dermatitis.

Diagnosis

Patients with otitis externa typically present with ear discomfort varying from mild itching to severe pain associated with gentle traction of the external ear or with chewing. The ear canal is usually tender, erythematous, and swollen, with a foul-smelling discharge. The otorrhea and swelling often obscures the tympanic membrane, making it difficult to exclude an accompanying otitis media with perforation. In younger children, it is important to look for a foreign body that may be the inciting event.

Treatment

The treatment of otitis externa consists of removing the debris and draining the infection, controlling the pain, reestablishing the normal acidic environment, and using topical antimicrobials if needed.[52] If possible, the ear canal should be cleansed by suctioning under direct visualization with a 5- or 7-French Frazier malleable tip attached to low suction.[51] Alternatively, liquid debris may be gently removed using a cotton swab with the cotton fluffed out.[51] Hydrogen peroxide may be used to soften thick or crusted debris. Do not flush the ear canal unless the tympanic membrane can be fully seen and found to be without perforation; doing so may damage the inner ear and cause hearing loss, tinnitus, and vertigo. Analgesics such as acetaminophen, a nonsteroidal antiinflammatory, and/or codeine are often required.

The first-line treatment for otitis externa is a topical antibiotic; systemic antibiotics are rarely indicated except when a concomitant acute otitis media is present or if there has been local spread of the infection (see below).[55] Simple acidification of the ear canal with 2% acetic acid is often effective, but a wide variety of other agents is available (Table 11.2). The addition of hydrocortisone may resolve symptoms more quickly by decreasing the edema of the ear canal. The most commonly used topical antibiotic in the United States is polymyxin B-neomycin-hydrocortisone (Cortisporin), although the recently available quinolone preparations have been found to be just as effective and free from ototoxic effects, and applied twice daily as opposed to the four times daily for other preparations.[40,56] Typically three to four drops are placed in the affected ear up to 3 days beyond the cessation of symptoms (usually for 5–7 days), although

TABLE 11.2. Topical Agents Commonly Used to Treat Otitis Externa[40,51,56]

Agent	Advantages	Precautions
2% Acetic acid otic solution (VoSol) + Hydrocortisone (VoSol HC Otic) + Aluminum acetate (Otic Domeboro)	Inexpensive; effective against most infections; rarely causes sensitization	Occasionally irritating; possibly ototoxic
Neomycin otic solutions and suspensions + Polymyxin B-hydrocortisone (Cortisporin) + Hydrocortisone-thonzonium (Coly-Mycin S)	Effective; generic is inexpensive	May cause contact dermatitis in up to 15% of patients; potentially ototoxic if tympanic membrane ruptured and use is for 14 days or more
Polymyxin B-hydrocortisone (Otobiotic)	Avoids potential dermatitis; also *indicated for acute otitis media with perforation*	Inactive against *Staphylococcus and other gram positives*
Quinolones Otic preparations + Ofloxacin 0.3% solution (Floxin Otic) + Ciprofloxacin 0.3% and hydrocortisone suspension (Cipro HC Otic) Ophthalmic solutions + Ofloxacin 0.3% (Ocuflox) + Ciprofloxacin 0.3% (Ciloxan)	Highly effective, no local irritation, no risk of ototoxicity, twice-daily dosing; also indicated for acute otitis media with perforation, and for chronic suppurative otitis media	Expensive, potential development of resistance
Aminoglycoside ophthalmic solutions + Gentamicin sulfate 0.3% (Garamycin) + Tobramycin sulfate 0.3% (Tobrex)	Less locally irritating	Potentially ototoxic if tympanic membrane ruptured and use is for 14 days or more; moderately expensive

more severe infections may require up to 14 days of therapy. Warming the bottle of drops in the hands before installation minimizes discomfort.[51] For those times that the ear canal is quite swollen, placing a wick of quarter-inch cotton sterile gauze or using a Pope ear wick facilitates drainage and helps draw the topical medication into the affected canal.[52] This wick can usually be removed within 2 days as the edema resolves. Patients should abstain from water sports such as swimming and diving for at least 7 to 10 days, or until the symptoms have completely resolved.

Prevention

Avoid trauma (e.g., use of cotton swabs or other items used to remove cerumen) to the ear canal. For those prone to developing otitis externa (e.g., swimmers), a hair dryer set on the lowest heat setting can be used to dry the external auditory. Ear drops containing equal portions of white vinegar and rubbing alcohol or an over-the-counter preparation containing acid and alcohol (e.g., Swim Ear) is effective for prophylaxis.[56] Persons who swim frequently should use a barrier to protect their ears from water.

Necrotizing (Malignant) Otitis Externa

Necrotizing otitis externa is a severe form of external otitis with a mortality rate up to 53%.[51] Most often due to *P. aeruginosa* osteomyelitis of the mastoid or temporal bones, it affects elderly patients with diabetes mellitus, and those who are immunocompromised, especially due to human immunodeficiency (HIV) infection. Suspect this condition if pain is constant and disproportionately more severe than the clinical signs would suggest.[52] Examination of the ear canal reveals granulation tissue at the bony cartilaginous junction. Either computed tomography or magnetic resonance imaging confirms the diagnosis. Treatment should be aggressive and include intravenous antipseudomonal antibiotics initially, followed by ofloxacin 400 mg or ciprofloxacin 750 mg orally twice a day for up to 3 months. Consult an otolaryngologist to assist in the care, especially since debridement of granulation or osteitic bones may be needed.

References

1. Coyte P, Croxford R, McIsaac W, Feldman W, Friedberg J. The role of adjuvant adenoidectomy and tonsillectomy in the outcome of the insertion of tympanostomy tubes. N Engl J Med 2001;344:1188–95.
2. Albrant D. APhA drug treatment protocols: management of pediatric acute otitis media. J Am Pharm Assoc 2000;40:599–608.
3. McConaghy JR. The evaluation and treatment of children with acute otitis media. J Fam Pract 2001;50:457–65.
4. Daly K, Giebink G. Clinical epidemiology of otitis media. Pediatr Infect Dis J 2000;19:S31–6.

5. Finkelstein J, Metlay J, Davis R, Rifas-Shiman S, Dowell S, Platt R. Antimicrobial use in defined populations of infants and young children. Arch Pediatr Adolesc Med 2000;154:395–400.

6. Gates G. Cost-effectiveness considerations in otitis media treatment. Otolaryngol Head Neck Surg 1996;114:525–30.

7. Eskola J, Kilpi T, Palmu A, et al. Efficacy of a pneumococcal conjugate vaccine against acute otitis media. N Engl J Med 2001;344:403–9.

8. Berman S. Otitis media in children. N Engl J Med 1995;332:1560–5.

9. O'Neill P. Acute otitis media. BMJ 1999;319:833–5.

10. Pichichero M, Reiner S, Brook I, et al. Controversies in the medical management of persistent and recurrent acute otitis media. Recommendations of a clinical advisory committee. Ann Otol Rhinol Laryngol 2000;183(suppl):1–12.

11. Koivunen P, Konitiokari T, Niemela M, Pokka T, Uhari M. Time to development of acute otitis media during an upper respiratory infection in children. Pediatr Infect Dis J 1999;18:303–5.

12. Uhari M, Mantysaari K, Niemela M. A meta-analytic review of the risk factors for acute otitis media. Clin Infect Dis 1996;22:1079–83.

13. Block S. Strategies for dealing with amoxicillin failure in acute otitis media. Arch Fam Med 1999;8:68–78.

14. Niemelä M, Pihakari O, Pokka T, Uhari M, Uhari M. Pacifier as a risk factor for acute otitis media: a randomized, controlled trial of parental counseling. Pediatrics 2000;106:483–8.

15. Heinig M. Host defense benefits of breastfeeding for the infant. Effect of breastfeeding duration and exclusivity. Pediatr Clin North Am 2001;48:105–23.

16. Heikkinen T, Thint M, Chonmaitree T. Prevalence of various respiratory viruses in the middle ear during acute otitis media. N Engl J Med 1999;340:260–4.

17. Pichichero M. Acute otitis media: part I. Improving diagnostic accuracy. Am Fam Physician 2000;61:2051–6.

18. Froom J, Culpepper L, Grob P, et al. Diagnosis and antibiotic treatment of acute otitis media: report from International Primary Care Network. BMJ 1990;300:582–6.

19. Jensen P, Lous J. Criteria, performance and diagnostic problems in diagnosing acute otitis media. Fam Pract 1999;16:262–8.

20. Heikkinen T, Ruuskanen O. Signs and symptoms predicting acute otitis media. Arch Pediatr Adolesc Med 1995;149:26–9.

21. DelMar C, Glasziou P, Hayem M. Are antibiotics indicated as initial treatment for children with acute otitis media? A meta-analysis. BMJ 1997;314:1526–9.

22. Glasziou P, DelMar C, Sanders S. Antibiotics for acute otitis media in children (Cochrane Review). The Cochrane Library, issue 3. Oxford, England: Update Software, 2000.

23. Little P, Gould C, Williamson I, Moore M, Warner G, Dunleavey J. Pragmatic randomized controlled trial of two prescribing strategies for childhood acute otitis media. BMJ 2001;322:336–42.

24. Damoiseaux R, vanBalen F, Hoes A, Verheij T, deMelker R. Primary care based randomized, double blind trial of amoxicillin versus placebo for acute otitis media in children aged under 2 years. BMJ 2000;320:350–4.

25. Klein J. Clinical implications of antibiotic resistance for management of acute otitis media. Pediatr Infect Dis J 1998;17:1084–9.

26. Dowell S, Butler J, Giebink G, et al. Acute otitis media—management and surveillance in an era of pneumococcal resistance: a report from the Drug-Resistant *Strep-*

tococcus pneumoniae Therapeutic Working Group (DRSPTWG). Pediatr Infect Dis J 1999;18:1–9.

27. Steele R, Thomas M, Begue R. Compliance issues related to the selection of antibiotic suspensions for children. Pediatr Infect Dis J 2001;20:1–5.

28. Hueston W, Ornstein S, Jenkins R, Wulfman J. Treatment of recurrent otitis media after a previous treatment failure. Which antibiotics work best? J Fam Pract 1999;48:43–6.

29. Pichichero M, Marsocci S, Murphy M, Hoeger W, Francis A, Green J. A prospective observational study of 5-, 7-, and 10-day antibiotic treatment for acute otitis media. Otolaryngol Head Neck Surg 2001;124:318–7.

30. Kozyrskyj A, Hildes-Ripstein E, Longstaffe S, et al. Treatment of acute otitis media with a shortened course of antibiotics—a meta-analysis. JAMA 1998;279:1736–42.

31. Kozyrskyj A, Hildes-Ripstein G, Longstaffe S, et al. Short course antibiotics for acute otitis media. Cochrane Database Syst Rev 2000(2);CD001095.

32. Cohen R, Levy C, Boucherat M, et al. Five vs. ten days of antibiotic therapy for acute otitis media in young children. Pediatr Infect Dis J 2000;19:471–3.

33. Zempsky W, Schechter N. Office-based pain management. The 15-minute consultation. Pediatr Clin North Am 2000;47:601–15.

34. Culpepper L. Tympanocentesis: to tap or not to tap. Am Fam Physician 2000;61: 1987,90–2.

35. Bernard P, Stenstrom R, Feldman W, Durieux-Smith A. Randomized, controlled trial comparing long-term sulfonamide therapy to ventilation tubes for otitis media with effusion. Pediatrics 1991;88:215–22.

36. Williams R, Chalmers T, Stange K, Chalmers F, Bowlin S. Use of antibiotics in preventing recurrent acute otitis media and in treating otitis media with effusion: a meta-analytic attempt to resolve the brouhaha. JAMA 1993;270:1344–51.

37. Erramouspe J, Heyneman C. Treatment and prevention of otitis media. Ann Pharmacother 2000;34:1452–68.

38. Paradise J, Bluestone C, Colborn D, et al. Adenoidectomy and adenotonsillectomy for recurrent acute otitis media. Parallel randomized clinical trials in children not previously treated with tympanostomy tubes. JAMA 1999;282:945–53.

39. Acuin J, Smith A, Mackenzie I. Interventions for chronic suppurative otitis media. Cochrane Database Syst Rev 2000(2);CD000473.

40. Morgen N, Berke E. Topical fluoroquinolones for eye and ear. Am Fam Physician 2000;62:1870–6.

41. Gates G. Otitis media—the pharyngeal connection. JAMA 1999;282:987–9.

42. Butler C, vanderVoort J. Steroids for otitis media with effusion—a systematic review. Arch Pediatr Adolesc Med 2001;155:641–7.

43. Stool S, Berg A, Berman S, et al. Managing otitis media with effusion in young children. Quick reference guide for clinicians. AHCPR publication 94-0623. Rockville, MD: Agency for Health Care Policy and Research, Public Health Service, U.S. Department of Health and Human Services, July 1994.

44. Paradise J, Feldman H, Campbell T, et al. Effect of early or delayed insertion of tympanostomy tubes for persistent otitis media on developmental outcomes at the age of three years. N Engl J Med 2001;344:1179–87.

45. Rovers M, Straatman H, Ingels K, vanderWilt Gv, Broek Pv, Zielhuis G. The effect of ventilation tubes on language development in infants with otitis media with effusion: a randomized trial. Pediatrics 2000;106:E42.

46. Rovers M, Straatman H, Ingels K, vanderWilt G, vandenBroek P, Zielhuis G. The

effect of short-term ventilation tubes versus watchful waiting on hearing in young children with persistent otitis media with effusion: a randomized trial. Ear Hear 2001;22:191–9.
47. Rovers M, Krabbe P, Straatman H, Ingels K, vanderWilt G, Zielhuis G. Randomized controlled trial of the effect of ventilation tubes (grommets) on quality of life at age 1–2 years. Arch Dis Child 2001;84:45–9.
48. Morris M. Tympanostomy tubes: types, indications, techniques, and complications. Otolaryngol Clin North Am 1999;32:385–90.
49. Perrin J. Should we operate on children with fluid in the middle ear? N Engl J Med 2001;344:1241–2.
50. Kay D, Nelson M, Rosenfeld R. Meta-analysis of tympanostomy tube sequelae. Otolaryngol Head Neck Surg 2001;124:374–80.
51. Sander R. Otitis externa: a practical guide to treatment and prevention. Am Fam Physician 2001;63:927–36.
52. Holten K, Gick J. Management of the patient with otitis externa. J Fam Pract 2001;50:353–60.
53. Clark W, Brook I, Bianki D, Thompson D. Microbiology of otitis externa. Otolaryngol Head Neck Surg 1997;116:23–5.
54. Halpern M, Palmer C, Seidlin M. Treatment patterns for otitis externa. J Am Board Fam Pract 1999;12:1–7.
55. Hannley M, Denneny J, Holzer S. Use of ototopical antibiotics in treating 3 common ear diseases. Otolaryngol Head Neck Surg 2000;122:934–40.
56. Schohet J, Scherger J. Which culprit is causing your patient's otorrhea? Postgrad Med 1998;104:50–5.

CASE PRESENTATION

Subjective

PATIENT PROFILE

Jason Harris is a 4-year-old male child.

PRESENTING PROBLEM

Earache.

PRESENT ILLNESS

For 2 days, Jason has complained of a left earache. There has been a low-grade fever, sore throat, and nasal congestion. Jason has had three prior episodes of earache over the past 6 months.

PAST MEDICAL HISTORY

No serious illness or hospitalization since birth.

SOCIAL HISTORY

Jason attends day care 5 mornings per week.

FAMILY HISTORY

His parents are both living and well. There is a 1-year-old sibling.

- What other historical information might be pertinent, and why?
- What might be the significance of having had three prior episodes of ear infection?
- What—if anything—might be pertinent about the child's day-care experience?
- What more might you like to know about the family history, and why?

Objective

VITAL SIGNS

Pulse, 78; respirations, 22; temperature, 38.0°C.

EXAMINATION

Patient is alert but in pain with a left earache. The left tympanic membrane is injected but not retracted or bulging. There is mild injection of the pharynx without tonsillar swelling or exudate. There are few enlarged left cervical lymph nodes. The chest is clear, and the heart is normal.

- What more—if anything—would you include in the physical examination, and why?
- How might you evaluate the child's hearing?
- What—if any—laboratory tests might you order today?
- If there were thick purulent drainage from the ear, what would be its significance?

Assessment

- What is the probable diagnosis? Describe the likely etiologic agent(s).
- How would you explain this diagnosis to the family?
- The parents ask if Jason needs a referral to an ear, nose, and throat specialist. How would you respond?
- What are the family implications of this illness?

Plan

- What therapeutic recommendations would you make regarding medication for relief of pain?
- When can Jason return to day care? What might influence your decision?
- If Jason's mother calls tonight to report that there is purulent drainage from the left ear, what would you advise?
- What follow-up would you advise for this illness?

12

Ischemic Heart Disease

Jim Nuovo

Cardiovascular disease remains the most significant cause of morbidity and mortality in the United States. In 1998 approximately 1.3 million Americans experienced a myocardial infarction (MI) and 700,000 of them died.[1] It is estimated that 12.4 million Americans are alive today with a history of MI, angina, or both. The financial impact of this disease is enormous. The cost estimate for cardiovascular disease in 1998 was over $110 billion. It is important for all primary care providers to implement screening and preventive care programs to reduce the burden of cardiovascular disease. Because of the high morbidity and mortality it is also important to recognize the early manifestations of this disease.

Unfortunately, in up to 20% of patients the first manifestation of ischemic heart disease (IHD) is sudden cardiac arrest.[2] Most deaths from IHD occur outside the hospital and within 2 hours of the onset of symptoms. Since the 1960s a great deal of effort has been directed toward the practice of cardiopulmonary resuscitation and emergency cardiac care. These efforts have been directed toward minimizing the number of cardiac deaths. Recently revised evidence-based guidelines present a summary of the collaborative effort of the American Heart Association and the International Liaison Committee on Resuscitation.[2] Furthermore, there has been a substantial undertaking to identify and treat individuals with significant cardiovascular risk factors with the goal of lowering morbidity and mortality (see Chapter 2). This effort has been successful as noted by the decline in death rates from myocardial ischemia and its complications. This chapter discusses three issues, relevant to the family physician, regarding IHD: the evaluation of patients with chest pain, the diagnosis and management of angina pectoris, and the diagnosis and management of MI.

Chest Pain

Chest pain is one of the common reasons for patients visiting primary care physicians.[3] The major diagnostic considerations for chest pain are listed in Table 12.1. Of the diagnostic considerations, which are the most commonly seen by family physicians? A Family Practice Research Network investigated this issue. Over 1 year the Michigan Research Network (MIRNET) prospectively collected infor-

TABLE 12.1. Common Causes of Chronic and Recurrent Chest Pain

Cardiac causes	**Neurologic causes**
Hypertrophic cardiomyopathy	Radiculopathy
Ischemic heart disease	Zoster (postherpetic neuralgia)
Mitral valve prolapse	
Pericarditis	**Psychiatric causes**
	Anxiety
Chest wall problems	Depression
Costochondritis	Hyperventilation
Myofascial syndrome	Panic disorder
Gastrointestinal causes	
Esophageal motility disorders	
Gastroesophageal reflux	

mation on 399 patients with episodes of chest pain. The most common diagnostic findings were (1) musculoskeletal pain (20.4%); (2) reflux esophagitis (13.4%); (3) costochondritis (13.1%); and (4) angina pectoris (10.3%).[4] The highest priority is generally given to distinguishing cardiac from noncardiac chest pain. Of the many diseases listed, the most common differential diagnostic considerations are of esophageal and psychiatric etiologies.

Noncardiac Chest Pain

Noncardiac chest pain remains a complex diagnosis and management problem. Studies have demonstrated that 10% to 30% of patients with chest pain who undergo coronary arteriography have no arterial abnormalities.[5,6] Follow-up studies of these patients have shown that the risk of subsequent myocardial infarction is low.[7,8] Fifty to seventy-five percent of these patients have persistent complaints of chest pain and disability.[9,10] The most common noncardiac problems in the differential are esophageal disorders, hyperventilation, panic attacks, and anxiety disorders (see Chapters 14 and 22).

ESOPHAGEAL CHEST PAIN

Of the patients who have undergone coronary arteriography and have been found to have normal coronary arteries, as many as 50% have demonstrable esophageal abnormalities.[11] Richter et al[12] critically reviewed 117 articles on recurring chest pain of esophageal origin to clarify issues related to this disease. They paid specific attention to the following controversial issues: potential mechanisms of esophageal pain, differentiation of cardiac and esophageal causes, evaluation of esophageal motility disorders, use of esophageal tests for evaluating noncardiac chest pain, usefulness of techniques for prolonged monitoring of intraesophageal pressure and pH, and the relation of psychological abnormalities to esophageal motility disorders. They concluded that (1) specific mechanisms that produce chest pain are not well understood; (2) esophageal chest pain has usually been attributed to the stimulation of chemoreceptors (acid and bile) or mechanoreceptors (spasm and distention); and (3) studies done to confirm direct associations between these factors and pain have not been consistent in their findings.

It appears that the triggers for esophageal chest pain are multifactorial and often idiosyncratic to the individual. Differentiating cardiac from esophageal disease can be frustrating. As many as 50% of patients with coronary disease have esophageal disease.[13] There are many esophageal disorders that produce pain mimicking myocardial ischemia. Areskog et al[14] have shown that esophageal abnormalities are common in patients who are admitted to a coronary care unit and are later found to have no evidence of cardiac disease. The clinical history frequently does not differentiate between cardiac and esophageal chest pain, although features may be helpful in this process. Features suggesting esophageal origin include pain that continues for hours, pain that interrupts sleep or is meal-related, pain relieved by antacids, or the presence of other esophageal symptoms (heartburn, dysphagia, regurgitation). Conversely, it is well documented that gastroesophageal reflux may be triggered by heavy exercise and may produce exertional chest pain mimicking angina even during treadmill testing.

Tests that can be done to determine the presence of esophageal disease include esophageal motility testing, continuous ambulatory esophageal pH monitoring, and provocative testing (e.g., acid perfusion and balloon distension).[15] Although findings from these tests have produced a better understanding of the pathologic conditions leading to the development of chest pain with esophageal disorders, there is no consensus as to the usefulness of these tests for the specific patient with chest pain. As noted by Pope,[16] "What is needed is a simple and safe provocative esophageal maneuver to turn on chest pain that possesses a high degree of sensitivity."

There is clearly an interaction between psychological abnormalities and esophageal disorders. Patients with esophageal disorders have been shown to have significantly higher levels of anxiety, somatization, and depression.[17] It is not clear if there is a cause-and-effect relation. Given the aforementioned difficulties in the diagnosis of esophageal chest pain, the differentiation of this pain from cardiac disease, and the close relation between cardiac, esophageal, and psychiatric disease, it is wise to maintain a consistent approach to the evaluation of these patients. Richter et al[12] developed a stepwise approach for patients with recurring chest pain. They recommended exclusion of cardiac disease, with the subsequent evaluation to rule out structural abnormalities of the upper gastrointestinal (GI) tract (barium swallow, upper GI series, and endoscopy). Also recommended is a trial of antireflux therapy for 1 to 2 months. In those patients who fail to respond, specialized testing may then be appropriate (esophageal motility, 24-hour pH monitoring, provocative testing, and psychological evaluation).[15]

PSYCHIATRIC ILLNESS

There has long been a connection between psychiatric disorders and noncardiac chest pain. Katon et al[18] reported the results of an evaluation of 74 patients with chest pain and no history of organic heart disease. Each patient underwent a structured psychiatric interview immediately after coronary arteriography. Patients with chest pain and negative coronary arteriograms were significantly younger, more likely to be female, more apt to have a higher number of autonomic symptoms (tachycardia, dyspnea, dizziness, paresthesias) associated with chest pain, and more likely to describe atypical chest pain. These patients also had significantly higher scores on indices of anxiety and depression that met *Diagnostic and Statistical Manual of Mental Disorders*, 3rd edition (DSM-III) criteria for panic disorder, major depression, and phobias.

The strong association between anxiety and depression disorders in patients with noncardiac chest pain has been observed in many other studies. Specific medical therapy directed at anxiety and depression may help some of these patients. Cannon et al[19] reported a study on a group of patients with chest pain despite normal coronary angiograms. Imipramine was shown to improve their symptoms. Patients who were given 50 mg nightly had a statistically significant reduction (52%) in episodes of chest pain.

Cardiac Chest Pain: Angina Pectoris

Angina is not simply one type of pain; it is a constellation of symptoms related to cardiac ischemia. The description of angina may fit several patterns:

1. *Classic angina.* Classic angina presents as an ill-defined pressure, heaviness (feeling like a weight), or squeezing sensation brought on by exertion and relieved by rest. The pain is most often substernal and left-sided. It may radiate to the jaw, interscapular area, or down the arm. Angina usually begins gradually and lasts only a few minutes.
2. *Atypical angina.* Similar symptoms are experienced but with the absence of one or more of the criteria for classic angina. For example, the pain may not be consistently related to exertion or relieved by rest. Conversely, the pain may have an atypical character (sharp, stabbing), but the precipitating factors are clearly anginal.
3. *Anginal equivalent.* The sensation of dyspnea is the sole or major manifestation.
4. *Variant (Prinzmetal's) angina.* This angina occurs at rest and may manifest in stereotyped patterns, such as nocturnal symptoms or symptoms that appear only after exercise. It is thought to be caused by coronary artery spasm. Its symptoms often occur periodically, with characteristic pain-free intervals, and are associated with typical electrocardiographic (ECG) changes, most commonly ST segment elevation.
5. *Syndrome X (microvascular angina).* Some patients with the clinical diagnosis of coronary artery disease have no evidence of obstructive atherosclerosis. Several reports investigating this population have found a subset with metabolic evidence for ischemia (myocardial lactate during induced myocardial stress as evidence for ischemia). The term *syndrome X* has been pro-

posed.[20] It has been suggested that some of these patients have microvascular angina.

It is important for clinicians to recognize the factors that may confound the clinical diagnosis of angina pectoris: (1) The severity of pain is not necessarily proportional to the seriousness of the underlying illness. (2) The physical examination is not generally helpful for differentiating cardiac from noncardiac disease. A normal examination cannot be counted on to rule out significant cardiac disease. (3) The ECG is normal in more than 50% of patients with IHD. A normal ECG cannot be used to rule out significant cardiac disease. (4) Denial is a significant component in the presentation of chest pain caused by MI. (5) Some of the diseases common in the differential diagnosis of chest pain may present concurrently. Major depressive disorder and panic disorder are known to be prevalent in patients with esophageal disorders. Colgan et al[21] reported that of 63 patients with chest pain and normal angiograms 32 (51%) had evidence of an esophageal disorder, and 19 of the 32 (59%) had a current psychiatric disorder (anxiety or depression). Patients with concurrent disorders are particularly challenging to the clinician sorting out the cause of the chest pain.

Clinical Tools Used to Distinguish Cardiac from Noncardiac Chest Pain

Despite the difficulties noted above, there are important clinical tools that can be used to distinguish cardiac from noncardiac chest pain.

HISTORY

Despite the cited difficulties, the history is key to distinguishing cardiac from noncardiac etiologies of chest pain. Noncardiac chest pain is often fleeting, brief, sharp, or stabbing. The pain may be reproduced by palpating the chest wall. The duration of pain is also important. Symptoms that last many hours or days are not likely to be anginal. A great deal of work has been done to assess the probability of IHD in a given patient based on the clinical presentation. In 1979 Diamond and Forrester[22] presented such an approach. Using data from the clinical presentation correlated with autopsy and angiographic information, they presented a pretest likelihood of coronary artery disease in symptomatic patients according to age, sex, and type of chest pain (nonanginal, atypical angina, or typical angina). Several observations can be made from this chart (Table 12.2): Men have a substantially greater risk than women for any given type of chest pain and at any given age. A middle-aged man with atypical chest pain is at high risk for having significant coronary artery disease. Young women (ages 30–40 years) with classic angina have a relatively low risk of having significant coronary artery disease.

TABLE 12.2. Pretest Likelihood of Significant Ischemic Heart Disease (IHD) Based on Symptoms

Age (years)	Likelihood of IHD, M/F (%)		
	Nonanginal	Atypical angina	Typical angina
30–39	5.0/0.8	22/4	69/26
40–49	14/3	46/13	87/55
50–59	21/8	59/32	92/79
60–69	28/18	67/54	94/90

Source: Diamond and Forrester[22] Copyright© 1979 Massachusetts Medical Society. Reprinted with permission. All rights reserved.

DIAGNOSTIC TESTING

After establishing a pretest probability of IHD, there are a variety of tests available to help establish an accurate diagnosis. Although many tests are now firmly established in clinical practice, none is particularly suited to wide-scale, cost-effective application because each has limitations concerning sensitivity and specificity.

Exercise Tolerance Testing. In 1997 the American College of Cardiology and the American Heart Association Task Force on Assessment of Cardiovascular Procedures set guidelines for exercise treadmill testing (ETT).[23] For patients with symptoms suggestive of coronary artery disease there are five basic indications for undertaking exercise stress testing: (1) as a diagnostic test for patients with suspected IHD, (2) to assist in identifying those patients with documented IHD who are potentially at high risk due to advanced coronary disease or left ventricular dysfunction, (3) to evaluate patients after coronary artery bypass surgery, (4) to quantify a patient's functional capacity or response to therapy, and (5) to follow the natural course of the disease at appropriate intervals. The purpose of ETT for the patient with chest pain is to help establish whether the pain is indeed due to IHD.

Although there are many exercise protocols available, the protocols proposed by Bruce in 1956 remain appropriate. A review of the ETT for family physicians has been published.[24,25] In the standard ETT (Bruce protocol) the patient is asked to exercise for 3-minute intervals on a motorized treadmill device while being monitored for the following: heart rate and blood pressure response to exercise, symptoms during the test, ECG response (specifically ST segment displacement), dysrhythmias, and exercise capacity. Contraindications to ETT include unstable angina, MI, rapid atrial or ventricular dysrhythmias, poorly controlled congestive heart failure (CHF), severe aortic stenosis, myocarditis, recent significant illness, and an uncooperative patient. A significant (positive) test includes an ST segment depression of 1.0 mm below the baseline. Many factors influence the results of an ETT and can lead to false-positive or false-negative findings. Factors leading to false-positive results include (1) the use of medications such as

digoxin, estrogens, and diuretics; and (2) conditions such as mitral valve prolapse, cardiomyopathy, and hyperventilation. Factors leading to false-negative
results include (1) the use of medications such as nitrates, beta-blockers, calcium
channel blockers; and (2) conditions such as a prior MI or a submaximal effort.[26]
The sensitivity of the ETT has been estimated to range from 56% to 81% and
the specificity from 72% to 96%.[26] The key point is that given the vagaries of
the ETT for diagnosing IHD (generally low sensitivity and specificity) a patient
with a high pretest likelihood of IHD (e.g., a 50-year-old man with typical angina)
still has a high probability of having significant disease even in the face of a normal (negative) test. Furthermore, a patient with a low probability of IHD (e.g.,
a 40-year-old woman with atypical chest pain) still has a low chance of significant disease even if the test is positive.[22] The optimal use of diagnostic testing
is for those patients with moderate pretest probabilities (e.g., a 40- to 50-year-
old man with atypical pain).

In addition to the diagnostic implications of an ETT, there are prognostic implications. The following are considered to be parameters associated with poor
prognosis or increased disease severity: failure to complete stage 2 of a Bruce
protocol, failure to achieve a heart rate over 120 bpm (off beta-blockers), onset
of ST segment depression at a heart rate of less than 120 bpm, ST segment depression over 2.0 mm, ST segment depression lasting more than 6 minutes into
recovery, ST segment depression in multiple leads, poor systolic blood pressure
response to exercise, ST segment elevation, angina with exercise, and exercise-
induced ventricular tachycardia.[26]

Radionuclide Perfusion Imaging. There are patients in whom the standard ETT
is not a useful diagnostic tool and in whom a radionuclide procedure would be
more appropriate. Patients with baseline ECG abnormalities due to digitalis or
left ventricular hypertrophy with strain or those with bundle branch block (especially left bundle branch block) cannot have proper evaluation of the ST segment for characteristic ischemic changes. In these patients a radionuclide stress
test is appropriate. The principle behind radionuclide testing is as follows: Myocardial thallium 201 chloride uptake is proportional to the coronary blood flow.
A myocardial segment supplied by a stenotic coronary artery receives less flow
relative to normal tissue, causing a thallium perfusion defect. Thallium washout
is also slower in stenotic areas. With perfusion imaging, both stress and rest images are compared for perfusion. As a general rule, a defect is visible on thallium imaging if there is 50% or greater stenosis in a coronary artery. In the standard exercise thallium test, repeat imaging is performed 3 to 4 hours after
completion of the ETT. Some investigators advocate 24-hour imaging in patients
with perfusion defects to look for delayed reversibility.

For patients unable to exercise, thallium imaging can be performed using
dipyridamole (Persantine) as a coronary vasodilator. Adenosine may also be used.
Its advantages over dipyridamole include an ultrashort half-life (less than 10 seconds) and better coronary vasodilation. Two technetium radiopharmaceuticals
[technetium sestamibi (Cardiolyte) and technetium teboroxime (Cardiotec)] have

been approved for myocardial perfusion imaging. These agents may eventually replace thallium because of more favorable imaging characteristics.[27]

Compared to the standard ETT, the thallium 201 ETT has the advantage of increased sensitivity (80–87%) and specificity (85–90%).[27] Dipyridamole, adenosine, and technetium perfusion testing has a sensitivity ranging from 70% to 95% and specificity from 60% to 100%. Unfortunately, the cost of these procedures is more than five times as great as a standard ETT ($1000–$1400 versus $175–$250).[25]

Stress Echocardiography.   Ischemic heart disease can be detected with stress echocardiography. During stress-induced myocardial ischemia, the affected ventricular walls become hypokinetic. Studies suggest that physical exercise and dobutamine may be the preferable means of provoking ischemia in patients undergoing stress echocardiography.[28,29] Preliminary data suggest a higher sensitivity and specificity than for the standard ETT and increased usefulness for predicting subsequent myocardial events; however, the primary utility of this test appears to be for detection of ischemia in patients who are unable to exercise adequately. Similar values for sensitivity and specificity between stress echocardiography and perfusion imaging have been reported. Stress echocardiography may be particularly valuable in patients who have a questionable defect on perfusion imaging.

The advantages and disadvantages of each of these diagnostic tests for IHD, as well as gender-specific issues, are presented in a summary by Redberg.[30]

Response to Nitroglycerin.   Another approach employs clinical information to determine the probability of coronary artery disease based on response to treatment. One such study involved the use of sublingual nitroglycerin to determine the likelihood of disease. Horwitz et al[31] evaluated the usefulness of nitroglycerin as a diagnostic aid for IHD. They found a sensitivity of 76% and a specificity of 80% in 70 patients with chest pain of anginal type. It was concluded that 90% of patients with recurrent, angina-like chest pain who exhibit a prompt response to nitroglycerin (within 3 minutes) have IHD; however, a delayed or absent response paradoxically indicates either an absence of IHD or unusually severe disease. Therefore failure to respond to nitroglycerin should not be used to exclude the diagnosis of IHD.

Angina Pectoris

Once the diagnosis of angina is established, there are several important management considerations for this disease. The first is related to disease prognosis, the second to drug therapy, and the third to further investigative tests and invasive therapeutic interventions. Comprehensive management guidelines were prepared in 1999 by the American College of Cardiology and American Heart Association Task Force.[32]

Prognosis

Three major factors determine the prognosis of patients with angina pectoris: the amount of viable but jeopardized left ventricular myocardium, the percentage of irreversibly scarred myocardium, and the severity of underlying coronary atherosclerosis. A number of studies were reported before invasive therapies were available that assess the prognosis of patients with stable angina. Most of them appeared between 1952 and 1973 and reported an annual mortality of 4%. Since cardiac catheterization has come into general use, the prognosis has been modified and is based on the number of diseased vessels. Currently, the annual mortality rates for patients with one-vessel disease, two-vessel disease, three-vessel disease, and left main coronary artery disease (CAD) are 1.5%, 3.5%, 6.0%, and 8.0% to 10.0%, respectively.[33]

Exercise tolerance testing has been used to establish the prognosis in patients with symptomatic IHD. The exercise test parameters associated with a poor outcome have been described above.[26]

When does angina signal severe coronary disease? Pryor et al[34] developed a nomogram based on a point scoring system to help answer this question. They based the nomogram on the following factors: type of chest pain (typical, atypical, nonanginal), sex, selective cardiovascular risk factors (hypertension, smoking, hyperlipidemia, diabetes mellitus), anginal duration (months), and the presence of carotid bruits. By applying the nomogram for the individual patient one can determine the probability of severe disease (i.e., 75% narrowing of the left main coronary artery or three-vessel disease).

Drug Therapy

In patients with stable exertional angina who do not have severe disease, the goal of therapy is to abolish or reduce anginal attacks and myocardial ischemia and to promote a normal lifestyle. For the relief of angina, the treatment strategy is to lower myocardial oxygen demand and increase coronary blood flow to the ischemic regions.

Patients are screened for the presence of significant cardiovascular risk factors and are advised to modify any that are present. Three classes of antianginal drugs are commonly used: nitrates, beta-blockers, and calcium channel blockers. Each reduces myocardial oxygen demand and may improve blood flow to the ischemic regions. The mechanisms by which these agents reduce myocardial oxygen demand or increase coronary blood flow to ischemic areas differ from one class of drug to another. No greater efficacy in relieving chest pain or decreasing exercise-induced ischemia has been shown for one or another group of drugs.

Nitrates

Nitrates are potent venous and arterial dilators. At low doses venous dilation predominates, and at higher doses arterial dilation occurs as well. Nitrates decrease myocardial oxygen demand in the following ways: Decreased venous return reduces left ventricular end-diastolic volume and ventricular wall stress. Increased arterial compliance and cardiac output lowers systolic blood pressure and decreases peripheral resistance (afterload). It also enhances myocardial oxygen supply by preventing closure of stenotic coronary arteries during exercise, dilating epicardial coronary arteries, and decreasing left ventricular end-diastolic pressure, thereby enhancing subendocardial blood flow and inhibiting coronary artery spasm. Nitrates are inexpensive and have a well documented safety record. Both short- and long-acting nitrates are available. Short-acting preparations are used for relief of an established attack, whereas long-acting nitrates are used for prevention. The most significant concern about the long-acting nitrates is tolerance. Most studies have shown that tolerance develops rapidly when long-acting nitrates are given for anginal prophylaxis.[34]

With nitroglycerin patches tolerance can develop within 24 hours, and further therapy can lead to complete loss of the antianginal effect.[35] Various dosing strategies with oral and transdermal formulations have been used to overcome the development of nitroglycerin tolerance. Patch-free intervals of 10 to 12 hours are commonly used to retain the antianginal effectiveness. For oral administration, nitroglycerin isosorbide dinitrate three times daily at 7 A.M., noon, and 5 P.M. appears to prevent the development of tolerance. Because of the concern for intervals during which patients remain unprotected, it is common to add another antianginal agent to the nitroglycerin regimen. Other problems with nitroglycerin include the fact that 10% of patients do not respond and 10% have associated intolerable headaches that may necessitate discontinuation.[35]

BETA-BLOCKERS

The antianginal effect of beta-blockers is well established.[36] These agents improve exercise tolerance and reduce myocardial ischemia. The effect produces a reduction in myocardial oxygen demand through a reduction in heart rate and contractility. Many beta-blockers are available. They may be divided into those that are nonselective (β_1 and β_2) (i.e., propranolol, timolol, nadolol), those that are β_1 selective (i.e., atenolol, metoprolol, acebutolol), and those that are nonselective and produce vasodilatory effects through the ability to block α_1-receptors and dilate blood vessels directly (i.e., labetalol). All beta-blockers, irrespective of their selective properties, are equally effective in patients with angina.[36]

Some 20% of patients do not respond to beta-blockers. Those who do not respond are more likely to have severe IHD. Furthermore, some patients do not tolerate the adverse side effects, such as fatigue, depression, dyspnea, and cold extremities. Other concerns include a small but significant aggravation of hyperlipidemia and precipitation of CHF and bronchospasm in susceptible individuals. Generally, beta-blockers are dose-adjusted to achieve a heart rate of 50 to 60 bpm. Patients should be cautioned to not stop beta-blockers abruptly, thereby avoiding a rebound phenomenon.

CALCIUM CHANNEL BLOCKERS

Calcium channel blockers are a diverse group of compounds, all of which impede calcium ion influx into the myocardium and smooth muscle cells. These agents relieve myocardial ischemia by reducing myocardial oxygen demand secondary to decreased afterload and myocardial contractility. In addition, they dilate coronary arteries. There are three classes of calcium channel blockers: papaverine derivatives (verapamil), dihydropyridines (nifedipine, nicardipine), and benzothiazepines (diltiazem). Each of the drugs in the three classes has different effects on the atrioventricular (AV) node, heart rate, coronary vasodilation, diastolic relaxation, cardiac contractility, systemic blood pressure, and afterload. All three classes are effective for the management of patients with stable angina.[37] Most studies have shown them to have effects equal to those of beta-blockers. Calcium channel blockers may be preferred in patients with obstructive airway disease, hypertension, peripheral vascular disease, or supraventricular tachycardia. In general, they are well tolerated. The most troublesome side effects include constipation, edema, headache, and aggravation of congestive heart failure.

Concern has developed that short-acting calcium channel blockers may be associated with an increased risk of MI. There has been evidence of a 58% to 70% increase in risk of MI compared to that in patients on beta-blockers or diuretics. The phenomenon has been noted to be dose-related. At present the National Heart, Lung, and Blood Institute has issued a statement recommending caution with the use of short-acting calcium channel blockers.[38]

COMBINATION THERAPY

It is important to maximize therapy with any one class of antianginal drug before considering it a failed trial. If monotherapy fails, it is appropriate to add another agent. Generally beta-blockers and nitrates or calcium channel blockers and nitrates complement each other. Calcium channel blockers and beta-blockers can be used together. Combination therapy may be more effective than either agent alone. It is important to be cautious, as some combinations produce deleterious effects. For example, verapamil and beta-blockers may produce extreme bradycardia or heart block.

ASPIRIN

Aspirin is effective for primary and secondary prevention of MI, presumably by inhibiting thrombosis. Although there is controversy as to the ideal therapeutic dose, low-dose therapy (81–325 mg) is generally recommended.[39] Alternative antiplatelet regimens to aspirin include ticlopidine and clopidogrel. A 1994 review found no evidence that any antiplatelet regimen was more effective than medium-dose aspirin alone in the prevention of vascular events.[40] Another review of randomized trials comparing either ticlopidine or clopidogrel with aspirin found several trials showing a small additional benefit of these two drugs over aspirin in reducing the odds of a vascular event.[41]

Invasive Testing

Cardiac catheterization is not routinely recommended for initial management of patients with stable angina. Patients who warrant such an evaluation are those who exhibit evidence of severe myocardial ischemia on noninvasive testing or who have symptoms refractory to antianginal medications. In patients who undergo catheterization, the most important determinant of survival is left ventricular function followed by the number of diseased vessels. Patients with left main artery disease or three-vessel disease with diminished left ventricular function are candidates for a coronary artery bypass graft procedure. Others (those with one- or two-vessel disease) are managed medically or considered for percutaneous transluminal coronary angioplasty (PTCA).

Unstable Angina Pectoris

Unstable angina manifests clinically either as an abrupt onset of ischemic symptoms at rest or as an intensification or change in the pattern of ischemic symptoms in a patient with a history of IHD. This intensification may be manifested by an increase in the frequency, severity, and duration of symptoms as well as an increasing ease of provocation (symptoms at rest or with minimal effort). Recurrence of ischemic symptoms soon after an MI (usually within 4 weeks) is also considered a sign of unstable angina. Unstable angina is generally diagnosed on clinical grounds alone. Because of the episodic nature of ischemia in unstable angina, however, transient ECG abnormalities (ST segment depression or elevation or T wave abnormalities, i.e., inversion, flattening, or peaking) may not be documented in 50% to 70% of patients with the clinical diagnosis of unstable angina. In studies in which prolonged Holter monitoring was used during the in-hospital phase of unstable angina, transient ischemic ST segment deviations have been described in 60% to 70% of cases, more than 70% of them being clinically unsuspected or silent.[42]

Prognosis

The prognosis of patients with unstable angina is not as good as those with chronic stable angina. Mortality is increased in those who fail to respond to initial therapy, who have severe left ventricular dysfunction, and who have multivessel CAD (particularly left main artery disease).

Management Strategy

An important development in the management of unstable angina was the 1994 report of the Agency for Health Care Policy and Research.[43] This report includes clinical practice guidelines that are based on a consensus panel of experts. The guidelines allow physicians to consider outpatient management for a select sub-group of patients with unstable angina, specifically those who are thought to be at low risk for MI. According to the report, in the initial management physicians should use the information in Table 12.3 to determine whether a particular patient has high, intermediate, or low likelihood of having significant CAD. For example, the patient with low likelihood might be nondiabetic, have atypical chest pain, be younger (<60 years for men, <70 years for women), and have a normal ECG. The next step is to determine the level of risk for MI. The information in Table 12.4 allows a similar stratification of risk. For example, a low-risk patient is one with a history of angina that is now provoked at a lower threshold but not at rest, and the ECG is normal or unchanged. Low-risk patients may be treated with aspirin, nitroglycerin, beta-blockers, or a combination. Follow-up should be no later than 72 hours. High- or moderate-risk patients should be admitted for intensive medical management. Intensive medical management includes consideration of aspirin, heparin, nitrates, beta-blockers, calcium channel blockers (if the patient is already on adequate doses of nitrates and beta-blockers or unable to tolerate them), and morphine sulfate.

Once patients are stable, they should be considered for noninvasive exercise testing to further define the prognosis and direct the treatment plan. Low-risk patients can be managed medically. Those at intermediate risk should be considered for additional testing (either a cardiac catheterization, radionuclide stress test, or echocardiographic stress test). Those at high risk should be referred for cardiac catheterization.[43]

Since the publication of the 1994 report, efforts have been directed at the use of markers of cardiac injury, i.e., cardiac troponins (troponin T and troponin I). Their detection, even at low levels, is highly sensitive and specific for injury. Troponin elevation in patients otherwise considered to have unstable angina identifies a subset of patients requiring more aggressive intervention. Hamm and Braunwald[44] have proposed a risk-stratification algorithm that incorporates troponin testing.

ANTIPLATELET THERAPY

Antiplatelet therapy is an important addition for patients with unstable angina. A number of studies have demonstrated that a common cause of crescendo angina is platelet aggregation and thrombus formation on the surface of an ulcerated plaque. In the Veterans Administration Cooperative Study, men with unstable angina who received aspirin (325 mg/day) had a 50% reduction in subsequent death from MI.[45] As noted previously, ticlopidine and clopidogrel are alternative antiplatelet regimens to aspirin.

PERCUTANEOUS TRANSLUMINAL CORONARY ANGIOPLASTY

There has been a marked increase in the use of angioplasty over the past 20 years. The American College of Cardiology and the American Heart Association Task

TABLE 12.3. Likelihood of Significant Coronary Artery Disease (CAD) in Patients with Symptoms Suggesting Unstable Angina

High likelihood (any of the listed features)	Intermediate likelihood (absence of high-likelihood features and any of the listed features)	Low likelihood (absence of high- or intermediate-likelihood features but may have the listed features)
Known history of CAD	Definite angina: men <60, women <70	Chest pain, probably not angina
Definite angina: men ≥60 women ≥70	Probable angina: men >60 or women >70	One risk factor but not diabetes
Hemodynamic changes or ECG changes with pain	Probably not angina in diabetics or in nondiabetics with ≥two other risk factors[a]	T wave flat or inverted <1 mm in leads with dominant R waves
Variant angina	Extracardiac vascular disease	Normal ECG
ST increase or decrease ≥1 mm	ST depression 0.05 to 1.00 mm	
Marked symmetric T wave inversion in multiple precordial leads	T wave inversion ≥1 mm in leads with dominant R waves	

Source: Braunwald et al.[43]

[a]CAD risk factors include diabetes, smoking, hypertension, and elevated cholesterol.

Table 12.4. Short-Term Risk of Death or Nonfatal Myocardial Infarction in Patients with Symptoms Suggesting Unstable Angina

High risk (at least one of the listed features must be present)	Intermediate risk (no high-risk feature but must have any of the listed features)	Low risk (no high- or intermediate-risk feature but may have any of the listed features)
Prolonged ongoing (>20 min) rest pain	Rest angina now resolved but not low likelihood of CAD	Increased angina frequency, severity, or duration
Pulmonary edema	Rest angina (>20 min or relieved with rest or nitroglycerin)	Angina provoked at a lower threshold
Angina with new or worsening mitral regurgitation murmurs	Angina with dynamic T wave changes	New-onset angina within 2 weeks to 2 months
Rest angina with dynamic ST changes ≥1 mm	Normal or unchanged ECG	Nocturnal angina
Angina with S_3 or rales	New onset of CCSC III or IV angina during past 2 weeks but not low likelihood of CAD	
Angina with hypotension	Q waves or ST depression ≥1 mm in multiple leads	
Age >65 years		

Source: Braunwald et al.[43]
CCSC = Canadian Cardiovascular Study Class.

Force have published guidelines for the selection of patients for coronary angioplasty.[46] Among patients with unstable angina, PTCA is recommended for those who do not show an adequate response to medical treatment (continued chest pain or evidence of ongoing ischemia during ECG monitoring) or who are intolerant of medical therapy because of uncontrollable side effects.

The long-term outcome after successful angioplasty has been reported to be excellent even when compared with patients undergoing bypass surgery.[47] Further research is important in the areas of long-term outcome for multiple lesions, extensive disease, and avoidance of complications. Technologies such as stents, laser angioplasty, and atherectomy await further evaluation.

CORONARY ARTERY BYPASS GRAFT

Large randomized trials have shown that surgical revascularization is more effective than medical therapy for relieving angina and improving exercise tolerance for at least several years. Development of atherosclerosis in the coronary artery bypass graft resulting in angina generally occurs within 5 to 10 years. However, patients with internal mammary artery grafts have substantially fewer problems with graft occlusion (90% patency rate at 10 years). Improved survival with surgical versus medical therapy is seen only in the subset of patients with severe CAD or left ventricular dysfunction.[48]

Silent Ischemia

Many investigations have established that most ischemic episodes in patients with stable angina are not accompanied by chest pain (silent ischemia). What remains unclear is the precise nature of events that accompany ischemic events that do or do not produce pain. Patients with predominantly silent ischemia may be hyposensitive to pain in general; denial may play a role, or they may experience pain but attribute the symptoms to a less significant event. It is well documented that personality-related, emotional, and social factors can modulate the perception of pain. It is not surprising that the symptoms among cardiac patients with the same degree of disease vary greatly. Personality inventory studies have shown that patients with reproducible angina have higher scores on indices of nervousness and excitability than do those who are free of symptoms. Many studies have shown that stress of various types can influence the frequency and duration of ischemic episodes in patients with angina.[49]

Silent ischemia is prevalent. Seventy percent of ischemic episodes in patients with IHD are estimated to be asymptomatic. Among patients with stable angina who undergo 24-hour Holter monitoring, 40% to 72% of the episodes are painless. Among patients with unstable angina, more than half manifest painless ST segment depression.

In 1988 Cohn[50] proposed classifying silent ischemia into three clinical types to help clarify the prevalence, detection, prognosis, and management of this syndrome. Type 1 includes persons with ischemia who are asymptomatic, never having had any signs or symptoms of cardiovascular disease. Type 2 includes persons who are asymptomatic after an MI but still show painless ischemia. Type 3 includes patients with both angina and silent ischemia. From Cohn's data 2.5% to 10.0% of middle-aged men have type 1 silent ischemia. Among middle-aged men known to have CAD, 18% have type 2 and 40% have type 3.

Methods of Detection

Certain tests can be used to assess the presence of silent ischemia: ETT, ambulatory ECG for ST segment changes (Holter monitor), radionuclide tests including thallium scintigraphy and gated pooled [multiple gated acquisition (MUGA)] scan, and stress echocardiography. Of these tests, the most commonly considered are ETT and Holter monitoring.

For Holter monitoring, when ST segment changes that meet strict criteria are seen in a patient with known IHD, it is generally accepted that they represent episodes of myocardial ischemia. Ischemic criteria include at least 1.0 mm of horizontal or down-sloping ST segment depression that lasts for at least 1 minute and is separated from other discrete episodes by at least 1 minute of a normal baseline. The methodology has limitations, including difficulty reading ST segment changes in patients with an abnormal baseline (left ventricular hypertrophy with strain) or in those with a left bundle branch block.

It is not thought at this time that any of the methods to detect silent ischemia are useful for screening for the presence of IHD in apparently healthy populations. Although this subject remains controversial, it may be wise to screen those patients at high risk (i.e., diabetics or patients with two or more cardiac risk factors).

Prognostic Implications

The presence of frequent, prolonged ischemic episodes despite medical therapy in patients with stable and unstable angina has been associated with a poor prognosis. Using Cohn's classification system, those patients with type 2 silent ischemia have the worst prognosis, especially those with left ventricular dysfunction and three-vessel disease. Exercise tests done 2 to 3 weeks after an MI have shown an adverse 1-year prognosis associated with silent ischemia.[50] It is unclear whether those with type 3 have a worse prognosis.

Management

Antiischemic medical and revascularization therapies have been shown to reduce asymptomatic ischemia. It is prudent to consider patients with persistent asymptomatic ischemia to be at higher risk for subsequent events and therefore to warrant more aggressive therapy. Patients with type 1 are advised to modify risk factors and avoid activities known to produce ischemia. Those with strongly positive tests can be considered for angiography. For patients with types 2 or 3, treatment with beta-blockers for a cardioprotective effect should be considered. It remains unresolved whether asymptomatic ischemia has a causal relation with subsequent MI and cardiac death or is merely a marker of high risk.[51]

Myocardial Infarction

Clinical Presentation

The classic initial manifestations of an acute MI include prolonged substernal chest pain with dyspnea, diaphoresis, and nausea. The pain may be described as a crushing, pressing, constricting, vise-like, or heavy sensation. There may be radiation of the pain to one or both shoulders and arms or to the neck, jaw, or interscapular area. Only a few patients have this classic overall picture. Although 80% of patients with an acute MI have chest pain at the time of initial examination, only 20% describe it as crushing, constricting, or vise-like.[52] The pain may also be described atypically, such as sharp or stabbing, or it can involve atypical areas such as the epigastrium or the back of the neck. "Atypical" presentations are common in the elderly.

Pathy[53] found that the initial manifestations of an acute MI were more likely to include symptoms such as sudden dyspnea, acute confusion, cerebrovascular events (e.g., stroke or syncope), acute CHF, vomiting, and palpitations. There is strong evidence that a substantial proportion of MIs are asymptomatic. In an update of the Framingham Study, Kannel and Abbott[54] reported that 28% of infarcts were discovered only through the appearance of new ECG changes (Q waves or loss of R waves) observed on a routine biennial study. These infarctions had been previously unrecognized by both patient and physician.

Physical Examination

For the patient with an "uncomplicated MI" there are few physical examination findings. The main purpose of the examination is to assess the patient for evidence of complications from the MI and to establish a baseline for future comparisons. Signs of severe left ventricular dysfunction include hypotension, peripheral vasoconstriction, tachycardia, pulmonary rales, an S_3, and elevated jugular venous pressure. Preexisting murmurs should be verified. A new systolic murmur can result from a number of causes: papillary muscle dysfunction, mitral regurgitation as a result of ventricular dilatation, ventricular septal rupture, and acute severe mitral regurgitation due to papillary muscle rupture.

Electrocardiography

The classic ECG changes of acute ischemia are peaked, hyperacute T waves, T wave flattening or inversion with or without ST segment depression, horizontal

ST segment depression, and ST segment elevation. Changes associated with an infarction are (1) the fresh appearance of Q waves or the increased prominence of preexisting ones; (2) ST segment elevations; and (3) T wave inversions. It is important to recognize that with acute MI the ECG may be entirely normal or contain only "soft" ECG evidence of infarction.

In the past infarcts were classified as transmural or subendocardial, depending of the presence of Q waves. This terminology has now been replaced by the terms *Q-wave* and *non–Q-wave* MI. This distinction has more clinical relevance, as several studies have indicated differences in etiology and outcome. The key differences between these two groups are as follows: (1) Q-wave infarctions account for 60% to 70% of all infarcts and non–Q-wave infarctions for 30% to 40%. (2) ST segment elevation is present in 80% of Q-wave infarctions and 40% of non–Q-wave infarctions. (3) The peak creatine kinase tends to be higher in Q-wave infarctions. (4) Postinfarction ischemia and early reinfarction are more common with non–Q-wave infarctions. (5) In-hospital mortality is greater with Q-wave infarctions (20% versus 8% for non–Q-wave infarctions). In general, it is thought that the non–Q-wave infarction is a more unstable condition because of the higher risk of reinfarction and ischemia.

Laboratory Findings

Elevation of the creatine kinase muscle and brain subunits (CK-MB) isoenzyme is essential for the diagnosis of acute MI. In general, acute elevations of this enzyme are accounted for by myocardial necrosis. Detectable CK-MB from noncardiac causes is rare except during trauma or surgery. The peak level appearance of CK-MB is expected within 12 to 24 hours after the onset of symptoms; normalization is expected in 2 to 3 days. Therefore patients should have a CK-MB level determined on admission and every 8 to 12 hours thereafter (repeated twice). Reliance on a single CK assay in an emergency room setting to rule out MI is not sensitive and should be discouraged. Cardiac troponins (T and I) are newer markers for cardiac injury. The troponins first become detectable after the first few hours following the onset of myocardial necrosis, and they peak after 12 to 24 hours. Normalization of troponin T levels requires 5 to 14 days; troponin I levels requires 5 to 10 days.[55]

Management Guidelines

Comprehensive management guidelines were prepared in 1999 by the American College of Cardiology and American Heart Association Task Force.[46] The main priority for patients with an acute MI is relief of pain. The frequent clinical observation of rapid, complete relief of pain after early reperfusion with thrombolytic therapy has made it clear that the pain of an acute MI is due to continuing ischemia of living jeopardized myocardium rather than to the effects of completed myocardial necrosis.

Effective analgesia should be administered at the time of diagnosis. Analgesia can be achieved by the use of sublingual nitroglycerin or intravenous morphine (or both). Sublingual nitroglycerin is given immediately unless the systolic blood pressure is less than 90 mm Hg. If the systolic blood pressure is under 90 mm Hg, nitroglycerin may be used after intravenous access has been obtained. Long-acting oral nitrate preparations are avoided for management of early acute MI. Sublingual or transdermal nitroglycerin can be used, but intravenous infusion of nitroglycerin allows more precise control. The intravenous dose can be titrated by frequently measuring blood pressure and heart rate. Morphine sulfate is also highly effective for the relief of pain associated with an acute MI. In addition to its analgesic properties, morphine exerts favorable hemodynamic effects by increasing venous capacitance and reducing systemic vascular resistance. The result is to decrease myocardial oxygen demand. As with nitroglycerin, hypotension may occur. The hypotension may be treated with intravenous fluids or leg elevation.

OXYGEN

Supplemental oxygen is given to all patients with an acute MI. Hypoxemia in a patient with an uncomplicated infarction is usually caused by ventilation-perfusion abnormalities. When oxygen is used it is administered by nasal cannula or mask at a rate of 4 to 10 L/min. In patients with chronic obstructive pulmonary disease it may be wise to use lower flow rates (see Chapter 13).

THROMBOLYTIC THERAPY

In addition to relieving pain and managing ischemia, thrombolytic therapy must be considered. Thrombosis has a major role in the development of an acute MI. Approximately 66% of patients with MIs have ST segment elevation, making it likely that the process is caused by an occlusive clot. The goal of thrombolytic therapy is reperfusion with a minimum of side effects. The most commonly used thrombolytic agents are streptokinase, anisoylated plasminogen streptokinase activator complex (APSAC), recombinant tissue-type plasminogen activator (rt-PA), urokinase, and pro-urokinase.

Early administration of thrombolytic therapy, within 6 to 12 hours from the onset of symptoms, has been associated with a reduction in mortality. Indications for thrombolytic therapy include typical chest pain >30 minutes but <12 hours that is unrelieved by nitroglycerin, and ST segment elevation in more than two contiguous leads (>1 mm in limb leads or >2 mm in chest leads) or ST segment depression in only V_1 and V_2 or a new left bundle branch block. Relative contraindications for thrombolytic therapy include history of stroke, active bleeding, blood pressure >180 mm Hg systolic, major surgery/trauma in the last 3 to 6 months, recent noncompressible vascular puncture, and possible intracranial event/unclear mental status.[56] Wright and colleagues[56] present a summary of the major thrombolytic trials. Advances in this therapeutic modality during the past

5 years include new third-generation fibrinolytic agents and various strategies to enhance administration and efficacy of these agents. A number of ongoing trials are attempting to determine whether the combination of fibrinolytic therapy with low molecular weight heparin enhances coronary reperfusion and reduces mortality and late reocclusion. Also presented is a dose and cost summary of the available fibrinolytic agents.[56]

Complications (Mechanical)

The most common complications of an acute MI are mechanical and electrical. Mechanical complications include those that are quickly reversible and those that are clearly life-threatening. Reversible causes of hypotension include hypovolemia, vasovagal reaction, overzealous therapy with antianginal or antiarrhythmic drugs, and brady- and tachyarrhythmias. Other, more serious etiologies include primary left ventricular failure, cardiac tamponade, rupture of the ventricular septum, acute papillary muscle dysfunction, and mitral regurgitation.

Killip and Kimball[57] developed a classification of patients with acute MI.

Class 1: Patients with uncomplicated infarction without evidence of heart failure as judged by the absence of rales and an S_3.
Class 2: Patients with mild to moderate heart failure as evidenced by pulmonary rales in the lower half of the lung fields and an S_3.
Class 3: Patients with severe left ventricular failure and pulmonary edema.
Class 4: Patients with cardiogenic shock, defined as systolic blood pressure less than 90 mm Hg with oliguria and other evidence of poor peripheral perfusion.

Cardiogenic shock has emerged as the most common cause of in-hospital mortality of patients with an acute MI. Despite advances in medical therapy, cardiogenic shock has a dismal prognosis (80–90% mortality). The management of patients with cardiogenic shock includes adequate oxygenation, reduction in myocardial oxygen demands, protection of ischemic myocardium, and circulatory support. The potential for myocardial salvage with emergency reperfusion should be considered in all cases.

Complications (Electrical)

The past 30 years has seen major developments in the recognition and treatment of arrhythmias. The most common include the brady- and tachyarrhythmias, AV conduction disturbances, and ventricular arrhythmias. Organized treatment protocols have been developed for each of these dysrhythmias.[58]

Post-MI Evaluation

Recommendations for pre- and postdischarge evaluations of patients with an acute MI have been outlined by the American College of Cardiologists, the American

Heart Association, and the American College of Physicians.[46] They include recommendations for testing exercise tolerance and strategies to determine those who would benefit from medical or surgical intervention. These recommendations include a submaximal ETT at 6 to 10 days and at 3 weeks to determine functional capacity.

Rehabilitation

The goal of cardiac rehabilitation includes maintenance of a desirable level of physical, social, and psychological functioning after the onset of cardiovascular illness.[59] Specific goals of rehabilitation include risk stratification, limitation of adverse psychological and emotional consequences of cardiovascular disease, modification of risk factors, alleviation of symptoms, and improved function. Risk stratification is accomplished by exercise tolerance testing. Additionally, high-risk patients include those with CHF, silent ischemia, and ventricular dysrhythmias. All patients should undergo an evaluation to reduce risk factors (smoking, hyperlipidemia, and hypertension) (see Chapter 2). Risk modification of these factors has been associated with significant reduction in subsequent cardiac events. Enrollment in a cardiac rehabilitation program with particular emphasis on exercise has been shown to reduce cardiovascular mortality.[60]

References

1. 2001 Heart and Stroke Statistical Update. American Heart Association. *http:// www.americanheart.org.*
2. Guidelines 2000 for cardiopulmonary resuscitation and emergency cardiovascular care. An international consensus on science. The American Heart Association in Collaboration with the International Liaison Committee on Resuscitation. *http://www. americanheart.org/ECC/index.html.*
3. Fulp SR, Richter JE. Esophageal chest pain. Am Fam Physician 1989;40:101–16.
4. Klinkman MS, Stevens D, Gorenflo DW. Episodes of care for chest pain: a preliminary report from MIRNET. J Fam Pract 1994;38:345–52.
5. Kemp HG, Vokonas PS, Cohn PF, Gorlin R. The anginal syndrome associated with normal coronary arteriograms: report of a six-year experience. Am J Med 1973;54:735–42.
6. Marchandise B, Bourrassa MG, Chairman BR, Lesperance J. Angiographic evaluation of the natural history of normal coronary arteries and mild coronary atherosclerosis. Am J Cardiol 1978;41:216–20.
7. Proudfit WL, Bruschke AVG, Sones FM. Clinical course of patients with normal or slightly or moderately abnormal coronary arteriograms: 10-year follow-up of 521 patients. Circulation 1980;62:712–17.
8. Kemp HG, Kronmal RA, Vlietstra RE, Frye RL. Seven year survival of patients with normal or near normal coronary arteriograms: a CASS registry study. J Am Coll Cardiol 1986;7:479–83.
9. Ockene IS, Shay MJ, Alpert JS, Weiner BH, Dalen JE. Unexplained chest pain in patients with normal coronary arteriograms: a follow-up study of functional status. N Engl J Med 1980;303:1249–52.

10. Lavey EB, Winkle RA. Continuing disability of patients with chest pain and normal coronary arteriograms. J Chronic Dis 1979;32:191–6.

11. Davies HA, Jones DB, Rhodes J. Esophageal angina as the cause of chest pain. JAMA 1982;248:2274–8.

12. Richter JE, Bradley LA, Castell DO. Esophageal chest pain current controversies in pathogenesis, diagnosis and therapy. Ann Intern Med 1989;110:66–78.

13. Schofield PM, Bennett DH, Whorwell PJ, et al. Exertional gastro-oesophageal reflux: a mechanism for symptoms in patient with angina pectoris and normal coronary angiograms. BMJ 1987;294:1459–61.

14. Areskog M, Tibbling L, Wranne B. Noninfarction in coronary care unit patients. Acta Med Scand 1981;209:51–7.

15. Glade MJ. Continuous ambulatory esophageal pH monitoring in the evaluation of patients with gastrointestinal reflux: Diagnostic and therapeutic technology assessment (DATTA). JAMA 1995;274:662–8.

16. Pope CE. Chest pain: heart? gullet? both? neither? [editorial]. JAMA 1992;248:2315.

17. Clouse RE, Lustman PJ. Psychiatric illness and contraction abnormalities of the esophagus. N Engl J Med 1983;309:1337–42.

18. Katon W, Hall ML, Russo J, et al. Chest pain: relationship of psychiatric illness to coronary arteriographic results. Am J Med 1988;84:1–9.

19. Cannon RO, Quyyumi AA, Mincemoyer R, Stine AM, Gracely RH, Smith WB. Imipramine in patients with chest pain despite normal coronary angiograms. N Engl J Med 1994;330:1411–17.

20. Cannon RO. Angina pectoris with normal coronary angiograms. Cardiol Clin 1991;9:157–66.

21. Colgan SM, Schofield PJ, Whorwell DH, Bennett DH, Brook NH, Jones PE. Angina-like chest pain: a joint medical and psychiatric investigation. Postgrad Med J 1988;64:743–6.

22. Diamond GA, Forrester JS. Analysis of probability as an aid in the clinical diagnosis of coronary-artery disease. N Engl J Med 1979;300:1350–8.

23. ACC/AHA guidelines for exercise testing: a report of the American College of Cardiology/American Heart Association Task Force on Practice Guidelines (Committee on Exercise Testing). J Am Coll Cardiol 1997;30:260–311.

24. Evans CH, Karunaratne HB. Exercise stress testing for the family physician. Part 1. Performing the test. Am Fam Physician 1992;45:121–32.

25. Evans CH, Karunaratne HB. Exercise stress testing for the family physician. Part 2. Am Fam Physician 1992;45:679–88.

26. Ellestad MH. Stress testing: principles and practice, 4th ed. Philadelphia: FA Davis, 1995.

27. Botvinick EH. Stress imaging: current clinical options for the diagnosis, localization, and evaluation of coronary artery disease. Med Clin North Am 1995;79:1025–61.

28. Afridi I, Quinones MA, Zoghbi WA, Cheirif J. Dobutamine stress echocardiography: sensitivity, specificity, and predictive value for future cardiac events. Am Heart J 1994;127:1510–15.

29. Beleslin BD, Ostojic M, Stepanovic J, et al. Stress echocardiography in the detection of myocardial ischemia: head-to-head comparison of exercise, dobutamine, and dipyridamole tests. Circulation 1994;90:1168–76.

30. Redberg RF. Diagnostic testing for coronary artery disease in women and gender differences in referral for revascularization. Cardiol Clin 1998;16:67–77.

31. Horwitz LD, Herman MV, Gorlin R. Clinical response to nitroglycerin as a diagnostic test for coronary artery disease. Am J Cardiol 1972;29:149–53.

32. 1999 update: ACC/AHA guidelines for the management of patients with chronic stable angina. A report of the American College of Cardiology/American Heart Association Task Force on Practice Guidelines (Committee on Management of chronic stable angina). J Am Coll Cardiol 1999;33:2092–197.

33. Hilton TC, Chaitman BR. The prognosis in stable and unstable angina. Cardiol Clin 1991;9:27–39.

34. Pryor DB, Shaw L, Harrell FE, et al. Estimating the likelihood of severe coronary artery disease. Am J Med 1991;90:553–62.

35. Bomber JW, Detullio PL. Oral nitrate preparations: an update. Am Fam Physician 1995;52:2331–6.

36. Howard PA, Ellerbeck EF. Optimizing beta-blocker use after myocardial infarction. Am Fam Physician 2000;62:1853–60.

37. Opie LH. Calcium channel antagonists. Part II. Use and comparative properties of prototypical calcium antagonists in ischemic heart disease, including recommendations based on analysis of 45 trials. Rev Cardiovasc Drug Ther 1987;1:4461–75.

38. Psaty BM, Heckbert ER, Koepsell TD, et al. The risk of myocardial infarction associated with antihypertensive drug therapies. JAMA 1995;274:670–5.

39. Hennekens CH, Buring JE. Aspirin in the primary prevention of cardiovascular disease. Cardiol Clin 1994;12:443–50.

40. Antiplatelet Trialists' Collaboration. Collaborative overview of randomized trials of antiplatelet therapy—I. Prevention of death, myocardial infarction, and stroke by prolonged antiplatelet therapy in various categories of patients. BMJ 1994;308:81–106.

41. Hankey GJ, Sudlow CLM, Dunbabin DW. Thienopyridine derivatives (ticlopidine, clopidogrel) versus aspirin for preventing stroke and other serious vascular events in high vascular risk patients. In: The Cochrane Library, issue 1. Oxford: Cochrane Library, 2000.

42. Shah PK. Pathophysiology of unstable angina. Cardiol Clin 1991;9:11–26.

43. Braunwald E, Mark DB, Jones RH, et al. Diagnosing and managing unstable angina: quick reference guide for clinicians, number 10. AHCPR publication no. 94-0603. Rockville, MD: US Department of Health and Human Services, Public Health Service, Agency for Health Care Policy and Research and National Heart, Lung, and Blood Institute, 1994.

44. Hamm CW, Braunwald E. A classification of unstable angina revisited. Circulation 2000;102:118–22.

45. Lewis HD, Davis JW, Archibald DG, et al. Protective effects of aspirin against acute myocardial infarction and death in men with unstable angina: results of a Veterans Administration cooperative study. N Engl J Med 1983;309:396–403.

46. 1999 update: ACC/AHA guidelines for the management of patients with acute myocardial infarction. A report of the American College of Cardiology/American Heart Association Task Force on Practice Guidelines (Committee of Management of Acute Myocardial Infarction). J Am Coll Cardiol 1999;34:890–911.

47. Faxon DP. Percutaneous coronary angioplasty in stable and unstable angina. Cardiol Clin 1991;9:99–113.

48. Sherman DL, Ryan TJ. Coronary angioplasty versus bypass grafting: cost-benefit considerations. Med Clin North Am 1995;79:1085–95.

49. Barsky AJ, Hochstrasser B, Coles A, et al. Silent myocardial ischemia: is the person or the event silent? JAMA 1990;264:1132–5.

50. Cohn PF. Silent myocardial ischemia. Ann Intern Med 1988;109:312–17.
51. Gottlieb SO. Asymptomatic or silent myocardial ischemia in angina pectoris: patho-physiology and clinical implications. Cardiol Clin 1991;9:49–61.
52. Lavie CJ, Gersh BJ. Acute myocardial infarction: initial manifestations, management, and prognosis. Mayo Clin Proc 1990;65:531–48.
53. Pathy MS. Clinical presentation of myocardial infarction in the elderly. Br Heart J 1967;29:190–9.
54. Kannel WB, Abbott RD. Incidence and prognosis of unrecognized myocardial in-farction: an update on the Framingham study. N Engl J Med 1984;311:1144–7.
55. Mair J, Morandell D, Genser N. Equivalent early sensitivities of myoglobin, creatine kinase MB mass, creatine kinase isoform ratios, and cardiac troponins I and T for acute myocardial infarction. Clin Chem 1995;41:1266–72.
56. Wright, RS, Kopecky SL, Reeder GS. Update on intravenous fibrinolytic therapy for acute myocardial infarction. Mayo Clin Proc 2000;75:1185–92.
57. Killip T, Kimball JT. Treatment of myocardial infarction in a coronary care unit: a two-year experience with 250 patients. Am J Cardiol 1967;20:457–61.
58. Guidelines 2000 for cardiopulmonary resuscitation and emergency cardiovascular care. International consensus on science. Circulation 2000;102:1–384.
59. Squires RW, Gau GT, Miller TD, Allison TG, Lavie CJ. Cardiovascular rehabilita-tion: status 1990. Mayo Clin Proc 1990;65:731–55.
60. O'Connor GT, Buring JE, Yusuf S, et al. An overview of randomized trials of reha-bilitation with exercise after myocardial infarction. Circulation 1989;80:234–44.

Case Presentation

Subjective

Patient Profile

John McCarthy is a 54-year-old married male restaurant operator.

Presenting Problem

"Chest pain, getting worse."

Present Illness

This is the second visit to the office for Mr. McCarthy, who is a well-controlled type 2 diabetic with angina pectoris for 1 year. His coronary artery disease has been stable, and he used three to four nitroglycerin tablets per month—especially after exertion and cold exposure—until the past week. He is now using three to five nitroglycerin tablets per day and has angina with mild exertion or when bending over. His pain radiates to the chin and to the left arm, which it seldom did before.

Past Medical History

No change since the past medical history recorded on his initial "get acquainted" office visit 6 months ago.

Social History

His restaurant business has been struggling recently; otherwise, no change since his last visit.

Habits

Stopped smoking 1 year ago. No alcohol use.

Family History

He is especially concerned about his son Mark, aged 28, who has been found to be HIV-positive.

REVIEW OF SYSTEMS

No other pertinent symptoms noted.

- What further information regarding Mr. McCarthy's chest pain would you like to know? Why?
- What more would you like to know about the current status of his diabetes mellitus?
- What might have caused his chest pain to become worse, and how would you inquire about these possibilities?
- What might this change in symptoms mean to the patient, and how would you ask about this?

Objective

GENERAL

The patient appears apprehensive and describes his pain by holding his clenched fist to the midchest.

VITAL SIGNS

Height, 6 ft; weight, 194 lb; blood pressure, 152/100; pulse, 82; respirations, 22; temperature, 37.2°C.

EXAMINATION

The eyes, ears, nose, and throat are normal. The neck and thyroid gland are unremarkable, and there is no cervical bruit. The chest is clear to percussion and auscultation. The heart has a regular sinus rhythm of 82. There is no cardiac enlargement, rub, or murmur.

LABORATORY

An ECG performed in the office today is normal for age.

- What additional data from the physical examination are likely to be pertinent? Explain.
- What—if any—findings on physical examination might increase or ease your concerns regarding the patient's history today?
- What—if any—laboratory tests would you obtain today? Why?
- What other tests—diagnostic imaging, treadmill ECG, or radionuclide scan—might be important in making a diagnosis today? Explain.

Assessment

- Based on the data available and pending further tests, what is your tentative diagnosis? How would you explain this to Mr. McCarthy and his family?
- What are the implications of this diagnosis for the patient?
- The family asks about the long-term prognosis. How would you respond?
- What symptoms or physical findings—if present—would you consider especially worrisome in this clinical setting? Explain.

Plan

- What are your therapeutic recommendations, and how would you explain them to the patient?
- Is a subspecialist consultation needed? Explain your reasoning.
- The patient wishes to know how soon he can return to work. How would you respond?
- If you decide to admit the patient to the hospital, what is your role in hospital care?

13
Obstructive Airway Disease

HOWARD N. WEINBERG

Obstructive airway disease includes two entities that share many common characteristics, asthma and chronic obstructive pulmonary disease (COPD). Chronic cough, a prominent symptom of both ailments, is also discussed in this chapter.

Background

Asthma

Asthma is a disorder of the pulmonary airways characterized by reversible obstruction, inflammation, and hyperresponsiveness.[1] Approximately 9 million to 12 million Americans are affected by this disease, with an annual mortality of 4000 to 5000.[2] Initial onset can be at any age, in either sex, and in every race. The severity of this illness is difficult to predict; some victims suffer a rapidly worsening course, whereas others appear to "outgrow" the disease.

The bronchospasm and inflammation may be triggered by allergens, infection, and psychophysiologic stressors. Allergens include inhaled substances such as molds, pollens, dust, animal danders, industrial pollutants, tobacco smoke, smoke from wood stoves, and cosmetics. Oral inducers may be food preservatives containing sulfiting agents and medications, especially aspirin and β-adrenergic antagonists (including selective agents and topical preparations).

Respiratory infections, particularly viral, are also major stimulators.[3] Occasionally a virus, such as the respiratory syncytial virus, induces bronchospasm in nearly all patients. Some patients have attacks only with infections.

Psychological factors certainly play a role in inducing asthma episodes. These triggers may be difficult to recognize and may manifest as part of a panic attack, as fear of the disease itself, or as a symptom of abuse. Panic attacks can also be confused with and misdiagnosed as asthma (see Chapter 22).

Chronic Obstructive Pulmonary Disease (COPD)

Chronic obstructive pulmonary disease is characterized by abnormal expiratory flow that does not change significantly over time. This delineation was intended to exclude asthma as well as specific upper airway diseases such as cancers and conditions affecting the lower airways such as bronchiectasis, sarcoidosis, and cystic fibrosis.[4] Traditionally included in this category has been chronic bronchitis and emphysema. In some patients, however, the overlap with asthma is so strong that a significant distinction cannot be made. Indeed, the term COPD was developed in recognition of the tremendous overlap between asthma, chronic bronchitis, and emphysema.

Chronic bronchitis is defined as a cough that occurs at least 3 months a year for 2 consecutive years and involves excess mucous secretion in the large airways. A malady of adults, chronic bronchitis affects about 20% of men and is primarily caused by smoking. Unfortunately, the incidence in women is increasing as the percentage of women smokers increases. Other contributing factors include air pollution, occupational exposures, and infection.[5]

Emphysema is defined as a permanent enlargement of distal air spaces with destruction of the acinar walls without fibrosis. This entity can be further subdivided into centriacinar, panacinar, and distal acinar types.[6] Like chronic bronchitis, this illness is found primarily in smokers. There is, however, a rare type of congenital emphysema and also a genetic syndrome associated with the lack of α_1-antitrypsin.

Chronic Cough

Although cough is an essential component of the presentation of both COPD and asthma, there are many other entities that can cause chronic coughing. The four most common causes are postnasal drip syndrome, COPD, asthma, and gastroesophageal reflux.[7] Other causes include acute and chronic infection, other lung diseases (embolism, cancer), aspiration, psychogenic factors, and cardiac failure. Cough can also result from medications, such as angiotensin-converting enzyme (ACE) inhibitors. Also, a significant number of patients have two or more causes for cough.

Clinical Presentation

Asthma

The classic symptoms of asthma are cough, dyspnea, and wheezing. The wheezing may be audible or require auscultation. Infrequently, a patient may be so "tight" that wheezing is detected only after initial therapy. The patient might be resting comfortably or be in extreme respiratory distress. At such times there may be accessory muscle movement (subcostal, intercostal, or supraclavicular), nasal flaring (particularly in children), cyanosis, or altered mental status. Auscultation often reveals rhonchi, wheezing, and a reversal of the normal 2:1 inspiratory/expiratory ratio. An increase in respiratory rate, independent of fever, is also a cardinal sign.

Sometimes, especially in children, the only presentation of asthma is a chronic night cough. Another symptom complex includes wheezing and shortness of breath that occurs following exercise. This entity is known as exercise-induced asthma (EIA) or bronchospasm (EIB). Many Olympic-caliber athletes have EIB.

COPD

The typical picture of COPD is prominent cough, dyspnea, and often wheezing. In severe situations tachypnea, accessory muscle movement, breathing through pursed lips, cyanosis, and agitation are present. Long-standing disease may be indicated by a pronounced barrel chest (i.e., an increase in the anterior-to-posterior dimension). Copious sputum production may also be noted. Chest auscultation may reveal wheezes, rales, or rhonchi in varying intensity, or it can be normal. Heart sounds might be distant, or a gallop indicative of secondary heart disease may be detected. Examination of the extremities might reveal cyanosis of the nailbeds or clubbing of the fingers.

Cough

Clinical presentation of cough is self-explanatory: the patient is coughing. It is important to note whether the cough is dry or productive of sputum (thick, thin, purulent, bloody). The time of day or night often provides a clue to the extensive differential diagnosis as can evidence of allergy such as rhinitis, allergic shiners, or a transverse nose crease (the allergic salute). Of particular note are symptoms related to gastro-esophageal reflux (e.g., heartburn, water brash, or increased belching). Finally, these patients may present with the signs and symptoms of a multitude of underlying diseases.

Diagnosis

Asthma and COPD

The diagnosis of asthma or COPD should be fairly evident after the history and physical examinations are completed. Laboratory and radiographic data by themselves usually cannot establish the diagnosis of either disorder but may provide confirmatory information and assist in the assessment of severity.

PULMONARY FUNCTION TESTS

Although extensive pulmonary testing may be indicated in the occasional patient, the most useful information is obtained from evaluating the forced expiratory volume in 1 second (FEV_1), the forced vital capacity (FVC), the FEV_1/FVC ratio, and the peak expiratory flow rate (PEFR). Obstructive disease is indicated by a reduced FEV_1 in the presence of a normal FVC, which also causes a reduction in the FEV_1/FVC ratio. Restrictive diseases (pure emphysema), on the other hand, show a normal FEV_1, a decreased FVC, and an increased FEV_1/FVC ratio.

With asthma a useful test is to observe the change in FEV_1 following treatment with a bronchodilator. An increase of 15% is indicative of reversible airway disease.[4] Three stimulators—exercise, histamine, methacholine—may be used for provocative testing. A decrease in FEV_1 of 20% is considered positive. The PEFR may be obtained using a peak flowmeter and can be measured in the office or at home. It provides a quick, objective indication of the severity of an episode and can serve as a signal to start certain treatments. It is also a measure of the response to therapeutic intervention. It is highly recommended that patients be provided with peak flowmeters and instructed about how to use them. These devices must be demonstrated and practiced. Many patients have trouble mastering the technique. To be fully effective, this device must be used when patients are feeling well in order to define a personal "best" for later comparison. With COPD the spirometric abnormalities may be a mixture of obstructive and restrictive diseases. In asymptomatic patients, especially smokers, abnormal results can serve as an indicator of early illness and, it is hoped, as a stimulus to quit smoking. In symptomatic patients, these measurements can serve as a sign of progression. Finally, the FEV_1 or PEFR may be used to evaluate the asthmatic component in the COPD patient.

ARTERIAL BLOOD GASES

Evaluation of the severity of disease may be assisted by the measurement of arterial blood gases (ABGs). Severe hypoxemia in the asthmatic or hypercapnia in the chronic lung patient might serve as an important factor in the decision to hospitalize a patient. Most outpatients do not need ABG measurements.

OTHER LABORATORY TESTS

Useful tests in ill patients include measurement of blood leukocytes as a sign of acute infection, and hematocrit as indicative of an additional reason for hypoxemia if it is low or as a sign of long-standing hypoxemia if polycythemia is noted. Sputum evaluation is useful for identifying the pathogen in an acute infection.

CHEST RADIOGRAPHY

It is not necessary to obtain a chest radiograph on every patient with asthma or COPD. A radiograph may be useful in the undiagnosed patient with chronic cough and may help to identify complications in patients with obstructive disease. These problems might include pneumonia, pneumothorax, pneumomediastinum, or subcutaneous emphysema. In the newly discovered asthmatic (especially children) radiography should be done if foreign body aspiration is suspected. The chest radiograph of the COPD patient may be normal; show a mild increase in lung markings; demonstrate the hyperlucency, overinflation, and bullae often seen with emphysema; or show an enlarged heart or the pulmonary congestion seen with heart failure. On occasion, a chest film holds the key to differentiating congestive heart failure with wheezing (cardiac asthma) from asthma. Other radiologic procedures, such as lung scans, computed tomography (CT) scans, and angiography have a role only in the management of complications.

Chronic Cough

The diagnosis and workup of chronic cough is often difficult, time-consuming, and expensive. Irwin and associates[7] presented a schema for evaluating previously undiagnosed patients. Their suggestions, in decreasing order of usefulness, include the history, physical examination, pulmonary function tests, methacholine challenge, upper gastrointestinal radiology, measurement of esophageal pH, sinus and chest radiography, and bronchoscopy. Following this approach a diagnosis is possible in 99% of patients.

Management

The management of asthma and COPD is best viewed from a standpoint of both disease complexes. It includes avoidance, immunotherapy, exercise, drug treatment, and psychosocial support (Fig. 13.1).

Avoidance

The lifestyle of the patient with pulmonary problems may be drastically affected by environmental factors: climate, outdoor air pollution, and indoor air pollution.

CLIMATE

Both asthmatic and COPD sufferers may be affected by changes in wind velocity, humidity, and temperature. Low wind velocity allows accumulation of allergens; high humidity leads to an increase in pollen-producing plants and molds; and sudden temperature drops cause a fall in airway conduction.[8] Barometric pressure changes are also associated with exacerbations of asthma and COPD. Extremes in climatic events, such as prolonged heat waves or air inversions, often result in increased mortality among COPD patients. Although patients cannot avoid climatic changes, they can stay inside on particularly bad days and can minimize the effects by using filtered air-conditioning and heating systems maintained at fairly constant temperature year round.

OUTDOOR AIR POLLUTION

Potential allergens include man-made (e.g., smoke and chemical fumes) and natural substances (e.g., pollens, dusts, and molds). Although difficult to avoid, some

Asthma Maintenance

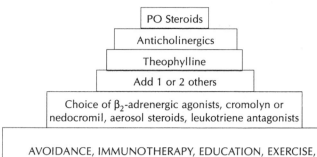

PO Steroids

Anticholinergics

Theophylline

Add 1 or 2 others

Choice of β_2-adrenergic agonists, cromolyn or nedocromil, aerosol steroids, leukotriene antagonists

AVOIDANCE, IMMUNOTHERAPY, EDUCATION, EXERCISE, FAMILY INVOLVEMENT

Acute Asthma

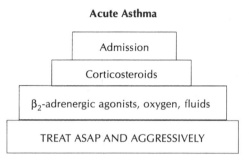

Admission

Corticosteroids

β_2-adrenergic agonists, oxygen, fluids

TREAT ASAP AND AGGRESSIVELY

COPD

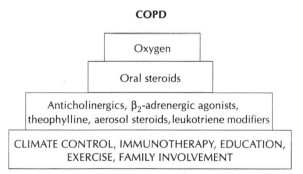

Oxygen

Oral steroids

Anticholinergics, β_2-adrenergic agonists, theophylline, aerosol steroids, leukotriene modifiers

CLIMATE CONTROL, IMMUNOTHERAPY, EDUCATION, EXERCISE, FAMILY INVOLVEMENT

FIGURE 13.1. Recommended step treatment plan for asthma and chronic obstructive pulmonary disease (COPD). ASAP = as soon as possible.

factors can be minimized by controlling the type of grass, ornamental shrubs, and flowering vegetation around the home.

INDOOR AIR POLLUTION

Fortunately, indoor allergens are much more readily controlled. It is of paramount importance to eliminate tobacco smoke. Other potential irritants include building materials, cleaning agents, air fresheners, pest control chemicals, decorative plants, dried flowers, cockroachs, scented candles, and cosmetics. The bedroom is a critical room to allergy-proof. Attention is directed to pillows, mattresses, carpets, drapes, blankets, shelf ornaments, and stuffed animals (especially in the bed). Wood stoves and kerosene heaters have been shown to aggravate respiratory problems. Sometimes families must give up their pets. This entire aspect of avoidance must be stressed to all patients and may obviate the need for further treatment.

Education of patients is essential regarding all aspects of management. Excellent material is available from the National Asthma Education Program.[9]

Immunotherapy

DESENSITIZATION

If avoidance fails, allergic patients should be tried on antihistamines and nasal sprays and considered for allergy desensitization.[10]

IMMUNIZATION

Influenza and pneumococcal vaccines should be given to all patients with significant respiratory illness. Influenza vaccine is administered yearly about 2 to 3 months prior to anticipated outbreaks. October and November are the prime times to immunize in the United States. If a patient misses the vaccine, consideration should be given to prophylaxis with antiviral medications. Pneumococcal vaccine should be supplemented with booster injections once after 5 years, although this recommendation may change.

Exercise

Aerobic exercise is important for both asthmatics and COPD patients. Proper and consistent exercise at least three times a week can lead to improved tolerance and endurance and an increase in the feeling of wellness.[11] Consider ordering pulmonary rehabilitation.

Drug Treatment

The choice of medication for these illnesses has greatly expanded since the 1980s and is presently continuing to undergo rapid changes in philosophy. It is especially true for asthma, where emphasis has shifted from treating just bronchospasm to treating inflammation as well.[1] Unfortunately, those who suffer with COPD have not experienced as great a revolution in drug treatment.

β_2-Adrenergic Agonists

The β_2-adrenergic agonist class of medication (beta-2s) is now the first step for treating bronchospasm. Available as liquids, short- and long-acting tablets, metered-dose inhalers (MDIs), dry powder inhalers, nebulizable solutions, and injectables, these agents have many potential uses. Available in the United States are albuterol (Proventil, Ventolin), bitolterol (Tornalate), metaproterenol (Alupent, Metaprel), pirbuterol (Maxair), terbutaline (Brethaire, Brethine), and salmeterol (Serevent) (Table 13.1).

The choice of preparation depends on the patient's age and the acuteness of the situation. MDIs and nebulizers have an almost instantaneous onset of action, and sustained-released tablets offer assistance with nocturnal symptoms. Oral forms have their greatest use in young children. It is rarely necessary to use both the oral and inhalation route at the same time, a situation that leads to increased toxicity with little gain in benefit.

Table 13.1. Recommended Dosages for Theophylline, β_2-Adrenergic Agonists and Corticosteroids

Medication	Age group (years)	Route	Usual dosage
Theophylline	<1	po	Varies
	1–9	po	24 mg/kg/day
	9–12	po	20 mg/kg/day
	12–16	po	18 mg/kg/day
	>16, smoker	po	18 mg/kg/day
	>16, nonsmoker	po	13 mg/kg/day
Albuterol	>2	po	0.1 mg/kg/tid–qid, max 2 mg tid
	>2	MDI	1–2 inhal q4h
	>12	Nebulizer	2.5 mg q4h
Bitolterol	>12	MDI	2 inhal q4h or 3 inhal q6h
Metaproterenol	<6	po	1.3–2.6 mg/kg/day tid–qid
	>6	po	10–20 mg tid/qid
	>2	MDI	1–2 inhal q4h
	>12	Nebulizer	0.2–0.3 ml q4h
Pirbuterol	>12	MDI	1–2 inhal q4h
Salmeterol	>12	MDI	2 inhal q12h
Terbutaline	>12	po	1.25–5.00 mg tid
	>12	MDI	2 inhal q4h
Beclomethasone	>6	MDI	2–4 inhal bid/qid, max 20/day
Budesonide	>6	MDI	1–2 inhal bid, max 8/day
Flunisolide	>6	MDI	2 inhal bid, max 8/day
Fluticasone	>6	MDI	Three different strengths
Triamcinolone	>6	MDI	1–2 inhal tid/qid, max 16/day
Prednisone	1–12	po	1–2 mg/kg/day, taper 5–10 days
	>12	po	40–80 mg/day, taper 5–10 days

Source: Data are from the Physicians' Desk Reference.[17]
MDI = Multiple-dose inhaler; inhal = inhalations.

Beta-2s are the treatment of choice for episodic or mild asthmatics and for EIB. Once the need is established for continual usage, as for moderate and severe asthmatics, some authorities use these agents as first-line treatment whereas others reserve their use for rescue efforts, preferring to use antiinflammatory drugs first. Certainly, every patient with significant obstructive disease should always have this medication on hand.

The newest member of this class, salmeterol, is unique in its 12-hour action. It is indicated for maintenance and nocturnal symptoms of both asthma and COPD. Shorter-acting agents may still be used between doses if rescue is needed, although tolerance may become a problem.[12]

In the near future, dry-powder forms of MDIs should be available. It is hoped this advance will reduce the problems associated with propellant gases and also be more compatible with the environment.

For the treatment of acute situations, beta-2s are the agents of choice. They can be administered by nebulizer (and repeated at 60- to 90-minute intervals if needed[13]) or by MDI using an InspirEase at the rate of one inhalation per minute for 5 minutes. The use of these agents has supplanted the need for older agents such as ephedrine, isoproterenol, and epinephrine. Even in the emergency situation, beta-2s have been found to be equally effective with significantly less toxicity when compared to subcutaneous epinephrine.[14]

Some patients experience great trouble utilizing an MDI. Proper technique must be taught and observed. For those too young or who cannot master the MDI, the following spacer devices are available: InspirEase, Inhal-aid, Paper tube, and Aerochamber.[15] Home-made alternatives are the inside of a paper towel roll or a small paper lunch bag. Any of these devices should work with all inhalers.

In the COPD patient these drugs have less application but are still valuable when bronchospasm is present. Pulse and blood pressure should be monitored.

CORTICOSTEROIDS

The use of steroids for asthma has received considerable impetus in recent years. Traditionally thought to be too strong for chronic use, the advent of MDI preparations has minimized side effects and pushed corticosteroids to the forefront. In addition, recognition of the importance of inflammation in the pathophysiology of asthma has made many authorities advocate corticosteroids as first-line treatment.[16] Unfortunately, the probably unfounded fear of the effect of steroids on growth and adrenal function has caused a reluctance to utilize this medication. For the moderate to severe asthmatic, for the unstable patient, and during an acute crisis, however, there should be no hesitancy to use steroids.

Aerosol preparations include beclomethasone (Beclovent, Vanceril), budesonide (Pulmicort), flunisolide (AeroBid), fluticasone (Flovent), and triamcinolone (Azmacort). The effect of these medications may not be fully seen for up to 4 to 8 weeks and are therefore not effective for the acute attack. They also do not protect against adrenal insufficiency. Oral medication must be tapered when switching to an aerosol (Table 13.1).[17]

A new product combining fluticasone and salmeterol (Advair) in three dosage strengths was released in April 2001. Initial reports show significant advantages over either medication used alone.[18] Oral steroids, usually in the form of prednisone, are essential for use during the acute exacerbation or for the severe, chronic patient with asthma or COPD. When used early during an episode, steroids may prevent a relapse[19] or the need for hospitalization. Some physicians prescribe oral steroids to any patient needing treatment in an emergency setting. Patients with long-standing disease often develop recognizable patterns of deterioration, such as with acute upper respiratory infections. These patients can be instructed to use steroids early to prevent exacerbations. Dosage varies with age and weight. For chronic treatment, every-other-day administration is preferred, whereas multiple daily dosing may be most effective in the acute situation.

Corticosteroids are also available for intravenous use, which is indicated whenever hospitalization is being considered. Unfortunately, there is no definitive proof as to the effectiveness of intravenous steroids for preventing hospitalization. In addition, their onset of action is at least 4 hours.

CROMOLYN AND NEDOCROMIL

Primarily used as prophylactic agents for asthma, cromolyn and nedocromil are antiinflammatory and, due to their almost complete lack of side effects, represent a significant therapeutic advantage. Unfortunately, not all patients respond to them.

Cromolyn (Intal) is available for MDI or nebulizer. Its onset of action can be as long as 1 to 2 months. Dosage is two inhalations qid; tapering to less frequent dosage can be attempted. Once it is begun, this medication should be used throughout an acute episode so as not to lose the prophylaxis. Along with beta-2s and inhaled steroids, cromolyn is useful for EIB.

Nedocromil (Tilade) is the newer of the two agents, and its safety is comparable to that of cromolyn. Dosage recommendations are also similar. In addition, nedocromil may be effective in preventing the cough caused by ACE inhibitors.

LEUKOTRIENE MODIFIERS

This is a new class of medications consisting of three agents: montelukast (Singulair), 10 mg in the evening, 4 or 5 mg for children; zafirlukast (Accolate), 20 mg bid avoiding food, 10 mg in children; and zileuton (Zyflo), rarely used due to qid dosing and the need to monitor liver enzymes. The first two products are occasionally also of benefit in COPD.[20]

THEOPHYLLINE

Long the cornerstone of asthma treatment, theophylline is no longer the initial drug of choice. A bronchodilator, theophylline is best utilized for patients needing more than one maintenance drug and for those with pronounced nocturnal symptoms. It is also worth a trial in COPD patients.

There are various formulations of theophylline: liquid, capsule, tablet, slow-release products, and the intravenous form. Most patients require several days of continuous usage to reach maximal effectiveness. Once a steady state is reached, it is best to maintain the same brand, as bioavailability may vary from product to product. Smokers and children tend to need higher doses due to rapid metabolism. Significant interactions are possible with erythromycins, fluoroquinolones, cimetidine, phenytoin, and oral contraceptives. Also, dosages need to be closely monitored in patients with liver failure or congestive heart failure. Serum theophylline levels are recommended for all the above situations and in difficult patients where fine-tuning is needed. The serum therapeutic level has been changed from 10 to 20 μg/mL to 5 to 15 μg/mL.[21] Older preparations that contain subtherapeutic doses of theophylline, Marax and Tedral, are no longer considered appropriate therapy (Table 13.1).

Children require close monitoring. As they grow, their dosage requires constant readjustment. Theophylline has come under scrutiny with regard to potential interference with school performance, but no significant effect has been established.

In the acute situation (office or emergency room) theophylline (as aminophylline) is no longer considered appropriate for intravenous usage as it does not represent a therapeutic advantage but does significantly increase toxicity.[22] It may be useful, however, in hospitalized patients.

Anticholinergics

The current choice of anticholinergic drug is ipratropium (Atrovent) for MDI or nebulizer. For COPD, because of fewer side effects, ipratropium may well be the preferred bronchodilator. The usual dosage is two inhalations qid, but this dosage can be exceeded in COPD patients.[21] For asthma, use ipratropium if other treatment is not effective. Several studies combining nebulized ipratropium with a β_2-agonist have produced unclear results when used in severe asthma.[23]

Calcium Channel Blockers

Calcium channel blockers have been suggested to have a mild bronchodilatory effect, but it has not been clinically demonstrated. They are, however, effective for the treatment of hypertension in obstructive disease, especially compared to beta-blockers and ACE inhibitors.

Antibiotics

For acute bacterial infections in patients with asthma and COPD, antibiotics are essential. There has been debate concerning when to treat the COPD-afflicted patient. The use of broad-spectrum antibiotics appears to be indicated when COPD sufferers have at least two of the following three symptoms: an increase in dyspnea, an increase in sputum production, and an increase in sputum purulence.[24]

MUCOLYTICS AND EXPECTORANTS

The value of mucolytics and expectorants has not been demonstrated in objective studies.

OXYGEN

Except in the acute situation, oxygen should be reserved for chronic patients who are in distress when breathing room air. With COPD patients who retain high levels of carbon dioxide, the only functioning respiratory drive may be related to hypoxia. It is therefore critical to adjust the oxygen to a level where the hypoxic drive is not lost.

PREGNANCY AND BREAST-FEEDING

Pregnancy is complicated by asthma about 1% of the time, with a potentially large risk to the fetus if hypoxia develops. The use of theophylline, beta-2s, cromolyn, Singulair, Accolate, and steroids is generally considered safe.[20] Some antibiotics and decongestants, live virus vaccines, and iodides must be avoided.

For lactating mothers the same medications considered safe during pregnancy are acceptable. Breast-feeding should be strongly encouraged, as studies suggest it delays the onset of allergies and asthma in the infant.[1,19]

PSYCHOSOCIAL SUPPORT

Psychosocial support is a critical component in any management plan and is addressed later in the chapter.

Prevention

Asthma and COPD are at opposite extremes when it comes to treatment and prevention. Whereas there are several fine alternatives for asthma treatment, management of COPD is at best symptomatic. On the other hand, asthma is essentially unpreventable, whereas COPD should not exist.

Smoking cessation is the key to relegating COPD to medical history. Except for a rare genetic or occupational case (which should also be preventable with good industrial hygiene), most COPD is directly related to smoking. The United States is moving in the direction of encouraging nonsmokers' rights, but unfortunately children have ready access to tobacco products and are still starting to smoke in large numbers. Physicians therefore must remind every smoker at every appointment to begin the process of cessation.

Control of smoking is also key to decreasing the morbidity of asthma. Even side-stream smoke has been shown to result in more attacks, more complications, and more frequent need for emergency services. It is critical that the parents of asthmatic children never smoke in the house or car. Prevention of death has always been a priority within the medical profession. It is certainly appropriate for asthma and COPD.

Asthma is usually viewed as a nonfatal disease, but it does carry the potential for death. Most studies show that preventable deaths and hospitalizations have been the result of delayed treatment due primarily to two factors: the patient's or family's inability to recognize the severity of an attack, and the physician's poor assessment of the severity of an attack.[25,26] Suggestions for prevention include frequent use of peak flowmeters as an objective guide to severity, establishing effective maintenance therapy, and emphasizing patient and family education. Education is aimed at recognizing an attack, knowing what measures to take at home, and learning to call for help early. The material provided in the national education program is superb and should be made available to all patients.[9]

On the other hand, COPD is a highly fatal disease, the fourth leading cause of mortality in the United States and still increasing.[27] Although little can be done to reverse this disease, good management of the environment, appropriate medication, and smoking cessation aid in improving the quality of life for the affected individual. Extremely severe cases may be considered for lung volume reduction surgery or transplantation.[11]

Family and Community Issues

Family support is an essential factor in the successful treatment of chronic lung disease. This point is especially true for children and the debilitated, who might be unable to care for themselves.

Asthma

Patient and family attitudes are critical in the patient's acceptance of this disease. Several factors have been identified with regard to poor patient attitude: the unpredictable nature of asthma leading to a feeling of "beyond my control"; a feeling of stigmatization; a false perception that asthma is psychogenic and therefore "in my head"; a tendency to deny the disease; and the fear elicited by an experience of being unable to breathe.[28] These attitudes may handicap all attempts at treatment and should be addressed via thorough patient and family education.

Also important is the tendency for families to label their asthmatics as ill. It is best to view the patient as a person with asthma and not as an asthmatic person. All activities should be continued, especially sports and physical education. It is far better to use an MDI and run than to sit on the sidelines and watch.

COPD

Emotional difficulties are common in COPD sufferers. The dyspnea and fatigue of this disease often leads to depression and fear. Quality of life may be reduced in all areas, including social, sexual, vocational, and recreational activities, leading to further loss of self-esteem and isolation.[29] Patients should be encouraged to do as much as possible for themselves and must be given every opportunity to participate in the usual family and community events, even if a wheelchair and oxygen are needed. When the illness becomes terminal, patients should be counseled to keep control of their own lives by participating in the decisions of how and where to die. They can be encouraged to make living wills or execute powers of attorney. If appropriate, patients should be allowed to die at home, and physicians should be willing to make house calls. This measure improves the final quality of life by affording the patient the comfort of dying in a familiar setting, surrounded by family and friends.

References

1. Guidelines for the diagnosis and management of asthma. National Asthma Education Program, expert panel report 2. NIH publ. no. 97-4051. Bethesda: National Heart, Lung and Blood Institute, 1997.
2. Shuttari MF. Asthma: diagnosis and management. Am Fam Physician 1995;52: 2225–35.
3. Johnston SL, Pattemore PK, Sanderson G, et al. Community study of role of viral infections in exacerbations of asthma in 9–11 year old children. BMJ 1995;310:1225–9.
4. American Thoracic Society. Standards for the diagnosis and care of patients with chronic obstructive pulmonary disease (COPD) and asthma. Am Rev Respir Dis 1987;136:225–44.
5. Ingram RH. Chronic bronchitis, emphysema, and airways obstruction. In: Harrison's principles of internal medicine, 15th ed. New York: McGraw-Hill, 2001;1456-63, 1491–99.
6. Snider GL, Kleinerman J, Thurlbeck WM, Bengali ZH. The definition of emphysema: report of a National Heart, Lung and Blood Institute, Division of Lung Diseases workshop. Am Rev Respir Dis 1985;132:182–5.
7. Irwin RS, Curley FJ, French CL. Chronic cough, the spectrum and frequency of causes, key components of the diagnostic evaluation, and outcome of specific therapy. Am Rev Respir Dis 1990;141:640–7.
8. Kemp JP, Metzer EO. Getting control of the allergic child's environment. Pediatr Ann 1989;18:801–8.
9. Teach your patients about asthma: a clinician's guide. NIH publ. no. 92-2737. Washington, DC: National Institutes of Health, 1992.
10. Abramson MJ, Puy RM, Weiner JM. Is allergen immunotherapy effective in asthma? A meta-analysis of randomized controlled trials. Am J Respir Crit Care Med 1995;151:969–74.
11. Ries AL, Kupferberg DH, What's new in COPD: the latest treatment options. J Respir Dis 2000;21:304–20.
12. Anderson CJ, Bardana EJ. Asthma in the elderly: interactions to be wary of. J Respir Dis 1995;16:965–76.
13. Fanta CH, Israel E, Sheffer AL. Managing—and preventing—severe asthma attacks. J Respir Dis 1992;13:94–108.
14. Becker AB, Nelson NA, Simons FER. Inhaled salbutamol (albuterol) vs. injected epinephrine in the treatment of acute asthma in children. J Pediatr 1983;102:465–9.

15. Plaut TF. Holding chambers for aerosol drugs. Pediatr Ann 1989;18:824–6.
16. Szefler SJ. A comparison of aerosol glucocorticoids in the treatment of chronic bronchial asthma. Pediatr Asthma Allergy Immunol 1991;5:227–35.
17. Physicians' desk reference, 55th ed. Oradell, NJ: Medical Economics, 2001.
18. Kavura M. Salmeterol and fluticasone propionate combined in a new powder inhalation device for the treatment of asthma: a randomized, double-blind, placebo controlled trial. J Allergy Clin Immunol 2000;105:1108–16.
19. Chapman KR, Verbeck PR, White JG, Rebeeck AS. Effect of a short course of prednisone in the prevalence of early relapse after the emergency room treatment of acute asthma. N Engl J Med 1991;324:788–94.
20. The Medical Letter on Drugs and Therapeutics 2000(6 March);42:19–24.
21. Gross NJ. COPD management: achieving bronchodilatation. J Respir Dis 1996; 17:183–95.
22. Seigel D, Sheppard D, Gelb A, Weinberg PF. Aminophylline increases the toxicity but not the efficacy of an inhaled beta-adrenergic agonist in the treatment of acute exacerbations of asthma. Am Rev Respir Dis 1985;132:283–6.
23. Herner SJ, Seaton TL, Mertens MK. Combined ipratropium and $\beta2$ adrenergic receptor agonist in acute asthma. J Am Board Fam Pract 2000;13:1:55–65.
24. Anthonisen NR, Manfreda J, Warren CPW, Hershfield EJ, Harding GKM, Nelson NA. Antibiotic therapy in exacerbation of COPD. Ann Intern Med 1987;106:196–204.
25. Morray B, Redding G. Factors associated with prolonged hospitalization of children with asthma. Arch Pediatr Adolesc Med 1995;149:276–9.
26. Strunk RC. Death caused by asthma: minimizing the risks.J Respir Dis 1989;10:21–36.
27. Fraser KL, Chapman KR. Chronic obstructive pulmonary disease, prevention, early detection, and aggressive treatment can make a difference. Postgrad Med 2000;108: 103–16.
28. Dirks JF. Patient attitude as a factor in asthma management. Pract Cardiol 1986;12(1): 84–98.
29. Dowell AR. Quality of life: how important is managing COPD? J Respir Dis 1991; 12:1057–72.

CASE PRESENTATION

Subjective

PATIENT PROFILE

Samuel Nelson is a 48-year-old single male farm worker.

PRESENTING PROBLEM

"My breathing is worse."

PRESENT ILLNESS

For the past 5 years, Mr. Nelson has had gradually progressive cough, shortness of breath on exertion, and occasional wheezing. He has continued to smoke and does not take his medication regularly. When worse, he returns to the physician to refill his beta-2-agonist inhaler for use as needed.

PAST MEDICAL HISTORY

He had pneumonia 3 years ago that did not require hospitalization.

SOCIAL HISTORY

Samuel was a high school dropout at age 16. He has never married and lives with his parents. He has no close friends.

HABITS

He has smoked two packs of cigarettes daily since age 15. He uses no alcohol or recreational drugs.

FAMILY HISTORY

His father, aged 76, has diabetes mellitus and osteoarthritis. His mother, aged 71, has high blood pressure. Three siblings are living and well.

- What additional information would you like about the history of present illness?

- What might be Mr. Nelson's reasons for the visit today? How would you inquire about this?
- What information about Mr. Nelson's work might be useful, and how would you ask about this?
- What more would you like to know about the patient's adaptation to his illness? Why might this be important?

Objective

VITAL SIGNS

Height, 5 ft, 10 in; weight 180 lb; blood pressure, 140/80; pulse, 76; respirations, 22; temperature, 37.2°C.

EXAMINATION

The patient is not in acute distress but has an occasional cough while talking. The head, eyes, ears, nose, and throat are normal. The neck and thyroid gland are normal. The chest has an increased anteroposterior diameter, and there are distant breath sounds throughout. No rales are present, but there are occasional faint wheezes on forced expiration. The heart has a regular sinus rhythm, and no murmurs are present.

- What more—if anything—might be included in the physical examination? Why?
- What—if any—laboratory tests would you order today? Why?
- What—if any—diagnostic imaging would you order today? Why?
- If, in addition to the symptoms described above, Mr. Nelson had lost 12 lb since a previous visit 6 months ago, what might you do differently? Explain.

Assessment

- What is your diagnostic impression today, and how would you explain this to the patient?
- How would you assess the meaning of the illness to Mr. Nelson?
- What is the apparent contribution of smoking to the patient's disease, and how would you describe this to him?
- The patient's employer calls to ask you about how Mr. Nelson is doing? How would you respond?

Plan

- What would be your therapeutic recommendations to the patient regarding medication, activity, and life style? How would you explain this to the patient?
- How might you persuade Mr. Nelson to stop smoking?
- What are the implications of this illness for the family and community?
- What continuing care would you advise? Explain.

14

Gastritis, Esophagitis, and Peptic Ulcer Disease

ALAN M. ADELMAN AND PETER R. LEWIS

Dyspepsia/Epigastric Pain

Gastritis, esophagitis, and peptic ulcer disease present commonly with epigastric pain, or dyspepsia. Dyspepsia refers to upper abdominal pain or discomfort and may be associated with fullness, belching, bloating, heartburn, food intolerance, nausea, or vomiting. Dyspepsia is a common problem. Despite discoveries about the cause and treatment of peptic ulcer disease, dyspepsia remains a challenging problem to evaluate and treat.

Epidemiology

Dyspepsia is a common problem, with an annual incidence of 1% to 2% in the general population and a prevalence that may reach 20% to 40%. The four major causes of dyspepsia are nonulcer dyspepsia (NUD), peptic ulcer disease (PUD), gastroesophageal reflux disease (GERD), and gastritis. NUD, PUD, GERD, and gastritis account for more than 90% of all causes of dyspepsia. Other, less common causes of dyspepsia are cholelithiasis, irritable bowel disease, esophageal or gastric cancer, pancreatitis, pancreatic cancer, Zollinger-Ellison syndrome, and abdominal angina. Patients who seek medical attention for dyspepsia are more likely to be concerned about the seriousness of the symptom, worried about cancer or heart disease, and experiencing more stress than individuals who do not seek medical attention for dyspepsia.

Presentation

No single symptom is helpful for distinguishing between the causes of dyspepsia, but some patient characteristics are predictive of serious disease. For example, as single symptoms, nocturnal pain, relief of pain by antacids, worsening of pain by food, anorexia, nausea, and food intolerance are not helpful for distinguishing the causes of dyspepsia. Patients older than 45 years or with alarm symptoms (i.e., weight loss, dysphagia, persistent vomiting, gastrointestinal bleeding, hematemesis, melena) are more likely to have serious underlying disorder. With the possible exceptions of peptic ulcer disease and duodenitis, there is no association of clinical value between endoscopic findings and dyspeptic symptoms. It is important to inquire about the use of nonsteroidal antiinflammatory drugs (NSAIDs), as their use is a frequent cause of peptic ulcer disease. To summarize, symptoms are not useful for differentiating the causes of dyspepsia.

General Approach

Individuals with evidence of complications of PUD (e.g., gastric outlet obstruction or bleeding) or systemic disease (e.g., weight loss, anemia) should be promptly evaluated. Because age is the strongest predictor of finding "organic" disease on endoscopy, individuals over the age of 45 years should be thoroughly evaluated. For the remaining patients there are three commonly used strategies for the evaluation and management of dyspeptic symptoms: (1) empiric therapy; (2) evaluation, usually with endoscopy, for a specific cause of the dyspeptic symptoms; and (3) test for *Helicobacter pylori* and treat if positive (test and treat).

Empiric treatment for dyspepsia consists of standard antiacid therapy (Table 14.1). Histamine-2 receptor antagonists (H_2RA) are available over-the-counter. If an H_2RA or proton pump inhibitor (PPI) fails to relieve symptoms, further workup should be undertaken. A recent review showed that PPIs, while more costly, are more effective than other anti-acid agents in relieving symptoms.[1]

The second approach to the patient with dyspepsia is thorough evaluation for a specific cause of the dyspeptic symptoms. When available, upper endoscopy

TABLE 14.1. Usual Daily Dosage of Antiacid Medications

Generic (brand) name	Usual daily dosage	Average wholesale price (AWP)[a] ($)[b]
Antacids (Maalox, Mylanta)	15–30 mL 0.5 hour and 2 hours after meals and at bedtime	30–60
Histamine-2 receptor antagonists		
Cimetidine (Tagamet)	800 mg hs	62
Famotidine (Pepcid)	20 mg bid	104
Nizatidine (Axid)	150 mg bid	94
Ranitidine (Zantac)	150 mg bid	89
Sucralfate	1 qid	88
Proton pump inhibitors		
Omeprazole (Prilosec)	20–40 mg qd	125–178
Lansoprazole (Prevacid)	15–30 mg qd	114–116
Rabeprazole (Aciphex)	20 mg qd	114
Esomeprazole (Nexium)	20–40 mg qd	120
Pantoprazole (Protonix)	40 mg qd	90

[a]Source for AWP: Red Book. Montvale, NJ: Medical Economics Company, Inc. Accessed Internet version at *http://physician.pdr.net/physician/static.htm?path=controlled/searchredbook.htm* on July 11, 2001. Where multiple generic equivalents are available, the least expensive AWP is listed.
[b]Amount rounded to the nearest dollar.

is the preferred procedure. Although an upper gastrointestinal (UGI) series is less expensive and may be more readily available, it has a false-negative rate that exceeds 18% in some studies and a false-positive rate of 13% to 35%. In addition, the UGI series is poor for diagnosing GERD and gastritis, two of the most common causes of dyspepsia. A negative UGI does not rule out disease, and if indicated, further evaluation with upper endoscopy should be pursued. Although more expensive, upper endoscopy has lower false-positive and false-negative rates, biopsies can be undertaken, and testing for *H. pylori* can be performed.

The third common approach to the evaluation of patients with dyspepsia is to test for *H. pylori* and treat if positive. (For further information on the evaluation and treatment of *H. pylori*, on Peptic Ulcer Disease, below.) This approach is favored by recently published American and Canadian guidelines.[2,3] Several decision analyses also support this approach.[4,5] And finally, several reviews[6,7] and clinical trials also favor the test-and-treat approach for the patient with dyspepsia.[8–11]

The eradication of *H. pylori* in patients with NUD (with negative endoscopy) is controversial. A meta-analysis by Moayyedi et al[12] showed a small but statistically significant benefit to eradication, while a more recent meta-analysis by Laine et al[13] showed no benefit.

Gastroesophageal Reflux Disease

Gastroesophageal reflux disease (GERD) is a common problem. About 10% of the general population report heartburn daily and 15% to 40% experience it monthly. Lifetime estimates of GERD symptoms in the general population may be greater than 50%.[14] The incidence of GERD increases during pregnancy and with obesity and tobacco use. Several factors may lead to GERD including hiatal hernia, incompetence of the lower esophageal sphincter (LES), inappropriate LES relaxation, impaired esophageal peristalsis and acid clearance, impaired gastric emptying, and repeated vomiting. Exposure to excessive acid or pepsin can lead to damage of the esophageal mucosa, resulting in inflammation and ultimately scarring and stricture formation. Medications (e.g., theophylline, calcium channel blockers, and β-adrenergic agonists), foods (e.g., caffeine and chocolate), and alcohol may lower LES pressure and lead to GERD. Medications such as alendronate (Fosamax) may cause local irritation of the esophagus. GERD may occur as an isolated entity or as part of a systemic disorder such as scleroderma. GERD is a risk factor for esophageal adenocarcinoma, one of the fastest growing cancers in the United States.

Presentation

The most reliable symptom of GERD is heartburn, a retrosternal burning sensation that may radiate from the epigastrium to the throat. Patients may also complain of pyrosis or water brash, the regurgitation of bitter-tasting material into the mouth. Belching is frequently described. Symptoms may be worse after eating, bending over, or lying down. Nocturnal symptoms may awaken the patient. GERD can cause respiratory problems including laryngitis, chronic cough, aspiration pneumonia, and wheezing. Atypical chest pain can also be caused by GERD (see Chapter 12). Finally, patients may complain of hoarseness, a globus sensation, odynophagia (pain with swallowing), or dysphagia.

Diagnosis

A young patient with no evidence of systemic illness requires no further workup and can be treated empirically. Older patients, particularly those with the complaint of odynophagia or dysphagia, require evaluation to rule out tumor or stricture. Upper endoscopy is the evaluation of choice. Ambulatory 24-hour pH monitoring is the most sensitive test for demonstrating reflux if endoscopy is negative. A barium swallow study or esophageal manometry may be necessary if a motility disorder is suspected, as endoscopy is often normal in patients with this problem.

Management

GERD is treated by both nonpharmacologic and pharmacologic means.[15,16] It is important to note that whereas patients with mild disease may respond to nonpharmacologic treatment, patients with moderate to severe symptoms or recurrent disease must continue to observe lifestyle changes while drug therapy is added or intensified.

All patients with GERD should be advised to reduce weight (if over their ideal body weight), avoid large meals (especially several hours before going to sleep), refrain from lying down after meals, and refrain from wearing tight clothing around the waist. Patients who experience nocturnal symptoms often find relief by putting the head of the bed on blocks 4 to 6 inches in height. Sleeping on more pillows or on a wedge may be less effective because of nocturnal movements. Because nicotine lowers LES pressure, smoking cessation is recommended. Medications and foods that can lower LES pressure as well as alcohol should be avoided.

Patients who do not respond to lifestyle and medication changes alone are treated with pharmacologic agents. The pharmacologic treatment of GERD can be approached as a stepwise process. For mild, intermittent symptoms, antacids or over-the-counter H_2RAs can be used. For persistent or severe symptoms, prescription-strength H_2RAs or PPIs are the mainstay of treatment, although other agents are available. H_2RAs can be tried first and, if ineffective, PPIs can be substituted. Once a patient's symptoms are controlled, a trial of decreasing the dose of medication (e.g., from twice daily to once daily) or switching from the more expensive PPIs to less expensive H_2RAs may be warranted.

H_2RAs suppress acid secretion by competing with histamine, thereby blocking its effect on parietal cells of the stomach. H_2RAs are effective, but both daytime and nocturnal acid production must be inhibited; therefore, twice-daily dosing is recommended rather than just nocturnal dosing. If symptoms are controlled for 6 to 8 weeks, just nocturnal dosing to control symptoms can be tried. For severe or refractory GERD, doubling the standard dose of H_2RAs may be effective. Combining H_2RAs with a prokinetic agent may be better than using either agent alone.

PPIs irreversibly block the final step in parietal cell acid secretion and are the most potent antisecretory agents available. In more severe GERD, PPIs are more efficacious than H_2RAs for symptom control including extraesophageal manifestations, esophageal healing, and reducing the risk of stricture formation and recurrence.[17] PPIs are less effective when taken on an as-needed basis. They are effective when dosed daily before breakfast, although some patients may require twice daily (before meals) dosing to achieve symptom control and/or esophageal healing. PPIs are the treatment of choice for erosive esophagitis. Side effects (chiefly headache and diarrhea) resulting in medication discontinuation are rare. As is true for H_2RAs, different PPIs, while having different pharmacokinetic properties at equivalent doses, are roughly comparable in terms of clinical efficacy. Patients unresponsive to one H_2RA or PPI may be responsive to another agent within the same medication class. Rarely, patients unresponsive to PPIs may respond to H_2RAs.

Prokinetic agents can increase esophageal contraction amplitude, increase LES pressure, and accelerate gastric emptying, three of the most significant motility problems in the pathogenesis of GERD. Metoclopramide, the only prokinetic drug available, is a dopamine antagonist that can cause extrapyramidal symptoms and, rarely, tardive dyskinesia. It is considered a second-line agent for GERD.

Sucralfate has also been shown to be efficacious for mild to moderate GERD. Sucralfate is a sulfated disaccharide that appears to protect against acid by local effects on the mucosa.

For the minority of patients with GERD who require maintenance medication, periodic examination, coupled with efforts to try to reduce medication, is warranted. A concern in patients with chronic GERD is Barrett's esophagus. Barrett's esophagus is metaplasia of the cells of the distal esophagus and is considered a precancerous lesion. The risk of development of adenocarcinoma of the esophagus may be as high as 2%. Unfortunately, neither aggressive medical therapy nor surgical therapy for GERD has been shown to alter the progression between Barrett's esophagus and esophageal adenocarcinoma.[18] There is uncertainty as to the efficacy and optimal frequency of endoscopic surveillance of patients with Barrett's esophagus. When dysplasia, the stage between metaplasia and adenocarcinoma, is identified, the recommended frequency of surveillance with esophagogastroduodenoscopy (EGD) and repeat biopsy varies, depending on the severity of dysplasia.

Individuals who are intolerant or unresponsive to optimal medical therapy are suitable operative candidates. Other indications for surgery are young age, nonadherence to medical therapy, or complications of GERD, such as recurrent esophageal strictures or bleeding. Surgical approaches to GERD attempt to create a more functional LES, limiting the potential for pathologic reflux of gastric contents. Although a VA Cooperative Trial comparing medical to surgical therapy reported improved results for the surgical cohort, a 10-year follow-up to this study showed no difference between the groups in terms of patient satisfaction, symptoms, and complications, including cancer.[19] Of note, 62% of the surgery group reported regular use of antireflux medications. Laparoscopic procedures provide effective treatment without the morbidity of open procedures. A case series of patients treated with laparoscopic surgery reported rare postoperative medication use.[20]

Peptic Ulcer Disease

Most peptic ulcers are caused by either *H. pylori* or NSAIDs. Although infection with *H. pylori* appears to be common, most individuals with *H. pylori* do not develop ulcers. Peptic ulcers may involve any portion of the UGI tract, but ulcers are most often found in the stomach and duodenum. Duodenal ulcers are approximately three times as common as gastric ulcers. About 10% of the population suffers from duodenal ulcers at some time in their lives. In the past, PUD was marked by periods of healing and recurrence. Successful treatment of ulcers associated with *H. pylori* infection greatly diminishes recurrences.

Presentation

Epigastric pain is the most common presenting problem of both duodenal and gastric ulcer disease. The pain may be described as gnawing, burning, boring, aching, or severe hunger pains. Patients with duodenal ulcers typically experience pain within a few hours after meals and complete or partial relief of pain with ingestion of food or antacids. Pain in gastric ulcer patients is more variable; pain may worsen with eating. Both duodenal and gastric ulcers may occur and recur in the absence of pain. Pain is variable among patients with both kinds of ulceration and correlates poorly with ulcer healing. Physical examination usually reveals epigastric tenderness midway between the xiphoid and umbilicus, but maximal tenderness is sometimes to the right of midline. Other findings may include a succussion splash due to a mixture of air and fluid in the stomach when gastric outlet obstruction results from an ulcer in the duodenum or pyloric channel or abdominal rigidity is apparent in the presence of perforation.

Diagnosis

There are two ways that PUD may be diagnosed. First, an ulcer may be diagnosed by either radiographic studies or endoscopy. Although duodenal and gastric ulcers can be diagnosed by UGI studies, when available, upper endoscopy is the investigation of first choice. Gastric ulcers more than 3 cm in diameter or without radiating mucosal folds are more likely to be malignant. In addition to the indications listed earlier in the chapter, endoscopy should be considered in patients with negative radiographic studies, those with a history of deformed duodenal bulbs (thus making radiographic examination difficult), and in patients with GI bleeding. If an ulcer is diagnosed endoscopically, a rapid *Campylobacter*-like organism urease test (CLOtest) is a quick, sensitive test for determining the presence of *H. pylori*. False positives are uncommon, and false negatives occur in approximately 10% of cases. The presence of *H. pylori* can also be determined histologically and by culture. Culture with drug sensitivities is important when drug resistance is suspected.

In the second approach, test and treat, a patient is tested for *H. pylori* and if positive, antibiotic therapy can be initiated without documenting an ulcer. There are several ways that *H. pylori* infection can be documented. Both qualitative (sensitivity 71%, specificity 88%) and quantitative [enzyme-linked immunosorbent assay (ELISA): sensitivity 85%, specificity 79%] serology tests are available. The stool antigen test is more accurate than serology tests (sensitivity 92%, specificity 88%). Urea breath test, using a carbon isotope (^{13}C or ^{14}C), is the most accurate noninvasive test (sensitivity 95%, specificity 96%).[21] The use of proton pump inhibitors, bismuth preparations, and antibiotics can suppress *H. pylori* and lead to false-negative results.

Most patients, especially those who are asymptomatic posttreatment, do not require documentation of eradication of *H. pylori*. If one wishes to test for cure, a urea breath test (4 weeks after therapy) or stool antigen test can be performed. A falling ELISA titer (1, 3, and 6 months after therapy) may also be used to document eradication. If a repeat endoscopy is performed, a CLOtest may be used.

Treatment

All patients with PUD who smoke should be advised to stop. Smoking can delay the rate of healing of ulcers. If PUD is associated with the use of an NSAID, the NSAID should be discontinued and traditional antiulcer therapy begun with either an H_2RA or PPI. If the NSAID cannot be stopped, then a PPI or misoprostol should be started. For patients who test positive for *H. pylori*, antibiotic treatment should be given. A number of drug regimens have been shown to be effective (Table 14.2).[22] If not part of the antibiotic regimen, a H_2RA or PPI should be added to hasten pain relief. Patients with *H. pylori*–negative ulcers are treated with traditional antiacid agents alone for 4 to 6 weeks. There is no evidence that the use of two or more antiacid agents (e.g., sucralfate and an H_2RA) offers any advantage over the use of a single antiacid agent.

There are a number of problems with the current antibiotic regimens. First, compliance may be a problem because of cost, duration of therapy, and side effects. GI side effects can occur with metronidazole, amoxicillin, and clarithromycin. There is a trade-off between better compliance with the shorter duration of therapy and better eradication rate with longer duration of therapy. A

TABLE 14.2. Treatment for Eradication of *Helicobacter pylori*-Associated Peptic Ulcer Disease[a22]

Therapies with proton pump inhibitor (PPI)[b]
PPI + metronidazole 250 mg qid + clarithromycin 500 mg bid–tid
PPI + amoxicillin 1000 mg bid or 500 mg qid + clarithromycin 500 mg bid–tid[c]
PPI + bismuth subsalicylate 2 tablets qid + metronidazole 250 mg qid + tetracycline hydrochloride 500 mg qid
Other
Bismuth subsalicylate 2 tablets qid + metronidazole 250 mg qid + tetracycline hydrochloride 500 mg qid[d]

[a]All regimens are given for 14 days.
[b]Continue PPI for total of 28 days
[c]Lansoprazole/clarithromycin/amoxicillin available as Prevpac.
[d]Available as Helidac; in addition, give H_2-receptor blocker for 28 days.

second problem is the emergence of antibiotic resistance against both metronidazole and clarithromycin, which favors the use of triple-drug regimens.

All H_2RAs effectively heal ulcers in equipotent doses (Table 14.1). About 75% to 90% of ulcers are healed after 4 to 6 weeks of therapy. The PPIs heal ulcers more quickly than H_2RAs, but healing rates at 6 weeks are not significantly improved over those with H_2RAs. PPIs should be considered for patients with severe symptoms, gastric ulcers, a potential for complications, or with refractory disease. Healing rates with sucralfate (Carafate) are comparable to those with H_2RAs. There are no significant side effects.

Prostaglandins protect the gastric mucosa, possibly by enhancing mucosal blood flow. Misoprostol, a prostaglandin E_1 analogue, can be used to prevent ulcers due to NSAIDs. Misoprostol also heals ulcers at approximately the same rate as H_2RAs, but severe diarrhea may limit patient compliance. Stimulation of uterine contractions and induction of abortions are the most serious side effects of misoprostol.

Dietary therapy is now limited to the elimination of foods that exacerbate symptoms and the avoidance of alcohol and coffee (with or without caffeine) because alcohol and coffee increase gastric acid secretion.

Refractory Ulcers and Maintenance Therapy

Most duodenal ulcers heal within 4 to 8 weeks of the start of therapy. After 12 weeks of therapy, 90% to 95% of ulcers are healed. Higher doses of H_2RAs (e.g., ranitidine 600–1200 mg/day) or PPIs may be used to heal refractory ulcers. Gastric ulcers heal more slowly than duodenal ulcers, but 90% are healed after 12 weeks of therapy. PPIs are the drug of choice for gastric ulcers.

Individuals with persistent or recurrent symptoms after therapy should be reevaluated. Compliance with previous recommendations and a search for NSAID use should be reviewed. Endoscopy should be performed to document healing. Drug resistance may be a factor in persistence of ulcers secondary to *H. pylori*. Gastric cancer should be excluded by biopsy if a gastric ulcer remains unhealed (see Gastric Cancer, below). Zollinger-Ellison syndrome is also considered in the case of refractory ulcers.

In patients successfully treated for *H. pylori* or who have discontinued the use of NSAIDs, maintenance treatment with H_2RAs or PPIs should not be needed. Patients with ulcers in the absence of *H. pylori*, complicated PUD (e.g., bleeding or perforation), a history of refractory ulceration, age greater than 60 years, or a deformed duodenum are candidates for at least 1 year of maintenance therapy with H_2RAs or PPIs.

Gastritis/Gastropathy

Gastritis represents a group of entities characterized by histologic evidence of inflammation. Gastropathy is characterized by the absence of histologic evidence of inflammation of the gastric mucosa. Both gastritis and gastropathy may be either acute or chronic. It may be difficult to distinguish the two entities by clinical, radiographic, and visual endoscopic examinations. Gastritis and gastropathy may occur simultaneously and/or overlap with conditions such as GERD or PUD, or may be a manifestation of less common conditions such as Crohn's or celiac disease or sarcoidosis.

Acute gastritis may be due to infections (mainly *H. pylori*; less commonly viral, fungal, mycobacterial, or parasitic causes), autoimmune conditions (e.g., pernicious anemia), and chronic acid suppression. Histologic variants of uncertain cause include lymphocytic and eosinophilic gastritis. Gastropathy is commonly due to medications [e.g., NSAIDs including aspirin and cyclooxygenase-2 (COX-2) inhibitors, bisphosphonates, potassium, and iron], alcohol, refluxed bile, ischemia, "stress" (as is seen in patients with shock, sepsis, trauma, or burns), or vascular congestion (as in portal hypertension or congestive heart failure).

Chronic gastritis may be preceded by episodes of symptomatic acute gastritis (e.g. *H. pylori*) or present without prior warning, with dyspepsia and constitutional symptoms. *H. pylori* is the most common cause of chronic gastritis, this effect may be accentuated in patients receiving chronic PPI therapy. Pernicious anemia may be associated with chronic gastritis.

Taken together these conditions range in presentation from asymptomatic to life threatening. Of particular interest to the clinician are acute and chronic erosive changes that may be complicated by symptomatic anemia or frank hemorrhage (presenting with melena or hematemesis—see Upper Gastrointestinal Bleed, below) and chronic atrophic changes that may progress to gastric cancer. Treatment consists of managing the underlying disease and removing gastric irritants.

Upper Gastrointestinal Bleed

Upper gastrointestinal bleed is defined as GI blood loss above the ligament of Treitz. If the bleeding is clinically evident, it may present in one of three ways.

Hematemesis may be bright red or coffee-grounds–appearing material and usually means active bleeding. Melena signifies that the blood has transited through the GI tract, causing digestion of blood. Melena may also be caused by lower GI bleeding. And finally, although uncommon, an UGI bleed may present as hematochezia if bleeding is brisk. If subacute or chronic, the UGI bleed may be discovered during the workup of iron-deficiency anemia or Hemoccult—positive stools.

Causes

The four most common causes of UGI bleeding are peptic ulceration, gastritis/gastropathy, esophageal varices, and esophagogastric mucosal tear (Mallory-Weiss syndrome). The causes of gastritis/gastropathy are described above. Bleeding due to varices is usually abrupt and massive. Varices may be due to alcohol cirrhosis or any other cause of portal hypertension such as portal vein thrombosis. Mallory-Weiss syndrome classically presents with retching followed by hematemesis. Other causes of UGI bleeding include gastric carcinoma, lymphoma, polyps, and diverticula.

Diagnosis and Management

The diagnosis and management of the patient with UGI bleeding depends on the site and extent of bleeding. Vomitus and stool should be tested to confirm the presence of blood. Initial management for all patients includes assessment of vital signs including orthostatic changes. Patients with significant blood loss should be typed and matched for blood replacement and large-bore intravenous lines placed for fluid and blood replacement.

A nasogastric tube should be placed and the aspirate tested for blood. Absence of blood may mean that the bleeding has ceased. If the aspirate consists of red blood or coffee-grounds material, the stomach is lavaged with saline.

Once the patient is hemodynamically stable, upper endoscopy can be performed. Rapid upper endoscopy upon presentation of patients in stable condition may hasten diagnosis and limit hospitalization.[23] Endoscopy may not reveal an obvious source of bleeding in cases of resolved blood loss due to Mallory-Weiss tears or vascular malformations, or distal duodenal lesions. Massive hemorrhage from varices can make endoscopy useless. The other more common causes will be readily apparent. If the patient continues to bleed and a source has not been identified, a tagged red blood cell scan or angiography may be used to identify the source of bleeding. Upper endoscopy can be therapeutic as well as diagnostic. Sclerotherapy or ligation of esophageal varices can be performed through the endoscope. A variety of endoscopic treatments are available for bleeding peptic ulcers including thermal coagulation, injection therapy with alcohol or epinephrine, and endoclips.

When bleeding is refractory to medical and endoscopically administered therapies, interventional radiological (e.g., embolization or transjugular intrahepatic portasystemic shunt, TIPS) or surgical (resection or shunting) interventions should be considered.

There are two additional therapies for bleeding varices. Peripherally administered somatostatin or balloon tamponade are effective alternative treatments for bleeding varices.

Prevention of GI bleeding is more effective than treatment. Treatment of *H. pylori*–positive PUD or maintenance therapy for *H. pylori*–negative PUD may decrease subsequent bleeding episodes. Nonselective beta-blockers (propranolol or nadolol) can prevent and reduce the mortality rate associated with GI bleeding in patients with cirrhosis and varices.

Gastric Cancer

While the incidence of distal gastric cancer has declined significantly in the United States since the 1930s, there has been an increase of proximal stomach cancers. African-American males have a higher incidence of gastric adenocarcinoma. Individuals moving from Japan to the United States lower their risk of gastric cancer, suggesting that dietary and environmental factors play roles in the pathogenesis of this disorder. Additional risk factors include gastric polyps, Barrett's esophagus, subtotal gastric resection, and chronic gastritis. Ninety percent of the gastric cancers are adenocarcinomas; lymphomas (the stomach is the most common extranodal site of lymphoma) and leiomyosarcomas comprise the remainder.

Early gastric cancers are usually asymptomatic. As the cancer grows, patients may complain of anorexia or early satiety, vague discomfort, or steady pain. Weight loss, nausea and vomiting, and dysphagia (more common with proximal cancers) may also be present. Rarely, paraneoplastic manifestations occur. The physical examination is usually normal in patients with early disease, but a palpable abdominal mass or supraclavicular nodes, enlarged liver, or ascites may be present with advanced or metastatic disease. Patients with gastric cancer may present with GI bleeding, overt or otherwise occult, although this represents a minority of presentations.

Upper gastrointestinal (UGI) x-ray studies can usually detect gastric cancer. In younger patients (<45 years) without alarming symptoms, UGI is adequate to diagnose a benign gastric ulcer. These patients should be followed radiographically to ensure healing of the ulcer. Benign gastric ulcers should heal within 6 to 12 weeks. If an ulcer is suspicious in appearance, alarming symptoms are present, or the patient is >45 years of age, EGD with biopsy is the preferred procedure. If the initial biopsies are benign, then endoscopy should be repeated at 12 weeks to ensure that the ulcer has healed completely.

While surgical treatment is the only definite chance for a cure, unfortunately only one third of patients present early enough to achieve a surgical cure. Despite advanced surgical treatments 5-year survival rates remain low. Postoperative (adjuvant) chemotherapy with or without radiation for patients undergoing tumor resection may be recommended.

References

1. Delaney BC, Innes MA, Deeks J, et al. Initial management strategies for dyspepsia. The Cochrane Library, Oxford, England: Updated February 23, 2000.
2. American Gastroenterological Association. American Gastroenterological Assoication medical position statement: evaluation of dyspepsia. Gastroenterology 1998; 114:579–81.
3. Hunt RH, Fallone CA, Thomson ABR, Canadian *Helicobacter Pylori* Study Group. Canadian *Helicobacter Pylori* Consensus Conference update: infection in adults. Can J Gastroenterol 1999;13:213–17.
4. Fendrick AM, Chernow ME, Hirth RA, Bloom BS. Alternative management strategies for patients with suspected peptic ulcer disease. Ann Intern Med 1995;123:260–8.
5. Ebell MH, Warbasse L, Brenner C. Evaluation of the dyspeptic patient: a cost-utility study. J Fam Pract 1997;44:545–55.
6. Smucny J. Evaluation of the patient with dyspepsia. J Fam Pract 2001;50:538–43.
7. Ofman JJ, Rabeneck L. The effectiveness of endoscopy in the management of dyspepsia: a qualitative systematic review. Am J Med 1999;106:335–46.
8. Lassen AT, Pedersen FM, Bytzer P, de Muckadell OBS. *Helicobacter pylori* test-and-eradicate versus prompt endoscopy for management of dyspeptic patients: a randomized trial. Lancet 2000;356:455–60.
9. Jones R, Tait C, Sladen G, Weston-Backer J. A trial of test-and-treat strategy for *Helicobacter pylori*-positive dyspeptic patients in general practice. Int J Clin Pract 1999;53:413–16.
10. Heaney A, Collins JSA, Watson RGP, McFarland RJ, Bamford KB, Tham TCK. A prospective randomised trial of a "test and treat" policy versus endoscopy based management in young *Helicobacter pylori* positive patients with ulcer-like dyspepsia, referred to a hospital clinic. Gut 1999;45:186–90.
11. Delaney BC, Wilson S, Roalfe A, et al. Randomised controlled trial of *Helicobacter pylori* testing and endoscopy for dyspepsia in primary care. BMJ 2001;322:1–5.
12. Moayyedi P, Soo S, Deeks J, et al, on behalf of the Dyspepsia Review Group. Systematic review and economic evaluation of *Helicobacter pylori* eradication treatment for non-ulcer dyspepsia. BMJ 2000;321:659–64.
13. Laine L, Schoenfeld P, Fennerty MB. Therapy for *Helicobacter pylori* in patients with nonulcer dyspepsia: a meta-analysis of randomized, controlled trials. Ann Intern Med 2001;134:361–9.
14. Locke GR 3rd, Talley NJ, Fett SL, Zinsmeister AR, Melton LJ 3rd. Prevalence and clinical spectrum of gastroesophageal reflux; a population-based study in Olinsted County, Minnesota. Gastroenterology 1997;112:1448–56.
15. DeVault KR, Castell DO. Updated guidelines for the diagnosis and treatment of gastroesophageal reflux disease. The Practice Parameters Committee of the American College of Gastroenterology. Am J Gastroenterol 1999;94:1434–42.
16. Scott M, Gelhot AR. Gastroesophageal reflux disease: diagnosis and management. Am Fam Physician 1999;59:1161–9.
17. Chiba N, DeGara CJ, Wilkinson JM, Hunt RH. Speed of healing and symptoms of

relief in grade II to IV gastroesophageal reflux disease: a meta-analysis. Gastroen-terology 1997;112:1798–810.

18. Kahrilas PJ. Management of GERD: medical versus surgical. Semin Gastrointest Dis 2001;12:3–15.

19. Spechler SJ, Lee E, Ahnen D, et al. Long-term outcome of medical and surgical ther-apies for gastroesophageal reflux disease: follow-up of a randomized controlled trial. JAMA 2001;285:2331–8.

20. Peters JH, DeMeester TR, Crookes P, et al. The treatment of gastroesophageal reflux disease with laparoscopic Nissen fundoplication: prospective evaluation of 100 pa-tients with "typical" symptoms. Ann Surg 1998;228:40–50.

21. Vairea D, Vakil N. Blood, urine, stool, breath, money, and *Helicobacter pylori*. Gut 2001;48:287–9.

22. Howden CW, Hunt RH. Guidelines for the management of *Helicobacter pylori* in-fection. Am J Gastroenterol 1998;93:2330–8.

23. Lee JG, Turnipseed S, Romano PS, et al. Endoscopy-based triage significantly re-duces hospitalization rates and costs of treating upper GI bleeding: a randomized con-trolled trial. Gastrointest Endosc 1999;50:755–61.

Case Presentation

Subjective

Patient Profile

Ralph Martino is a 45-year-old divorced male attorney.

Presenting Problem

"Heartburn."

Present Illness

For the past 6 weeks, Mr. Martino has had a recurrent burning sensation in the upper abdomen, worse after meals, especially if the food is spicy or "acid." Antacids and milk afford some relief. There has been no nausea, vomiting, constipation, or diarrhea. He notes occasional upper abdominal pain that seems different from the "heartburn." Similar heartburn has occurred several times in the past, especially at the time of his divorce 10 years ago.

Past Medical History

The patient had hepatitis and a fractured femur as a teenager.

Social History

He is divorced and lives alone with two dogs. He is a partner in a law firm and specializes in labor relations.

Habits

He smokes one pack of cigarettes daily and takes one to two drinks of vodka each evening. He uses six to eight cups of coffee daily but takes no recreational drugs.

Family History

His father died at age 66 of colon cancer. His mother, aged 78, has had gallbladder surgery. One sister, aged 47, has Crohn's disease.

REVIEW OF SYSTEMS

He has a long history of recurrent headache and low back pain.

- What additional information regarding the medical history would you like to know? Why?
- What might the patient be trying to tell you?
- What questions might you ask to learn more about current stressors in his life?
- What is likely to be the patient's adaptation to his illness? Why might this be pertinent?

Objective

VITAL SIGNS

Height, 5 ft 11 in; weight 186 lb; blood pressure, 138/90; pulse, 70; respirations, 18.

EXAMINATION

The patient appears tense and "worried." The chest is clear to percussion and auscultation. The heart has a regular sinus rhythm, and no murmurs are heard. The abdomen is scaphoid, and active bowel sounds are present. There is mild epigastric tenderness, but no mass is found. On rectal examination, the prostate is normal and no rectal mass is palpable. There is a positive test for occult blood in the feces.

- What more data—if any—might be derived from the physical examination? Explain.
- Are there specific diagnostic maneuvers that might be helpful today?
- What—if any—laboratory studies might be useful in making the diagnosis?
- What—if any—diagnostic imaging or endoscopy would you recommend today? Why?

Assessment

- What is your diagnostic assessment at this time? How would you explain this to Mr. Martino?
- What is likely to be the meaning of this illness to Mr. Martino? Explain.
- What is the significance of the positive test for occult blood in feces?

- What are the possible contributions of alcohol and tobacco use to his current illness?

Plan

- Pending the results of further tests, what therapeutic recommendations would you make to Mr. Martino regarding diet, life style, and medication?
- Is consultation likely to be necessary? Under what circumstances? Explain.
- If the patient calls tonight describing the passage of large quantities of dark red blood from the rectum, what would be your concern? What would you do?
- What follow-up would you recommend for this patient?

15
Urinary Tract Infections

BOYD L. BAILEY, JR.

Urinary tract infection (UTI) is a cause of significant discomfort, acute and long-term morbidity, and loss of productivity, resulting in over 7 million office visits with an estimated 1 million episodes annually of UTI-related illness requiring hospitalizations.[1] Among children, 1 in 20 girls and 1 in 50 boys have a UTI each year.[2]

Four major risk groups[3] for community-acquired UTIs have been identified: school-age girls, young women in their sexually active years (including pregnancy), males with prostate obstruction, and the elderly. This chapter discusses important clinical issues in the following categories: UTI in children, UTI in pregnancy, acute uncomplicated lower UTI in young women, recurrent infection in women, acute uncomplicated pyelonephritis in young women, complicated UTIs, UTIs in young men, catheter-associated UTIs, asymptomatic bacteriuria without a catheter, chronic UTI in the elderly, UTIs with spinal cord injuries, and fungal UTIs. The primary aim of UTI diagnosis and management is the prevention of long-term complications of progressive events that affect later-life morbidity or mortality.

UTIs in Children

For boys and girls the incidence of symptomatic infection during the first 6 months of life is similar, but after 6 months to a year it falls off rapidly for boys. Among girls, the first-year incidence is more evenly distributed through the year. During the first 3 months, boys are infected more often, presumably related to the uncircumcised susceptibility.[2] In neonates the prevalence is threefold higher among premature infants.[4] For girls the incidence steadily rises with a small transient increase at preschool time and then remains level until sexual activity becomes a factor. Asymptomatic bacteriuria is absent in boys until later in adult life when obstructive problems occur. In girls asymptomatic bacteriuria is present early in infancy and remains fairly constant until the late teens.[1]

The primary host-related factors that lead to the development of UTI include infancy, female sex, abnormal defense mechanisms, the presence of urinary tract abnormalities, sexual activity, and instrumentation.[4] In children without urinary tract abnormalities, periurethral bacterial colonization, for unclear reasons, is a risk factor for UTI.[5] Voiding dysfunction (urgency, frequency, dysuria, hesitancy, dribbling of urine, and overt incontinence) can be recognized with an eye toward modification.[6]

Escherichia coli accounts for as much as 80% of cases of UTI.[2,4] In neonates and complicated cases, *Proteus mirabilis* (mainly in boys), *Klebsiella pneumoniae*, *Pseudomonas aeruginosa*, Enterobacter species, *Staphylococcus aureus* (mainly in older children), *Streptococcus viridans*, enterococci, and *Candida albicans* are to be considered.[4]

Diagnosis

URINALYSIS AND CULTURE

In any febrile infant or child the differential diagnosis should include UTI. Screening by urinalysis for pyuria and bacteriuria is not adequately sensitive to allow UTI to be ruled out without a culture.[4,7] In a properly collected specimen (urethral catheterization or suprapubic aspiration in infants), a presumptive diagnosis can be made with the presence of any bacteria and five leukocytes per high-power field (hpf).[8]

IMAGING EVALUATION

Imaging tests should be conducted after the first episode of UTI in girls younger than 5 years, boys of any age, older sexually inactive girls with recurrent UTI, and any child with pyelonephritis.[8] Debate continues about the best radiologic approach for evaluating of UTI.[7,9] The issue centers around the role of radionuclide scans, and how these methods may replace or be used in conjunction with traditional ultrasonography (US), voiding cystourethrography (VCUG), intravenous pyelography (IVP), and spiral computer-assisted tomography (CT).

Radionuclide cystography, a method using scintigraphic imaging, gives accurate information similar to that of contrast based VCUG, with the possible advantage of significantly less radiation exposure.[10] The scintigraphic study using 99m-technetium dimercaptosuccinic acid (DMSA) has become a leading choice for gauging renal function and identifying renal cortical defects. The DMSA scan is quickly becoming a gold standard for diagnosis of acute pyelonephritis. When applied at 6 to 12 months after cortical defects have first developed, the DMSA scan may be the best test for renal scarring. US has the obvious advantage of being a noninvasive test that is strong at ruling out obstruction. IVP gives comprehensive structural information, and is very good for detecting kidney stones, but transient swelling during infection weakens the predictive capability of the test. The spiral CT is becoming the first choice for the presence of obstructive stone disease. VCUG gives comprehensive lower tract information and allows grading the severity of reflux.[7]

An imaging strategy can be summarized this way. Use renal/bladder US to look for obstruction; use a DMSA scan to identify cortical defects and assess differential function; use a VCUG to detect bladder anomalies, neurogenic defects, residual urine, and urethral abnormalities such as posterior valves, urethral strictures, and the presence of vesicoureteral reflux; and use spiral CT to determine the presence of stones.[7]

Management

Early diagnosis and prompt treatment of UTI in infants and young children are crucial. With vesicoureteral reflux, or other urinary tract abnormalities, immediate treatment reduces the risk of renal scarring. In the history, inquire about the defecation pattern and preceding use of antibiotics such as amoxicillin or a cephalosporin. Physical examination should include a rectal examination to detect a large fecal reservoir.[6]

Symptomatic neonates should be treated for 7 to 10 days with a parenteral combination of ampicillin and gentamicin. Young infants with UTI, children with clinical evidence of acute pyelonephritis, and children with upper tract infection associated with urologic abnormalities or surgical procedures can be treated with a combination of an aminoglycoside and ampicillin, or an aminoglycoside and a cephalosporin.[4] Duration of therapy remains unsettled. For complicated infection, 7 to 14 days has been arbitrarily recommended; for uncomplicated infection, 3 to 5 days has shown adequacy.[7]

For uncomplicated UTI, oral agents may include amoxicillin, ampicillin, sulfisoxazole acetyl, trimethoprim-sulfamethoxazole, nitrofurantoin, or cephalosporins for a duration of 5 to 10 days.[7] Antibiotic treatment of asymptomatic bacteriuria in children is controversial based on certain issues: there is limited evidence that renal damage is prevented or loss of function reduced; replacement of a low-virulence organism with a more virulent one may occur; and the child may experience unknown long-term side effects of antibiotics.[4] A reasonable approach with asymptomatic bacteriuria is to treat children younger than 5 years or those who have urinary tract structural abnormalities.

UTIs During Pregnancy

Pregnant women with UTIs are at greater risk of delivering infants with low birth weight, premature infants, preterm infants with low birth weight, and infants small for gestational age. In addition, the likelihood is greater for premature labor, hypertension/preeclampsia, anemia, and amnionitis. There is strong evidence that UTI causes low birth weight through premature delivery rather than growth retardation.[11]

The risk of pyelonephritis from antepartum bacteriuria may be as high as 30%. Identification and eradication reduces this risk to less than 5%. Antepartum bacteriuria has an estimated prevalence of 2% to 12%, with an increasing relation to age, parity, and lower socioeconomic status.[12]

An optimal time for screening all pregnancies has been suggested to be around 16 weeks (see Chapter 3). Although often the first prenatal visit is before 16 weeks, a practical approach to screening is to obtain a culture at this first visit. If negative, no further cultures are necessary unless there is a history of prior UTI, or the patient becomes symptomatic. If the screening culture result is 10^5 colony-forming units (CFU)/mL or higher, the test should be repeated to improve on the specificity of a single culture. If the repeat culture is positive, treatment for asymptomatic bacteriuria follows.[12]

As in nonpregnant females, *E. coli* is the most common cause of UTI during pregnancy, accounting for more than 80% of isolates. Other organisms include *Enterobacter* species, *Klebsiella* species, *Proteus* species, enterococci, and *Staphylococcus saprophyticus*.

The first concern regarding treatment during pregnancy is the safety of antibiotics. Considered reasonably safe are penicillins, cephalosporins, and methenamine. Cautious use can be considered with sulfonamides [allergic reaction, kernicterus, glucose-6-phosphate dehydrogenase (G6PD) deficiency], aminoglycosides (eighth nerve and renal toxicity), nitrofurantoin (neuropathy, G6PD deficiency), clindamycin (allergic reaction, pseudomembranous colitis), and erythromycin estolate (cholestatic hepatitis).[12,13]

For asymptomatic bacteriuria, a regimen of 3 to 7 days is used with antibiotics chosen with safety in mind. There is little support for single-dose therapy, although for a pregnant female with a history of recurrent UTIs, or who develops a UTI early in pregnancy, a single postcoital prophylactic dose may be considered. Appropriate postcoital single oral doses are either cephalexin 250 mg or nitrofurantoin 50 mg.[14] Pyelonephritis is managed the same as with nonpregnant females.[12]

Acute Uncomplicated Lower UTI In Young Women

The risk for UTI is increased by sexual intercourse, delayed postcoital voiding (although controversial[15]), diaphragm and spermicidal gel, and a history of recurrent UTIs.[16] One of three types of infection can account for these infections: acute cystitis, acute urethritis, or vaginitis.[17]

Cystitis pathogens include *E. coli*, *S. saprophyticus*, *Proteus* species, or *Klebsiella* species. Symptoms are abrupt in onset, severe, and usually multiple; they include dysuria, increased frequency, and urgency. Suprapubic pain and tenderness and sometimes low back pain also occur. Pyuria is usually present and occasionally hematuria.

Urethritis pathogens include *Chlamydia trachomatis*, *N. gonorrhoeae*, and herpes simplex virus. Symptoms are more likely to be gradual in onset and mild (including dysuria and possibly vaginal discharge and bleeding from a concomitant cervicitis), and include lower abdominal pain. Suspicion is raised if the patient has a new sexual partner or evidence of cervicitis on examination. Pyuria is usually present.

Vaginitis pathogens include *Candida* species and *Trichomonas vaginalis*. Symptoms include vaginal discharge or odor, pruritus, dyspareunia, and external dysuria without increased frequency or urgency. Pyuria and hematuria are rarely present (see Chapter 16).

With no complicating clinical factors, reasonable empiric treatment for presumed cystitis, prior to organism identification, is a 3-day regimen of any of the following: oral trimethoprim-sulfamethoxazole (TMP-SMX), trimethoprim, norfloxacin, ciprofloxacin, ofloxacin, lomefloxacin, or enoxacin (Table 15.1). With the complicating factors of diabetes, symptoms for more than 7 days, recent UTI, use of a diaphragm, or age over 65 years, a 7-day regimen can be considered using these same antibiotics.[17]

For cystitis during pregnancy, consider a 7-day regimen that includes oral amoxicillin, macrocrystalline nitrofurantoin, cefpodoxime proxetil, or TMP-SMX. Avoid using fluoroquinolones in pregnant women, and use gentamicin cautiously because of fetal eighth nerve threat. TMP-SMX has not been approved for use during pregnancy but is widely used. Once the causative organisms have been identified, the antibiotics can be modified.[17]

Recurrent Infections (Cystitis) in Women

Recurrent cystitis can be termed relapse or reinfection. Relapse is defined as a recurrence within 2 weeks of completing therapy for the same pathogen. Reinfection is defined as a recurrence more than 2 weeks after completing therapy for a different species or strain. For relapse, efforts should be made to rule out a urologic abnormality and to treat for an extended time, such as 2 to 6 weeks. For reinfection, the following strategy is useful: If a spermicide and diaphragm are being used, changing the contraceptive method is recommended. For two or fewer incidents of UTI per year, physician- or patient-initiated therapy can be started, based on symptoms, using either single-dose or 3-day therapy. For three or more UTIs per year, the relation to coitus must be considered. If the UTI is not related to coitus, a low-dose antibiotic, daily or three times weekly, is recommended. This regimen is commonly continued for 3 to 6 months.[15,17] If the recurrent UTIs are related to coitus, a single low-dose postcoital treatment may be preferable (Table 15.1).

Usually not attributable to predisposing anatomic defects, recurrent UTIs in women most likely are related to an underlying biologic predisposition or to behavior promoting UTI.[18]

Although perineal cleansing methods are partially protective, oral antimicrobial therapy is probably most effective. It can be accomplished as chronic prophylaxis, postcoital prophylaxis, or intermittent self-administered therapy.

TABLE 15.1. Antibiotic Regimens for Adult Cystitis, Pyelonephritis, and Prophylaxis

Antibiotic	Oral (cystitis)	Oral (pyelonephritis and complicated UTIs)	Parenteral	Daily prophylaxis	Single-dose postcoital
Amoxicillin	250 mg every 8 h	500 mg every 8 h			
Ampicillin			1 g every 6 h		
Trimethoprim	100 mg every 12 h			100 mg every 24 h	
Trimethoprim-sulfamethoxazole	160 plus 800 mg every 12 h	160 plus 800 mg every 12 h	160 plus 800 mg every 12 h	40 plus 200 mg every 24 h	40 plus 200 mg
Norfloxacin	400 mg every 12 h	400 mg every 12 h		200 mg every 24 h	
Ciprofloxacin	250 mg every 12 h	500 mg every 12 h	200 to 400 mg every 12 h		
Ofloxacin	200 mg every 12 h	200 mg followed by 300 mg every 12 h			
Lomefloxacin	400 mg every day	400 mg every day			
Enoxacin	400 mg every 12 h	400 mg every 12 h			
Macrocrystalline nitrofurantoin	100 mg four times a day			100 mg every 24 h	50 to 100 mg
Cephalexin				250 mg every 24 h	250 mg
Cefpodoxime proxetil	100 mg every 12 h	200 mg every 12 h			
Cefixime	400 mg every day	400 mg every day			
Ceftriaxone			1 to 2 g every day		
Gentamicin			1 mg/kg of body weight every 8 h, or 3 to 5 mg/kg every 24 h		
Imipenem-cilastatin			250 to 500 mg every 6 to 8 h		
Ampicillin-sulbactam			1.5 g every 6 h		
Ticarcillin-clavulanate			3.2 g every 6 to 8 h		
Piperacillin-tazobactam			3.375 g every 6 to 8 h		
Aztreonam			1 g every 8 to 12 h		

Sources: Data sources include Pfau and Sacks,[14] Stamm and Hooten,[17] and Johnson.[18]

Acute Uncomplicated Pyelonephritis in Young Women

Uncomplicated pyelonephritis exhibits findings suggestive of upper tract tissue penetration and inflammation, such as fever and flank pain. Underlying factors that impede the response to natural host responses are minimized. The infecting organism should be highly susceptible to most antibiotics.

Characteristic pathogens in acute uncomplicated pyelo-nephritis in young women include *E. coli, Proteus mirabilis, K. pneumoniae,* and *S. saprophyticus.* Outpatient management is reasonable for mild to moderate illness without nausea and vomiting. A 10- to 14-day regimen of the following is appropriate: oral TMP-SMX, norfloxacin, ciprofloxacin, ofloxacin, lomefloxacin, or enoxacin (Table 15.1). For severe illness or possible urosepsis requiring hospitalization, the following regimen can be followed: parenteral TMP-SMX, ceftriaxone, ciprofloxacin, gentamicin (with or without ampicillin), or ampicillin-sulbactam until afebrile then oral TMP-SMX, norfloxacin, ciprofloxacin, ofloxacin, lomefloxacin, or enoxacin (Table 15.1) to complete a 14-day course of therapy.[17]

During pregnancy hospitalization is the optimal course with the following suggested regimen: parenteral ceftriaxone, gentamicin (with or without ampicillin), aztreonam, ampicillin-sulbactam, or TMP-SMX until afebrile, then oral amoxicillin, amoxicillin-clavulanate, a cephalosporin, or TMP-SMX to complete a 14-day course of therapy.[17]

Complicated UTIs

Clinically, a complicated UTI may present in the same way as an uncomplicated one. A complicated infection occurs in urinary tracts that have a functional, metabolic, or anatomic derangement predisposing to a more difficult infectious process including more resistant organisms.

Characteristic organisms present in complicated urinary tract infections include *E. coli, Proteus* species, *Klebsiella* species, *Pseudomonas* species, *Serratia* species, enterococci, and staphylococci. Outpatient management is reasonable for mild to moderate illness without nausea or vomiting. The best oral antibiotic course, administered for 10 to 14 days, is norfloxacin, ciprofloxacin, ofloxacin, lomefloxacin, or enoxacin. TMP-SMX, amoxicillin, or cefpodoxime proxetil could also be used. For severe illness or possible urosepsis, hospitalization is necessary with treatment by parenteral ampicillin and gentamicin, ciprofloxacin, ofloxacin, ceftriaxone, aztreonam, ticarcillin-clavulanate, piperacillin-tazobactam, or imipenem-cilastatin until afebrile, then oral TMP-SMX, norfloxacin, ciprofloxacin, ofloxacin, lomefloxacin, or enoxacin for a total of 14 to 21 days.[17]

UTIs in Younger Men

Without underlying structural urologic abnormalities, risk factors for UTIs in young men include homosexuality, lack of circumcision,[19] and a sex partner colonized with uropathogens.[17]

Management of symptomatic cystitis without obvious complicating factors requires a urine culture to establish the pathogen. This step establishes sensitivity and helps define relapse or reinfection in the event of recurrence. Once the culture is obtained, a 7-day course of TMP-SMX, trimethoprim, or a fluoroquinolone is initiated.

The traditional approach of undertaking a thorough post-UTI evaluation to rule out a urologic abnormality has been disputed.[20,21] If pursued in young men who have responded to treatment, the chance of finding a urinary tract defect is low.[18]

Catheter-Associated UTIs

Mortality from UTIs is increased threefold in hospitalized patients with an indwelling catheter. Catheterization is associated with a 5% to 10% incidence of UTI per day of catheterization. A 3-day presence of an indwelling catheter has been identified as a risk factor for UTI. Catheter-associated UTI (CAUTI) is the most common acquired infection in long-term-care facilities. Complications include catheter obstruction, fever, stones, pyelonephritis, chronic interstitial nephritis, bacteremia, renal failure, and death. In the intensive care setting, 95% of nosocomial UTIs are CAUTI.[22]

With short-term catheterization, *E. coli* is the most common organism, followed by *Pseudomonas aeruginosa, K. pneumoniae, Proteus mirabilis, Serratia marcescens, Citrobacter* spp., *Staphylococcus epidermidis*, and enterococci.[23] With long-term catheterization, significant infection may be due to the ordinarily nonuropathogenic *Providencia stuartii* or *Morganella morganii*. Yeast may become an isolated pathogen when antibiotics are in use.[22,23]

Treatment revolves around three modes of action: prevention, antimicrobials for acquired asymptomatic bacteriuria and symptomatic lower UTI, and antimicrobials for a symptomatic (complicated) upper UTI. Prevention focuses on avoiding catheterization if possible. If catheterization is mandatory, minimize the duration and use a closed drainage system. Short-term use of silver alloy catheters in hospitalized patients reduces the incidence of symptomatic UTI and bacteremia, and is likely to result in cost savings.[24] For short-term catheterization of 3 to 14 days, daily prophylactic norfloxacin, ciprofloxacin, or amoxicillin has shown benefit.[18] For acquired asymptomatic bacteriuria and symptomatic lower UTI after short-term catheter use, a single-dose of TMP-SMX (320–1600 mg) has been shown to be as effective as a 10-day course.[25]

Asymptomatic Bacteriuria in Patients Without a Catheter

With the exception of pregnancy and prior to urologic surgery, screening for asymptomatic bacteriuria has no apparent value. Even among the elderly where there may be an association between asymptomatic bacteriuria and mortality, a causal link has not been demonstrated.[17]

Chronic UTIs in the Elderly

Among males the incidence of bacteriuria essentially disappears after infancy and reappears during later adulthood as obstructive elements come into play. With aging, both symptomatic infection and asymptomatic bacteriuria occur. The incidence of UTI in both sexes steadily rises with age during the elderly years.[1] The place of residence helps predict incidence. For those over age 65, estimates of incidence are as follows: (1) at home—women 20%, men 10%; (2) in nursing homes—women 25%, men 20%. In hospitals the incidence is high for both sexes.[26] The elderly behave in a dynamic fashion, with high turnover of those with bacteriuria and those with a UTI.[26]

Many factors come into play for elderly men and women that balance the incidence of UTI: lack of estrogen in women, and prostatic secretion in men,[27] and bacterial adhesion factors in both sexes[26] (see Chapter 5).

Whereas *E. coli* and *S. saprophyticus* are the most common cause of UTI in young adults, some significant shifts in causative organism occur with the elderly. For nursing homes, *E. coli* remains the most common causative organism, and *Enterococcus* organisms have become the second most common. For the most part, *S. saprophyticus* does not occur in this setting. *E. coli* drops in frequency for women, and gram-positive organisms can dominate among men.[28] This shift to non–*E. coli* organisms can easily be attributed to an increased rate of hospitalization of the elderly.[26]

A debatable issue that has become somewhat clearer is that asymptomatic bacteriuria does not seem to influence mortality in elderly women.[29] Previous studies have pointed in both directions,[30] with some clearly showing increased functional disability even if an effect on mortality is not clear.[31]

Basically, a lower UTI presents with dysuria, urgency, and frequency. An upper UTI may present with clear signs of fever, chills, and flank pain with tenderness. In a fair percentage of cases, possibly 20%, these signs and symptoms can be absent or obscured by a presentation that might include fever, altered mental status (confusion) with variable gastrointestinal symptoms and signs (nausea and vomiting, abdominal tenderness), apathy, incontinence, and even respiratory symptoms.[26] Alternatively, not all nonspecific "mental status" changes can be attributed to a UTI, and focusing on antibiotic therapy alone is inappropriate.[27] A difficult question is whether bacteriuria is really asymptomatic in the elderly.[32]

Laboratory screening is a little more direct in men than women, but does not, unfortunately, substitute for a culture in the elderly, as it can in younger people.

The management of UTIs in the elderly was addressed in specific areas of this chapter (see Recurrent Infections (Cystitis) in Women, Complicated UTIs, and Catheter-Associated UTIs, above). In the elderly, antibiotics in general require minimal dose adjustment. Consider total body weight and renal function. Duration of treatment is similar to that in other age groups.[24] Antibiotic choices are shown in Table 15.1. Regular use of cranberry juice (300 mL/day) appears to reduce both bacteriuria and pyuria, and leads to fewer symptomatic infections and less antibiotic use.[33]

UTI in Spinal Cord Injuries

Special considerations for increased risk of UTI with spinal cord injuries include bladder overdistention, vesicoureteral reflux, high-pressure voiding, large postvoid residuals, stones in the urinary tract, and outlet obstruction.[34]

Management of infection risks focuses primarily on proper drainage of the bladder. A turning point that occurred during the 1960s was the understanding of the value of intermittent catheterization in reducing the risk of significant bacteriuria.[35] Development of bacteriuria is certain with an indwelling catheter and suprapubic catheter. Although not fully understood, bacteriuria and the incidence of symptomatic UTIs are reduced by intermittent catheterization. In addition, intermittent catheterization performed by the affected person is preferable to having it done by a caregiver.[34] There are many variations in the technique of intermittent catheterization. The critical predictor for improved outcome is intermittent catheterization rather than having an indwelling catheter.

Diagnostic signs and symptoms are poorly sensitive and specific.[34] Estimation of pyuria is generally considered the best indication of UTI.

Fungal UTIs

Fungal UTI is most commonly caused by *Candida*, and occasionally by *Cryptococcus neoformans*, *Aspergillus* species, and the endemic mycoses. Clinical clues are CAUTI, obstructed urinary tracts, especially in diabetics, and immunosuppressive therapy. Antibiotics, and none are exempt, can play a role in the emergence of candiduria upon use or immediately following.

For asymptomatic colonization with *Candida* (except following renal transplant, and in whom urologic instrumentation or surgery is planned), no specific antifungal therapy is required.

Candida cystitis is best treated with amphotericin B bladder instillation (50 μg/mL), systemic therapy (single-dose intravenous 0.3 mg/kg), or fluconazole 200 mg po for 14 days.

Ascending pyelonephritis and *Candida* urosepsis require systemic antifungal therapy with IV amphotericin B at 0.6 mg/kg/day, duration depending on severity but in general involving a total dose of 2 g. An alternative is fluconazole at 5 to 10 mg/kg/day (IV or po).[36]

Laboratory Guides and Interpretation

The organisms that cause UTIs are few in number, but there are growing pressures for more efficient and timely screening measures to determine the likelihood of a UTI. Ideal screening for a UTI would involve a highly sensitive test that confidently excludes the disease, thereby eliminating the need to proceed to more costly follow-up tests of culturing and antibiotic sensitivity. The ideal screening test would be highly specific for detecting or identifying the disease for which empiric treatment has been initiated while uropathogen identity and antimicrobial sensitivity are pending. Unfortunately, the ideal screening test does not exist.

Pyuria

From a practical standpoint, pyuria represents readily measurable evidence of host injury. The most accurate method, or gold standard, of defining significant pyuria is the leukocyte excretion rate. There is evidence that the significant rate is 400,000 white blood cells (WBC)/hour.[37] This measurement is cumbersome—hence the popularity of quicker, simpler, but less accurate screening tests. They include microscopic examination of unspun urine in a counting chamber (WBC/mm³), spun urine under a coverslip (WBC/hpf), and leukocyte esterase.[38] In general, the WBC/hpf is approximately 11% of the WBC/cubic mm³.[39] Diagnostic information related to these tests is displayed in Table 15.2.[38–46]

Bacteriuria

A UTI can be defined as the presence of significant numbers of pathogenic bacteria in appropriately collected urine.[38] Urine culture is considered the gold standard for defining significant bacteriuria. All other tests are simply screening devices chosen to balance immediate, simple results with accuracy. The most common tests are direct microscopy and the dipstick (nitrite and leukocyte esterase). Many methods have been used with variable accuracy.[45] Commonly used screening tests with approximated diagnostic information are shown in Table 15.2.

Urine Culture

It is important to realize that even though the culture is universally used as a gold standard for significant bacteriuria in UTIs against which other tests are meas-

Table 15.2. Diagnostic Information on Common Urine Screening Tests, Individually and in Various Combinations[a]

Screening test	Sensitivity	Specificity	Positive likelihood ratio	Negative likelihood ratio
Nitrite (present or absent)	0.5	0.95	10.00	0.53
Bacteria				
Unstained, spun				
(2+ on scale of 4+)	0.75	0.8	3.75	0.31
Gram stain, unspun (1/hpf)	0.8	0.85	5.33	0.24
Microscopic pyuria				
Spun (5 WBCs/hpf)	0.6	0.85	4.00	0.47
Unspun (50 WBC/mm^3)	0.65	0.9	6.50	0.39
WBCs + bacteria				
Standard spun[b]	0.66	0.99	66.00	0.34
Enhanced unspun[c]	0.85	0.98	42.50	0.15
Leukocyte esterase				
(present or absent)	0.2	0.95	4.00	0.84
Leukocyte esterase + nitrite	0.5	0.98	25.00	0.51
Methylene blue	0.6	0.98	30.00	0.41
Uriscreen	0.9	0.9	9.00	0.11
Bac-T-screen	0.9	0.7	3.00	0.14
Chemstrip LN	0.9	0.7	3.00	0.14

[a]Values have been taken from several sources,[39–41] rounded by the author, and represent reasonable numbers to use in clinical practice.
[b]5 WBCs/hpf + any bacteria in spun urinalysis.
[c]10 WBCs/mm^3 + any bacteria by Gram stain.
hpf = high-power field; WBC = white blood cell count.

Table 15.3. Suggested Culture Colony Count Thresholds for Significant Bacteriuria

Various clinical settings	Significant bacteriuria (CFU/mL)
Infants and children	
Voided	$\geq 10^3$
Catheter	$\geq 10^3$
Suprapubic aspirate (SPA)	$\geq 10^3$
External collection devices	$\geq 10^4$
Adult	
Midstream, clean-catch	
Female	
Asymptomatic	$\geq 10^5$
Symptomatic	$\geq 10^2$
Male	$\geq 10^3$
In-and-out (straight) catheterization	$\geq 10^2$
Chronic indwelling catheter	$\geq 10^2$
Indwelling catheter or SPA in spinal injuries	Any detectable colony count
External collection devices	$\geq 10^5$
Condom collection device in spinal injuries	$\geq 10^4$

Sources: Data are from Cardenas and Hooton[34] and Eisenstadt and Washington.[46]

ured, it is not the perfect test and falls short of being 100% sensitive and specific. Bacterial culture methods include, in order of decreasing predictive accuracy, the quantitative culture (pour plate method), semiquantitative culture (surface streak procedure), and miniaturized culture (filter paper, roll tube, and dipslide methods). The colony count that represents significant bacteriuria varies with factors that include age, sex, anatomic location of the infection, and symptoms. Although the urine culture is considered the gold standard for defining significant bacteriuria, the level of significance is not uniform across the clinical spectrum of disease. Colony counts of what can currently be considered as significant bacteriuria for infection are shown in Table 15.3.[34,46]

References

1. Warren JW. Clinical presentations and epidemiology of urinary tract infections. In: Mobley LT, Warren JW, eds. Urinary tract infections: molecular pathogenesis and clinical management. Washington, DC: ASM Press, 1996;3–28.
2. Stull TL, LiPuma JJ. Epidemiology and natural history of urinary infections in children. Med Clin North Am 1991;75(2):287–98.
3. Stamm WE, Hooton TM, Johnson JR, et al. Urinary tract infections: from pathogenesis to treatment. J Infect Dis 1989;159(3):400–6.
4. Zelikovic I, Adelman RD, Nancarrow PA. Urinary tract infections in children. An update. West J Med 1992;157(5):554–61.
5. Shortliffe LM. The management of urinary tract infections in children without urinary tract abnormalities. Urol Clin North Am 1995;22(1):67–73.
6. Hellerstein S. Urinary tract infections in children: Why they occur and how to prevent them. Am Fam Physician 1998;57(10):2440–6.
7. Linshaw MA. Controversies in childhood urinary tract infections. World J Urol 1999;17(6):383–95.
8. Carmack MA, Arvin AM. Urinary tract infections—navigating complex currents [editorial]. West J Med 1992;157(5):587–8.
9. Hellerstein S. Evolving concepts in the evaluation of the child with a urinary tract infection [editorial comment]. J Pediatr 1994;124(4):589–92.
10. Conway JJ, Cohn RA. Evolving role of nuclear medicine for the diagnosis and management of urinary tract infection [editorial comment]. J Pediatr 1994;124(1):87–90.
11. Schieve LA, Handler A, Hershow R, et al. Urinary tract infection during pregnancy: its association with maternal morbidity and perinatal outcome. Am J Public Health 1994;84(3):405–10.
12. Zinner SH. Management of urinary tract infections in pregnancy: a review with comments on single dose therapy. Infection 1992;20(suppl 4):S280.
13. Chow AW, Jewesson PJ. Use and safety of antimicrobial agents during pregnancy. West J Med 1987;146:761–4.
14. Pfau A, Sacks TG. Effective prophylaxis for recurrent urinary tract infections during pregnancy. Clin Infect Dis 1992;14:810.
15. Madersbacher S, Thalhammer F, Marberger M. Pathogenesis and management of recurrent urinary tract infection in women. Curr Opin Urol 2000;10(1):29–33.
16. Hooton TM, Hillier S, Johnson C, et al. Escherichia coli bacteriuria and contraceptive method. JAMA 1991;265(1):64–9.

17. Stamm WE, Hooton TM. Management of urinary tract infections in adults. N Engl J Med 1993;329:1328.
18. Johnson JR. Treatment and prevention of urinary tract infections. In: Mobley LT, Warren JW, eds. Urinary tract infections: molecular pathogenesis and clinical management. Washington, DC: ASM Press, 1996;95–118.
19. Spach DH, Stapleton AE, Stamm WE. Lack of circumcision increases the risk of urinary tract infection in young men. JAMA 1992;267:679.
20. Krieger JN, Ross SO, Simonsen JM. Urinary tract infections in healthy university men. J Urol 1993;149(5):1046–8.
21. Pfau A. Re: urinary tract infections in healthy university men [letter]. J Urol 1994;151(3):705–6.
22. Burrows LL, Khoury AE. Issues surrounding the prevention and management of device-related infections. World J Urol 1999;17(6):402–9.
23. Warren JW. The catheter and urinary tract infection. Med Clin North Am 1991;75:481–95.
24. Saint S, Veenstra DL, Sullivan SD, Chenoweth C, Fendrick AM. The potential clinical and economic benefits of silver alloy urinary catheters in preventing urinary tract infection. Arch Intern Med 2000;160(17):2670–5.
25. Harding GKM, Nicolle LE, Ronald AR, et al. How long should catheter-acquired urinary infection in women be treated? A randomized controlled study. Ann Intern Med 1991;114:713.
26. Baldassarre JS, Kaye D. Special problems in urinary tract infection in the elderly. Med Clin North Am 1991;75(2):375–90.
27. Nicolle LE. Urinary tract infections in long-term care facilities. Infect Control Hosp Epidemiol 1993;14(4):220–5.
28. Lipsky BA, Ireton RC, Gihn SD, et al. Diagnosis of bacteriuria in men: specimen collection and culture interpretation. J Infect Dis 1987;155:847–54.
29. Abrutyn E, Mossey J, Berlin JA, et al. Does asymptomatic bacteriuria predict mortality and does antimicrobial treatment reduce mortality in elderly ambulatory women? Ann Intern Med 1994;120(10):827–33.
30. Nordenstam GR, Brandberg CA, Oden AS, et al. Bacteriuria and mortality in an elderly population. N Engl J Med 1986;314:1152–6.
31. Nicolle LE, Henderson E, Bjornson J, et al. The association of bacteriuria with resident characteristics and survival in elderly institutionalized men. Ann Intern Med 1987;106:682–6.
32. Hamilton-Miller JMT. Issues in urinary tract infections in the elderly. World J Urol 1999;17:396–401.
33. Avorn J, Monane M, Gurwitz JH, et al. Reduction of bacteriuria and pyuria after ingestion of cranberry juice. JAMA 1994;271(10):751–4.
34. Cardenas DD, Hooton TM. Urinary tract infection in persons with spinal cord injury. Arch Phys Med Rehabil 1995;76(3):272–80.
35. Ronald AR, Pattullo ALS. The natural history of urinary tract infection in adults. Med Clin North Am 1991;75(2):299–312.
36. Sobel JD, Vazquez JA. Fungal infections of the urinary tract. World J Urol 1999;17(6):410–4.
37. Stamm WE. Measurement of pyuria and its relation to bacteriuria. Am J Med 1983;75(1B):53–8.
38. Pappas PG. Laboratory in the diagnosis and management of urinary tract infections. Med Clin North Am 1991;75(2):313–26.

39. Alwall N. Pyuria: deposit in high-power microscopic field—wbc/hpf—versus wbc/mm^3 in counting chamber. Acta Med Scand 1973;194:537–40.
40. Bailey BL. Urinalysis predictive of urine culture results. J Fam Pract 1995;40 (1):45–50.
41. Hoberman A, Wald ER, Penchansky L, Reynolds EA, Young S. Enhanced urinalysis as a screening test for urinary tract infection. Pediatrics 1993;91(6):1196–9.
42. Bachman JW, Heise RH, Naessens JM, Timmerman MG. A study of various tests to detect asymptomatic urinary tract infections in an obstetric population. JAMA 1993;270(16):1971–4.
43. Lockhart GR, Lewander WJ, Cimini DM, Josephson SL, Linakis JG. Use of urinary gram stain for detection of urinary tract infection in infants. Ann Emerg Med 1995; 25(1):31–5.
44. Carroll KC, Hale DC, Von Boerum DH, et al. Laboratory evaluation of urinary tract infections in an ambulatory clinic. Am J Clin Pathol 1994;101(1):100–3.
45. Jenkins RD, Fenn JP, Matsen JM. Review of urine microscopy for bacteriuria. JAMA 1986;255(24):3397–403.
46. Eisenstadt J, Washington JA. Diagnostic microbiology for bacteria and yeasts causing urinary tract infections. In: Mobley LT, Warren JW, eds. Urinary tract infections: molecular pathogenesis and clinical management. Washington, DC: ASM Press, 1996;29–68.

CASE PRESENTATION

Subjective

PATIENT PROFILE

Nancy Nelson is a 40-year-old married female accountant.

PRESENTING PROBLEM

"It hurts when I pass urine."

PRESENT ILLNESS

For 2 days, Mrs. Nelson has had urinary burning, frequency, urgency, and nocturia. She reports some mild left flank pain. She has felt warm but has not taken her temperature.

PAST MEDICAL HISTORY

She has had two urinary tract infections over the past 18 months, and both responded promptly to medication.

SOCIAL HISTORY

She works 3 days a week as a bookkeeper in a large firm. Her husband, Ken, is a home builder, and they have two teenage children.

HABITS

She uses no tobacco and takes alcohol occasionally. She drinks six cups of coffee daily.

FAMILY HISTORY

Her father, aged 71, is living and well. Her mother died at age 68 of breast cancer. She has no siblings.

REVIEW OF SYSTEMS

She has occasional pain in the joints of her hands and low back pain after lifting and carrying.

- What additional medical history would be helpful? Why?
- What symptoms or past history—if present—would you consider especially worrisome? Explain.
- Might a vulvovaginitis be part of her problem? How would you inquire about this possibility?
- What are Mrs. Nelson's possible concerns about her symptoms? How would you address this issue?

Objective

VITAL SIGNS

Blood pressure, 112/64; pulse, 68; respirations, 18; temperature, 37.4°C.

EXAMINATION

The patient is ambulatory and does not appear acutely ill. There is no mass or organ enlargement in the abdomen. There is moderate suprapubic tenderness without bladder distension. There is equivocal left costovertebral angle tenderness. The examination of the vagina, cervix, fundus, and adnexa are normal except for a thin watery vaginal discharge.

LABORATORY

There is a positive nitrite reaction on urinary dipstick. Red blood cells, bacteria, and many white blood cells are present on microscopic examination of a spun urine specimen.

- What additional data—if any—from the physical examination might be useful, and why?
- What—if any—laboratory tests would you obtain today? Why?
- What—if any—diagnostic imaging would you obtain today?
- If the patient had a thick purulent vaginal discharge, what might you do differently? Explain.

Assessment

- What is the probable diagnosis? What is the likely etiologic cause?
- How would you explain your assessment to the patient and her husband?
- What is the possible significance of the prior urinary tract infections?
- What is the possible meaning of this illness to the patient? To her husband?

Plan

- Describe your therapeutic recommendations for the patient. How would you explain this plan to the patient?
- What is your advice regarding work, household duties, and sexual relations?
- Might this patient benefit from consultation with a urologist? Explain.
- What follow-up would you advise?

16
Vulvovaginitis and Cervicitis

Mary Willard

Although modern medical practice has often relegated vaginal symptoms to the realm of the specialist gynecologist, the range of symptoms and diagnoses covered under this category with the concomitant preventive health and risk management issues is ideally suited to the expertise of the family physician. Excellence in the diagnosis and management of these diseases is the standard of care and can be achieved with a minimal investment of equipment, time (a 1-minute slide examination), and cost to the patient. Patients with vaginal complaints account for an estimated 10% of office visits each year,[1] and many more may be inaccurately diagnosed by phone. This chapter reviews the systematic approach to the evaluation and treatment of vaginal diseases as well as issues of particular interest to family physicians.

Diagnostic Assessment

It is critical for the family physician to remember that few complaints are more annoying to the female patient than vaginal itching and discharge. Tolerance of low-grade symptomatology is the norm for some patients until a flare turns the problem into a midnight emergency. Although the history and physical examination are helpful, only appropriate testing can make the diagnosis.

Laboratory Equipment and Technique

The equipment needed for accurate diagnosis of vaginal complaints is simple: saline in small containers, nonsterile cotton-tipped applicators, slides, coverslips, a good microscope with 10× and 40× capacity (i.e., low- and high-dry power), 10% potassium hydroxide solution (KOH) preparation, diagnostic tests for *Chlamydia* and gonococci, and a small magnifying lens. Vaginal fluid should be examined as soon as possible after the fluid is obtained, as *Trichomonas vaginalis* is fragile and may die quickly.

The technique of examining vaginal fluid is straightforward. After inserting the vaginal speculum, a plain cotton-tipped applicator is swept into the vaginal fluid, withdrawn (preferably with a "clump" of discharge), and placed immedi-

322

ately into a small container with only 1 mL of saline. Small pediatric red-topped tubes containing saline can be kept in all rooms where pelvic examinations may be performed so they are immediately available. For maximal results, the smallest amount of saline and the largest sample of vaginal fluid should be used. Once the sample of vaginal fluid is obtained, cervical cultures can be prepared if necessary, the pelvic examination completed, and the saline examined.

The vaginal fluid in saline is examined microscopically using gloves as per universal precautions. Take the cotton applicator from the tube and place a drop of fluid on two slides, one for the saline examination and one for a KOH preparation. If a diagnosis of yeast is being entertained, it is critical to try to get a "clump" of the discharge onto the designated KOH slide. A drop of a 10% KOH solution (made by mixing 90 mL distilled water with 10 g KOH) is dropped on it and immediately smelled for a fishy odor, which may be an indicator of bacterial vaginosis. If further evaluation for hyphae is to be done, place a coverslip and allow the slide to sit until the saline slide is examined. The KOH destroys some of the vaginal epithelial and white blood cells (WBCs), leaving only hyphae for inspection.

Next examine the saline slide with coverslip under low power. Search for motion of cells, sheets of epithelial cells compatible with denuding of mucosa, or "clue cells." The latter are vaginal epithelial cells "studded" with bacteria that adhere for unknown reasons. These epithelial cells look dense and tend to glitter when the focus is varied. Although clue cells are present normally in up to 10% of the field, a preponderance of them, especially when combined with a fishy odor on the KOH preparation, supports the diagnosis of bacterial vaginosis.[2]

Once the examination under low power is completed, it is appropriate to scan the field under high-dry power to check for *T. vaginalis* and to better examine the epithelial cells. Trichomonads appear as motile triangular cells, somewhat larger than WBCs, with long moving tails. Because many bacteria are part of the normal vaginal ecosystem and are nonpathogenic,[3] Gram stains and routine cultures are not first-line tests for diagnosing vaginal diseases. If the high-power field has more than 10 WBCs, consider the possibility of an upper genital tract infection.

If an examination for yeast is necessary, place the KOH preparation under the microscope. Hyphae and spores are best seen on this specimen by focusing under low power to find a "clumped" area and then going immediately to high-dry power and focusing on the edges of the clump. The clumped material usually represents epithelial cells and hyphae tissue not desiccated by the KOH preparation; the edge of the clump is the best place to identify the hyphae. Certainly if the history so warrants and the cervical os reveals discharge from above, appropriate tests for *Chlamydia*, gonococci, or both are performed.

When analyzing vaginal complaints, few tests other than those noted above are needed except in specific circumstances or in refractory cases (which are discussed in relevant sections). One area of controversy is the role of vaginal pH tests. Because the premenopausal vaginal ecosystem keeps the pH under 4.5, assessment of change might be of some value. Although sensitive, this test is not specific and can be influenced greatly by fluids from the cervix, by semen, or by douching. It has, therefore, limited application in the office. There is also investigation into the use of monoclonal antibodies and DNA analysis. Unfortunately, none of these tests is of sufficient reliability to replace the simple slide evaluations.

History

As with any clinical problem, the history is a critical clue to diagnosis and must be obtained methodically from each patient. The ambiguous nature of the problem, however, means that the diagnosis cannot be made solely on historical clues, such as a "cheesy" discharge. Most women can, with minimal clarification by the physician, reveal a clear history of their complaint. Because there is individual variation in the amount and character of the vaginal discharge that is "normal," the family physician role is to help patients distinguish a change from that pattern. Ask about skin lesions, internal or external itching, odor, dyspareunia, and the use (and frequency) of douching, new soaps, or deodorant sprays. Always inquire about previous similar episodes, but ask how these diagnoses were made, especially in the patient treated over the phone. Many patients who state that they "always get yeast infections" have never had an accurate diagnosis made, and any vaginal cream has the potential of calming an inflamed mucosa (thereby diminishing the symptoms until the next flare).

One of the most commonly missed presentations of vaginitis is the complaint of dysuria (see Chapter 15). Treating all patients with dysuria as cystitis results in the inevitable phone call 48 to 72 hours later from a patient who is no better. Because women with vulvitis complain of pain externally with urination, clarification of the type of dysuria at the initial encounter assists in determining which patients require additional evaluation for vaginitis.

It is essential that the family physician obtain a complete sexual history from these patients and assess them for risk of sexually transmitted diseases. If the patient is sexually active, the physician should inquire about any new spermicidal agents or condoms, symptom complaints from a partner(s), a new sexual partner, and sexual practices. Moreover, the patient should be educated about sexual practices that minimize risk of disease.

Physical Examination

Although the pelvic examination can be tailored by the history, patients with vaginal complaints must be evaluated systematically. The external genitalia are thoroughly assessed for clues using a hand-held magnifying lens if necessary. The urethra, labia, and vulvae are completely checked for ulcerations, warts, tears, cysts, abscesses, erythema, and edema. Additionally, the vaginal mucosa itself must be inspected for color, lesions, and edema. Normal vaginal mucosa is pink with moist folds. A fiery red or weepy mucosa is a sign of inflammation. Any plaque-type lesions are scraped for adherence to vaginal mucosa, a sign of possible candidiasis.

As part of the complete evaluation, observe the cervical os for pus as a cause of discharge. Using a large cotton swab (e.g., one used for proctoscopic examinations), clean the cervix of all discharge, and observe the os for a short time, usually 10 seconds. If purulent fluid appears at the os opening from above, it is an indicator of upper pelvic infection for which *Chlamydia* and gonococci must be tested. At this point, a bimanual examination should also be performed to assess adnexal tenderness or masses.

Clinical Presentation

It is impossible, given the constraints of space, to discuss all possible forms of vaginitis or other vaginal diseases. Instead, the focus here is on the more common etiologies and important vaginal skin diseases that may masquerade as "itch." This approach assists in clarifying most vaginal complaints.

Traditional medical training clearly defined the classic presentations for vaginitis. Unfortunately, this "eyeball" method correctly diagnoses only one third of the cases,[4] making thorough clinical evaluation necessary (Fig. 16.1). Nevertheless, an appreciation of the textbook presentations is necessary when teasing apart the significant historical details given by the patient. It is equally important to realize the change in epidemiology of vaginitis since the 1970s. The most common cause of vaginitis is now bacterial vaginosis, followed by mycotic diseases (e.g., *Candida* sp.), and then trichomoniasis.[5] Whatever the reason for this shift, knowledge of the probabilities is useful.

Contact and Chemical Dermatitides

Contact and chemical dermatitides are much overlooked diagnoses for the patient with vulvitis. Any topical agent used in the genital area (including nonoxynol-9 and rubber in condoms) can be an allergen. A reddened, swollen vulva or a vaginal mucosa exuding a clear exudate characterizes this problem. Equally important is the patient who has been douching repeatedly and with increasing frequency. This practice sets up a denuding phenomenon that inflames and strips the mucosa. The appropriate treatment for this category of inflammation is to discontinue the product and consider using a short-term course of topical external steroids for symptomatic relief.[6]

Mycotic Diseases

Although the incidence is rising,[5] contrary to popular belief among patients and physicians, true fungal infections probably account for approximately one third of all vaginal infections. The textbook presentation is a patient complaining of a vaginal itch and cheesy exudate, with white plaques adherent to the vaginal wall and a KOH preparation showing multiple hyphae. The diagnosis should not be made unless hyphae are seen on the slide. Because as many as 20% of asymptomatic women have positive cultures,[7] it is obvious that culture methods are too sensitive and should be reserved for refractory cases,[8] frequent relapses, or when yeast is suspected clinically but the KOH preparation is negative. In this case, suspect *Candida glabrata*, which may present with vaginal burning and, as a spore former, can be diagnosed only on Gram stain. This infection is often refractory to the standard duration of treatment and may require protracted therapy.[6]

Yeast infections typified by *Candida albicans* have been erroneously ascribed to many causes. For example, yeast infections probably do not occur any more frequently in diabetic women but may be more difficult to eradicate.[6] Therefore, consider diabetes in the patient with chronic infections, not frequent ones. There is also little proved association between yeast infection and use of birth control pills.[9] For frequent relapses, consider treating the sexual partner(s) to achieve full eradication and changing the patient's diet, as high calories and crude fiber have been associated with susceptibility to infection.[10] Remember, too, that women with human immunodeficiency virus (HIV) disease may manifest persistent or diffuse candidiasis as a presenting symptom (see Chapter 21).

Treatment is straightforward and consists of either topical azole applications or an oral one-time dose of fluconazole (Diflucan).[11] To date, no data prove oral routes to be superior and they are associated with side effects such as headache, drug reactions, and gastrointestinal (GI) toxicity.[11] Additionally, there is no proved superiority of one drug over another or of creams over tablets, although general data show the azoles to be slightly more efficacious than nystatin.[12] Use of a cream allows external and internal application and may be more soothing acutely. Most of these are now available in over-the-counter (OTC) formulations that have similar costs to prescription items. Physician and patient preferences dictate the specific drug and route, and there is no risk associated with treatment during pregnancy. Truly refractory cases may require longer treatment courses, and the patient with frequent relapses may benefit from oral ketoconazole (Nizoral) 100 mg/day or oral fluconazole (Diflucan) 150 mg every week or month except during pregnancy.[12,13]

Trichomoniasis

The syndrome caused by *T. vaginalis* may cause severe itching or pain often accompanied by frequency of urination because of concomitant cystitis from the organism. On examination the vulva and the vaginal mucosa is fiery red with cervical petechiae ("strawberry cervix"). The typical discharge is yellow-green and bubbly in nature, but any range of color and texture may be seen, making slide examination critical. As noted above, the diagnosis is made by finding motile trichomonads on the saline smear. Because of the low positive predictive value of *Trichomonas* reported on Papanicolaou smears,[7] all of these results should be confirmed by a wet preparation before therapy is initiated. Although the culture methodology for *T. vaginalis* may have better sensitivity and specificity in theory, there is still debate over the ideal medium and methods, so the technique is not useful.

The drug of choice in therapy is metronidazole (Flagyl), with the best response noted after a 2-g single dose.[13] An alternative regimen of 500 mg bid for 7 days is best used for refractory cases only, as it produces no higher an initial cure than the one-time dose. Metronidazole has a significant Antabuse-type reaction, so patients must be cautioned to use no alcohol, including cough medicine, during the treatment. As a sexually transmitted disease, it is critically important for the patient's sexual partner(s) to be treated concurrently to prevent reinfection, and although there are some resistant cases, resistance is not an all-or-none phenomenon. Rather, resistance may range from mild (where treatment is effective) to severe, necessitating a treatment dose of 2.5 g/day in divided doses for 7 to 10 days.[14] At this time, no other medication available in the United States provides better therapeutic results.

Trichomoniasis during pregnancy is difficult to treat. Although the literature is scant, oral metronidazole may be teratogenic during the first trimester and is therefore contraindicated until the second trimester and reserved for severe infections only. Both intravaginal clotrimazole and clindamycin may be effective in controlling the symptoms during the first trimester, although they may not produce eradication.[6,13]

Bacterial Vaginosis

Formerly known as *Gardnerella* or nonspecific vaginitis, bacterial vaginosis has been credited with as many as 50% of all diagnoses of vaginitis.[15] It represents an overgrowth in the vagina of anaerobic organisms classically known as *Gardnerella vaginalis* and now noted to be multiple organisms. It produces no vulvar symptoms, no change in vaginal mucosa, little itching, and no pain, unless the discharge is so profuse the vulvae are simply macerated. Because its course is usually indolent, it does not cause an acute change in symptoms. The patient may note only a slight change in normal discharge and an odor that may be more pronounced after intercourse. Patients are frequently inured to the symptoms until treatment is finished and the discharge gone. There may not be an odor immediately on examination, but KOH releases the amines in the epithelial cells and produces the classic fishy odor that is diagnostic when clue cells are present. Because *Gardnerella* bacteria may be a normal inhabitant of the vagina, culture of the organism for a diagnosis has poor specificity and so has not been recommended.[7]

Treatment for this syndrome is metronidazole 500 mg po bid for 7 days or metronidazole gel 0.75% 5 g intravaginally bid for 5 days (Fig. 16.1).[13] Alternatively, clindamycin 2% vaginal cream can be used for 7 days. Unfortunately, the one-time dose used to treat trichomoniasis is insufficient for bacterial vaginosis. For refractory cases or as an alternate, oral clindamycin 300 mg bid for 7 days can be used.[13]

Because some association has been noted between bacterial vaginosis and premature rupture of membranes or postpartum endometriosis, therapy should be considered during pregnancy.[16] The recommended drug during pregnancy is a 2% clindamycin vaginal cream at night for 7 days or oral metronidazole 250 mg tid for 7 days[16] (see above).

At this time, the role of sexual transmission of this disorder is unclear. Studies can be found to support either opinion, and partner therapy has not produced an improved cure rate, at least at conventional dosage.[16] Equally unclear is the role of treatment in the asymptomatic patient, but it may be considered in someone undergoing vaginal surgery because of a potential role in pelvic inflammation.[16]

Atrophic Vaginitis

A common cause of vaginal symptoms in the postmenopausal woman, atrophic vaginitis should be considered concomitantly with the evaluation for other etiologies. Lack of estrogen produces thin vaginal epithelium and cells deficient in the acids that provide the premenopausal woman with a balanced vaginal ecosystem. Therefore, the mucosa easily denudes and becomes traumatized. Thus presenting symptoms may include lack of vaginal lubrication with coitus, pruritus, and dyspareunia, with or without discharge.

On examination the vaginal folds are flattened, and the mucosa is pale pink and shows lack of lubrication. The cervix is usually atrophic and frequently friable, and the wet preparation is negative. Hormone replacement therapy is the treatment of choice, but vaginal estrogen creams used nightly can provide short-term relief.[17] The patient must be reminded that a vaginal discharge may recur as the cells mature back to a premenopausal pattern.

Chlamydia *Infection*

Even though *Chlamydia* does not produce vaginitis (except in adolescents), it does cause mucopurulent cervicitis. On examination, the cervix may be eroded and present a mucopurulent discharge that when wiped quickly re-forms at the os. When this condition is seen, the alert clinician performs appropriate tests, examining wet preparations for concomitant vaginal infections, as patients with one STD are at high risk of having more.

Once a diagnosis of *Chlamydia* is suspected, empiric treatment is warranted, especially in a high-risk patient (defined as sexually active, nonmonogamous, and young). The standard treatment is doxycycline (Vibramycin) 100 mg po bid for 7 days or azithromycin (Zithromax) 1 g po once.[13] If the patient is allergic to tetracycline (rare) or pregnancy is suspected, an appropriate alternative is erythromycin 500 mg po qid for 7 days. Partners should be treated aggressively, but a test of patient cure is considered unnecessary.

Herpesvirus Infection

Especially in the case of recurrences, patients with herpesvirus infection may present only with symptoms of external burning and minimal liquid discharge. Without ulcerations externally or on the cervix, this diagnosis should not be entertained unless there is a known history of a positive culture.

Human Papillomavirus Infection

Current trends indicate that most human papillomavirus (HPV) disease presents as warts either externally or internally. Therefore, HPV is unlikely to be a cause of any symptoms unless the growth is large enough to cause an exudative process. Because HPV is associated with cervical dysplasia, a Papanicolaou smear must be examined regularly. No form of treatment has proved to be superior or to eradicate the virus. Topical podophyllin externally and cryotherapy internally remain standard options. Both podofilox (0.5% solution) and an immunomodulating agent, Aldara (imiquimod), are available by prescription for patient home use.[13] Neither is superior to office treatment, but both offer the advantage of patient home use. A self-administered regimen of 5% imiquimod cream applied externally overnight three times a week for 16 weeks will produce no more toxicity than podophyllin and may be the best initial choice.[18]

Leukorrhea Secondary to Birth Control Pills

On some occasions, the only cause of leukorrhea is an eroded cervix secondary to the use of birth control pills. The hormones in birth control pills cause more endocervix to be exposed to the environment of the vagina, producing irritation and weeping of the mucosa. It is usually asymptomatic. If a patient is having symptoms, this diagnosis is excluded.

Vulvar Diseases

It is critical to remember that many skin diseases manifest with vaginal symptoms. Most, such as seborrheic dermatitis, psoriasis, tinea, and pediculosis, have unique characteristics that are obvious. Without these unique characteristics, diagnosis and appropriate therapy may best be achieved by performance of a simple punch biopsy or referral to dermatology. Patients must be told that the treatment effect may take months to realize. In addition, any pigmented lesion should be biopsied and the patient referred if indicated by biopsy results.

Vestibulitis

With vestibulitis there is variable redness and edema of the vestibular glands, frequently with a lesion. The number of glands involved can range from 1 to 100, and the symptoms are vulvar pain with dyspareunia. The etiology is still

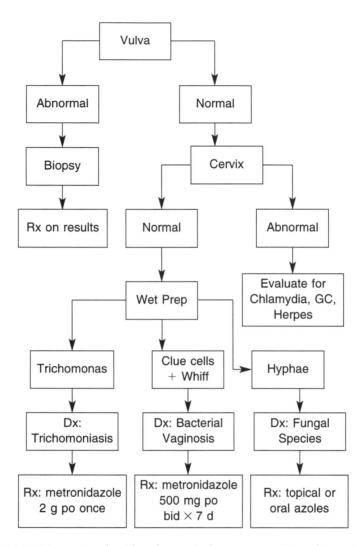

FIGURE 16.1. Diagnostic algorithm for vaginal symptoms. Dx = diagnosis; GC = gonococcus; Rx = treatment.

hotly debated, but probably HPV is involved. Treatment results are best with vestibular resection or intralesional interferon, but no therapy is 100% effective.[19]

Lichen Sclerosis

Lichen sclerosis is a hyperplastic condition with a white lesion seen predominantly in women over age 50. There is a typical "keyhole" pattern on both sides of the vulva. The lesion may eventually cover the entire vulva with adhesion and eventual obliteration of the labia minora to the majora. Treatment is a topical testosterone ointment (30 mL of testosterone in oil with 120 g petrolatum) twice a day for 4 to 6 months and then one or two times a week for life.[17] If the patient cannot tolerate the side effects, alternative therapy of progesterone cream can be used. There is a high recurrence rate, even with surgery or laser, so dramatic treatment is best avoided.

Lichen Simplex Chronicus

Caused by chronic itching or irritation, lichen simplex chronicus is a thick, scaly condition with localized vulvar lesions without adhesions. Treatment is symptomatic with topical steroids for 1 to 2 months. Because the only recurrences are seen in patients treated by surgery, this intervention is no longer acceptable.[20]

Lichen Planus

Lichen planus may involve mucous membranes in other organ systems. There is vulvar burning, leukorrhea, and redness of the inner labia. Patients may have violaceous papules externally and small, lacy, gray, reticular patterns on the inner labia. Without these identifying marks, this lesion may appear similar to that of atrophic vaginitis; it should be entertained as a diagnosis whenever therapy for atrophic vaginitis fails. Treatment is topical with either a potent fluorinated steroid or a medium potency steroid under occlusion.[20] The patient must be reminded that this condition flares and remits over long periods.

When the Tests Are Negative

A dilemma ensues when, despite the best efforts of the clinician, the examination and tests reveal no reason for the patient's symptoms. In such cases, the clinician should review the history, the adequacy of specimen collection, the performance of the laboratory tests, and the possibility of *Chlamydia*, and should obtain any history previously overlooked and consider the diagnosis of an acid-base change in the vaginal environment known as cytolytic vaginosis. Although not easily diagnosed, this entity is caused by an overgrowth of acidophilic Döderlein's lactobacilli, producing an increase in enzymes that degrade intracellular glycogen to lactic acid and causing massive desquamation and cytolysis and a watery discharge. Because the luteal phase epithelial cells are richer in lactic acid, this syndrome may be cyclic in nature. The hallmark for diagnosis is epithelial cells that have a moth-eaten appearance, often called pseudo-clue cells, and a few WBCs on the wet preparation. In addition, because this process is driven by an acidic environment, the symptoms worsen with douching using conventional acidic agents. Instead, these patients can be treated with a douching mixture of sodium bicarbonate and water (1–2 tablespoons in 500 mL water) used three times a week while symptomatic.[4]

If the workup was adequate, the clinician should resist the urge to perform "shotgun" or even empiric treatment, as such treatment perpetuates old myths, and instead be supportive and understanding of the symptoms and encourage the patient to be checked for subsequent recurrences.

Special Considerations for the Family Physician

Much of the success of therapy depends on the unique relationship between the family physician and the patient.

Compliance

The trusting relationship between the patient and the family physician enhances compliance with often distasteful regimens. The patient is encouraged to finish the full course of therapy despite symptom resolution, and when the therapy demands partner compliance, the patient must be instructed to abstain from intercourse until therapy is completed. Role-playing this partner discussion with the patient may help allay anxiety. Choose the shortest regimen possible and make sure the patient understands side effects (including local irritation), route of usage, and use of medication during menses. Negotiate with the patient the best time to begin treatment and inform her of the possibility of recurrence or treatment failure. In addition, it is critical to assess the patients' attribution of disease in this condition. Clarity about sexual transmission is important; if possible, use printed information for the patient to read and give to her partner(s).

Issues of self-support and control of symptoms can be critical to compliance as well. These points can be reinforced through good patient education. Sources of self-help for the patient can be found in women's health literature such as *Our Bodies, Our Selves* or its revision.[21] These references may provide the patient with more detailed information on hygiene, as well as alternative remedies. The physician, however, should first read the relevant sections to be sure that the information is consonant with good care and to explain areas of disagreement. (For example, there is scant scientific evidence for the use of intravaginal yogurt.) Some patients work best with a combination of conventional medical therapy and time-honored suggestions.

Recurrent or Persistent Vaginitis

Nothing is more frustrating to the patient or physician than recurrence (defined as symptoms recurring after a 1-month disease-free interval) or persistence of symptoms. In this situation the physician should start over with the history, emphasizing compliance with previous therapy and focusing attention on details of diet, clothing, and irritants. Question the patient about high dairy intake, increased simple sugars, use of new deodorant tampons or pads, or other topical agents such as perfumes or home remedies. Explore the relation to tight clothing, exercise gear, the use of dildos or vibrators, and the use of hot tubs or pools.

The examination and basic tests should be repeated, but if the history reveals no further clues, culture the cervix for *Chlamydia* and the vaginal vault for bacteria and *Candida* and perform any necessary vulvar biopsies. In the diabetic patient the blood glucose must be controlled concomitantly while reinstituting therapy.

Results of the tests dictate therapy. Persistent *Candida* or *Trichomonas* infection may need prolonged (*Candida*) or increased (*Trichomonas*) therapy. Consider treating according to the results of the bacterial culture using an antibiotic[6] targeted to the dominant organism.

If tests are negative, provide support and sympathy, educate the patient about good hygiene and sexual behaviors that minimize risk, and proscribe anything that might exacerbate symptoms. Encourage the patient to return to be examined when symptoms recur.

Management of the HIV-Positive Patient

Other than the fact that patients who are HIV-seropositive may have problems with HPV, treatment of vaginal disorders follows the same recommendations as for nonpositive patients. Although refractory candidiasis may be a clue for the physician to check a patient for HIV status, a "normal" vaginal infection should not be of concern.[22]

Role of Colposcopy

The role of colposcopy is not well defined regarding vaginal symptoms. It may be a useful tool in the future, but its current usage is in the evaluation of an abnormal Papanicolaou smear or cervix. Therefore, use it in a patient with persistent cervicitis only to screen for abnormal areas to biopsy. Additionally, conventional wisdom dictates that patients with HPV undergo colposcopy to detect a precancerous state of the cervix.

Prevention of Vaginitis

When an STD has caused the vaginitis, the family physician must educate the patient about the difference between a disease that can arise de novo and then be propagated between partners and one acquired from someone else. Patients are understandably concerned about where they got the disease, but the clinician can help focus the patient on treatment, give basic relevant information, and plan a subsequent visit to continue pursuing their concerns. Clarity about sexual transmission is important, as the patient may also need to be concerned about hepatitis and HIV risk. Acquisition of an STD is certainly threatening to partners who thought of themselves as mutually monogamous, and relationship issues are frequently topics for subsequent visits.

In addition to concerns about sexual transmission, the physician should educate the patient about the causative or associative factors found to be significant in the history. Use of local irritants, clothing, and other offending behaviors must be discouraged. Above all, encouraging the patient to come in for evaluation of subsequent infections is critical, as the etiology may differ from the current one.

References

1. Paavonen J, Stamm WE. Lower genital tract infections in women. Infect Dis Clin North Am 1987;1179–98.
2. Bump RC, Zuspan FP, Buesching WJ, Ayers LW, Stephens T. The prevalence, six-month persistence and predictive values of laboratory indicators of bacterial vaginosis (nonspecific vaginitis). Am J Obstet Gynecol 1984;150:917–23.
3. Faro S. Bacterial vaginitis. Obstet Gynecol 1991;34:582–6.
4. Cibley LJ, Cibley LJ. Cytolytic vaginosis. Am J Obstet Gynecol 1991;165:1245–8.
5. Kent HL. Epidemiology of vaginitis. Am J Obstet Gynecol 1991;165:1168–76.
6. Horowitz BJ, Mardh PA, eds. Vaginitis and vaginosis. New York: Wiley Liss, 1991.
7. Eschenbach DA, Hiller SL. Advances in diagnostic testing for vaginitis and cervicitis. J Reprod Med 1989;34(suppl 18):555–64.
8. Horowitz BJ. Mycotic vulvovaginitis: a broad overview. Am J Obstet Gynecol 1991;165:1188–92.
9. Roy S. Vulvovaginitis: causes and therapies: nonbarrier contraceptives and vaginitis and vaginosis. Am J Obstet Gynecol 1991;165:1240–4.
10. Reed B, Slatery M, French T. Diet and vaginitis. J Fam Pract 1989;29:509–15.
11. Drugs for vulvovaginal candidiasis. Med Lett Drugs Ther 2001;43:3,4.
12. Watson MC, Grimshaw JM, Bond CM, et al. Oral versus intra-vaginal imidazole and triazole anti-fungal treatment of uncomplicated vulvovaginal candidiasis. Cochrane Review. The Cochrane Library 2001;1.
13. Drugs for sexually transmitted infections. Med Lett Drugs Ther 1999;41:85–90.
14. Forna F, Gulmezoglu AM. Interventions for treating trichomoniasis in women. Cochrane Review. The Cochrane Library 2001;1.
15. Eschenbach DA, Hiller S, Critchlow C, Stevens C, DeRowen T, Holmes KK. Diagnosis and clinical manifestations of bacterial vaginosis. Am J Obstet Gynecol 1988;158:819–23.
16. Joesoef MR, Schmid GP, Hillier SL. Bacterial vaginosis: review of treatment options and potential clinical indications for therapy. CID 1999;28(suppl 1):S57–S65.
17. Byyny RL, Speroff L. A clinical guide for the care of older women. Baltimore: Williams & Wilkins, 1990.
18. Gall SA. Female genital warts: global trends and treatments. Infect Dis Obstet Gynecol 2001;9(3):149–54.
19. McKay M, Frankman O, Horovitz BJ, Lecart C, Micheletti L, Ridley C. Vulvar vestibulitis and vestibular papillomatoses: report of the ISSVD committee on vulvodynia. J Reprod Med 1991;36:413–5.
20. McKay M. Vulvar dermatoses. Clin Obstet Gynecol 1991;34:614–29.
21. Boston Women's Health Book Collective. The new our bodies, ourselves. New York: Simon & Schuster, 1992.
22. Hammill HA, Murtagh CP. Gynecologic care of the human immunodeficiency virus-positive woman. Clin Obstet Gynecol 1991;34:599–604.

Case Presentation

Subjective

Patient Profile

Ellen McCarthy Harris is a 26-year-old married female secretary.

Presenting Problem

Vaginal discharge.

Present Illness

There is a 10-day history of vaginal discharge with intense itching that began after her last menstrual period. The symptoms have not responded to an over-the-counter vaginal cream.

Past Medical History

No serious illnesses or hospitalizations.

Social History

She has worked at her secretarial job for 4 years. She and her husband, Andrew, have two children.

Habits

She does not use tobacco, coffee, or recreational drugs.

Family History

Her father has diabetes mellitus and coronary artery disease. Her mother is living and well. Her brother, aged 28, is HIV-positive.

Review of Systems

No symptoms in other areas.

- What additional information regarding the history of present illness might be important? Explain.
- Why might the over-the-counter medication not have worked?

- Over the past 10 days, what might the patient be doing differently because of her illness? Why might this be pertinent?
- What might the patient be trying to tell you today?

Objective

VITAL SIGNS

Blood pressure, 112/64; pulse, 68; temperature, 37.0°C.

EXAMINATION

The abdomen is scaphoid with no mass, tenderness, or organ enlargement. The vaginal introitus is moderately inflamed. There is a frothy vaginal discharge. The cervix is mildly injected, and there are a few punctate hyperemic areas. The fundus and adnexa are normal. The rectal examination is normal, and the test for occult blood in the feces is negative.

- What other data—if any—regarding the physical examination might be important?
- What office diagnostic test(s) might you perform, and what are you likely to find?
- What specimens—if any—might you send to the laboratory?
- If the vaginal discharge were thick and purulent, what might you do differently? Explain.

Assessment

- What is the probable etiologic diagnosis? How will you explain this to the patient?
- What—if any—is the likely relationship to her menses?
- What are some concerns that the patient might like to address? How would you give "permission" to address these issues?
- What are the possible family issues in this case? How might you address these?

Plan

- What are your specific therapeutic recommendations? How will you explain these to Mrs. Harris?
- What is your advice regarding her activities, including sexual intercourse?
- Mrs. Harris asks what she can do to prevent recurrence. How would you reply?
- What follow-up would you advise?

17
Disorders of the Back and Neck

WALTER L. CALMBACH

Disorders of the Back

Low back pain is a common and costly medical problem. The lifetime prevalence of low back pain is estimated to be 70% to 85%, while the point prevalence is approximately 30%.[1] Each year, 2% of all American workers have a compensable back injury, and 14% lose at least one workday due to low back pain.[2] Among chronic conditions, back problems are the most frequent cause for limitation of activity (work, housekeeping, school) among patients under 45 years of age.[3] Acute low back pain is the fifth most common reason for a visit to the physician, accounting for 2.8% of all physician visits.[4] And nonsurgical low back pain is the fourth most common admission diagnosis for patients over 65.[5] Although difficult to estimate, the direct medical costs due to back pain totaled $33.6 billion in 1994. Indirect costs (i.e., lost productivity and compensation) are estimated to be as high as $43 billion.[6] In most cases, low back pain is treated successfully with a conservative regimen, supplemented by selective use of neuroradiologic imaging, and appropriate surgical intervention for a small minority of patients.[7]

Background

EPIDEMIOLOGY

Low back pain affects men and women equally, with the onset of symptoms between the ages of 30 and 50 years. It is the most common cause of work-related disability in people under 45 years of age, and is the most expensive cause of work-related disability.[8] Risk factors for the development of low back pain include heavy lifting and twisting, bodily vibration, obesity, and poor conditioning; however, low back pain is common even among patients without these risk factors.[1]

In cases of more severe back pain, occupational exposures are much more significant, including repetitive heavy lifting, pulling, or pushing, and exposures to industrial and vehicular vibrations. If even temporary work loss occurs, additional important risk factors include job dissatisfaction, supervisor ratings, and job environment (i.e., boring, repetitive tasks).[1] Factors associated with recurrence of low back pain include traumatic origin of first attack, sciatic pain, radiographic changes, alcohol abuse, specific job situations, and psychosocial stigmata.

Of patients with acute low back pain, only 1.5% develop sciatica (i.e., painful paresthesias and/or motor weakness in the distribution of a nerve root). However, the lifetime prevalence of sciatica is 40%, and sciatica afflicts 11% of patients with low back pain that lasts for more than 2 weeks.[9,10] Sciatica is associated with long-distance driving, truck driving, cigarette smoking, and repeated lifting in a twisted posture. It is most common in the fourth and fifth decades of life, and peaks in the fourth decade. Most patients with sciatica, even those with significant neurologic abnormalities, recover without surgery.[11] Only 5% to 10% of patients with persistent sciatica require surgery.[5,12]

Despite the incidence and prevalence of low back pain and sciatica, the major factor responsible for its societal impact is disability.[12] The National Center for Health Statistics estimates that 5.2 million Americans are disabled with low back pain, of whom 2.6 million are permanently disabled.[13] Between 70% and 90% of the total costs due to low back pain are incurred by the 4% to 5% of patients with temporary or permanent disability.[12] Risk factors for disability due to low back pain include poor health habits, job dissatisfaction, less appealing work environments, poor ratings by supervisors, psychologic disturbances, compensable injuries, and history of prior disability.[12] These same factors are associated with high failure rates for treatments of all types.

NATURAL HISTORY

Recovery from nonspecific low back pain is usually rapid. Approximately one third of patients are improved at 1 week, and two thirds at 7 weeks. However, recurrences are common, affecting 40% of patients within 6 months. Thus, "acute low back pain" is increasingly perceived as a chronic medical problem with intermittent exacerbations.[14]

Low back pain may originate from many structures, including paravertebral musculature, ligaments, the annulus fibrosus, the spinal nerve roots, the facet joints, the vertebral periosteum, fascia, or blood vessels. The most common causes of back pain include musculoligamentous injuries, degenerative changes in the intervertebal discs and facet joints, spinal stenosis, and lumbar disc herniation.[14]

The natural history of herniated lumbar disc is usually quite favorable. Only about 10% of patients who present with sciatica have sufficient pain at 6 weeks that surgery is considered. Sequential magnetic resonance imaging (MRI) shows gradual regression of the herniated disc material over time, with partial or complete resolution in two thirds of patients by 6 months.[14] Acute disc herniation has changed little from its description in the classic article of Mixter and Barr: the annulus fibrosus begins to deteriorate by age 30, which leads to partial or complete herniation of the nucleus pulposus, causing irritation and compression of adjacent nerve roots.[5,15,16] Usually this herniation is in the posterolateral position, producing unilateral symptoms. Occasionally, the disc will herniate in the midline, and a large herniation in this location can cause bilateral symptoms. More than 95% of lumbar disc herniations occur at the L4–L5 or L5–S1 levels.[10] Involvement of the L5 nerve root results in weakness of the great toe extensors and dorsiflexors of the foot, and sensory loss at the dorsum of the foot and in the first web space. Involvement of the S1 nerve root results in a diminished ankle reflex, weakness of the plantar flexors, and sensory loss at the posterior calf and lateral foot.

Among patients who present with low back pain, 90% recover within 6 weeks with or without therapy.[17] Even in industrial settings, 75% of patients with symptoms of acute low back pain return to work within 1 month.[17] Only 2% to 3% of patients continue to have symptoms at 6 months, and only 1% at 1 year. However, symptoms of low back pain recur in approximately 60% of cases over the next 2 years.

Demographic characteristics such as age, gender, race, or ethnicity do not appear to influence the natural history of low back pain. Obesity, smoking, and occupation, however, are important influences.[18] Adults in the upper fifth quintile of height and weight are more likely to report low back pain lasting for 2 or more weeks.[9,18] Occupational factors that prolong or delay recovery from acute low back pain include heavier job requirements, job dissatisfaction, repetitious or boring jobs, poor employer evaluations, and noisy or unpleasant working conditions.[16] Psychosocial factors play an important role in the natural history of low back pain, modulating response to pain, and promoting illness behavior. The generally favorable natural history of acute low back pain is significantly influenced by a variety of medical and psychosocial factors that the practicing physician must be familiar with in order to counsel patients regarding prognosis and treatment.

Clinical Presentation

HISTORY

Low back pain is a symptom that has many causes. When approaching the patient with low back pain, the physician should consider three important issues: Is a systemic disease causing the pain? Is the patient experiencing social or psychosocial stresses that may amplify or prolong the pain? Does the patient have signs of neurologic compromise that may require surgical evaluation?[14] Useful items on medical history include: age, fever, history of cancer, unexplained weight loss, injection drug use, chronic infection, duration of pain, presence of nighttime pain, response to previous therapy, whether pain is relieved by bed rest or the supine position, persistent adenopathy, steroid use, and previous history of tuberculosis.[14] Factors that aggravate or alleviate low back pain should also be elicited. Nonmechanical back pain is usually continuous, while mechanical back pain is aggravated by motion and relieved by rest. Low back pain that worsens with cough has traditionally been associated with disc herniation, although recent data indicate that mechanical low back pain also worsens with cough. The presence of leg weakness or leg paresthesias in a nerve root distribution is consistent with disc herniation. Bowel or bladder incontinence with or without saddle paresthesias suggests the cauda equina syndrome; this is a surgical emergency and requires immediate referral to a surgeon. Hip pain can mimic low back pain, and is often referred to the groin, the anterior thigh, or the knee, and is worsened with ambulation. Patients with osteoarthritis or degenerative joint disease report morning stiffness, which improves as the day progresses. Patients with spinal stenosis report symptoms suggestive of spinal claudication, that is, neurologic symptoms in the legs that worsen with ambulation. Spinal claudication is differentiated from vascular claudication in that the symptoms of spinal claudication have a slower onset and slower resolution. A history of pain at rest, pain in the recumbent position, or pain at night suggests infection or tumor as a cause for low back pain. Osteoporosis is a consideration among postmenopausal women or women who have undergone oophorectomy. These patients report severe, localized, unrelenting pain after even "minor" trauma. Patients who present writhing in pain suggest the presence of an intraabdominal process or vascular cause for the pain, such as abdominal aortic aneurysm.

PHYSICAL EXAMINATION

The initial examination is fairly detailed. With the patient standing and appropriately gowned, the examining physician notes the stance and gait, as well as the presence or absence of the normal curvature of the spine (e.g., thoracic kyphosis, lumbar lordosis, splinting to one side, scoliosis). The range of motion of the back is documented, including flexion, lateral bending, and rotation. Intact dorsiflexion and plantar flexion of the foot is determined by observing heel-walk and toe-walk. Intact knee extension is determined by observing the patient squat and rise, while keeping the back straight.

With the patient seated, a distracted straight-leg raising test is applied. With the hip flexed at 90 degrees, the flexed knee is brought to full extension. A positive straight-leg raising test reproduces the patient's paresthesias in the distribution of a nerve root at <60 degrees of knee extension. Sensation to light touch and pinprick are examined and motor strength of hip and knee flexors is tested. The deep tendon reflexes are tested [knee jerk (L4), ankle jerk (S1)] and long tract signs are elicited by applying Babinski's maneuver (Table 17.1).

With the patient in the supine position, the straight-leg raising test is repeated. With the hip and knee extended, the leg is raised (i.e., the hip is flexed). A positive test reproduces the patient's paresthesias in the distribution of a nerve root. Isolated low back pain does not indicate a positive straight-leg raising test. The crossed straight-leg raising test (i.e., reproduction of the patient's symptoms by straight-leg raising of the contralateral leg) is very specific for acute disc herniation, and suggests a large central disc herniation. The examining physician should realize that the straight-leg raising test is sensitive but not specific, while

TABLE 17.1. Motor, Sensory, and Deep Tendon Reflex Patterns Associated with Commonly Affected Nerve Roots

Nerve root	Motor reflexes	Sensory reflexes	Deep tendon reflexes
C5	Deltoid	Lateral arm	Biceps jerk (C5,C6)
C6	Biceps, brachioradialis, wrist extensors	Lateral forearm	Brachioradialis
C7	Triceps, wrist flexors, MCP extensors	Middle of hand, middle finger	Triceps jerk
C8	MCP flexors	Medial forearm	—
T1	Abductors and adductors of fingers	Medial arm	—
L4	Quadriceps	Anterior thigh	Knee jerk
L5	Dorsiflex foot and great toe	Dorsum of foot	Hamstring reflex (L5, S1)
S1	Plantarflex foot	Lateral foot, posterior calf	Ankle jerk

MCP = metacarpophalangeal.

the crossed straight-leg raising test is specific but not sensitive.[14] Hip range of motion is then tested, and pain radiation to the groin, anteromedial thigh, or knee is documented.

A more detailed examination may be necessary in selected patients. If significant pathology is suspected in a male patient, the cremasteric reflex is tested, i.e., application of a sharp stimulus at the proximal medial thigh should normally cause retraction of the ipsilateral scrotum. With the patient in the prone position, the femoral stretch test is applied. While the hip and knee are in extension, the knee is flexed, placing increased stretch on the femoral nerve, which includes elements from the L2, L3, and L4 nerve roots (i.e., the prone knee-bending test). The hamstring reflex is tested by striking the semitendinosus and semimembranosus tendons at the medial aspect of the popliteal fossa. The hamstring reflex involves both the L5 and S1 nerve roots. Thus, an absent or decreased hamstring reflex in the presence of a normal ankle jerk response (S1) implies involvement of the L5 nerve root (Table 17.1). Sensation in the area between the upper buttocks is tested, as well as the anal reflex and anal sphincter tone (S2, S3, S4).

The clinical diagnosis of acute disc herniation requires repeated physical examination demonstrating pain or paresthesias localized to a specific nerve root, with reproduction of pain on straight-leg raising tests, and muscle weakness in the nerve appropriate root distribution.

Diagnosis

RADIOLOGY

Plain Radiographs. Plain radiographs are usually not helpful in diagnosing acute low back pain, because they cannot demonstrate soft tissue sprains and strains, or an acute herniated disc. However, plain radiographs are useful in ruling out conditions such as vertebral fracture, spondylolisthesis, spondylolysis, infection, tumor, or inflammatory spondyloarthropathy[5,19] (Fig. 17.1). In the absence of neurologic deficits, plain radiographs in the evaluation of low back pain should be reserved for patients over 50 years of age, patients with a temperature >38°C, patients with anemia, a history of trauma, previous cancer, pain at rest, or unexplained weight loss, drug or alcohol abuse, steroid use, diabetes mellitus, or any other reason for immunosuppression.[20] For selected patients, initial plain radiographs of the spine in the early evaluation of acute low back pain should include anteroposterior and lateral views of the lumbar spine.[15] Oblique views are used to rule out spondylolysis, particularly when evaluating acute low back

A

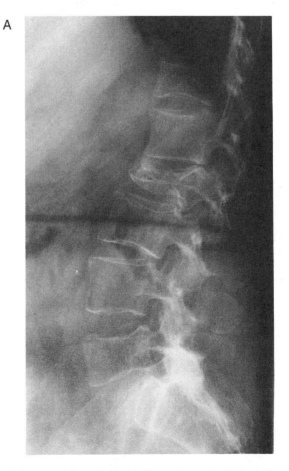

FIGURE 17.1. Radiologic studies of the lumbar spine. (A) Plain radiograph demonstrating a compression fracture of the L2 vertebral body due to multiple myeloma. (B) CT scan demonstrating nucleus pulposus herniating posteriorly into the spinal canal. (C) MRI demonstrating an enhancing intramedullary metastatic lesion in the cauda equina at the L1 level.

B

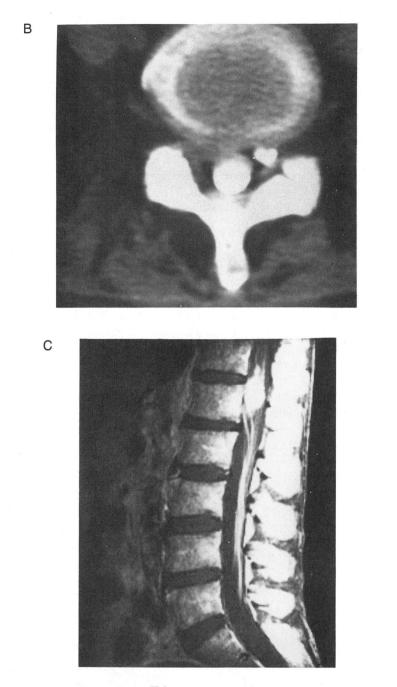

C

FIGURE 17.1. (*Continued*)

pain in young athletic patients active in sports such as football, wrestling, gymnastics, diving, figure skating, or ballet.[21] If the patient's pain fails to improve after 4 to 6 weeks of conservative therapy, radiographs should be obtained; such patients may be at risk for vertebral infection, cancer, or inflammatory disease.[22]

For patients 65 years of age and older, diagnoses such as cancer, compression fracture, spinal stenosis, and aortic aneurysm become more common. Osteoporotic fracture may occur even in the absence of trauma. Because hormone replacement therapy and other medications may prevent further fractures, early radiography is recommended for older patients with back pain.[14]

Radiographic abnormalities are nonspecific and are observed equally in patients with and without symptoms of low back pain.[23] Clinical correlation is essential before symptoms of low back pain can be attributed to radiographic abnormalities.

CT, MRI, and Myelogram.   Computed tomography (CT), myelogram, and magnetic resonance imaging (MRI) each has a specific role in evaluating a select subset of patients with low back pain. Physicians must be aware that many asymptomatic patients demonstrate disc bulging, protrusion, and even extrusion.[5,24] For example, 30% to 40% of CT scans and 64% of MRIs demonstrate abnormalities of the intervertebral disc in asymptomatic patients.[7,24]

CT or MRI should be reserved for patients in whom there is strong clinical suggestion of underlying infection or cancer, progressive or persistent neurologic deficit, or cauda equina syndrome.[5,14] CT or MRI should be considered for patients who show no response to a 4- to 6-week course of conservative therapy.[5] CT and MRI are equally effective in detecting disc herniation and spinal stenosis, but MRI is more sensitive in detecting infection, metastatic cancer, and neural tumors.[14] Myelography is useful in differentiating significant disc herniation from incidental disc bulging not responsible for the patient's signs or symptoms, but has largely been replaced by noninvasive techniques such as MRI or CT.[15] CT myelography is sometimes used in planning surgery.[14]

ANCILLARY TESTS

Because plain radiographs are not highly sensitive for detection of early cancer or vertebral infection, tests such as erythrocyte sedimentation rate (ESR) and complete blood count (CBC) should be obtained for selected patients.[14,25]

Differential Diagnosis

OSTEOARTHRITIS

Osteoarthritis of the vertebral spine is common in later life, and is especially prevalent in the cervical and lumbar spine (also see Chapter 18). Typically, the pain of osteoarthritis of the spine is worse in the morning, increases with motion, but is relieved by rest. It is associated with morning stiffness, and a decreased range of motion of the spine in the absence of systemic symptoms. The severity of symptoms does not correlate well with radiographic findings, and patients with severe degenerative changes on plain radiographs may be asymptomatic, while patients with symptoms suggestive of osteoarthritis of the spine may have minimal radiologic findings. In some patients, extensive osteophytic changes may lead to compression of lumbar nerve roots or may even cause cauda equina syndrome.

SPINAL STENOSIS

Spinal stenosis is a common cause of back pain among older adults. Symptoms usually begin in the sixth decade, and over time the patient's posture becomes progressively flexed forward. The mean age of patients at the time of surgery for spinal stenosis is 55 years, with an average symptom duration of 4 years.[10] The symptoms of spinal stenosis are often diffuse because the disease is usually bilateral and involves several vertebrae. Pain, numbness, and tingling may occur in one or both legs. Pseudoclaudication is the classic symptom of spinal stenosis. Pseudoclaudication is differentiated from vascular claudication in that pseudoclaudication has a slower onset and a slower resolution of symptoms.[7]

Symptoms are usually relieved with flexion (e.g., sitting, pushing a grocery cart) and exacerbated by back extension. Plain radiographs often show osteophytes at several levels, but as mentioned earlier, caution must be used in ascribing back pain to these degenerative changes. CT or MRI may be used to confirm the diagnosis. Electromyography (EMG) or somatosensory evoked potentials may be used to differentiate the pain of spinal stenosis from peripheral neuropathy. The natural history of spinal stenosis is such that patients tend to remain stable or slowly worsen. Symptoms evolve gradually, but about 15% of patients improve over a period of about 4 years, 70% remain stable, and 15% experience worsening symptoms.[14] Nonoperative therapy for spinal stenosis includes leg strengthening and avoidance of alcohol to reduce the risk of falls, and physical activity such as walking or using an exercise bicycle is also recommended.[27] Decompressive laminectomy may be necessary for selected patients with spinal stenosis who have persistent severe pain. Although treatment for spinal stenosis must be individualized, recent reports suggest that patients treated surgically have better outcomes at 4 years than patients treated nonsurgically, even after adjusting for differences in baseline characteristics.[28] However, at 4-year follow-up, 30% of patients still have severe pain and 10% have undergone reoperation.[28]

OSTEOPOROSIS

Osteoporosis is a common problem among seniors, affecting up to 25% of women over 65. Decreased bone mineral density in the vertebral body is associated with an increased risk for spinal compression fractures. In primary care settings, 4% of patients who present with acute low back pain have compression fractures as the cause.[14] Pain symptoms are worse with prolonged sitting or standing, and usually resolve over 3 to 4 months as compression fractures heal.[6] African-

American and Mexican-American women have only one fourth as many compression fractures as European-American women.[5] Patients with compression fractures due to osteoporosis usually have no neurologic complaints and do not suffer from neural compression. Plain radiographs document a loss of vertebral body height due to compression fractures. Laboratory tests are normal in primary osteoporosis, and any abnormalities should prompt a search for secondary causes of osteoporosis. The diagnosis of primary osteoporosis is made on clinical grounds, i.e., diffuse osteopenia, compression fractures, and normal laboratory findings.[29,30]

NEOPLASIA

Multiple myeloma is the most common primary malignancy of the vertebral spine. However, metastatic lesions are the most common cause of cancers of the spine, arising from breast, lung, prostate, thyroid, renal, or gastrointestinal tract primary tumors. Both Hodgkin's and non-Hodgkin's lymphomas frequently involve the vertebral spine. Because the primary site of the tumor is often overlooked, back pain is the presenting complaint for many cancers. In primary care settings, 0.7% of patients who present with low back pain have cancer as the cause.[10,25] Findings significantly associated with cancer as the cause of low back pain include age >50 years, previous history of cancer, pain lasting >1 month, failure to improve with conservative therapy, elevated ESR, and anemia.[25] Patients report a dull constant pain that is worse at night, and not relieved by rest or the recumbent position. Typical radiographic changes may be absent early in the course of vertebral body tumors. A technetium bone scan is usually positive due to increased blood flow and reactive bone formation; however, in multiple myeloma and metastatic thyroid cancer, the bone scan may be negative.[31] Greater diagnostic specificity and improved cost-effectiveness can be achieved by using a higher cut-off point for the ESR (e.g., >50 mm/hr) combined with either a bone scan followed by MRI as indicated, or MRI alone.[32] Symptomatic cancer of the lumbar spine is an ominous sign with a potential for devastating morbidity due to spinal cord injury.[33] Early recognition and treatment are essential if irreversible cord damage is to be avoided.

POSTERIOR FACET SYNDROME

The posterior facet syndrome is caused by degenerative changes in the posterior facet joints. These are true diarthrodial joints that sometimes develop degenerative joint changes visible on plain radiographs. Degenerative changes in the posterior facet joints cause a dull achy pain that radiates to the groin, hip, or thigh, and is worsened with twisting or hyperextension of the spine.[34] Steroid injection into the posterior facet joints to relieve presumed posterior facet joint pain is a popular procedure, but the placebo effect of injection in this area is significant and controlled studies have failed to demonstrate benefit from steroid injections.[35,36] The presence of degenerative changes in the facet joints on plain radiographs does not imply that the posterior facets are the cause of the patient's pain. Caution must be used in ascribing the patient's symptoms to these degenerative changes. Historically, the posterior facet syndrome was diagnosed by demonstrating pain relief after injection of local anesthetic into the posterior facet joints, but recent studies cast doubt on the validity of this procedure.[7,34] Several factors have been proposed to identify subjects who might benefit from lidocaine injection into lumbar facet joints: pain relieved in the supine position, age >65, and low back pain not worsened by coughing, hyperextension, forward flexion, rising from flexion, or extension-rotation.[37] However, a recent systematic review concluded that while facet joint injection provided some short-term relief, this benefit was not statistically significant; therefore, convincing evidence is lacking regarding the effects of facet joint injection therapy on low back pain.[38]

ANKYLOSING SPONDYLITIS

Ankylosing spondylitis is a spondyloarthropathy most commonly affecting men under 40 years of age. Patients present with mild to moderate low back pain that is centered in the back and radiates to the posterior thighs. In its initial presentation, the symptoms are vague and the diagnosis is often overlooked. Pain symptoms are intermittent, but decreased range of motion in the spine remains constant. Early signs of ankylosing spondylitis include limitation of chest expansion, tenderness of the sternum, and decreased range of motion and flexion contractures at the hip. Inflammatory involvement of the knees or hips increases the likelihood of spondylitis.[39] The radiologic hallmarks of ankylosing spondylitis include periarticular destructive changes, obliteration of the sacroiliac joints, development of syndesmophytes on the margins of the vertebral bodies, and bridging of these osteophytes by bone between vertebral bodies, the so-called bamboo spine. Laboratory analysis is negative for rheumatoid factor, but the ESR is elevated early in the course of the disease. Tests for human leukocyte antigen (HLA)-B27 are not recommended because as many as 6% of an unselected population test positive for this antigen.[15]

VISCERAL DISEASES

Several visceral diseases may present with back pain as a chief symptom.[5] These include nephrolithiasis, endometriosis, and abdominal aortic aneurysm. Abdominal aortic aneurysm causes low back pain by compression of surrounding tissues or by extension or rupture of the aneurysm. Patients report dull steady back pain unrelated to activity, which radiates to the hips or thighs. Patients with an acute rupture or extension of the aneurysm report severe tearing pain, diaphoresis, or syncope, and demonstrate signs of circulatory shock.[29]

CAUDA EQUINA SYNDROME

The cauda equina syndrome is a rare condition caused by severe compression of the cauda equina, usually by a large midline disc herniation or a tumor.[14] The patient may report urinary retention with overflow incontinence, as well as bilateral sciatica, leg weakness, and sensory loss in a saddle distribution. Patients with these findings represent a true surgical emergency, and should be referred immediately for surgical treatment and decompression.

PSYCHOSOCIAL FACTORS

Psychological factors are frequently associated with complaints of low back pain, influencing both patient pain symptoms and therapeutic outcome.[40] Features that suggest psychological causes of low back pain include nonorganic signs and symptoms, dissociation between verbal and nonverbal pain behaviors, compensable cause of injury, joblessness, disability-seeking, depression, anxiety, requests for narcotics or other psychoactive drugs, and repeated failure of multiple treatments.[41] Prolonged back pain may be associated with failure of previous treatment, depression, or somatization.[14] Substance abuse, job dissatisfaction, pursuit of disability compensation and involvement in litigation are also associated with persistent unexplained symptoms.[8]

Management

NONSPECIFIC LOW BACK PAIN

For most patients, the best recommendation is rapid return to normal daily activities. However, patients should avoid heavy lifting, twisting, or bodily vibration in the acute phase.[14] A 4- to 6-week trial of conservative therapy is appropriate in the absence of cauda equina syndrome or a rapidly progressive neurologic deficit (Table 17.2).

BED REST

Bed rest does not increase the speed of recovery from acute back pain, and sometimes delays recovery.[42,43] Symptomatic relief from back pain may benefit from 1 or 2 days of bed rest, but patients should be told that it is safe to get out of bed even if pain persists.[14]

MEDICATIONS

Antiinflammatories.   Nonsteroidal antiinflammatory drugs (NSAIDs) are effective for short-term symptomatic relief in patients with acute low back pain.[44] There does not seem to be a specific type of NSAID that is clearly more effective than others.[44] Therapy is titrated to provide pain relief at a minimal dose, and is continued for 4 to 6 weeks. NSAIDs should not be continued indefinitely, but rather prescribed for a specific period.[3]

Muscle Relaxants.   Although evidence for the effectiveness of muscle relaxants is scant, the main value of muscle relaxants is less for muscle relaxation than for their sedative effect. Diazepam (Valium), cyclobenzaprine (Flexeril), and metho-

TABLE 17.2. Nonoperative Treatment Considerations for Low Back Pain and Sciatica

Treatment	Acute low back pain	Acute sciatica	Subacute low back pain and leg pain	Chronic low back pain and leg pain
Bedrest	Avoid	Avoid	Avoid	Avoid, short-term for flare-ups only
NSAIDs	Symptomatic pain relief, time-limited	Symptomatic pain relief, time-limited	Selected cases if effective	Avoid long-term
Muscle relaxants	Optimal 1 week; maximum 2–4 weeks	Optimal 1 week; maximum 2–4 weeks	Selected cases if effective	Avoid long-term
Opioids	No	Optimal 1–3 days; maximum 2–3 weeks	Selected presurgical cases; avoid	Avoid
Antidepressants	No	No	Selected cases	Yes
Local injections	No	No	Selected cases as an adjunct	Flare-ups
Facet injections	No	No	No	Avoid; no long-term effect alone
Epidural corticosteroids	No	Yes	Flare-ups, if effective	Flare-ups only; avoid
Orthoses	Adjunctive	No	Adjunctive	Adjunctive
Cryotherapy (ice)	Adjunctive	Adjunctive	Flare-ups	Flare-ups; self-applied
Thermotherapy	Adjunctive	Adjunctive	Adjunctive	Flare-ups; self-applied
Traction	No	No	No	No
Joint manipulation	Not recommended for first 3–4 weeks	Not with neural signs	If effective; maximum 2–4 months	Flare-ups; time-contingent if effective
Joint mobilization	Yes, if effective	Yes, if effective	If effective; maximum 2–4 months	Flare-ups; time-contingent if effective

TABLE 17.2. Nonoperative Treatment Considerations for Low Back Pain and Sciatica (*Continued*)

Treatment	Acute low back pain	Acute sciatica	Subacute low back pain and leg pain	Chronic low back pain and leg pain
Soft tissue techniques (massage, myofascial release, mobilization)	Yes, if effective	Yes, if effective	If effective; maximum 2–4 months	Flare-ups; time-contingent if effective
McKenzie exercises	No	No	Flare-ups, if effective	Flare-ups, if effective
Dynamic lumbar stabilization	No	No	Yes	Yes
Back school	Yes	Yes	Yes	Yes
Functional restoration	No	No	Yes	Optimal 3–4 months; maximum 4–6 months
Pain clinic	No	No	No	Yes

NSAID = nonsteroidal antiinflammatory drug.
Source: Adapted from Wheeler,[41] with permission. Copyright © American Academy of Family Physicians. All rights reserved.

350

carbamol (Robaxin) are commonly used as muscle relaxants, and carisoprodol (Soma) has documented effectiveness.[3] Muscle relaxants should be prescribed in a time-limited fashion, usually less than 2 weeks. Muscle relaxants and narcotics are not recommended for patients who present with complaints of chronic low back pain (i.e., low back pain of greater than 3 months' duration).[5]

UNPROVEN TREATMENTS

Traction is not recommended for the treatment of acute low back pain.[45] No scientific evidence supports the efficacy of corsets or braces in the treatment of acute low back pain, and these treatments are not recommended.[5] Transcutaneous electrical nerve stimulation (TENS) is not effective in the treatment of low back pain.[46]

EXERCISE

Back exercises are not useful in the acute phase of low back pain, but are useful later for preventing recurrences.[14] Guidelines from the Agency for Health Care Policy and Research (AHCPR) stress aerobic exercise (e.g., walking, biking, swimming) especially during the first 2 weeks; continuing ordinary activities improves recovery and leads to less disability.[22] However, a recent systematic review concluded that specific back exercises do not improve clinical outcomes.[47] There is moderate evidence that flexion exercises are not effective in the treatment of acute low back pain, and strong evidence that extension exercises are not effective in the treatment of acute low back pain.

SPINAL MANIPULATION

Clinical trials suggest that spinal manipulation has some efficacy.[48,49] Current recommendations are that patients should not be referred for spinal manipulation unless pain persists for more than 3 weeks because half of patients spontaneously improve during this time frame.[14]

BACK SCHOOL

A recent systematic review concluded that there is moderate evidence that back schools are not more effective than other treatments for acute low back pain.[50]

ACUPUNCTURE

A recent systematic qualitative review concluded that there is no evidence to show that acupuncture is more effective than no treatment, moderate evidence to show that acupuncture is not more effective than trigger point injection or TENS, and limited evidence to show that acupuncture is not more effective than placebo or sham procedure for the treatment of chronic low back pain.[51] Therefore, acupuncture is not recommended as a regular treatment for patients with low back pain.

Herniated Intervertebral Disc

Early treatment resembles that for nonspecific low back pain, outlined above. However, for patients with suspected lumbar disc herniation, the role of spinal manipulation is not clear. Narcotic analgesics may be necessary for pain relief for some patients with herniated intervertebral disc, but these medications should be used in a time-limited (i.e., not symptom-limited) manner.[14] Epidural corticosteroid injection may offer temporary symptomatic relief for some patients.[52] However, this invasive procedure offers no significant functional improvement, and does not reduce the need for surgery.[52] If neuropathic pain persists and/or neurologic deficits progress, CT or MRI should be performed, and surgery should be considered.[14]

SURGERY

Background. The rate of lumbar surgery in the United States is 40% higher than in most developed nations, and five times higher than in England and Scotland.[53] The lifetime prevalence of lumbar spine surgery ranges between 1% and 3%, and 2% to 3% of patients with low back pain may be surgical candidates on the basis of sciatica alone.[12] Surgery rates vary widely by geographical region in the U.S., and have risen dramatically in the last 10 years.[54] Psychological factors influence postsurgical outcomes more strongly than initial physical examination or surgical findings. Prior to surgery, patients should be evaluated with standard pain indices, activities of daily living scales, and psychometric testing. Surgical results for treating symptomatic lumbar disc herniation unresponsive to conservative therapy are excellent in well-selected patients.[55]

Indications. There is no evidence from clinical trials or cohort studies that surgery is effective for patients who have low back pain unless they have sciatica, pseudoclaudication, or spondylolisthesis.[56] In the absence of cauda equina syndrome or progressive neurologic deficit, patients with suspected lumbar disc herniation should be treated nonsurgically for at least a month.[14] The primary benefit of discectomy is to provide more rapid relief of sciatica in patients who have failed to resolve with conservative management.[56] In well-selected patients, 75% have complete relief of sciatic symptoms after surgery and an additional 15% have partial relief. Patients with clear symptoms of radicular pain have the best surgical outcome, while those with the least evidence of radiculopathy have the poorest surgical outcome.[57] Relief of back pain itself is less consistent. Appropriate patient selection is key to successful surgical outcome.

Options. Standard discectomy is the most common procedure used to relieve symptomatic disc herniation. A posterior longitudinal incision is made over the involved disc space, a variable amount of bone is removed, the ligamentum flavum is incised, and herniated disc material is excised. This procedure allows adequate visualization and yields satisfactory results among 65% to 85% of patients.[11,58] Recent reports suggest that patients who undergo surgical therapy have greater improvement of their symptoms and greater functional recovery at 4 years than patients treated nonoperatively[59]; however, work status and disability status were similar between these two groups. Previous studies have shown that there is no clear benefit to surgery at 10-year follow-up.[11]

Microdiscectomy allows smaller incisions, little or no bony excision, and removal of disc material under magnification. This procedure has fewer complications, fewer unsuccessful outcomes, and permits faster recovery. However, rates of reoperation are significantly higher in patients initially treated with microdiscectomy, presumably due to missed disc fragments or operating at the wrong spinal level.[58] A recent systematic review concluded that the clinical outcomes for patients after microdiscectomy are comparable to those of standard discectomy.[56]

Percutaneous discectomy is an outpatient procedure performed under local anesthesia in which the surgeon uses an automated percutaneous cutting and suction probe to aspirate herniated disc material. This procedure results in lower rates of nerve injury, postoperative instability, infection, fibrosis, and chronic pain syndromes. However, patients undergoing percutaneous discectomy sustain unacceptably high rates of recurrent disc herniation. Only 29% of patients reported satisfactory results after percutaneous discectomy, while 80% of subjects were satisfied after microdiscectomy.[60] A recent systematic review concluded that only 10% to 15% of patients with herniated nucleus pulposus requiring surgery might be suitable candidates for percutaneous discectomy.[56] This procedure is not recommended for patients with previous back surgery, sequestered disc fragments, bony entrapment, or multiple herniated discs.[58,61]

For the time being, automated percutaneous discectomy and laser discectomy should be regarded as research techniques.[56] Arthroscopic discectomy is an emerging technique that shows promising results and effectiveness similar to that of standard discectomy.[62]

Chemonucleolysis is a procedure in which a proteolytic enzyme (chymopapain) is injected into the disc space to dissolve herniated disc material. A recent systematic review concluded that chemonucleolysis is effective for the treatment patients with low back pain due to herniated nucleus pulposus, and is more effective than placebo.[56] However, chemonucleolysis showed consistently poorer results than standard discectomy. Approximately 30% of patients undergoing chemonucleolysis had further disc surgery within 2 years. Proponents of chemonucleolysis have suggested that it may be associated with lower costs, but readmission for a second procedure negates this putative advantage. Chemonucleolysis may be indicated for selected patients as an intermediate stage between conservative and surgical management.[56]

Complications.   Complications of surgery on the lumbar spine are largely related to patient age, gender, diagnosis, and type of procedure.[63] Mortality rates increase substantially with age, but are <1% even among patients over 75 years of age. Mortality rates are higher for men, but morbidity rates and likelihood of discharge to a nursing home are significantly higher for women, particularly

women over 75. With regard to underlying diagnosis, complications and duration of hospitalization are highest after surgery to correct spinal stenosis, degenerative changes, or instability, and are lowest for procedures to correct herniated
disc. With regard to type of procedure, complications and duration of hospitalization are highest for procedures involving arthrodesis with or without laminectomy, followed by laminectomy alone or with discectomy, and are lowest for
discectomy alone. Other surgical complications include thromboembolism (1.7%)
and infection (2.9%).[5]

SUMMARY

The physician's goal in treating patients with low back pain is to promote activity and early return to work. While it is important to rule out significant pathology as the cause of low back pain, most patients can be reassured that symptoms
are due to simple musculoligamentous injury.[14] Patients should be counseled that
they will improve with time, usually quite quickly.

Bed rest is not recommended for the treatment of low back pain or sciatica;
rather, a rapid return to normal activities is usually the best course.[14] Nonsteroidal
antiinflammatory drugs can be used in a time-limited way for symptomatic relief.[44]
Back exercises are not useful for acute low back pain, but can help prevent recurrence of back pain and can be used to treat patients with chronic low back pain.[14]
Work activities may be modified at first, but avoiding iatrogenic disability is key
to successful management of acute low back pain.[5,41] Surgery should be reserved
for patients with progressive neurologic deficit or those who have sciatica or
pseudoclaudication that persists after nonoperative therapy has failed.[14]

Chronic Low Back Pain

Chronic low back pain (i.e., pain persisting for more than 3 months) is a special
problem that warrants careful consideration. Patients presenting with a history of
chronic low back pain require an extensive diagnostic workup on at least one occasion, including in-depth history, physical examination, and the appropriate imaging techniques (plain radiographs, CT, or MRI).

Management of patients with chronic back pain should be aimed at restoring
normal function.[47] Exercises may be useful in the treatment of chronic low back
pain if they aim at improving return to normal daily activities and work.[47] A recent systematic review concluded that exercise therapy is as effective as physiotherapy (e.g., hot packs, massage, mobilization, short-wave diathermy, ultrasound, stretching, flexibility, electrotherapy) for patients with chronic low back
pain.[47] And there is strong evidence that exercise is more effective than "usual
care." Evidence is lacking about the effectiveness of flexion and extension exercises for patients with chronic low back pain.[47]

Although one literature synthesis cast doubt on the effectiveness of antidepressant therapy for chronic low back pain,[64] it is widely used and recommended.[14] Antidepressant therapy is useful for the one third of patients with

chronic low back pain who also have depression. Tricyclic antidepressants may be more effective for treating pain in patients without depression than selective serotonin reuptake inhibitors.[65] However, narcotic analgesics are not recommended for patients with chronic low back pain.[14]

A recent systematic review concluded that there is moderate evidence that back schools have better short-term effects than other treatments for chronic low back pain, and moderate evidence that back schools in an occupational setting are more effective compared to placebo or "waiting list" controls.[50] Functional restoration programs combine intense physical therapy with cognitive-behavioral interventions and increasing levels of task-oriented rehabilitation and work simulation.[41] Patients with chronic low back pain may require referral to a multidisciplinary pain clinic for optimal management. Such clinics can offer cognitive behavioral therapy, patient education classes, supervised exercise programs, and selective nerve blocks to facilitate return to normal function.[14] Complete relief of symptoms may be an unrealistic goal; instead, patients and physicians should try to optimize daily functioning.

Prevention

Prevention of low back injury and consequent disability is an important challenge in primary care. Pre-employment physical examination screening is not effective in reducing the occurrence of job-related low back pain. However, active aerobically fit individuals have fewer back injuries, miss fewer workdays, and report fewer back pain symptoms.[66] Evidence to support smoking cessation and weight loss as means of reducing the occurrence of low back pain is sparse, but these should be recommended for other health reasons.[66] Exercise programs that combine aerobic conditioning with specific strengthening of the back and legs can reduce the frequency of recurrence of low back pain.[44,66] The use of corsets and education about lifting technique are generally ineffective in preventing low back problems.[67,68] Ergonomic redesign of strenuous tasks may facilitate return to work and reduce chronic pain.[69]

Disorders of the Neck

CERVICAL RADICULOPATHY

Cervical radiculopathy is a common cause of neck pain, and can be caused by a herniated cervical disc, osteophytic changes, compressive pathology, or hypermobility of the cervical spine. The lifetime prevalence of neck and arm pain among adults may be as high as 51%. Risk factors associated with neck pain include heavy lifting, smoking, diving, working with vibrating heavy equipment, and possibly riding in cars.[70]

Cervical nerve roots exit the spine above the corresponding vertebral body (e.g., the C5 nerve root exits above C5). Therefore, disc herniation at the C4-C5 interspace causes symptoms in the distribution of C5.[71] Radicular symptoms may be caused by a "soft disc" (i.e., disc herniation) or by a "hard disc" (i.e., osteophyte formation and foraminal encroachment).[71] The most commonly involved interspaces are C5-6, C6-7, C4-5, C3-4, and C7-T1.[70]

The symptoms of cervical radiculopathy may be single or multiple, unilateral or bilateral, symmetrical or asymmetrical.[72] Acute cervical radiculopathy is commonly due to a tear of the annulus fibrosus with prolapse of the nucleus pulposus, and is usually the result of mild to moderate trauma. Subacute symptoms are usually due to long-standing spondylosis accompanied by mild trauma or overuse. The majority of patients with subacute cervical radiculopathy experience resolution of their symptoms within 6 weeks with rest and analgesics. Chronic radiculopathy is more common in middle age or old age, and patients present with complaints of neck or arm pain due to heavy labor or unaccustomed activity.[72–74]

Cervical radiculopathy rarely progresses to myelopathy, but as many as two thirds of patients treated conservatively report persistent symptoms. In severe cases of cervical radiculopathy in which motor function has been compromised, 98% of patients recover full motor function after decompressive laminectomy.[75]

CLINICAL PRESENTATION

Among patients with cervical radiculopathy, sensory symptoms are much more prominent than motor changes. Typically, patients report proximal pain and distal paresthesias.[71] The fifth, sixth, and seventh nerve roots are most commonly affected. Referred pain caused by cervical disc herniation is usually vague, diffuse, and lacking in the sharp quality of radicular pain. Pain referred from a herniated cervical disc may present as pain in the neck, pain at the top of the shoulder, or pain around the scapula.[72]

On physical examination, radicular pain increases with certain maneuvers such as neck range of motion, Valsalva maneuver, cough, or sneeze. Active and passive neck range of motion is tested, examining flexion, rotation, and lateral bending. Spurling's maneuver is useful in assessing neck pain: the examining physician flexes the patient's neck, then rolls the neck into lateral bending, and finally extends the neck. The examiner then applies a compressive load to the vertex of the skull. This maneuver narrows the cervical foramina posterolaterally, and may reproduce the patient's radicular symptoms.

DIAGNOSIS

The differential diagnosis of cervical nerve root pain includes cervical disc herniation, spinal canal tumor, trauma, degenerative changes, inflammatory disorders, congenital abnormalities, toxic and allergic conditions, hemorrhage, and musculoskeletal syndromes (e.g., thoracic outlet syndrome, shoulder pain).[71,75] In cases of cervical radiculopathy unresponsive to conservative therapy, or in the presence of progressive motor deficit, investigation of other pathologic processes is indicated. Plain radiographs are usually not helpful because abnormal radiographic findings are equally common among symptomatic and asymptomatic patients. CT scan, myelography, and MRI each has a specific role to play in the diagnosis of cervical radiculopathy.[73,74] CT scan is especially useful in delineating bony lesions, CT myelography can effectively demonstrate functional stenoses of the spinal canal, and MRI is an excellent noninvasive modality for demonstrating soft tissue abnormalities (e.g., herniated cervical disc, spinal cord derangement, extradural tumor).

MANAGEMENT

Immobilization. The purpose of neck immobilization is to reduce intervertebral motion which may cause compression, mechanical irritation, or stretching of the cervical nerve roots.[76] The soft cervical collar or the more rigid Philadelphia collar both hold the neck in slight flexion. The collar is useful in the acute setting, but prolonged use leads to deconditioning of the paracervical musculature. Therefore, the collar should be prescribed in a time-limited manner, and patients should be instructed to begin isometric neck exercises early in the course of therapy.

Bed Rest. Bed rest is another form of immobilization that modifies the patient's activities and eliminates the axial compression forces of gravity.[76] Holding the neck in slight flexion is accomplished by arranging two standard pillows in a V shape with the apex pointed cranially, then placing a third pillow across the apex. This arrangement provides mild cervical flexion, and internally rotates the shoulder girdle, thereby relieving traction on the cervical nerve roots.

Medications. Nonsteroidal antiinflammatory drugs (NSAIDs) are particularly beneficial in relieving acute neck pain. However, side effects are common, and usually two or three medications must be tried before a beneficial result without unacceptable side effects is achieved. Muscle relaxants help relieve muscle spasm in some patients; alternatives include carisoprodol (Soma), methocarbamol (Robaxin), and diazepam (Valium). Narcotics may be useful in the acute setting, but should be prescribed in a strictly time-limited manner.[76] The physician should be alert to the possibility of addiction or abuse.

Physical Therapy. Moist heat (20 minutes, three times daily), ice packs (15 minutes, four times daily or even hourly), ultrasound therapy, and other modalities also help relieve the symptoms of cervical radiculopathy.[76]

Surgery. Surgical intervention is reserved for patients with cervical disc herniation confirmed by neuroradiologic imaging and radicular signs and symptoms that persist despite 4 to 6 weeks of conservative therapy.[71]

Cervical Myelopathy

The cause of pain in cervical myelopathy is not clearly understood but is presumed to be multifactorial, including vascular changes, cord hypoxia, changes in spinal canal diameter, and hypertrophic facets. Therefore, patients with cervical myelopathy present with a variable clinical picture. The usual course is one of increasing disability over several months, usually beginning with dysesthesias in the hands, followed by weakness or clumsiness in the hands, and eventually progressing to weakness in the lower extremities.[72]

CLINICAL PRESENTATION

In cases of cervical myelopathy secondary to cervical spondylosis, symptoms are usually insidious in onset, often with short periods of worsening followed by long periods of relative stability.[77] Acute onset of symptoms or rapid deterioration may suggest a vascular etiology.[71] Unlike cervical radiculopathy, cervical myelopathy rarely presents with neck pain; instead, patients report an occipital headache that radiates anteriorly to the frontal area, is worse on waking, but improves through the day.[72] Patients also report deep aching pain and burning sensations in the hands, loss of hand dexterity, and vertebrobasilar insufficiency, presumably due to osteophytic changes in the cervical spine.[71,72]

On physical examination, patients demonstrate motor weakness and muscle wasting, particularly of the interosseous muscles of the hand. Lhermitte's sign is present in approximately 25% of patients, i.e., rapid flexion or extension of the neck causes a shock-like sensation in the trunk or limbs.[71] Deep tendon reflexes are variable. Involvement of the anterior horn cell causes hyporeflexia, whereas involvement of the corticospinal tracts causes hyperreflexia. The triceps jerk is the reflex most commonly lost, due to frequent involvement of the sixth nerve root (i.e., the C5-6 interspace). Almost all patients with cervical myelopathy show signs of muscular spasticity.

DIAGNOSIS

Radiologic Diagnosis in Cervical Spondylosis
Intrathecal contrast-enhanced CT scan is a highly specific test that allows evaluation of the intradural contents and the disc margins, and helps differentiate an extradural defect due to disc herniation from that due to osteophytic changes.[73] MRI allows visualization of the cervical spine in both the sagittal and axial planes. Resolution with MRI is sharp enough to identify lesions of the spinal cord and differentiate disc herniation from spinal stenosis.[73] CT scan is preferred in evaluating osteophytes, foraminal encroachment, and other bony changes. CT and MRI complement one another, and their use should be individualized for each patient.[74] Clinical correlation of abnormal neuroradiologic findings is essential because degenerative changes of the cervical spine and cervical disc are common even among asymptomatic patients.[73,74]

MANAGEMENT

Conservative Therapy.   Most patients with cervical myelopathy present with minor symptoms and demonstrate long periods of non-progressive disability. Therefore, these patients should initially be treated conservatively: rest with a soft cervical collar, physical therapy to promote range of motion, and judicious use of NSAIDs. However, only 30% to 50% of patients improve with conservative management. A recent multicenter study comparing the efficacy of surgery versus conservative management demonstrated broadly similar outcomes with regard to activities of daily living, symptom index, function, and patient satisfaction.[77]

Surgery. Early surgical decompression is appropriate for patients with cervical myelopathy who present with moderate or severe disability, or in the presence of rapid neurologic deterioration.[78] Anterior decompression with fusion, posterior decompression, laminectomy, or laminoplasty is appropriate to particular clinical situations.[79] The best surgical prognosis is achieved by careful patient selection. Accurate diagnosis is essential, and patients with symptoms of relatively short duration have the best prognosis.[71] If surgery is considered, it should be performed early in the course of the disease, before cord damage becomes irreversible.

Surgical decompression is recommended for patients with severe or progressive symptoms; excellent or good outcomes can be expected for approximately 70% of these patients.[77]

Cervical Whiplash

Cervical whiplash is a valid clinical syndrome, with symptoms consistent with anatomic sites of injury, and a potential for significant impairment.[80] Whiplash injuries afflict more than 1 million people in the U.S. each year,[81] with an annual incidence of approximately 4 per 1000 population.[82] Symptoms in cervical whiplash injuries are due to soft tissue trauma, particularly musculoligamentous sprains and strains to the cervical spine. After a rear-end impact in a motor vehicle accident, the patient is accelerated forward and the lower cervical vertebrae are hyperextended, especially at the C5-6 interspace. This is followed by flexion of the upper cervical vertebrae, which is limited by the chin striking the chest. Hyperextension commonly causes an injury to the anterior longitudinal ligament of the cervical spine and other soft tissue injuries of the anterior neck including muscle tears, muscle hemorrhage, esophageal hemorrhage, or disc disruption. Muscles most commonly injured include the sternocleidomastoid, scalenus, and longus colli muscles.

Neck pain and headache are the cardinal features of whiplash injury.[83] Injury to the upper cervical segments may cause pain referred to the neck or the head and presents as neck pain or headache. Injury to the lower cervical segments may cause pain referred to shoulder and or arm. Patients may also develop visual disturbances, possibly due to vertebral, basilar, or other vascular injury, or injury to the cervical sympathetic chain.[81]

After acute injury most patients recover rapidly: 80% are asymptomatic by 12 months, 15% to 20% remain symptomatic after 12 months, and only 5% are severely affected.[83] However this last group of patients generates the greatest health care costs.

CLINICAL PRESENTATION

On history, patients describe a typical rear-end impact motor vehicle accident with hyperextension of the neck followed by hyperflexion. Pain in the neck may be immediate or may be delayed hours or even days after the accident. Pain is usually felt at the base of the neck and increases over time. Patients report pain and decreased range of motion in the neck, which is worsened by motion or activity, as well as paresthesias or weakness in the upper extremities, dysphagia, or hoarseness.

Physical examination may be negative if the patient is seen within hours of the accident. Over time, however, patients develop tenderness in the cervical spine area, as well as decreased range of motion and muscle spasm. Neurologic examination of the upper extremity should include assessment of motor function and grip strength, sensation, deep tendon reflexes, and range of motion (especially of the neck and shoulder).

DIAGNOSIS

Findings on plain radiographs are usually minimal. Five views of the cervical spine should be obtained: anteroposterior, lateral, right and left obliques, and the odontoid view. Straightening of the cervical spine or loss of the normal cervical lordosis may be due to positioning in radiology, muscle spasm, or derangement of the skeletal alignment of the cervical spine. Radiographs should also be examined for soft tissue swelling anterior to the C3 vertebral body, which may indicate an occult fracture. Signs of preexisting degenerative changes such as osteophytic changes, disc space narrowing, or narrowing of the cervical foramina are also common. Electromyography and nerve conduction velocity tests should be considered if paresthesias or radicular pain are present. Technetium bone scan is very sensitive in detecting occult injuries. However, whiplash injuries usually cause soft tissue injuries that are not demonstrable with most of these studies. For example, MRI of the brain and neck of patients within 2 days of whiplash injury shows no difference between subjects and controls.[84] Therefore, CT or MRI should be reserved for patients with neurologic deficit, intense pain within minutes of injury, suspected spinal cord or disc damage, suspected fracture, or ligamentous injury.[81,82]

MANAGEMENT

Many patients recover within 6 months without any treatment. However, treatment may speed the recovery process and limit the amount of pain the patient experiences during recovery.[82]

Rest. While rest in a soft cervical collar has been the traditional treatment for patients with whiplash injury, recent studies indicate that prolonged rest (i.e., 2 weeks or more) and/or excessive use of the soft cervical collar may be detrimental and actually slow the healing process.[85] Initially, patients should be treated with a brief period of rest and protection of the cervical spine, usually with a soft cervical collar for 3 or 4 days. The collar holds the neck in slight flexion; therefore, the widest part of the cervical collar should be worn posteriorly. The cervical collar is especially useful in alleviating pain if worn at night or when driving. If used during the day, it should be worn 1 or 2 hours and then removed for a similar period in order to preserve paracervical muscle conditioning. The soft cervical collar should not be used for more than a few days; early in the course of treatment, the patient should be encouraged to begin mobilization exercises for the neck.[81]

Medications. NSAIDs are effective in treating the pain and muscle spasm caused by whiplash injuries. Muscle relaxants are a useful adjunct, especially when used nightly, and should be prescribed in a time-limited manner. Narcotics are usually not indicated in the treatment of whiplash injuries.

Physical Therapy. A treatment protocol with proven success involves early active range of motion and strengthening exercises.[86] Patients are instructed to perform gentle rotational exercises 10 times an hour as soon as symptoms allow within 96 hours of injury. Patients who comply with early active treatment protocols report significantly reduced pain and a significantly improved range of motion.

Physical modalities alleviate symptoms of pain and muscle spasm. Early in the course of whiplash injuries, heat modalities for 20 to 25 minutes, every 3 to 4 hours, are useful. However, excessive use of heat modalities can actually delay recovery. Later in the course of whiplash injury, usually 2 to 3 days after injury, cold therapy is indicated to decrease muscle spasm and pain. Range of motion exercises followed by isometric strengthening exercises should be initiated early in the therapy of whiplash injuries, even immediately after injury. Patients should be given specific instructions regarding neck exercises and daily activities. Patient education programs regarding exercises, daily activities, body mechanics, and the use of heat and cold modalities, are also helpful. The patient should be encouraged to remain functional in spite of pain or other symptoms. Any increase in pain following exercise should not be seen as a worsening of the injury. Prolonged physiotherapy should be avoided, because it reinforces the sick role for the patient.[81]

Multimodal treatments maximize success rates after cervical whiplash injury.[82] The goals of therapy are to restore normal function and promote early return to work. Physical therapy is used to reduce inappropriate pain behaviors, strengthen neck musculature, and wean patients off use of a soft cervical collar. Occupational therapy is used to facilitate the patient's return to normal functioning in the workplace. Neuropsychological counseling may be helpful for some patients.

Intraarticular Corticosteroid Injection. Intraarticular injection of corticosteroids is not effective therapy for pain in the cervical spine following whiplash injury.[87]

PROGNOSIS

Most patients with whiplash injuries have negative diagnostic studies but improve, although slowly and irregularly. Patients benefit from a program of rest, immobilization, neck exercises, and return to function. At 2-year follow-up, approximately 82% of patients with whiplash injury can expect to be symptom-free. Patients with persistent symptoms are older, have more signs of spondylosis on cervical radiographs, and probably sustained more severe initial injuries. Patients symptomatic at 2-year follow-up initially reported more pain, a greater variety of pain symptoms, had higher rates of pretraumatic headache, and had more rapid onset of postinjury symptoms. Symptomatic and asymptomatic patients were similar with regard to gender, vocation, and psychological variables.[88] Some patients who sustain a whiplash injury never recover completely, probably due to a combination of the severity of the injury, underlying cervical abnormalities, and psychosocial factors.[81]

References

1. Anderson GBJ. The epidemiology of spinal disorders. In Frymoyer JW, ed. The adult spine: principles and practice, 2nd ed. Philadelphia: Lippincott-Raven, 1997;93–141.
2. Loeser JD, Volinn E. Epidemiology of low back pain. Neurosurg Clin North Am 1991;2:713–18.
3. Deyo RA. Conservative therapy for low back pain. JAMA 1983;250(8):1057–62.
4. Hart LG, Deyo RA, Cherkin DC. Physician office visits for low back pain: frequency, clinical evaluation, and treatment patterns from a U.S. national survey. Spine 1995;20:11–19.
5. Deyo RA, Loeser JD, Bigos SJ. Herniated lumbar inter-vertebral disc. Ann Intern Med 1990;112:598–603.
6. Frymoyer JW, Durett CL. The economics of spinal disorders. In: Frymoyer JW, ed. The adult spine: principles and practice, 2nd ed. Philadelphia: Lippincott-Raven, 1997;143–50.
7. Frymoyer JW. Back pain and sciatica. N Engl J Med 1988;318(5):291–300.
8. Anderson GBJ. Epidemiologic features of chronic low back pain. Lancet 1999;354:581–5.
9. Deyo RA, Tsui-Wu YJ. Descriptive epidemiology of low back pain and its related medical care in the United States. Spine 1987;12:264–8.
10. Deyo RA, Rainville J, Kent DL. What can the history and physical examination tell us about low back pain? JAMA 1992;268(6):760–5.
11. Weber H. Lumbar disc herniation: a controlled prospective study with ten years of observation. Spine 1983;8(2):131–40.
12. Frymoyer JW, Cats-Baril WL. An overview of the incidences and costs of low back pain. Orthop Clin North Am 1991;22(2):263–71.
13. National Center for Health Statistics. Prevalence of selected impairments. U.S., 1977, series 10, number 132. Hyattsville, MD. DHHS publication (PHS) 81–1562, 1981.
14. Deyo RA, Weinstein JN. Primary care: low back pain. N Engl J Med 2001; 344(5):363–70.
15. Wipf JE, Deyo RA. Low back pain. Med Clin North Am 1995;79(2):231–46.

16. Mixter WJ, Barr JS. Rupture of inter-vertebral disc with involvement of the spinal canal. N Engl J Med 1934;211(5):210–5.

17. Spitzer WO, LeBlanc FE, Dupuis M, et al. Scientific approach to the assessment and management of activity related spinal disorders. A monograph for clinicians. Report of the Quebec Task Force on Spinal Disorders. Spine 1987;12(suppl 1):S1–59.

18. Frymoyer JW, Nachemson A. Natural history of low back disorders. In: Frymoyer JW, ed. In: The adult spine: principles and practice. New York: Raven Press, 1991;1537–50.

19. Modic MT, Ross JS. Magnetic resonance imaging in the evaluation of low back pain. Orthop Clin North Am 1991;22(2):283–301.

20. Deyo RA, Diehl AK. Lumbar spine films in primary care: current use and effects of selective ordering criteria. J Gen Intern Med 1986;1:20–5.

21. Hensinger RN. Spondylolysis and spondylolisthesis in children and adolescents. J Bone Joint Surg 1989;71A(7):1098–107.

22. Bigos S, Bowyer O, Braen G, et al. Acute low back problems in adults. Clinical practice guideline no. 14. Rockville, MD: Agency for Health Care Policy and Research, December 1994. (AHCPR publication no. 95-0642.)

23. Frymoyer JW, Newberg A, Pope MH, Wilder DG, Clements J, MacPherson B. Spine radiographs in patients with low back pain: an epidemiological study in men. J Bone Joint Surg 1984;66A(7):1048–55.

24. Jensen MC, Brant-Zawadzki MN, Obuchowski N, Modic MT, Malkasian D, Ross JS. Magnetic resonance imaging in people without back pain. N Engl J Med 1994;331(2):69–73.

25. Deyo RA, Diehl AK. Cancer as a cause of back pain: frequency, clinical presentation, and diagnostic strategies. J Gen Intern Med 1988;3:230–8.

26. Garfin SR, Herkowitz HN, Mirkovic S. Spinal stenosis. Inst Course Lect 2000;49:361–74.

27. Hilibrand AS, Rand N. Degenerative lumbar stenosis: diagnosis and management. J Am Acad Orthop Surg 1999;7:239–49.

28. Atlas SJ, Keller RB, Robson D, Deyo RA, Singer DE. Surgical and nonsurgical management of lumbar spinal stenosis: four-year outcomes from the Maine Lumbar Spine Study. Spine 2000;25(5):556–62.

29. McCowin PR, Borenstein D, Wiesel SW. The current approach to the medical diagnosis of low back pain. Orthop Clin North Am 1991;22(2):315–25.

30. Barth RW, Lane JM. Osteoporosis. Orthop Clin North Am 1988;19(4):845–58.

31. Bates DW, Reuler JB. Back pain and epidural spinal cord compression. J Gen Intern Med 1988;3:191–7.

32. Joines JD, McNutt RA, Carey TS, Deyo RA, Rouhani R. Finding cancer in primary care outpatients with low back pain: a comparison of diagnostic strategies. J Gen Intern Med 2001;16(1):14–23.

33. Perrin RG. Symptomatic spinal metastases. Am Fam Physician 1989;39(5):165–72.

34. Jackson RP. The facet syndrome: myth or reality? Clin Orthop 1992;279:110–21.

35. Carette S, Marcoux S, Truchon R, et al. A controlled trial of corticosteroid injections into facet joints for chronic low back pain. N Engl J Med 1991;325(14):1002–7.

36. Lilius G, Laasonen EM, Myllynen P, Harilainen A, Gronlund G. Lumbar facet joint syndrome: a randomized clinical trial. J Bone Joint Surg 1989;71B(4):681–4.

37. Revel M, Poiraudeau S, Auleley GR, et al. Capacity of the clinical picture to characterize low back pain relieved by facet joint anesthesia. Proposed criteria to identify patients with painful facet joints. Spine 1998;23(18):1972–7.

38. Nelemans PJ, deBie RA, deVet HC, Sturmans F. Injection therapy for subacute and chronic benign low back pain. Spine 2001;26(5):501–15.
39. Gran JT. An epidemiological survey of the signs and symptoms of ankylosing spondylitis. Clin Rheumatol 1985;4:161–9.
40. Frymoyer JW, Rosen JC, Clements J, Pope MH. Psychologic factors in low back pain disability. Clin Orthop 1985;195:178–84.
41. Wheeler AH. Diagnosis and management of low back pain and sciatica. Am Fam Physician 1995;52(5):1333–41.
42. Waddell G, Feder G, Lewis M. Systematic reviews of bedrest and advice to stay active for acute low back pain. Br J Gen Pract 1997;47:647–52.
43. Malmivaara A, Hakkinen U, Aro T et al. The treatment of acute low back pain—bedrest, exercises, or ordinary activity? N Engl J Med 1995;332:351–5.
44. van Tulder MW, Scholten RJ, Koes BW, Deyo RA. Nonsteroidal anti-inflammatory drugs for low back pain: a systematic review with the framework of the Cochrane Collaboration Back Review Group. Spine 2000;25(19):2501–13.
45. Beurskens AJ, de Vet HC, Koke AJ, et al. Efficacy of traction for nonspecific low back pain: 12-week and 16-month results of a randomized clinical trial. Spine 1997;22:2756–62.
46. Deyo RA, Walsh NE, Martin DC, Schoenfeld LS, Ramamurthy S. A controlled trial of transcutaneous electrical nerve stimulation (TENS) and exercise for chronic low back pain. N Engl J Med 1990;322(23):1627–34.
47. van Tulder M, Malmivaara A, Esmail R, Koes B. Exercise therapy for low back pain: a systematic review with the framework of the Cochrane Collaboration Back Review Group. Spine 2000;25(21):2784–96.
48. Cherkin DC, Deyo RA, Battie M, Street J, Barlow W. A comparison of physical therapy, chiropractic manipulation, and provision of an educational booklet for the treatment of patients with low back pain. N Engl J Med 1998;339:1021–9.
49. Anderson GBJ, Lucente T, Davis AM, Kappler RE, Lipton JA, Leurgans S. A comparison of osteopathic spinal manipulation with standard care for patients with low back pain. N Engl J Med 1999;341:1426–31.
50. van Tulder MW, Esmail R, Bombardier C, Koes BW. Back schools for nonspecific low back pain (Cochrane Reivew). In: The Cochrane Library; issue 3. Oxford: Update Software, 1999.
51. van Tulder MW, Cherkin DC, Berman B, Lao L, Koes BW. The effectiveness of acupuncture in the management of acute and chronic low back pain. Spine 1999; 24(11):1113–23.
52. Carette S, Leclaire R, Marcoux S. Epidural corticosteroid injections for sciatica due to herniated nucleus pulposus. N Engl J Med 1997;336:1634–40.
53. Cherkin DC, Deyo RA, Loeser JD, Bush T, Waddell G. An international comparison of back surgery rates. Spine 1994;19(11):1201–6.
54. Taylor VM, Deyo RA, Cherkin DC, Kreuter W. Low back pain hospitalization: recent U.S. trends and regional variations. Spine 1994;19(11):1207–13.
55. Hurme M, Alaranta H. Factors predicting the results of surgery for lumbar inter-vertebral disc herniation. Spine 1987;12(9):933–8.
56. Gibson JNA, Grant IC, Waddell G. The Cochrane review of surgery for lumbar disc prolapse and degenerative lumbar spondylosis. Spine 1999;24(17):1820–32.
57. Abramovitz JN, Neff SR. Lumbar disc surgery: results of the prospective lumbar discectomy study. Neurosurgery 1991;29(2):301–8.

58. Hoffman RM, Wheeler KJ, Deyo RA. Surgery for herniated lumbar discs: a literature synthesis. J Gen Intern Med 1993;8:487–96.

59. Atlas SJ, Chang Y, Kamann E, Keller RB, Deyo RA, Singer DE. Long-term disability and return to work among patients who have a herniated disc: the effect of disability compensation. J Bone Joint Surg 2000;82A(1):4–15.

60. Chatterjee S, Foy PM, Findaly GF. Report of a controlled clinical trial comparing automated percutaneous lumbar discectomy and microdiscectomy in the treatment of contained lumbar disc herniation. Spine 1995;20:734–8.

61. Revel M, Payan C, Vallee C, et al. Automated percutaneous lumbar discectomy vs. chemonucleolysis in the treatment of sciatica. Spine 1993;18(1):1–7.

62. Hermantin FU, Peters T, Quartararo L, Kambin P. A prospective, randomized study comparing the results of open discectomy with those of video-assisted arthroscopic microdiscectomy. J Bone Joint Surg 1999;81A:958–65.

63. Deyo RA, Cherkin DC, Loeser JD, Bigos SJ, Ciol MA. Morbidity and mortality in association with operations on the lumbar spine: the influence of age, diagnosis, and procedure. J Bone Joint Surg 1992;74A(4):536–43.

64. Turner JA, Denny MC. Do antidepressant medications relieve chronic low back pain? J Fam Pract 1993;37(6):545–53.

65. Atkinson JH, Slater MA, Wahlgren DR, et al. Pain 1999;83:137–45.

66. Lahad A, Malter AD, Berg AO, Deyo RA. The effectiveness of four interventions for the prevention of low back pain. JAMA 1994;272(16):1286–91.

67. Von Poppel MN, Koes BW, van der Ploeg T, Smid T, Bouter LM. Lumbar supports and education for the prevention of low back pain in industry. JAMA 1998; 279:1789–94.

68. Daltroy LH, Iversen MD, Larson MG, et al. A controlled trial of an educational program to prevent low back injuries. N Engl J Med 1997;337:322–8.

69. Loisel P, Abenhaim L, Durand P, et al. A population-based, randomized clinical trial on back pain management. Spine 1997;22(24):2911–18.

70. Kelsey JL, Githens PB, Walter SD, et al. An epidemiological study of acute prolapsed cervical intervertebral disc. J Bone Joint Surg 1984;66A:907–14.

71. Clark CR. Degenerative conditions of the spine. In: Frymoyer JW, ed. The adult spine: principles and practice. New York: Raven Press, 1991;1145–64.

72. Lestini WF, Wiesel SW. The pathogenesis of cervical spondylosis. Clin Orthop 1989;239:69–93.

73. Jahnke RW, Hart BL. Cervical stenosis, spondylosis, and herniated disc disease. Radiol Clin North Am 1991;29(4):777–91.

74. Russell EJ. Cervical disc disease. Radiology 1990;177(2):313–25.

75. Dillin W, Booth R, Cuckler J, Balderston R, Simeone F, Rothman R. Cervical radiculopathy: a review. Spine 1986;11(10):988–91.

76. Murphy MJ, Lieponis JV. Non-operative treatment of cervical spine pain. In: Sherk HH, ed. The cervical spine. Philadelphia: Lippincott, 1989;670–7.

77. Sampath P, Bendebba M, Davis JD, Ducker TB. Outcome of patients treated for cervical myelopathy. Spine 2000;25(6):670–6.

78. La Rocca H. Cervical spondylotic myelopathy: natural history. Spine 1988;13(7):854–5.

79. White AA 3rd, Panjabi MM. Biomechanical considerations in the surgical management of cervical spondylotic myelopathy. Spine 1988;13(7):856–69.

80. Hirsch SA, Hirsch PJ, Hiramoto H, Weiss A. Whiplash syndrome: fact or fiction? Orthop Clin North Am 1988;19(4):791–5.

81. Carette S. Whiplash injury and chronic neck pain. N Engl J Med 1994;330(15): 1083–4.
82. Eck JC, Hodges SD, Humphreys SC. Whiplash: a review of a commonly misunderstood injury. Am J Med 2001;110(8):651–6.
83. Bogduk N, Teasell R. Whiplash: the evidence for an organic etiology. Arch Neurol 2000;57(4):590–1.
84. Borchgrevink G, Smevik O, Haave I, et al. MRI of cerebrum and spinal column within 2 days after whiplash neck sprain injury. Injury 1997;28:331–5.
85. Borchgrevink GE, Kaasa A, McDonagh D, et al. Acute treatment of whiplash neck sprain injuries. Spine 1998;23:25–31.
86. Rosenfeld M, Gunnarsson R, Borenstein P. Early intervention in whiplash-associated disorders. A comparison of two treatment protocols. Spine 2000;25:1782–7.
87. Barnsley L, Lord SM, Wallis BJ, Bogduk N. Lack of effect of intraarticular corticosteroids for chronic pain in the cervical zygapophyseal joints. N Engl J Med 1994;330(15):1047–50.
88. Radanov BP, Sturzenegger M, DiStefano G. Long-term outcome after whiplash injury: a 2-year follow-up considering features of injury mechanism and somatic, radiologic, and psychosocial findings. Medicine 1995;74(5):281–97.

Case Presentation

Subjective

Patient Profile

Andrew Harris is a 27-year-old male married truck driver.

Presenting Problem

"Back strain."

Present Illness

Mr. Harris describes a 4-day history of low back pain that began when he lifted a heavy box while unloading his truck. The pain occasionally radiates to the right leg and foot. He has difficulty walking and is unable to work despite 3 days of rest.

Past Medical History

He has had several episodes of back strain over the past 5 years, but none as severe as the current illness.

Social History

Mr. Harris has been employed by a national freight line for 8 years. He lives with his wife and their two young children.

Habits

He uses no alcohol, tobacco, or recreational drugs. He drinks four cups of coffee daily.

Family History

His father had surgery for prostate enlargement 2 years ago and is now living and well at age 61. His mother died at age 60 of a stroke. There is one 32-year-old brother who has had lumbar disc surgery.

REVIEW OF SYSTEMS

Mr. Harris has an occasional tension headache and some pain in his shoulders and knees during cold damp weather.

- Discuss the possible reasons for Mr. Harris' visit today.
- What additional historical information might be useful? Why?
- What more would you like to know about the previous instances of back strain?
- What further information about the patient's job might be useful? Explain.

Objective

VITAL SIGNS

Height, 5 ft 10 in; weight, 232 lb; blood pressure, 140/84; pulse, 74.

EXAMINATION

The patient is ambulatory but moves carefully owing to low back pain. He has difficulty climbing onto the examination table. There is mild tenderness of the lumbosacral spine with adjacent right paraspinal muscle tenderness. Straight leg raising is positive on the right but not on the left. Deep tendon reflexes are +2 and symmetrical. There is decreased perception of pinprick on the lateral right lower leg and foot.

- What further information obtained from the physical examination might be helpful? Why?
- What is the relationship of the patient's weight to his ideal weight and height?
- What—if any—diagnostic maneuvers might help clarify the problem?
- What—if any—diagnostic imaging would you obtain today?

Assessment

- Describe your diagnosis. What is the likely anatomical cause?
- How will you explain your assessment to Mr. Harris?
- What might be the meaning of this illness to the patient? How would you ask about this concern?
- What is the potential economic impact of this illness on the family? How would you address this issue?

Plan

- What would be your therapeutic recommendation? How would you explain this to the patient?
- What would you advise regarding Mr. Harris's weight? How might you persuade him to lose weight?
- Is a subspecialist consultation appropriate at this time? If so, how would you explain this to the patient?
- What follow-up would you plan for Mr. Harris?

18
Osteoarthritis

ALICIA D. MONROE AND JOHN B. MURPHY

Epidemiology

Arthritis affects an estimated 43 million persons in the United States.[1] Osteoarthritis (OA) is the most common rheumatic disease, and the third most common principal diagnosis recorded by family practitioners for office visits made by older patients.[2,3] Hip and knee OA are a leading cause of activity limitation, disability, and dependence among the elderly.[3,4] Population-based studies of OA demonstrate that the prevalence of radiographic OA is much higher than clinically defined or symptomatic OA, and there is a progressive increase in the prevalence of OA with advancing age.[3,5] The prevalence, pattern of joint involvement, and severity of OA has been observed to vary among populations by ethnicity and race, but some of the data are conflicting. [4,6] Europeans have higher prevalence rates of radiographic hip OA (7–25%), compared to Hong Kong Chinese (1%), and Caribbean and African black populations (1–4%).[4] The National Health and Nutrition Examination Survey (NHANES I) study showed higher rates of knee OA for U.S. black women, but no racial differences in hip OA. In the Johnson County Arthritis Study, African Americans and whites showed similar high rates of radiographic hip OA (29.9% versus 26.4%) and knee OA (37.4% versus 39.1%).[7]

Pathophysiology

Systemic factors (age, sex, race, genetics, bone density, estrogen replacement therapy, and nutritional factors) may predispose joints to local biomechanical factors (obesity, muscle weakness, joint deformity, injury) and the subsequent development of OA.[4,6] The degenerative changes seen in osteoarthritic cartilage are clearly distinct from those seen with normal aging.[8] The pathologic changes in OA cartilage appear to be mediated by complex interactions between mechanical and biologic factors including excessive enzymatic degradation, decreased synthesis of cartilage matrix, increased levels of cytokines and other inflammatory molecules, and dysregulation of OA chondrocytes. The net result includes disorganization of the cartilage matrix and fibrillation.[8,9] As the disease advances, disorganization gives way to fissures, erosion, ulceration, and eventually cartilage is irreversibly destroyed. As the cartilage degenerates, joint stresses are increasingly transmitted to the underlying bone, initiating the bony remodeling process, which results in marginal osteophytes, subchondral sclerosis, and cysts.

Clinical Presentation and Diagnosis

Signs and Symptoms

Osteoarthritis, classified as primary (idiopathic) or secondary, represents a "final common pathway" for a number of conditions of diverse etiologies.[6] Primary OA is further classified as localized (e.g., hands, feet, knees, or other single sites) or generalized including three or more local areas. Secondary OA is classified as (1) posttraumatic, (2) congenital or developmental, (3) metabolic, (4) endocrine, (5) other bone and joint diseases, (6) neuropathic, and (7) miscellaneous. Commonly affected joints include the interphalangeal, knee, hip, acromioclavicular, subtalar, first metatarsophalangeal, sacroiliac, temporomandibular, and carpometacarpal joint of the thumb. Joints usually spared include the metacarpophalangeal, wrist, elbow, and shoulder. Early during the symptomatic phase, OA pain is often described as a deep, aching discomfort. It occurs with motion, particularly with weight-bearing, and is relieved by rest. As the disease progresses, pain can occur with minimal motion and at rest. OA pain is typically localized to the joint, although pain associated with hip OA is often localized to the anterior inguinal region, and the medial or lateral thigh, but it may also radiate to the buttock, anterior thigh, or knee. OA pain of the spine may be associated with radicular symptoms including pain, paresthesias, and muscle weakness. Although joint stiffness can occur, it is usually of short duration (<30 minutes).

Physical examination of an affected joint may show decreased range of motion, joint deformity, bony hypertrophy, and occasionally an intraarticular effusion. Crepitance and pain on passive and active movement and mild tenderness may be found. Inflammatory changes including warmth and redness are usually absent. During late stages there may be demonstrable joint instability. Physical findings associated with hand OA include Heberden's nodes of the distal interphalangeal joints, representing cartilaginous and bony enlargement of the dorsolateral and dorsomedial aspects. Bouchard's nodes are similar findings at the proximal interphalangeal joints. Physical findings of knee OA can also include quadriceps muscle atrophy, mediolateral joint instability, limitation of joint motion, initially with extension, and varus angulation resulting from degenerative cartilage in the medial compartment of the knee. The patient with OA of the hip often holds the hip adducted, flexed, and internally rotated, which may result in functional shortening of the leg and the characteristic limp (antalgic gait).

Radiographic Features and Laboratory Findings

During early stages of OA plain radiographs may be normal. As the disease progresses, joint space narrowing becomes evident as articular cartilage is lost. Marginal osteophyte formation is seen as a result of bone proliferation. Subchondral bony sclerosis appears radiographically as increased bone density. Subchondral bone cysts develop and vary in size from several millimeters to several centimeters, appearing as translucent areas in periarticular bone. Bony deformity, joint subluxation, and loose bodies may be seen in advanced cases. Computed tomography, magnetic resonance imaging, and ultrasonography provide powerful tools for the assessment of OA, although the diagnosis of OA rarely requires such expensive modalities. There are no specific laboratory tests for OA. Unlike with the inflammatory arthritides, with OA the erythrocyte sedimentation rate (ESR) and hemogram are normal and autoantibodies are not present. If there is joint effusion, the synovial fluid is noninflammatory, with fewer than 2000 white blood cells (WBCs), a predominance of mononuclear WBCs, and a good mucin clot. The diagnosis of OA is usually based on clinical and radiologic features, with the laboratory assessment being useful for excluding other arthritic conditions or secondary causes of OA.

Management

The goals of OA management are pain control, prevention of joint damage, maximizing function and quality of life, and minimizing therapeutic toxicity.[10] An appropriate treatment plan for OA combines oral medications, exercise, and patient education. Nonpharmacologic management strategies for OA include periods of rest (1–2 hours) when symptoms are at their worst, avoidance of repetitive movements or static body positions that aggravate symptoms, heat (or cold) for the control of pain, weight loss if the patient is overweight, adaptive mobility aids to diminish the mechanical load on joints, adaptive equipment to assist in activities of daily living (ADL), range of motion exercises, strengthening exercises, and endurance exercises.[11,12] Immobilization should be avoided. The use of adaptive mobility aids (e.g., canes, walkers) is an important strategy, but care must be taken to ensure that the mobility aid is the correct device, properly used, appropriately sized, and in good repair. Medial knee taping to realign the patella in patients with patellofemoral OA, and the use of wedged insoles for patients with medial compartment OA and shock absorbing footwear may help reduce joint symptoms.[10,13]

Pharmacologic approaches to the treatment of OA include acetaminophen, salicylates, nonselective nonsteroidal anti-inflammatory drugs (NSAIDs), cyclooxygenase-2 (COX-2) specific inhibitors, topical analgesics, and intraarticular steroids.[14,15] Acetaminophen is advocated for use as first-line therapy for relief of mild to moderate pain, but it should be used cautiously in patients with liver disease or chronic alcohol abuse. Salicylates and NSAIDs are commonly used as first-line medications for the relief of pain related to OA. Compliance with salicylates can be a major problem given their short duration of action and the need for frequent dosing; thus NSAIDs are preferable to salicylates. There is no justification for choosing one nonselective NSAID over another based on efficacy, but it is clear that a patient who does not respond to an NSAID from one class may well respond to an NSAID from another. The choice of a nonselective NSAID versus a COX-2 specific inhibitor should be made after assessment of risk for GI toxicity (e.g., age 65 or older, history of peptic ulcer disease, previous GI bleeding, use of oral corticosteroids or anticoagulants). For patients at increased risk for upper GI bleeding, the use of a nonselective NSAID and gastroprotective therapy or a COX-2 specific inhibitor is indicated. NSAIDs should be avoided or used with extreme caution in patients at risk for renal toxicity [e.g., intrinsic renal disease, age 65 or over, hypertension, congestive heart failure, and concomitant use of diuretics or angiotensin-converting enzyme (ACE) inhibitors].[10]

Topical capsaicin may improve hand or knee OA symptoms when added to the usual treatment; however, its use may be limited by cost and the delayed onset of effect requiring multiple applications daily and sustained use for up to 4 weeks. Intraarticular steroids are generally reserved for the occasional instance when there is a single painful joint or a large effusion in a single joint, and the

TABLE 18.1 Pharmacologic Treatment of Osteoarthritis

Drug	Dosage range/frequency	Relative cost/ 30days
Acetaminophen	750–1000 mg qid	$
Aspirin, enteric coated	975 mg qid	$
Extended release aspirin	800 mg qid	$
Salicylsalicylic acid	3–4 g/day 2 or 3 doses	$
Choline magnesium trisalicylate	3 g/day in 1, 2, or 3 doses	$$
Celecoxib (Celebrex)	100–200 mg bid	$$$$
Diclofenac (Voltaren)	150–200 mg/day in 2 or 3 doses	$$
Diflunisal (Dolobid)	500–1000 mg/day in 2 doses	$$
Etodolac (Lodine)	300 mg bid–tid	$$
Fenoprofen (Nalfon)	300–600 mg tid–qid	$$
Flurbiprofen (Ansaid)	200–300 mg/day in 2, 3, or 4 doses	$$
Ibuprofen (Motrin)	1200–3200 mg/day in 3 or 4 doses	$
Indomethacin (Indocin)	25–50 mg tid–qid	$
Ketoprofen (Orudis)	50 mg qid or 75 mg tid	$$
Meclofenamate sodium	200–400 mg in 3 or 4 doses	$$$
Meloxicam (Mobic)	7.5–15 mg/day	$$$
Nabumetone (Relafen)	1000 mg once/day to 2000 mg/day	$$$
Naproxen (Naprosyn)	250–500 mg bid–tid	$
Naproxen sodium (Anaprox)	275–550 mg bid	$
Oxaprozin (Daypro)	600 mg once/day to 1800 mg/day	$$
Piroxicam (Feldene)	20 mg once/day	$$
Rofecoxib (Vioxx)	25–50 mg once/day	$$$
Sulindac (Clinoril)	150–200 mg bid	$
Tolmetin (Tolectin)	600–1800 mg/day in 3 or 4 doses	$$

$ = 18–35; $$ = 36–55; $$$ = 56–80; $$$$ = 81–145.

pain is unresponsive to other modalities. For patients who do not respond to
NSAIDs or acetaminophen, tramadol can be considered, but seizures have been
reported as a rare side effect. Narcotics should be avoided if at all possible, but
they may be considered in patients unresponsive to or unable to tolerate other
medications. Glucosamine sulfate, chondrotin sulfate, or acupuncture may be effective in reducing pain symptoms from OA, and glucosamine may prevent progression of knee OA.[10,16] Osteotomy, arthroscopy, arthrodesis, and total joint replacement are the primary surgical approaches for OA. Candidates for
arthroplasty are individuals with severe pain, impaired joint function, or those
who have experienced declines in functional status that do not improve with nonpharmacologic and pharmacologic measures.

The costs of OA can be substantial (Table 18.1). The direct costs for drug therapy (which can easily exceed $60 per month)[17] are added to lost income related
to time spent on physician and physical therapy visits, disability-related work absences, and absences related to surgery. The pain and functional disability associated with OA can contribute to social isolation and depression. Potentially modifiable risk factors include obesity, mechanical stress/repetitive joint usage, and
joint trauma.[4] Weight reduction, avoidance of traumatic injury, prompt treatment
of injury, and work-site programs designed to minimize work-related mechanical joint stress may be effective interventions for preventing OA.

References

1. CDC. Prevalence of arthritis—United States, 1997. MMWR 2001;50(17):334–6.
2. Facts about family practice. Kansas City, MO: AAFP, 1987;30–7.
3. Lawrence RC, Helmick CG, Arnett FC, et al. Estimates of the prevalence of arthritis and selected musculoskeletal disorders in the United States. Arthritis Rheum
1998;41(5):778–99.
4. Felson DT, Zhang Y. An update on the epidemiology of the knee and hip osteoarthritis
with a view to prevention. Arthritis Rheum 1998;41:1343–55.
5. Croft P. Review of UK data on the rheumatic diseases: osteoarthritis. Br J Rheumatol 1990;29:391–5.
6. Felson DT, conference chair. Osteoarthritis: new insights. Part I: The disease and its
risk factors. Ann Intern Med. 2000;133:635–46.
7. Jordan JM, Linder GF, Renner JB, Fryer JG. The impact of arthritis in rural populations. Arthritis Care Res 1995;8:242–50.
8. Hamerman D. The biology of osteoarthritis. N Engl J Med 1989;320:1322–30.
9. Piperno M, Reboul P, LeGraverand MH, et al. Osteoarthritic cartilage fibrillation is
associated with a decrease in chrondrocyte adhesion to fibronectin. Osteoarthritis Cartilage 1998;6:393–99.
10. Felson DT, conference chair. Osteoarthritis: new insights. Part 2: Treatment approaches. Ann Intern Med 2000;133:726–37.
11. Dunning RD, Materson RS. A rational program of exercise for patients with osteoarthritis. Semin Arthritis Rheum 1991;21(suppl 2):33–43.
12. Kovar PA, Allegrante JP, MacKenzie CR, Petersan MGE, Gutin B, Charlson ME.
Supervised fitness walking in patients with osteoarthritis of the knee: a randomized
controlled trial. Ann Intern Med 1992;116:529–34.

13. Brandt KD. Nonsurgical management of osteoarthritis, with an emphasis on non-pharmacologic measures. Arch Fam Med 1995;4:1057–64.
14. Bradley J, Brandt K, Katz B, Kalasinski L, Ryan S. Comparison of an anti-inflammatory dose of ibuprofen, an analgesic dose of ibuprofen and acetominophen in the treatment of patients with osteoarthritis. N Engl J Med 1991;325:87–91.
15. Griffin MR, Brandt KD, Liang MH, Pincus T, Ray WA. Practical management of osteoarthritis: integration of pharmacologic and nonpharmacolic measures. Arch Fam Med 1995;4:1049–55.
16. Reginster JY, Deroisy R, Rovati LC, et al. Long-term effects of glucosamine sulfate on osteoarthritis progression: a randomized, placebo-controlled clinical trial. Lancet 2001;357:251–56.
17. Med Lett 2000;42:57–64.

CASE PRESENTATION

Subjective

PATIENT PROFILE

Harold Nelson is a 76-year-old diabetic male retired welder.

PRESENTING PROBLEM

"My knees and hands hurt."

PRESENT ILLNESS

Mr. Nelson has a 20-year history of "arthritis" involving multiple joints, especially the hands and knees. The symptoms seem worse for the past 6 to 8 weeks, especially since the weather turned cold and snowy. He currently takes six to eight aspirin a day but is afraid to use other medication because of his diabetes, especially since he had an episode of incontinence after taking an over-the-counter cold remedy in the past.

PAST MEDICAL HISTORY, SOCIAL HISTORY, HABITS, AND FAMILY HISTORY

These are all unchanged since his previous visit 7 months ago (see Chapter 5).

REVIEW OF SYSTEMS

Mild constipation present for the past 4 to 6 weeks.

- What additional historical data might be useful? Why?
- What might be causing the increasing joint pain, and how would you inquire about these possibilities?
- What more would you like to know about his constipation? Why might this be significant?
- What might Mr. Nelson be doing differently because of his joint pain? How would you address this issue?

Objective

VITAL SIGNS

Height 5 ft 7 in; weight, 166 lb (This is a 10-lb weight gain in the past 7 months); blood pressure, 152/82; pulse, 72; temperature, 37.2°C.

EXAMINATION

There are Heberden's nodes of the distal joints of the fingers. There is a knobby deformity of multiple joints of the hands, wrists, and knees. The involved joints are not hot, but grip strength is decreased and the knees lack about 10 degrees of flexion and extension. The low back is not tender, and no muscle spasm is present. He lacks about 20 degrees of flexion at the waist.

LABORATORY

A blood glucose test performed in the office reveals a level of 110 mg/dl.

- What—if any—additional information might be derived from the physical examination? Why?
- What other areas of the body should be examined? Why?
- What—if any—laboratory determinations should be ordered today?
- What—if any—diagnostic imaging should be obtained?

Assessment

- What is your diagnostic assessment? How would you describe this to the patient?
- What might be the significance of the weight gain over the past 7 months?
- What might be the meaning of the joint pain to the patient? How would you ask about this?
- What would be your thoughts if the patient developed warm swollen tender joints? What would you do differently?

Plan

- What would be your therapeutic recommendation today? How would you explain this to Mr. Nelson?
- How would you approach the patient's concern about medication use?
- What life-style and activity recommendations would you make today?
- What continuing care would you advise?

19
Common Dermatoses

DANIEL J. VAN DURME

Acne Vulgaris

Acne is the most common dermatologic condition presenting to the family physician's office. There are an estimated 40 to 50 million people in the United States affected with acne, including about 85% of all adolescents between the ages of 12 and 25.[1] It can present with a wide range of severity and may be the source of significant emotional and psychological, as well as physical, scarring. As adolescents pass through puberty, and develop their self-image, the physical appearance of the skin can be critically important. Despite many effective treatments for this disorder, patients (and their parents) often view acne as a normal part of development and do not seek treatment. The importance of early treatment to prevent the physical and emotional scars cannot be overemphasized.

The multifactorial pathogenesis of acne is important to understand, as most treatments are not curative but rather are directed at disrupting selected aspects of development. Acne begins with abnormalities in the pilosebaceous unit. There are four key elements involved in acne development: (1) keratinization abnormalities, (2) increased sebum production, (3) bacterial proliferation, and (4) inflammation. Each may play a greater or lesser role and manifests as a different type or presentation of acne. Initially, there is an abnormality of keratinization and increased sebum. Cohesive hyperkeratosis of the cells lining the pilosebaceous unit combines with increased sebum to block the follicular canal with "sticky" cells and thus a microcomedo develops. This blocked canal leads to further buildup of sebum behind the plug. This sebum production can be increased by androgens and other factors as well. The plugged pilosebaceous unit is seen as a closed comedone ("whitehead"), or as an open comedone ("blackhead") when the pore dilates and the fatty acids in the sebaceous plug become oxidized. The normal bacterial flora of the skin, especially *Proprionybacterium acnes*, proliferates in this plug and releases chemotactic factors drawing in leukocytes. The plug may also lead to rupture of the pilosebaceous unit under the skin, which in turn causes an influx of leukocytes. The resulting inflammation leads to the development of papular or pustular acne. This process can be marked and accompanied by hypertrophy of the entire pilosebaceous unit, leading to the formation of nodules and cysts. There are also factors that can aggravate or trigger acne, such as an increase in androgens during puberty, cosmetics, mechanical trauma, or medications.[2,3]

Diagnosis

Diagnosis is straightforward and is based on the finding of comedones, papules, pustules, nodules, or cysts primarily on the face, back, shoulders, or chest, particularly in an adolescent patient. The presence of comedones is considered a necessity for the proper diagnosis of acne vulgaris. Without comedones, one must consider rosacea, steroid acne, or other acneiform dermatoses. It is important for choice of therapy and for long-term follow-up to describe and classify the patient's acne appropriately. Both the quantity and the type of lesions are noted. The number of lesions indicates whether the acne is mild, moderate, severe, or very severe (sometimes referred to as grades I–IV). The predominant type of lesion should also be noted (i.e., comedonal, papular, pustular, nodular, or cystic).[3] Thus a patient with hundreds of comedones on the face may have "very severe comedonal acne," whereas another patient may have only a few nodules and cysts and have "mild nodulocystic acne."

Management

Prior to pharmacologic management it is important to review and dispel some of the misperceptions that many patients (and parents) have about acne. This condition is not due to poor hygiene, nor are blackheads a result of "dirty pores." Aggressive and frequent scrubbing of the skin may actually aggravate the condition. Mild soaps should be used regularly, and the face should be washed gently and dried well prior to the application of topical medication. Several studies have failed to implicate diet as a significant contributor to acne,[4] and fatty foods and chocolate have not been found to be significant causative agents. Nevertheless, if patients are aware of something in their diet that triggers a flare-up, they should avoid it.

All patients should be taught that acne can be suppressed or controlled when medicines are used regularly, but that the initial therapy usually takes several weeks to show significant benefit. As the current lesions heal, the medications work to prevent the eruption of additional lesions. Typically, a noticeable response to medication is seen in about 6 weeks, and patients must be informed of this time lapse so they do not give up too soon. Some patients may have some initial worsening in the appearance of the skin when they first start treatment.

The treatment options for acne are based on several factors, including the predominant lesion and skin type, the distribution of lesions, individual patient preferences, and some trial and error. Benzoyl peroxide has both antibacterial and mild comedolytic activity and serves as the foundation of most acne therapy. This agent is available as cleansing liquids and bars and as gels or creams, with strengths ranging from 2.5% to 10%. The increase in strength increases the drying (and often the irritation) of the skin. It does not provide additional antibacterial activity. This agent can be used once or twice daily as basic therapy in most patients, although 1% to 2% of patients may have a contact allergy to it.[2]

Because all acne starts with some degree of keratinization abnormality and microcomedone formation, it is prudent to start with a comedolytic agent. Currently, the most effective agents are the topical retinoids—tretinoin (Retin-A, Avita), adapalene (Differin), and tazarotene (Tazorac). They are generally started at the lowest dose possible and thinly applied every night. Mild erythema and irritation are common at first. If they are severe, the frequency can be decreased to three times per week or less, and then slowly increased to every night. The strength of the preparation can also be gradually increased as needed and as tolerated over several weeks to months. Patients should be warned about some degree of photosensitivity with tretinoin and should use sun blocks as needed. Tazarotene is in pregnancy category X and must be avoided in pregnant women due to potential teratogenic effects. If benzoyl peroxide is also used, it is crucial to separate the application of these compounds by several hours. When applied close together, these preparations cause more irritation to the skin while inactivating each other, rendering treatment ineffective.

Antibiotics are recommended for papular or pustular (papulopustular) acne. They act by decreasing the proliferation of *P. acnes* and by inactivating the neutrophil chemotactic factors released during the inflammatory process. Topical agents include erythromycin (A/T/S 2%, Erycette solution), clindamycin (Cleocin T), tetracycline (Topicycline), and sodium sulfacetamide with sulfur (Novacet, Sulfacet-R). These agents are available in a variety of delivery vehicles and are applied once (sometimes twice) a day in conjunction with benzoyl peroxide. With both topical and oral antibiotics, some degree of trial and error is necessary. Some patients respond well to clindamycin, whereas another patient may respond only to erythromycin. Azelaic acid (Azelex) topical cream has been Food and Drug Administration (FDA) approved since 1996 for inflammatory acne and has some antibacterial and comedolytic activity. It should be used with caution in patients with a dark complexion, due to potential hypopigmentation. Additionally, benzoyl peroxide is available as a combination gel with erythromycin (Benzamycin) or with clindamycin (BenzaClin) and can be convenient and effective, but somewhat expensive.

Oral antibiotics are indicated for patients with severe or widespread papulopustular acne or patients with difficulty reaching the affected areas on their body (i.e., on the back). The most commonly used oral antibiotics are tetracycline and erythromycin, which are started at 1 g/day in divided doses. Tetracycline patients are warned of the photosensitivity side effect and advised to take the medicine on an empty stomach, without dairy products. Erythromycin patients should be warned of potential gastrointestinal (GI) upset. Other options for oral medications are doxycycline (50–100 mg twice a day), minocycline (50–100 mg twice a day), and occasionally trimethoprim-sulfamethoxazole (Bactrim DS or Septra DS 1 tablet once daily) for the refractory cases. As the acne improves, the dose of the oral medications can often be gradually decreased to about one-half the original dose for long-term maintenance therapy.[5,6]

Oral contraceptives have also been shown to have substantial benefits in many young women with acne. The non-androgenic progestins, norgestimate (Ortho-Cyclen, Ortho-TriCyclen) or desogestrel (Ortho-Cept, Desogen) should be used, and may take 2 to 4 months to show benefit.[6,7]

Nodulocystic acne requires initial therapy with benzoyl peroxide, tretinoin, and antibiotics. If these agents fail to control the acne adequately, oral isotretinoin (Accutane) may be used. This agent has been extremely effective in decreasing the production of sebum and shrinking the hypertrophied sebaceous glands of nodulocystic acne. In most patients it induces a remission for many months or cures the condition. If lesions remain, they are usually more susceptible to conventional therapy as described above. Accutane treatment consists of a 16- to 20-week course at 0.5 to 2.0 mg/kg/day. Although this medicine can be profoundly effective, it has "black box" warnings about its teratogenicity and its association with pseudotumor cerebri. There are also numerous less severe side effects, including xerosis, cheilitis, epistaxis, myalgias, arthralgias, elevated liver enzymes, and others. Liver function tests, triglyceride levels, and complete blood counts should be frequently monitored. The highly teratogenic potential must be made clear to all female patients, and this medication must be used with extreme caution in all women with childbearing potential. Patient selection guidelines for women include (negative) serum pregnancy tests before starting, maintenance of two highly effective methods of contraception throughout therapy and for 1 to 2 months after therapy, and signed informed consent by the patient.[7,8]

Atopic Dermatitis

Atopic dermatitis (AD) is a common, chronic, relapsing skin condition with an estimated incidence of 10% in the United States. It usually arises during childhood, with about 85% of patients developing it during the first 5 years of life.[9] The disease presents with severe pruritus, followed by various morphologic features. It has been described as "the itch that rashes." Although AD can be found as an isolated illness in some individuals, it is often a manifestation of the multisystemic process of atopy, which includes asthma, allergic rhinitis, and atopic dermatitis (see Chapter 13). A family or personal history of atopy can be a key element in making the diagnosis.

While there are questions as to the specifics of the role of the immune system and allergies in AD, there is some type of abnormality in the cell-mediated immune system (a T-cell defect) in these patients. They have an increased susceptibility to cutaneous viral (and fungal) infections, especially herpes simplex, molluscum contagiosum, and papillomavirus.[10,11] However, even though about 80% of patients with AD have an elevated immunoglobulin E (IgE) level, there is not enough evidence to conclude what specific role allergies play in the development of this disease.[12,13] Thus even though many people are under the misperception that their skin is allergic to just about everything, they should be taught that the process is not a true allergy but rather a reaction of genetically abnormal skin to environmental stressors.

The eruption is eczematous and usually symmetric. It is erythematous, may have papules and plaques, and often has secondary changes of excoriations and lichenification. The persistent excoriations can lead to secondary bacterial infection, which may be noted by more exudative and crusting lesions. In infants and children, AD is commonly seen on the face and the extensor areas, whereas in older children and adults it is more commonly seen in flexural areas of the popliteal and antecubital fossae and the neck and wrists (Fig. 19.1). Patients with AD may also have numerous other features including generalized xerosis, cheilitis, hand dermatitis, palmar hyperlinearity, and sensitivity to wool and lipid solvents (e.g., lanolin).[9,10]

Treatment of atopic dermatitis begins with attempts at moisturizing the skin. Bathing is done only when necessary and then with cool or tepid water and a mild soap (e.g., Dove or Purpose) or a soap substitute (e.g., Cetaphil). Immediately after bathing and gently patting the skin dry, an emollient is applied to the skin to help seal in the moisture. This emollient should have no fragrances, no alcohol, and no lanolin (e.g., Aquaphor, Keri lotion, Lubriderm) and should be used daily to maintain well-lubricated skin. If the affected areas are particularly severe in an acute outbreak, wet dressings with aluminum acetate solution (Burow's solution) can be applied two or three times daily. If the affected area has dry, noninflamed skin, a moisturizer with lactic acid (e.g., Lac-Hydrin) can be of such help that steroids can be avoided.

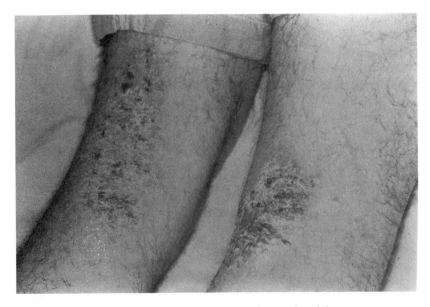

Figure 19.1. Atopic dermatitis in the popliteal fossae.

Controlling the intense pruritus is important. Keeping the nails trimmed short, and the use of mittens at night can decrease the excoriations in children. Topical steroids can control the inflammatory process. Generally the lowest possible potency should be used, but often high-potency creams may be needed on lichenified areas. In infants and children, one can often maintain good control with 0.25% to 2.5% hydrocortisone cream or ointment, applied two or three times a day. For more severe cases and in adults, 0.1% triamcinolone cream or ointment (or an equivalent-strength steroid) may be needed. Only rarely should fluorinated steroid preparations be used. While the underlying pathogenesis and the pruritus of AD are not primarily histamine mediated, many authors recommend the use of antihistamines that can be adjusted and titrated to balance the antipruritic effect with any potential sedating effects.[9–11] The more traditionally sedating antihistamines such as diphenhydramine (Benadryl) or hydroxyzine (Atarax, Vistaril) can be used at night and loratadine (Claritin) or cetirizine (Zyrtec) can be used during the day. Doxepin hydrochloride 5% cream (Zonalon) has both H_1 and H_2 blocking effects and may help to control pruritus without the problems of long-term topical steroid use; however, absorption of this agent leads to drowsiness in some patients, particularly if a large amount of the skin is treated. Tacrolimus ointment (Protopic) is an immunomodulating agent that was FDA approved for AD in 2001. It works similarly to cyclosporine and has been shown to be safe and effective for both long- and short-term use in AD.[14]

If the AD suddenly becomes much worse, development of a secondary infection or a possible contact dermatitis must be considered. If there is secondary infection, antibiotics directed at *Staphylococcus aureus* are used. Dicloxacillin, erythromycin, cephalexin, and topical mupirocin (Bactroban) are good choices. For patients prone to recurrent impetigo, it is reasonable to have a usual supply of mupirocin at home for any outbreaks. If these measures fail to provide adequate control, it is reasonable to pursue possible specific provocative factors such as foods, contact allergens or irritants, dust mites, molds, or possible psychological stressors.[9]

This condition can produce a great deal of anxiety and frustration in both patients and parents, and the stress can further aggravate the condition. Although psychological factors aggravate the condition, it is important to emphasize that the condition is not caused by "nerves." It is an inherited condition that can be aggravated by emotional stress. This supportive counseling for the patient and the family can be crucial. Furthermore, although affected children may appear "fragile," they are not, and they may desperately need some affectionate handling to help ease their own anxieties about their condition.[15]

Miliaria

Miliaria (heat rash) is a common condition resulting from the blockage of eccrine sweat glands. There is an inflammatory response to the sweat that leaks through the ruptured duct into the skin, and papular or vesicular lesions result.

It usually occurs after repeated exposure to a hot and humid environment. Miliaria can occur at any age but is especially common in infants and children.[16]

One of the most common forms of miliaria is miliaria crystallina, in which the blockage occurs near the skin surface and the sweat collects below the stratum corneum. A thin-walled vesicle then develops, but there is little to no erythema. This situation is often seen in infants or bedridden patients and can be treated with cool compresses and good ventilation to control perspiration.

Miliaria rubra (prickly heat or heat rash) is more commonly seen in susceptible patients of any age group when exposed to sufficient heat. In this case the occlusion is at the intraepidermal section of the sweat duct. As a result there is more erythema, sometimes a red halo, or just diffuse erythema with papules and vesicles. Occasionally, the eruptions become pustular, resulting in miliaria pustulosa. There is usually more of a mild stinging or "prickly" sensation than real pruritus. The condition is self-limited but can be alleviated by cool wet to dry soaks. A low-strength steroid lotion (e.g., 0.025% or 0.1% triamcinolone lotion) is often helpful for alleviating the symptoms in these patients.[10]

Pityriasis Rosea

Pityriasis rosea (PR) is a benign, self-limited condition primarily found in patients between the ages of 10 and 35. The cause is unknown, but a viral etiology is suspected as some patients have a prodrome of a viral-like illness with malaise, low-grade fever, cough, and arthralgias; there is an increased incidence in the fall, winter, and spring.[17]

This disorder typically starts with a single, 2- to 10-cm, oval, papulosquamous, salmon-pink patch (or plaque) on the trunk or proximal upper extremity. This "herald patch" is followed by a generalized eruption of discrete, small, oval plaques on the trunk and proximal extremities, sparing the palms and soles and oral cavity. These plaques align their long axis with the skin lines, thus giving the rash a characteristic "Christmas tree" appearance (Fig. 19.2). The plaques often have a fine, tissue-like "collarette" scale at the edges.

The differential diagnosis includes tinea corporis, as the initial herald patch can be confused with ringworm. The diffuse eruption of PR may resemble secondary syphilis but can often be distinguished by the sparing of the palms and soles in PR. It may also give the appearance of psoriasis (especially guttate psoriasis) but has much finer plaques that are not clustered on the extensor areas. Finally, the eruption may be confused with tinea versicolor. Skin scrapings for a potassium chloride (KOH) preparation should be strongly considered in any patient with apparent PR, as well as serologic testing for syphilis in any sexually active patient.

The management of PR is fairly easy. Pruritus is generally mild and can be controlled with oral antihistamines or topical low-potency steroid preparations. Patients can be reassured that the lesions will fade within about 6 weeks, but may last up to 10 weeks. They should be warned, however, that postinflammatory

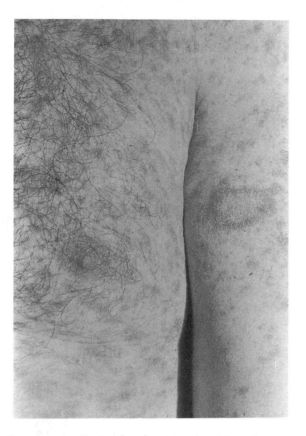

Figure 19.2. Pityriasis rosea. (Note herald patch on arm.)

hypo- or hyperpigmentation (especially in those with more darkly pigmented skin) is possible.[17]

Psoriasis

Psoriasis is a chronic, recurrent disorder characterized by an inflammatory, scaling, hyperproliferative papulosquamous eruption. Lesions are well-defined plaques with a thick, adherent, silvery white scale. If the scale is removed, pinpoint bleeding can be seen (Auspitz's sign). Psoriasis occurs in about 1% to 3% of the worldwide population.[18] The etiology is unknown, although some genetic link is suspected, as one third of patients have a positive family history for the disease. It may start at any age, with the mean age of onset during the late twenties.[19]

Lesions most commonly occur on the extensor surfaces of the knees and elbows but are also typically seen on the scalp and the sacrum and can affect the palms and soles as well. The nails may show pitting, onycholysis, or brownish macules ("oil spots") under the nail plate. Finally, up to 20% of these patients may develop psoriatic arthritis, which can be severe, even crippling.[20]

Although psoriasis is usually not physically disabling and longevity is not affected, the patient's physical appearance can be profoundly affected and may cause significant psychological stress as the patient withdraws from social activities. Attention to the psychosocial implications of this chronic disease is crucial for every family physician.

The classic presentation, chronic plaque psoriasis or psoriasis vulgaris, demonstrates erythematous plaques and silvery adherent scales on elbows, knees (Fig. 19.3), scalp, or buttocks. It is usually easy to diagnose when in the classic form, but there are numerous morphologic variants. Discoid, guttate, erythrodermic, pustular, flexural (intertriginous), light-induced, and palmar-plantar psoriasis are among the many clinical presentations of this condition. The plaques may be confused with seborrheic or atopic dermatitis, and the guttate variant may resemble pityriasis rosea or secondary syphilis. If the diagnosis is unclear, referral to a dermatologist or a biopsy (read by a dermatopathologist, if possible) is in order.

The lesions often appear on areas subjected to trauma (Koebner phenomenon). Other precipitating factors include infections, particularly upper respiratory infections, and stress. Several drugs, particularly lithium, beta-blockers, angiotensin-converting enzyme (ACE) inhibitors, and antimalarial agents are well known to trigger an outbreak or exacerbate existing psoriasis in some patients.[18,19]

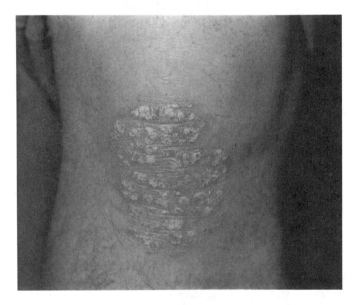

FIGURE 19.3. Typical psoriatic plaque.

The non-steroidal antiinflammatory drugs (NSAIDs) used for psoriatic arthritis may worsen the skin manifestations. Systemic corticosteroids can initially clear the psoriasis, but a "rebound phenomenon," or worsening of the lesions, even after slowly tapering the dose is common.

Management

Patients must understand that there is no cure for psoriasis. All treatments are suppressive (i.e., designed to control the manifestations, improve the cosmetic appearance for the patient, and, it is hoped, induce a remission). Therapy should start with liberal use of emollients and mild soaps. Moderate exposure to sunlight, while avoiding sunburn, can also improve the condition. After this start, treatment modalities are divided into topical agents and systemic therapies. The decision to use systemic agents is usually based on the percent of body surface area involved, with 20% often being used as the cutoff for changing to systemic treatment. In practice, however, the decision to use systemic therapy is based on the severity of the disease, the resistance to topical treatments, the availability of other agents, and a complex of social and psychological factors.[18–22] This decision is usually best made by an experienced dermatologist in consultation with the patient and the family physician.

Keratolytic preparations such as those with salicylic acid (Keralyt gel) or urea-based (Lac-Hydrin) can soften plaques and increase the efficacy of other topical agents. With the exception of emollients, the topical treatments for chronic plaque psoriasis should be applied to the lesions only and not the surrounding skin. It should be carefully explained to the patient that the medications that stop the overgrowth of the psoriatic skin have side effects on the normal surrounding skin and application should be done carefully.

Topical steroid preparations are a typical starting point for psoriasis, and while they can provide prompt relief, it is often temporary. Tolerance to these agents is common (tachyphylaxis), and one must remain vigilant for the long-term side effects of thinning of the skin, hypopigmentation, striae, and telangiectasia. The lowest effective strength is used, always using caution with higher strengths on the face, groin, and intertriginous areas. Increased efficacy is seen when ointments are used under occlusion, but this practice can also lead to enough systemic absorption to suppress the pituitary-adrenal system.[20]

The topical agent calcipotriene 0.005% (Dovonex) has shown good results with mild to moderate plaque psoriasis. It is a derivative of vitamin D and works by inhibiting keratinocyte and fibroblast proliferation. It is available as a cream, ointment, or scalp solution and is applied as a thin layer twice a day with most improvement noted within 1 month. Side effects include itching or burning in 10% to 20% of patients and rare cases of hypercalcemia (<1%), particularly when large amounts are used (>100 g/week).[21]

Tazarotene (Tazorac) is a topical retinoid gel that inhibits epidermal proliferation and inflammation in psoriasis (and is also FDA approved for acne vulgaris). Tazarotene alone has shown only modest benefit and can often cause irritation.

Optimal benefit from this agent is obtained by combining it with a medium-potency steroid, such that tazarotene is applied each night and the steroid is applied each morning. This drug must be avoided in pregnant women due to potential teratogenic effects.[21]

Chronic plaques can often be managed by using the antimitotic agents of anthralin or coal tar. Anthralin preparations (e.g., Anthra-Derm, Drithocreme, Dritho-Scalp) can be applied to thick plaques in the lowest dose possible for about 15 minutes a day and then showered off. Care must be taken to avoid the face, genitalia, and flexural areas. The duration and strength of the preparation is gradually increased as tolerated until irritation occurs. This preparation is messy and can stain normal skin, clothing, and bathroom fixtures. Coal tar preparations can be used alone or, more successfully, in combination with ultraviolet B (UVB) light therapy (Goeckerman regimen).[19] Coal tar may be found in both crude and refined preparations, such as bath preparations, gels, ointments, lotions, creams, solutions, soaps, and shampoos. In general, the treatment is similar to that with anthralin; progressively higher concentrations are used as needed until irritation or improvement results. The preparations are left on overnight, and staining can be a problem.

When systemic therapy is needed, treatment with ultraviolet (UV) light can be extremely effective. There are two basic regimens: One uses UVB (alone or with coal tar or anthralins) and the other uses UVA light therapy with oral psoralens (PUVA) therapy. The psoralen acts as a photosensitizer, and the UVA is administered in carefully measured amounts via a specially designed unit. Phototherapy and photochemotherapy can be expensive and carcinogenic. Thus they are administered only by an experienced dermatologist. Other systemic agents include the retinoid acitretin (Soriatane), methotrexate, etretinate (Tegison), and cyclosporine.[18–21] Due to the numerous side effects of these medicines, their use is generally best left to an experienced dermatologist and is beyond the scope of this text.

The lesions of psoriasis may disappear with treatment, but residual erythema, hypopigmentation, or hyperpigmentation is common. Patients must be instructed to continue treatment until there is near or complete resolution of the induration and not to always expect complete disappearance of the lesions.

Family and Community Issues

Proper patient and family education is crucial for managing the physical and psychosocial manifestations of this disease. The patient should be allowed to participate in the decision of which treatment modalities will be used and must be carefully instructed on the proper use of the one(s) chosen. The ongoing emotional support the family physician provides can help prevent the emotional scars that psoriasis may leave behind. The National Psoriasis Foundation (6600 SW 92nd, Suite 300, Portland, OR 97223; phone 800-723-9166, *www.psoriasis.org*) is a nonprofit organization dedicated to supporting research and education in this field. It provides newsletters and other educational material for patients and their families. A written prescription with the address and Web site can be one of the most effective long-term "treatments" for these patients.

Poison Ivy, Poison Oak, and Sumac (Rhus Dermatitis)

Plant-related contact dermatitis can be triggered by numerous plant compounds, but the most common allergen is the urishiol resin found in the genus *Toxicodendron* (formerly *Rhus*) containing the plants poison ivy, poison oak, and poison sumac. These three plants cause more allergic contact dermatitis than all other contact materials combined.[10] The oleoresin urishiol, which serves as the allergen (and rarely as a primary irritant), is located within all parts of the plant.[23]

The clinical presentation varies with the amount of the allergen and the patient's own degree of sensitivity. About 70% to 80% of Americans are mildly to moderately sensitive to the allergen, with about 10% to 15% at each end of the spectrum—either very sensitive or completely tolerant.[24] The eruption is erythematous with papules, wheals, and often vesicles. In severe cases, large bullae or diffuse urticarial hives are seen. The distribution is often linear or streak-like on exposed skin from either direct contact with the plant or by inadvertent spreading of the resin by the patient.

A history of exposure to the plant or to any significant activities outdoors helps in the diagnosis. It must be remembered, however, that the resin adheres to animal hair, clothing, and other objects and can then cling to the patient's skin after this indirect contact. Thus the patient may not be aware of any direct exposure. The thick, calloused skin on the hands often prevents eruption on the palms while the resin is transferred to another part of the body, where an eruption does occur. Outbreaks typically occur within 8 to 48 hours of the exposure. Alternatively, the initial exposure may sensitize the patient so the rash occurs a couple of weeks after exposure in response to the resin remaining on or in the skin.[23] The ability of the resin to remain on the skin (even after washing) and cause a later eruption has led to the mistaken belief that the fluid of the vesicles can cause spreading of the lesions.

Treatment begins with removal of any remaining allergen by thorough skin cleansing with soap and water as soon after exposure as possible. Rubbing (isopropyl) alcohol can be even more effective in dispersing the oily resin. Any clothing that may have come in contact with the plant should also be washed. If the affected area is small, and there is no significant vesicular formation, topical steroids (medium to high potency, such as triamcinolone 0.1–0.5%) are sufficient. The blisters can be relieved by frequent use of cool compresses with water or with Burow's solution (one packet or tablet of Domeboro in 1 pint of water). Oral antihistamines (e.g., diphenhydramine 25–50 mg or hydroxyzine 10–25 mg, four times a day) can help relieve the pruritus. If the outbreak is severe or widespread, or it involves the face and eyes, oral steroids may be needed. A tapering dose of prednisone (starting at 0.5–1.0 mg/kg/day) can be used over 5 to

7 days if the outbreak started a week or more after exposure. A longer, tapering course should be used (10–14 days) if treating an outbreak that started within 1 to 2 days of exposure. This regimen treats the lesions that are present and should suppress further development of lesions as the skin is sensitized.[24]

Prevention is best done by avoidance of the plants altogether or using clothing (that is then carefully removed to avoid rubbing the resin on the skin) as a barrier. The FDA has approved the first medication proved to prevent outbreak, bentoquatam (IvyBlock). This nonprescription lotion is applied before potential exposure and dries on the skin to form a protective barrier. This lotion does not irritate or sensitize the skin and provides 4 to 8 hours of protection. Desensitization attempts have not been successful and are not recommended.

Seborrheic Dermatitis

Seborrheic dermatitis, a chronic, recurrent scaling eruption, is common (incidence 3–5%) and typically occurs on the face, scalp, and the areas of the trunk where sebaceous glands are more prominent. It is usually seen in two age groups: infants during the first few months of life (may present as "cradle cap") and adults ages 30 to 60 (dandruff). It causes mild pruritus, is generally gradual in onset, and is fairly mild in its presentation. An increased incidence (up to 80%) has been described in patients with acquired immunodeficiency syndrome (AIDS), and these patients often present with a severe, persistent eruption[25] (see Chapter 21). The etiology is unknown, but there appears to be some link to the proliferation of the yeast *Pityrosporum ovale*, in the *Malassezia* genus. While this organism is present as normal flora for all people, the response of seborrheic dermatitis to antifungals agents strongly suggests a role for *P. ovale*.[26]

The lesions are scaling macules, papules, and plaques. They may be yellowish, thick and greasy, or sometimes white, dry, and flaky. Thick, more chronic lesions occasionally crust and then fissure and weep. Secondary bacterial infection leading to impetigo is not uncommon. The differential diagnosis includes atopic dermatitis, candidiasis, or a dermatophytosis. When the scalp is involved, the plaques are often confused with psoriasis, and the two conditions may overlap, referred to as seboriasis or sebopsoriasis. When the trunk is involved, the lesions may appear similar to those of pityriasis rosea.

Periodic use of shampoos containing selenium sulfide (Selsun, Selsun Blue), pyrithione zinc (Sebulon, Head and Shoulders), salicylic acid and sulfur combinations (Sebulex), or coal tar (Denorex, Neutrogena T-Gel) can be effective, not just on the scalp, but also on the trunk. The antifungal agent ketoconazole (Nizoral) is also available as a shampoo and can be highly effective. These shampoos are used two or three times a week and must be left on the skin (scalp) for about 5 to 10 minutes prior to rinsing. They are used alternating with regular soaps/shampoos as needed. This regimen may prevent the tachyphylaxis that can occur with daily use. After about 1 month the frequency of use can be decreased as tolerated to maintain control. Low-potency topical steroid creams or lotions such as 2.5% hydrocortisone or 0.01% fluocinolone (also available as a shampoo) can be used once or twice a day in the scalp or in other areas such as the face, groin, and chest. Topical ketoconazole cream (Nizoral) or terbinafine cream or spray (Lamisil) twice daily can also be helpful. Thick scales, such as may be found on the scalps of infants, can be gently scrubbed off with a soft toothbrush after soaking the area for 5 minutes with warm mineral oil or a salicylic acid shampoo. In severe and unresponsive cases, isotretinoin (Accutane) has been shown to be very effective in seborrheic dermatitis by markedly shrinking the size of the sebaceous glands and demonstrating some antiinflammatory effect. As compared to treatment for acne vulgaris, these patients often respond to lower doses (0.1 to 0.3 mg/kg/day) and shorter courses (4 weeks).[26] The same precautions, especially regarding pregnancy, that are described above must be observed.

Rosacea (Acne Rosacea)

A chronic facial dermatosis, acne rosacea typically appears in patients between the ages of 30 and 60. It is characterized by acneiform lesions such as papules, pustules, and occasionally nodules (Fig. 19.4). It is more common in those of

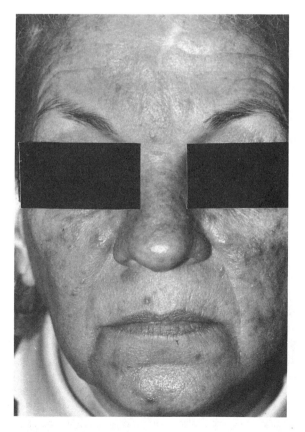

FIGURE 19.4. Acne rosacea.

Celtic, Scandinavian, or Northern European descent—those with fair skin who
tend to flush easily. In addition to the facial flushing, generalized erythema, and
telangiectasias, they may have moderate to severe sebaceous gland hyperplasia.
Ocular manifestations such as conjunctivitis, blepharitis, and episcleritis can be
found in more than half of the patients. Severe involvement of the nose can lead
to soft tissue hypertrophy and rhinophyma. Otherwise, most lesions are on the
forehead, cheeks, and nose. The pathogenesis is unknown, but increasing evidence suggests that it is primarily a cutaneous vascular disorder that leads to lymphatic damage followed by edema, erythema, and finally papules and pustules.[27]
Despite popular conception, alcohol is not known to play a causative role, but
the vasodilatory effects of alcohol may make the condition appear worse. There
is also some vasomotor instability in response to stress, sun exposure, hot liquids, and spicy foods, and these should be avoided.[28]

Treatment with oral erythromycin or tetracycline 1 g/day in divided doses or
with minocycline or doxycycline at 50 to 100 mg twice a day can help alleviate
both the facial and ocular manifestations of the disease. Response is variable,
with some patients showing a prompt response followed by weeks or months of
remission and others requiring long-term suppression with antibiotics. If long-
term treatment is needed, the dose is titrated down to the minimal effective
amount. Topical agents include clindamycin and erythromycin, but some of
the better responses are seen with metronidazole 0.75% gel, lotion or cream
(MetroGel, MetroLotion, Metrocream), or 1% cream (Noritate) in mild to moderate cases.[29] Topical sodium sulfacetamide and sulfur lotion is available in a
unique preparation (Sulfacet-R) that includes a color blender for patients to add
tint to the lotion to match their own skin coloration. This agent is popular with
women in particular who may wish to hide the erythema and lesions. Oral metronidazole (Flagyl) may be used with caution in resistant cases. Topical tretinoin
(Retin-A) and oral isotretinoin (Accutane) have shown promising results in patients with severe, refractory rosacea.[29–31]

Dyshidrotic Eczema (Pompholyx)

Dyshidrotic eczema, a recurrent eczematous dermatosis of the fingers, palms, and
soles, is more common in the young population (under age 40) and typically presents with pruritic, often tiny, deep-seated vesicles. The etiology is unknown, but
despite the name and the fact that many patients may have associated hyper-
hidrosis, it is not a disorder of sweat retention. Many of these patients have a
history of atopic dermatitis, and it is considered a type of hand/foot eczema. Emotional stress plays a role in some cases, as does ingestion of certain allergens
(e.g., nickel and chromate).[10]

The onset is typically abrupt and lasts a few weeks, but the disorder can become chronic and lead to fissuring and lichenification. Secondary bacterial infection can also occur. The vesicles are usually small but can be bullous and may
give the appearance of tapioca. The most common site is the sides of the fingers

in a cluster distribution (Fig. 19.5). The nails can also show involvement with dystrophic changes such as ridging, pitting, or thickening.

Controlling this disorder can be difficult and frustrating for the physician and patient alike. Attempts should be made to remove the inciting stressor whenever possible. Further treatment is similar to that for atopic dermatitis: Cool compresses may provide relief, and topical steroids can alleviate the inflammation and pruritus. It is one of the dermatoses in which high-potency fluorinated or halogenated steroids (in the ointment or gel formulation) are often needed to penetrate the thick stratum corneum of the hands. If secondary infection is present, erythromycin or cephalexin can be helpful. Rarely, oral steroids may be needed, but these drugs are reserved for the more severe, recalcitrant cases.

Drug Eruptions

Rashes of various types are common reactions to medications. The dermatologic manifestations can be highly variable: maculopapular (or morbilliform) eruptions;

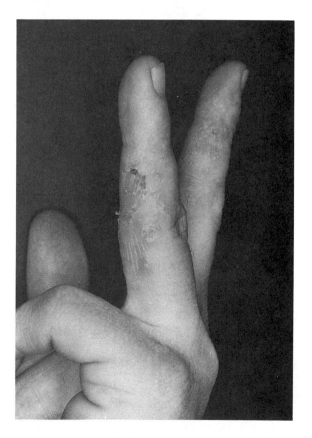

FIGURE 19.5. Dyshidrotic eczema (or pompholyx).

urticaria; fixed, hyperpigmented lesions; photosensitivity reactions; vesicles and bullae; acneiform lesions; and generalized pruritus, among others. Serious and even life-threatening dermatologic reactions can occur as well, such as Stevens-Johnson syndrome, toxic epidermal necrolysis, hypersensitivity syndrome, and serum sickness.[31,32]

Definitively assigning a diagnosis of a particular eruption to a single agent can be difficult, as patients may take multiple medications, they may have coexistent illnesses, and the drug eruption may not manifest until the patient has been taking it for several days (sometimes weeks). Only when the eruption follows the administration a particular agent, resolves with removal of the agent, recurs with readministration, and other causes have been excluded can one say that the eruption is definitely due to a specific drug. Caution must be used prior to any rechallenge with an agent, and so readministration is often not recommended. Subsequently, many patients mistakenly believe they have dermatologic reactions or allergies to certain medications when their rash may have had nothing to do with their medication.

Table 19.1 lists several of the typical drug reactions to some of the more common drugs in clinical practice.[10,15,24,32–34] Treatment consists of stopping the offending (or suspected) medication. Topical low- to mid-potency steroids and oral antihistamines can relieve the pruritus that accompanies many eruptions.

TABLE 19.1. Common Reactions to Common Drugs

Anaphylaxis	Maculopapular (morbilliform)	Serum sickness
Aspirin	Barbiturates	Aspirin
Sulfonamides	Isoniazid	Penicillin
NSAIDs	Phenothiazines	Sulfonamide
Serum (animal derived)	Sulfonamides and sulfonylureas	Urticaria
Penicillins	Lithium	Antibiotics
Fixed drug eruptions	NSAIDs	Opiates
Antibiotics—penicillins, sulfonamides, tetracyclines	Phenytoin	Blood products
	Thiazides	Radiocontrast agents
Phenolphthalein	Gentamicin	NSAIDs
Barbiturates	Penicillin compounds	Vesicular eruption
Dextromethorphan	Quinidine	Barbiturates
NSAIDs	Photosensitivity	Clonidine
Allopurinol	Carbamazepine	Naproxen
Lupus-like eruptions	Methotrexate	Sulfonamides
Hydralazine	Coal tar compounds	Captopril
Methyldopa	Oral contraceptives	Furosemide
Hydrochlorothiazide	Furosemide	Penicillin
Procainamide	NSAIDs	Cephalosporins
Isoniazid	Quinidine	Nalidixic acid
Quinidine	Tetracyclines	Piroxicam
	Griseofulvin	
	Phenothiazines	
	Sulfonamides and sulfonylureas	
	Thiazides	

NSAID = nonsteroidal antiinflammatory drug.

Contact Dermatitis

Contact dermatitis is the clinical response of the skin to an external stimulant. It is an extremely common condition. Chemically caused dermatitis is responsible for an estimated 30% of all occupational illness.[35] The condition is such a problem with a wide variety of mechanisms of pathogenesis and potential products involved that an international journal, *Contact Dermatitis*, is devoted specifically to this topic. By suspecting virtually everything and anything and taking a thorough history, the family physician nevertheless should be able to diagnose and manage most of these patients.

While some authors describe several different subtypes of contact dermatitis, the two most common types are irritant contact dermatitis and allergic contact dermatitis. Morphologically and histologically, they can appear identical, and the difference to the clinician is more conceptual.[36] Irritant contact dermatitis accounts for the majority of cases of contact dermatitis, and results from a break in the skin's integrity and subsequent local absorption of an irritant. There is no true demonstrable allergen present. A single exposure can induce an inflammatory response if the agent is caustic enough or if there is a marked degree of exposure. Often the response is the result of prolonged exposure with repeated minor damage to the skin, such as in those who must wash their hands frequently. Common offending agents include soaps, industrial solvents, and topical medications (e.g., benzoyl peroxide, tretinoin, lindane, benzyl benzoate, anthralin).[37,38]

The second most common type is allergic contact dermatitis. It is a delayed hypersensitivity reaction that occurs after the body is sensitized to the offending agent. The reaction is thus often delayed somewhat from the time of exposure. The response varies depending on the individual's sensitivity, the amount and concentration of the allergen, and the degree of penetration. Poison ivy dermatitis is perhaps the most common form of allergic contact dermatitis (discussed earlier in the chapter). Other common offenders are nickel, fragrances, rubber chemicals, neomycin, thimerosal, parabens (found in sunscreens and lotions), and benzocaine (topical anesthetic).[36–38] Even topical steroid preparations have been reported to cause allergic contact dermatitis in some patients.[39]

Physical findings may be identical or may vary somewhat with different forms of contact dermatitis. The irritant type often causes an erythematous scaling eruption with a typically indistinct margin (Fig. 19.6), whereas the allergic type may cause more erythema, edema, vesicular formation, and weeping. The offending agent is often identified more by the shape of the eruption than the appearance of the skin (e.g., a watchband or the elastic band of some article of clothing).

Treatment is symptomatic after removal of the irritant or allergen. Cool compresses can provide relief from the pruritus, particularly if there is any weeping. Oral antihistamines may be needed along with topical steroids. Ointment compounds are recommended, as they are less irritating and sensitizing than most creams or lotions. The patient should avoid any topical preparations with benzocaine or other -caines, as they may aggravate the condition. In severe cases a

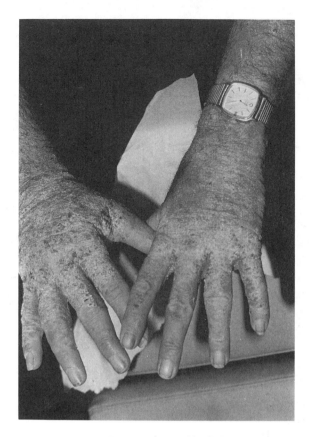

FIGURE 19.6. Contact dermatitis, irritant type.

tapering course of oral steroids over 1 to 2 weeks is necessary. Subacute and chronic cases may also be colonized with *Staphylococcus aureus*, and an oral antibiotic (e.g., dicloxacillin, erythromycin, or cephalexin) may speed resolution.

Avoidance of the irritant or allergen is sometimes difficult for patients. Their job may require some exposure, or it may be difficult to verify the specific agent. Testing with a commercially available patch test kit (T.R.U.E. Test Allergen Patch Test Panel) is the most reliable method of identifying a true allergic contact dermatitis and its causative agent.[39] This is particularly useful in developing a long-term plan of avoidance.

Urticaria

Urticaria, a common skin condition affecting about 20% of the population, is characterized by transient wheals or hives.[40] It is typically a type I immunologic reaction (mediated by IgE) but may be from physical or environmental exposure (pressure- or cold-induced). Urticaria can be acute (lasting less than 6 weeks) or chronic. Perhaps the most frustrating issue for the patient and physician faced with urticaria is that the underlying cause is often difficult to ascertain. In only about 20% of cases of chronic urticaria can the specific etiology be determined.[41,42]

A generalized eruption of pruritic wheals with erythema and localized edema and lesions lasting less than 24 hours establishes the diagnosis. Angioedema is a closely related process in which deeper tissues may be involved, particularly mucous membranes. Severe generalized urticaria can be a systemic illness leading to cardiac problems and even death.

One should search carefully to find the underlying etiology by doing a thorough comprehensive history and physical examination. Common causes include medications (antibiotics, NSAIDs, narcotics, radiocontrast dyes), illnesses (viral hepatitis, streptococcal, parasitic), connective tissue disorders (lupus, juvenile rheumatoid arthritis), endocrine disorders (hyper- or hypothyroidism), neoplastic disorders (lymphoma, leukemia, carcinoma), physical agents (pressure, cold, heat, exercise, menstruation), skin contacts (chemicals, fragrances, dyes, soaps, lotions, feathers, animal dander), insect bites and bee stings, foods (chocolate, shellfish, strawberries, nuts), and psychological stress.[10,15,40,41,43] The amount of laboratory work and other testing recommended can be highly variable and depends in part on the clinical utility of finding the underlying trigger(s). In general, an extensive workup is not advised during the first 6 weeks. Once the condition has persisted into chronic urticaria, a thorough history is as effective as an extensive and costly laboratory workup in finding the underlying cause.[40,44]

Treatment consists of avoidance of any known or suspected precipitant and the use of medications as needed for comfort. The H_1-blockers such as cetirizine (Zyrtec), loratadine (Claritin), diphenhydramine, or hydroxyzine can be used alone or in combination with an H_2-blocker such as cimetidine (Tagamet). Doxepin, a tricyclic antidepressant, can also be helpful at 25 mg once or twice a day. For severe, acute urticaria, a tapering dose of prednisone over 2 weeks can be helpful. Chronic urticaria may require a great deal of maintenance emotional support, as the condition can make normal activities difficult. Patients must be reassured, and medications may be needed on a long-term daily basis.

References

1. White GM Recent findings in the epidemiologic evidence, classification, and subtypes of acne vulgaris. J Am Acad Dermatol 1998;39:S34–7.
2. Russell JJ. Topical therapy for acne. Am Fam Physician 2000;61:357–66.
3. Leyden JJ. New understandings of the pathogenesis of acne. J Am Acad Dermatol 1995;32:S15–25.
4. Rosenberg EW. Acne diet reconsidered. Arch Dermatol 1981;117:193–5.
5. Johnson BA, Nunley JR. Use of systemic agents in the treatment of acne vulgaris. Am Fam Physician 2000;62:1823–30,1835–6.
6. Leyden JJ. Therapy for acne vulgaris. N Engl J Med 1997;336(16):1156–62.

7. Thiboutot D. New treatments and therapeutic strategies for acne. Arch Fam Med 2000;9:179–83.
8. Van Durme DJ. Family physicians and Accutane. Am Fam Physician 2000;62:1772–7.
9. Kristal L, Klein PA. Atopic dermatitis in infants and children. An update. Pediatr Clin North Am 2000;47:877–95.
10. Habif TP. Clinical dermatology: a color guide to diagnosis and therapy, 3rd ed. St. Louis: Mosby-Year Book, 1996.
11. Fleischer AB. Atopic dermatitis. Perspectives on a manageable disease. Postgrad Med 1999;106:49–55.
12. Borirchanyavat K, Kurban AK. Atopic dermatitis. Clin Dermatol 2000;18:649–55.
13. Halbert AR, Weston WL, Morelli JG. Atopic dermatitis: is it an allergic disease? J Am Acad Dermatol 1995;33:1008–18.
14. Leicht S, Hanggi M. Atopic dermatitis. Postgrad Med 2001;109(6):119–27.
15. Goldstein BG, Goldstein AO. Practical dermatology, 2nd ed. St. Louis: Mosby-Year Book, 1997.
16. Feng E, Janniger CK. Miliaria. Cutis 1995;55:213–6.
17. Bjornberg A, Tenger E. Pityriasis rosea. In: Freedberg IM, Eisen AZ, Wolff K, et al, eds. Dermatology in general medicine, 5th ed. New York: McGraw-Hill, 1999;541–6.
18. Greaves MW, Weinstein GD. Treatment of psoriasis. N Engl J Med 1995;332:581–8.
19. Christophers E, Moreweitz U. Psoriasis. In: Freedberg IM, Eisen AZ, Wolff K, et al, eds. Dermatology in general medicine. 5th ed. New York: McGraw-Hill, 1999;495–522.
20. Linden KG. Weinstein GD. Psoriasis: current perspectives with an emphasis on treatment. Am J Med 1999;107:595–605.
21. Pardasani AG, Feldman SR, Clark AR. Treatment of psoriasis: an algorithm-based approach for primary care physicians. Am Fam Physician 2000;61:725–33,736.
22. American Academy of Dermatology. Committee on Guidelines of Care, Task Force on Psoriasis. Guidelines of care for psoriasis. J Am Acad Dermatol 1993;28:632–7.
23. Tanner TL. Rhus (Toxicodendron) dermatitis. Prim Care 2000;27:493–502.
24. Pariser RJ. Allergic and reactive dermatoses. Postgrad Med 1991;89:75–85.
25. Janniger CK, Schwartz RA. Seborrheic dermatitis. Am Fam Physician 1995;52:149–59.
26. Johnson BA, Nunley JR. Treatment of seborrheic dermatitis. Am Fam Physician 2000;61:2703–10, 2713–14.
27. Wilkin JK. Rosacea: pathophysiology and treatment. Arch Dermatol 1994;130:359–62.
28. Zuber TJ. Rosacea. Prim Care 2000;27:309–18.
29. Thiboutot DM. Acne and rosacea. New and emerging therapies. Dermatol Clin 2000;18:63–71.
30. Ertl GA, Levine N, Kligman AM. A comparison of the efficacy of topical tretinoin and low dose oral isotretinoin in rosacea. Arch Dermatol 1994;130:319–24.
31. Hirsch RJ, Weinberg JM. Rosacea 2000. Cutis 2000;66:125–8.
32. Roujeau JC, Stern RS. Severe adverse cutaneous reactions to drugs. N Engl J Med 1994;33:1272–85.
33. Manders SM. Serious and life-threatening drug eruptions. Am Fam Physician 1995;51:1865–72.
34. Crowson AN. Recent advances in the pathology of cutaneous drug eruptions. Dermatol Clin 1999;17:537–60.

35. Anonymous. Contact dermatitis and urticaria from environmental exposures: Agency for Toxic Substances and Diseases Registry. Am Fam Physician 1993;48:773–80.
36. Rietschel RL. Comparison of allergic and irritant contact dermatitis. Immunol Allergy Clin North Am 1997;17:359–64.
37. Oxholm A, Maibach MI. Causes, diagnosis, and management of contact dermatitis. Compr Ther 1990;16:18–24.
38. Adams RM. Recent advances in contact dermatitis. Ann Allergy 1991;67:552–66.
39. Belsito DV. The diagnostic evaluation, treatment, and prevention of allergic contact dermatitis in the new millennium. J Allergy Clin Immunol 2000;105:409–20.
40. Greaves MW. Chronic urticaria. N Engl J Med 1995;332:1767–72.
41. Beltrani VS. Allergic dermatoses. Med Clin North Am 1998;82:1105–33.
42. Huston DP, Bressler RB. Urticaria and angioedema. Med Clin North Am 1992;76:805–40.
43. Mahmood T. Urticaria. Am Fam Physician 1995;51:811–6.
44. Kozel MM, Mekkes JR, Bossuyt PM, Bos JD. The effectiveness of a history-based diagnostic approach in chronic urticaria and angioedema. Arch Dermatol 1998;134:1575–80.

CASE PRESENTATION

Subjective

PATIENT PROFILE

Ruth Nelson McCarthy is a 51-year-old married female restaurant operator.

PRESENTING PROBLEM

"Rash on hands."

PRESENT ILLNESS

For 8 to 10 months, the patient has noticed a rash on her hands. It occurs especially between the fingers and, when present, is red, irritated, and scaling. The itching of the rash prompts scratching, especially during her sleep at night.

PAST MEDICAL HISTORY

She has been taking estrogen replacement therapy since her previous visit 8 months ago (see Chapter 2).

FAMILY HISTORY, SOCIAL HISTORY, AND HABITS

All are unchanged since her previous visit.

- What additional information would you like regarding the history of present illness? Explain.
- What more would you like to know about her work?
- What might the patient be doing to treat her rash? Why might this be important?
- What are possible reasons for the patient's visit today? How would you address this issue?

Objective

Vital Signs

Blood pressure, 136/88; pulse, 72; respirations, 18; temperature, 37°C.

Examination

There is dermatitis of both hands, worse on the right. The rash especially involves the fingers and the interdigital folds. The skin is cracked and bleeding in places, and there is evidence of excoriation.

- What additional data about the examination of the hands might be useful?
- Are there additional areas of the body that you might examine? Why?
- What—if any—laboratory tests might be useful? Why?
- What physical findings might suggest that the problem is other than a localized dermatitis? Explain.

Assessment

- What is the probable diagnosis and its cause? How will you explain this to the patient?
- How might this relate to activities in her life?
- What are some implications of the diagnosis for Mrs. McCarthy and her family?
- If a similar rash were also present on other areas of the body, what diagnostic possibilities would you consider?

Plan

- What specific therapy would you recommend? How would you explain this to Mrs. McCarthy?
- How might this problem be prevented in the future? What changes in her work would you advise?
- If the rash became infected, with purulent drainage and crusting, what might you do differently?
- What continuing care would you recommend?

20
Diabetes Mellitus

CHARLES KENT SMITH, JOHN P. SHEEHAN,
AND MARGARET M. ULCHAKER

Diabetes mellitus (DM) affects 12 million to 15 million individuals in the United States, incurring an immense cost in terms of morbidity and premature death. The most prevalent form, type 2 DM, previously called adult-onset DM, has racial preponderances, female predilection, and strong associations with obesity. During the 1980s there was a revolution in DM management with the advent of home blood glucose monitoring devices, human insulin, and reliable laboratory markers of long-term glycemic control. Additionally, published national and international standards of care have been disseminated directly to patients and physicians, heightening the importance of adequate care and glycemic control to minimize devastating long-term complications.[1,2] Table 20.1 describes diagnostic criteria for diabetes mellitus, impaired glucose tolerance, and gestational diabetes.

Heightened clinical awareness of the genetics and predisposing factors should foster early diagnosis and adequate metabolic control of the type 2 patient. In contrast, the type 1 DM patient generally presents with a more precipitous clinical picture of ketoacidosis. Declining islet cell secretory function is more gradual, however, and can evolve over a 10-year period. Understanding the autoimmune nature of islet destruction has led to experimental protocols attempting to interrupt this process. Occasionally, there is diagnostic confusion owing to a lack of a family history, the absence of significant ketosis, and the absence of significant obesity and other diagnostic hallmarks. The measurement of C-peptide levels, islet cell antibodies, and glutamic acid decarboxylase (GAD) antibodies provides useful diagnostic clarification.[3] C-peptide is the fragment produced when proinsulin, produced by the islets of Langerhans, is cleaved to produce insulin. For every molecule of insulin produced, a molecule of C-peptide has to exist; therefore, C-peptide is a marker of endogenous insulin production. Measurement of a C-peptide level is very useful in documenting insulin secretory capacity in the insulin-treated individual, in whom an insulin level would measure both endogenous and exogenous insulin. Careful clinical follow-up can clarify evolving absolute insulin deficiency even in the absence of these laboratory markers.

TABLE 20.1. Diagnostic Criteria for Diabetes Mellitus, Impaired Glucose Tolerance, and Gestational Diabetes

Nonpregnant adults

Criteria for diabetes mellitus: Diagnosis of diabetes mellitus in nonpregnant adults should be restricted to those who have one of the following:

Fasting plasma glucose ≥126 mg/dL. Fasting is defined as no caloric intake for at least 8 hours.

Symptoms of diabetes mellitus (such as polyuria, polydipsia, unexplained weight loss) coupled with a casual plasma glucose level of ≥200 mg/dL. Casual is defined as any time of day without regard to time interval since the last meal.

2-hour postprandial plasma glucose ≥200 mg/dL during an oral glucose tolerance test. The test should be performed by World Health Organization criteria using a glucose load containing the equivalent of 75 g anhydrous glucose dissolved in water.

Note: In the absence of unequivocal hyperglycemia with acute metabolic decompensation, these criteria should be confirmed by repeat testing on a second occasion. The oral glucose tolerance test is not recommended for routine clinical use.

Criterion for impaired glucose tolerance: 2-hour postprandial plasma glucose ≥140 mg/dL and ≤199 mg/dL during an oral glucose tolerance test. The test should be performed by World Health Organization criteria using a glucose load containing the equivalent of 75 g anhydrous glucose dissolved in water.

Pregnant Women

Criteria for gestational diabetes: After an oral glucose load of 100 g, gestational diabetes is diagnosed if two plasma glucose values equal or exceed:

Fasting: 105 mg/dL
1 Hour: 190 mg/dL
2 Hour: 165 mg/dL
3 Hour: 145 mg/dL

Source: Clinical practice recommendations: 2001.[1]

Pathophysiology

Previously, type 1 DM was considered to be an acute event. Viral associations were invoked with regard to the seasonal trends in its incidence. However, patients can have markers of islet destruction in the form of islet cell antibodies for up to 10 years prior to the development of overt DM. Islet cell, insulin, and GAD autoantibodies, along with the loss of first-phase insulin secretion in response to an intravenous glucose tolerance test, are highly predictive of evolving type 1 DM.[4] Attempts to interrupt this autoimmune process with immunosuppressive agents have been tried with some encouraging results, but toxicity remains a concern. Insulin has been given to experimental animals that have autoimmune islet destruction without overt DM in an attempt to suppress the autoimmune process. A pilot study of 12 patients demonstrated exciting promise for clinical applicability of this approach in humans.[5] However a nationwide clinical trial of prophylactic insulin in individuals at high risk to develop type 1 DM disappointingly showed no effect on the rate of progression to type 1 DM. A group of investigators in Edmonton, Alberta, Canada have treated seven patients with type 1 DM with islet cell transplantation. These patients, who are initially on triple immunosuppression therapy, have normal ambient glucose levels. However, on intravenous glucose tolerance testing, they have impaired glucose tolerance. The key to islet cell transplantation is developing safe immunosuppressives or modifying the process to eliminate the need for immunosuppressives.[6]

In contrast, type 2 DM is associated with genetic predispositions, advancing age, obesity, and lack of physical exercise. The importance of caloric intake and energy expenditure has been clearly established.[7] Although type 2 DM is a syndrome of insulin resistance and islet secretory defects, in any given individual it is not possible to define the degree of insulin resistance versus secretory defects with any precision. The earliest metabolic defect found in first-degree relatives of individuals with type 2 DM is defective skeletal muscle glucose uptake with later increased insulin resistance at the level of the liver and resultant uncontrolled hepatic glucose output. The ensuing hyperglycemia can have a toxic effect called glucotoxicity on the islets, resulting in secondary secretory defects with declining insulin secretion and self-perpetuating hyperglycemia. Hyperglycemia may also downregulate glucose transporters. To become hyperglycemic, insulin secretion must be insufficient to overcome the insulin resistance; it has been estimated that insulin secretory capacity is reduced by 50% at the time of diagnosis with type 2 DM.[8] It is unclear whether secretory defects or insulin resistance is the primary defect even for type 2 DM. Patients may exhibit many abnormalities, including loss of first-phase insulin secretion and loss of the pulsatility of insulin secretion.[9–12] Additionally, both men and women tend to have abdominal obesity, which is associated with hyperinsulinemia and insulin resistance.[13] Type 2 DM is a syndrome not only of disordered glucose metabolism but also of lipid metabolism; many patients have a concurrent dyslipidemia manifesting elevations in serum triglycerides, depressions in high-density lipoprotein (HDL) cholesterol, and marginal increases in total cholesterol. This dyslipidemia results from uncontrolled hepatic very low density lipoprotein (VLDL) secretion and defective clearance of lipoprotein molecules. The associations of hyperinsulinemia and insulin resistance with essential hypertension have been documented[14] along with the marked tendency for patients with essential hypertension to develop DM and the converse—patients with type 2 DM developing essential hypertension. A central unifying hypothesis focuses on hyperinsulinemia and insulin resistance being primary metabolic aberrations that result not only in hyperglycemia but also hypertension and dyslipidemia. Thus our current understanding of type 2 DM and the cardiodysmetabolic syndrome, formerly known as syndrome X[15] (hyperinsulinemia, dyslipidemia, hypertension, and hyperglycemia) highlights the important issue not only of primary prevention of type 2 DM but also secondary prevention.

Importance of Glycemic Control

The relation between microvascular complications of DM and glycemic control has been debated for decades. Many studies suggested an association between poor long-term glycemic control and retinopathy, neuropathy, and nephropathy.

Unfortunately, many of these studies were not randomized, and the role of genetic factors was unclear. However, positive trends with glycemic control had been described. Small human studies and several animal studies link sustained metabolic control to the prevention of complications. One study showed, however, that early poor control despite later good control results in diabetic complications.[16] The Diabetes Control and Complications Trial (DCCT) in individuals with type 1 DM proved the profound impact of intensive therapy on reducing the risk of microvascular complications.[17] Decades of questions about the glucose hypothesis are therefore finally answered, with the obvious recommendation that most individuals with type 1 DM be treated with intensive therapy. A potential negative aspect of attempts to achieve optimum glycemic control by intensive insulin therapy is the potential for severe hypoglycemia. An educated and motivated patient working with a multidisciplinary health care team can significantly reduce the risk of this. Glycemic goals may need to be modified in the individual with poor hypoglycemia awareness. The United Kingdom Prospective Diabetes Study (UKPDS), a 20-year prospective study in type 2 DM, demonstrated that both intensive glycemic control and intensive blood pressure control reduced the risk of microvascular and macrovascular complications of DM.[18–20] Excellent metabolic control, as defined by normal hemoglobin A_{1c} (HbA$_{1c}$) levels without significant hypoglycemia, is an achievable goal.

Defining Control

The definition of DM control has varied. During the bygone era of urine testing, predominantly negative urine tests were indicative of good glycemic control. However, because blood glucose can be twice normal in the absence of glycosuria, urine glucose monitoring is now outmoded. Home blood glucose monitoring (HBGM) provides positive feedback of daily glycemic control to patients and physicians. Patients engaged in intensive insulin therapy can monitor themselves four to ten times per day and make adjustments in their regimen to optimize blood glucose control. The precision and accuracy of the home units has improved considerably, as has the simplicity and duration of the test. Some systems enable users to obtain the blood sample from the forearm. Each system has its inherent weaknesses and limitations in such areas as blood volume, timing, hematocrit, temperature, and humidity. It is important that patients adhere strictly to the manufacturers' guidelines because attention to proper calibrations, strip handling, and ongoing maintenance are critical. Minimally invasive HBGM is the wave of the future, with the Glucowatch Biographer being the first to reach market. The HbA$_{1c}$, the marker of long-term glycemic control, measures the degree of glycosylation of the A_{1c} subfraction of hemoglobin and reflects the average blood glucose over the preceding 60 to 90 days. It also allows for identification of possible falsification of or errors in HBGM results. It is a useful motivating tool for patients; it often becomes a perceived challenge to reduce the result within the constraints of hypoglycemia. The National Glycosylated Hemoglobin Standardization Program is responsible for standardizing and correlating various assays to the DCCT methodology.[21]

Hemoglobinopathies can skew HbA_{1c} results, and can be detected via inspection of the chromatograms in the laboratory. The American Diabetes Association recommends that the HbA_{1c} be performed at least two to four times per year in all patients. Given that the DCCT demonstrated a linear relation between the HbA_{1c} (all the way into the normal, non-diabetic range) and microvascular complication risk, the ideal is therefore normalization of the HbA_{a1c} within the constraints of hypoglycemia. In addition to markers of glycemic control, it is critical to monitor other clinical parameters. Annual lipid profiles are an integral part of overall DM care in view of the high prevalence of dyslipidemia especially in the patient with type 2 DM. In type 1 DM patients, lipid disturbances are uncommon unless patients are in poor glycemic control, have a familial dyslipidemia, or have renal insufficiency. Markers of nephropathy are also important to measure. The earliest marker, microalbuminuria, is not only a forerunner of overt clinical nephropathy but also a marker for greatly increased cardiovascular risk in both type 1 and type 2 patients.[22,23] Microalbuminuria can be conveniently measured in spot urine specimens or by overnight albumin excretion rates,[24] rather than the more cumbersome 24-hour urine collection.

Patient Education

Patient attention to management principles decidedly affects short-term metabolic control and ultimately has an impact on long-term complications. The interactions of patients with registered nurses and dietitians (preferably certified diabetes educators) are critical. The presence of family members and significant others during the educational sessions is vital to a successful outcome. Education must encompass a comprehensive understanding of the pathophysiology of DM and its complications and the importance of attaining and sustaining metabolic control. Accurate HBGM is critical; after initial instruction, periodic reassessment of performance technique helps to ensure continued accuracy. The results stored in the memory of most meters can be downloaded to a computer, via a meter-specific computer program. However, the traditional written glucose log actually provides more information when an educated, motivated patient records glucose results, times of day, medication administered, and notes regarding activity and other variables. Education must also focus on dietary principles. For individuals with diabetes, the current dietary recommendations are a diet containing at least 50% of the calories from carbohydrate, less than 30% fat, and 20% or less protein. Caloric requirements are based on ideal body weight (IBW)—not actual body weight. We calculate IBW by the Hamwi formula.[25]

Women
  100 pounds for 5 feet
  5 pounds for every additional inch
  Example: Woman 5'3" = 115 pounds IBW

Men
  106 pounds for 5 feet
  6 pounds for every additional inch
  Example: Man 5'8" = 154 pounds IBW

Based on anthropometric measures, 10% may be subtracted or added based on small body frame or large body frame, respectively.

Basal caloric requirements then are as follows.

Woman 5'3": IBW = 115 pounds
115 × 10 kcal = 1150 kcal/day

Add 300 to 400 kcal/day for moderate to strenuous activity. Subtract 500 kcal/day for 1 pound per week weight loss.

Because individuals with DM type 2 are generally hyperinsulinemic, diet prescriptions for weight loss and maintenance require a lower caloric level than previously mentioned. The activity factor in kilocalories (300–400 kcal/day) can be modified in these individuals. For the type 2 DM patient, caloric restriction is of major importance. In contrast, diet for the type 1 DM patient should involve careful consistency of carbohydrate intake. Achieving this degree of dietary education generally requires several sessions with a dietitian/nutrition specialist. Dietary principles are an ongoing exercise, and eradication of myths and misconceptions is a major task. Unfortunately, many patients still perceive that "sugar-free" implies carbohydrate-free and that "sugar-free" foods cannot affect blood glucose control. This belief fails to recognize the monomer/polymer concept and the fact that most carbohydrates are ultimately digested into glucose. In addition to maintaining carbohydrate consistency, patients must learn carbohydrate augmentation for physical activity in the absence of insulin reduction. Patients also need instruction on carbohydrate strategies for dealing with intercurrent illness when the usual complex carbohydrate may be substituted with simple carbohydrate. Although it has long been said that diet is the cornerstone of DM management,[26] effective DM dietary education is still problematic owing to time constraints and reimbursement problems.

Insulin-treated patients must be aware of the many facets of insulin therapy. Accurate drawing-up and mixing of insulin is an assumption that is often not founded in reality. Site selection, consistency, and rotation are crucial. Insulin absorption is most rapid from the upper abdomen; the arms, legs, and buttocks, respectively, are next. We find that administering the premeal insulin in the abdomen optimizes postmeal control (assuming the use of lispro, insulin aspart, or regular insulin). In contrast, the buttocks, as the slowest absorption site, is not a good choice for premeal injections. However, the lower buttocks is an ideal site for bedtime injections of intermediate-acting insulin [neutral protamine Hagedorn (NPH)/lente] to minimize nocturnal hypoglycemia. Haphazard site selection and rotation can lead to erratic glycemic control. Because of the variability in absorption among sites, we suggest site consistency—using the same anatomic site at the same time of day (all breakfast injections in the abdomen, all dinner injections in the arms, all bedtime injections in the lower buttocks). Broad rotation within the sites is important to eliminate local lipohypertrophy.[27] The fast-acting insulin analogues, lispro with its peak action 1 hour postinjection and the new insulin aspart with its peak action 30 to 90 minutes postinjection, significantly improve postprandial glycemic control. This facilitates insulin injection timing as it is injected 0 to 10 minutes premeal. In contrast, regular insulin requires premeal timing of insulin injections (generally 30 minutes) to optimize postprandial glycemic control, as its peak effect is 3 to 4 hours after injection. Patients need a comprehensive perspective on insulin adjustments[28] for hyperglycemia, altered physical activity, illness management, travel, and alcohol consumption.

Patients need education on the pathophysiology, prevention, and treatment of microvascular complications. Education on macrovascular risk factors and their modification for prevention of cardiovascular, cerebrovascular, and peripheral vascular disease is also critical. Patients can have a considerable impact on decreasing foot problems and amputations with simple attention to hygiene (avoidance of foot soaks), daily foot inspection, and the use of appropriate footwear. These measures can greatly reduce the incidence of trauma, sepsis, and ultimately amputations.[29]

Diabetic Complications

Complications of DM include those that are specific to DM and those that are nonspecific but are accelerated by the presence of DM. The microvascular complications of DM are diabetes specific—the triad of retinopathy, neuropathy, and nephropathy. Macrovascular disease—atherosclerosis—a common complication in patients with DM, is not specific to DM but is greatly accelerated by its presence. A major misconception among patients and even physicians is that the complications of DM tend to be less severe in patients with type 2 DM. Patients with type 2 DM or impaired glucose tolerance have greatly accelerated macrovascular disease and also suffer significant morbidity from microvascular complications.

Retinopathy

Retinopathy, the commonest cause of new-onset blindness during middle life, is broadly classified as nonproliferative (background) and proliferative. In addition, macular edema may be present in either category. Macular edema is characterized by a collection of intraretinal fluid in the macula, with or without lipid exudates (hard exudates). In nonproliferative retinopathy, ophthalmoscopic findings may include microaneursyms, intraretinal hemorrhages, and macular edema. In more advanced nonproliferative retinopathy, cotton wool spots reflecting retinal ischemia can be noted. In proliferative retinopathy, worsening retinal ischemia results in neovascularization, preretinal or vitreous hemorrhage and fibrous tissue proliferation. Macular edema can also occur in proliferative retinopathy. Early diagnosis and treatment with laser therapy has been shown to be vision sparing in patients with macular edema and/or proliferative retinopathy. Several studies clearly document the importance of annual examinations by an ophthalmologist for all patients.[30] Good visual acuity does not exclude significant retinal pathology; unfortunately, many patients, and health care providers alike, believe good visual acuity implies an absence of significant retinal disease.

Neuropathy

The clinical spectrum of diabetic neuropathy is outlined in Table 20.2.

Nephropathy/Hypertension

Diabetic nephropathy may first manifest as microalbuminuria, detected on a spot urine determination or by the timed overnight albumin excretion rate. The presence of microalbuminuria should alert the patient and physician to the need for stringent glycemic control; such control has been shown to decrease the progression from microalbuminuria to clinical proteinuria and attendant evolution of hypertension. Hypertension increases the rate of deterioration of renal function in patients with DM, and aggressive treatment is mandatory. The Captopril Diabetic Nephropathy Study demonstrated that treatment with the angiotensin-converting enzyme inhibitor (ACEI) captopril was associated with a 50% reduction in the risk of the combined end points of death, dialysis, and transplantation in macroproteinuric (>500 mg/24 hr) type 1 DM patients. Overall, the risk of doubling the serum creatinine was reduced by 48% in captopril-treated patients. The beneficial effects were seen in both normotensive and hypertensive

TABLE 20.2. Classification of Diabetic Neuropathy

Type	Signs and symptoms
Sensory peripheral polyneuropathy	Pain and dysesthesia Glove and stocking sensory loss Loss of reflexes Muscle weakness/wasting

Autonomic	Orthostatic hypotension
	Gastroparesis, diarrhea, atonic bladder,
	   impotence, anhidrosis, gustatory sweating,
	   cardiac denervation on ECG

Mononeuropathy	Cranial nerve palsy Carpal tunnel syndrome Ulnar nerve palsy
Amyotrophy	Acute anterior thigh pain Weakness of hip flexion Muscle wasting
Radiculopathy	Pain and sensory loss in a dermatomal distribution

patients such that captopril at a dose of 25 mg po tid is approved for use in normotensive proteinuric (>500 mg/24 hr) type 1 DM patients.[31] In light of this and other studies in both type 1 and type 2 DM patients, the use of ACEI for prevention of progression of microalbuminuria and macroalbuminuria is recommended, unless there is a contraindication. For antihypertensive therapy ACEI is the antihypertensive of choice, unless contraindicated, given the data not only in nephropathy but also in retinopathy. The recent Heart Outcomes Prevention Evaluation (HOPE) study demonstrated a reduced risk of microvascular and macrovascular events in individuals with DM treated with the ACEI ramipril.[32,33]

Given the macrovascular benefits alone, we should probably be looking for reasons not to prescribe ACEIs, rather than reasons to prescribe them. In patients intolerant of ACEIs due to cough, angiotensin receptor blockers and calcium channel blockers are good alternatives in light of data that show decreasing proteinuria with many of these agents over and above that achievable with conventional antihypertensive therapy. Additionally, beta-blockers have a favorable metabolic and side-effect profile. Avoidance of excessive dietary protein intake is also important, as excessive dietary protein may be involved in renal hypertrophy and glomerular hyperfiltration. Strict glycemic control even over a 3-week period can decrease renal size (as seen on ultrasonography) and decrease the hyperfiltration associated with amino acid infusions to levels comparable to those of normal, non-DM individuals.[34] Nationwide clinical trials with pimagedine (an inhibitor of protein glycosylation and cross-linking) in diabetic nephropathy were discontinued due to adverse events and efficacy issues. Newer generation inhibitors of glycosylation and cross-linking are under clinical development.

Patients with DM in general are salt-sensitive, having diminished ability to excrete a sodium load with an attendant rise in blood pressure; therefore, avoidance of excessive dietary sodium intake is important. Hyperinsulinemia and insulin resistance are also important in the genesis of hypertension, with insulin-resistant patients having higher circu-lating insulin levels to maintain normal glucose levels. Associated with this insulin resistance and hyperinsulinemia is the occurrence of elevated blood pressures even in nondiabetic individuals. Insulin is antinatriuretic and stimulates the sympathetic nervous system; both mechanisms may be important in the genesis of hypertension. Hypertension exacerbates retinopathy, nephropathy, and macrovascular disease and must be diagnosed early and managed aggressively. When lifestyle modifications fail to control blood pressure, the pharmacologic agent chosen should be not only efficacious but kind to the metabolic milieu. Diuretics are very useful in edematous states. Beta-blockers have an important role in the post–myocardial infarction/anginal patient and in the heart failure patient. The benefits of beta-blockade in these patients outweigh the theoretical problems of masking of hypoglycemia, delay in recovery of hypoglycemia, and the worsening of insulin resistance. ACEIs inhibitors are a good choice in the proteinuric patient; calcium channel blockers are a good choice for the angina patient. Alpha-blockers are a good choice in the patient with benign prostatic hyperplasia, however, they are generally not used as monotherapy given the data suggesting increased risk of congestive heart failure.[35] Monotherapy of hypertension is frequently unsuccessful, especially in the setting of nephropathy, such that combination therapy is frequently needed with special attention to underlying concomitant medical problems (see Chapter 8).

Macrovascular Disease

Macrovascular disease is the major cause of premature death and considerable morbidity in individuals with DM, especially those with type 2 DM. Conventional risk factors for macrovascular disease warrant special attention in DM; they include smoking, lack of physical activity, dietary fat intake, obesity, hypertension, and hyperlipidemia. Correction and control of hyperlipidemia through improved metabolic control and the use of diet or pharmacotherapy are mandatory for the DM patient. The National Cholesterol Education Program guidelines[36] are of special importance to the diabetic, as are the American Diabetes Association guidelines[1] for the treatment of hypertriglyceridemia, with pharmacotherapy now being indicated for patients with persistent elevation in triglycerides above 200 mg/dL. LDL cholesterol lowering has been demonstrated to confer greater coronary event risk reduction and mortality reduction in diabetic patients than in nondiabetic patients. DM is one of the few diseases in which women have greater morbidity and mortality than men, especially in terms of macrovascular disease, with black women bearing the greatest load.

Foot Problems

Foot problems in the diabetic are a major cause of hospitalization and amputations. They generally constitute a combination of sepsis, ischemia, and neuropathy. The presence of significant neuropathy facilitates repetitive trauma without appropriate pain and ultimately nonhealing. Additionally, neuropathy may mask manifestations of peripheral vascular disease (PVD) (e.g., claudication and rest pain) such that patients may have critical ischemia with minimal symptoms. Therefore, PVD may be difficult to diagnose on the usual clinical grounds alone. Not only may neuropathy mask clinical symptoms, the clinical signs may be somewhat confusing. Patients with less severe neuropathy may exhibit cold feet related to arteriovenous shunting, and patients with more severe neuropathy may exhibit cutaneous hyperemia related to autosympathectomy. Noninvasive vascular testing along with clinical evaluation is helpful for the diagnosis and management of PVD. Calcific medial arterial disease is common and can cause erroneously high blood pressure recordings in the extremities, confusing the assessment of the severity of PVD. Severe ischemia with symptoms and nonhealing wounds generally requires surgical intervention. Milder symptoms and disease may respond favorably to enhanced physical activity and the use of one of the hemorheologic agents—pentoxifylline or cilostazol. Appropriate podiatric footwear and management are important to both ulcer healing and prevention of repetitive trauma.[29,37] Early PVD can readily be detected by ankle-brachial indices using a hand-held Doppler. A reduced ankle-brachial index at the posterior tibial artery in isolation has been demonstrated to be an important marker, conferring a 3.8-fold increased risk of cardiovascular death.

Achieving Glycemic Control

A recent consensus conference of the American College of Endocrinology issued revised goals for glycemic control focusing on an HbA$_{1c}$ <6.5% and a fasting blood glucose <110 mg/dL. These new goals are in line with the International Diabetes Federation standards, which in turn are in accord with the clinical trials data.

Type 1 DM

Optimal management of type 1 DM requires an educated, motivated patient and a physiologic insulin regimen. The major challenge is physiologic insulin replacement matched to dietary carbohydrate with appropriate compensation for variables such as exercise. Physiologic insulin replacement involves intensive insulin therapy with multiple injections (three or more per day) or the use of continuous subcutaneous insulin infusion (CSII) pumps. Several regimens have been utilized to achieve glycemic control (Table 20.3). The conventional split-mix regimen combining lispro/regular and an intermediate-acting insulin in the morning before breakfast and in the evening before supper is antiquated. Its major limitation is nocturnal hypoglycemia from the pre-supper intermediate-acting insulin when stringent control of the fasting blood glucose is sought. This regimen was one of those used in the conventional group in the DCCT and was inferior at reducing the risk of complications.

Taking the split-mix regimen and then dividing the evening insulin dose—delivering lispro/regular insulin before supper and the intermediate-acting insulin

TABLE 20.3. Commonly Used Physiologic Insulin Programs

Insulin program	Breakfast	Lunch	Dinner	Bed (10 P.M.–1 A.M.)
Basal-bolus humalog/regular and bid ultralente	H/R + U	H/R	H/R + U	0
Basal-bolus humalog and insulin glargine	H/R	H/R	H/R	G^a
Tid: Humalog and NPH/lente	H/R + N/L	—	H/R	N/L^b
Qid: Humalog/regular, ultralente and NPH/lente	H/R + U	H/R	H/R	N/L^b
Qid: regular and NPH/lente	R	R	R	N/L^b

^{a}Do not mix insulin glargine with any other insulin in a syringe.
^{b}Give injection in lower buttocks.
H = humalog; G = glargine; L = lente; N = NPH; R = regular; U = ultralente.

at bedtime—can afford a significant reduction in the risk of nighttime hypo-glycemia.[38] Most patients require 0.5 to 0.8 units/kg body weight to achieve ac-ceptable glycemic control. There are numerous options for dosing insulin in an intensive therapy regimen. One option is to distribute two thirds of the insulin in the morning and one third of the insulin in the evening, with (1) one third of the morning dose being lispro/regular and two thirds being intermediate-acting insulin; (2) 50% of the evening insulin as lispro/regular insulin before supper; and (3) the remaining 50% as intermediate-acting insulin at bedtime (10 P.M. to 1 A.M.). These doses are modified according to individual dietary preferences and carbohydrate distribution. See Table 20.3 for other options.

Additionally, patients need algorithms to adjust their insulin for hyperglycemia, varying physical activity, and intercurrent illnesses. These individualized algo-rithms are based on the unit/kg insulin dose. Many episodes of severe hypo-glycemia occur in the context of unplanned physical activity and dietary errors; likewise, many episodes of ketoacidosis occur during episodes of minor inter-current illness. For physical activity, a reduction in insulin dosage of 1 to 2 units per 20 to 30 minutes of activity generally suffices pending the intensity of the activity. The other option is to augment carbohydrate intake (i.e., 15 g carbohy-drate prior to every 20–30 minutes of activity). During illness it is important that patients appreciate the fact that illness is a situation of insulin resistance and that all of the routine insulin should be administered. Carbohydrate from meals and snacks may be substituted as simple carbohydrate in the form of liquids such as juices and regular ginger ale. It is important that the treatment regimen is indi-vidualized and that therapeutic options for insulin administration are discussed with each patient. In this way, patients' lifestyles can be accommodated and ap-propriate insulin regimens tailored.[28] For example, using a basal-bolus regimen with ultralente or insulin glargine, it is possible to delay the lunchtime injection pending the patient's time constraints; furthermore, the insulin dose can be ad-justed depending on carbohydrate intake and physical activity. Inhaled quick-acting insulin is under clinical investigation. Concerns exist, however, about the vasodilatory properties of insulin and the theoretical potential for pulmonary hypotension and pulmonary edema, especially in patients with cardiac dysfunc-tion.[39] In some individuals, a lunchtime injection is not feasible. A schoolchild or a person engaged in construction work might find it difficult to accommodate a prelunch insulin injection and might be better off with a morning intermedi-ate-acting insulin to cover the lunchtime carbohydrate intake, with lispro/regu-lar insulin being taken to cover the breakfast carbohydrate intake as a combined prebreakfast dose.

Severe hypoglycemia in the well-educated, adherent, motivated patient on a physiologic insulin regimen is uncommon. Most severe hypoglycemic episodes are explained on the basis of diet or exercise and insulin-adjustment errors.[40] The individual who is attempting to achieve true euglycemia, however, is at risk for periodic easily self-treated hypoglycemia. See Table 20.4 for management strate-gies. For the individual with type 1 DM who has been educated thoroughly, is on a physiologic insulin regimen with an agreed diet plan, and has algorithms

TABLE 20.4. Hypoglycemia Management Strategies

Causes	Signs and symptoms	Treatment
Insulin/OHA overdose	Sympathomimetic	Conscious—15 g
Carbohydrate omission	Coldness	Simple carbohydrate
Missed/late meal	Clamminess	Juice 4 oz
Missed/late snack	Shaking	Regular soda 6 oz
Uncompensated	Diaphoresis	3 B-D glucose tablets
activity/exercise	Headaches	7 Lifesavers
	Neuroglycopenic	Unconscious
	Confusion	Glucagon SC[a]
	Disorientation	D_{50} 50 cc IV
	Loss of consciousness	

[a]We do not recommend the use of gel products (e.g., Monojel) for treatment of unconscious hypoglycemia, as aspiration is a potential hazard.
OHA = oral hypoglycemic agent.

for illness and physical activity, failure to attain the desired degree of glycemic control is largely related to psychosocial variables or, occasionally, altered and unpredictable insulin kinetics.

Type 2 DM

In most instances, type 2 DM is a syndrome of insulin resistance coupled with variable secretory defects, both of which can be compounded by glucotoxicity. As insulin resistance is related to genetic factors, obesity, and sedentary lifestyle, the mainstay of treatment for the type 2 DM patient is correction of insulin resistance through diet and exercise and reversal of glucotoxicity acutely through reestablishment of euglycemia. Many patients still perceive themselves to be more absolutely insulin-deficient than insulin-resistant and are willing to accept insulin therapy as a compromise in the context of failed weight loss efforts. Additionally, many patients perceive pharmacotherapy to be equivalent to a diet and exercise regimen alone, assuming the desired degree of glycemic control is achieved. Chronic nonadherence to a diet regimen with resultant failure of weight loss or progressive obesity frequently leads to mislabeling the patient as a "brittle diabetic." It is important to avoid premature and unnecessary insulin therapy in these individuals and to stress to them the importance of diet and exercise as the most physiologic approach to controlling their metabolic disorder.

Pharmacotherapy for Type 2 DM

Pharmacotherapy for type 2 DM can be directed at (1) decreasing insulin resistance and increasing insulin sensitization (metformin hydrochloride and the thiazolidinediones), (2) interference with the digestion and absorption of dietary carbohydrate (α-glucosidase inhibitors), (3) augmentation of insulin secretion and action (sulfonylureas, repaglinide, and nateglinide), and (4) insulin therapy (Table 20.5).

Table 20.5. Oral Medications Commonly Used to Treat Type 2 DM

Parameter	Metformin	Pioglitazone	Rosiglitazone	Sulfonylurea
Mode of action	↓ Hepatic glucose ↑ Skeletal muscle glucose utilization	↑ Skeletal muscle glucose utilization ↓ Hepatic glucose	↑ Skeletal muscle glucose utilization ↓ Hepatic glucose	↑ Insulin secretion ↓ Hepatic glucose production
Glucose effects	Fasting and postprandial	Fasting and postprandial	Fasting and postprandial	Fasting and postprandial
Hypoglycemia as monotherapy	No	No	No	Yes
Weight gain	No	Possible	Possible	Possible
Insulin levels	→	↓	↓	↑
Side effects	GI (self-limiting symptoms of nausea, diarrhea, anorexia)	? Elevation in hepatic transaminases	? Elevation in hepatic transaminases	Potential allergic reaction if sulfa allergy Potential drug interactions (first-generation agents) SIADH
Lipid effects	→	↑ HDL, ↓ Trigs LDL concentration unaltered	Increase in total cholesterol, LDL and HDL concentration ? Change in particle composition	↑ or ↓
Usual starting dose for a 70-kg man	500 mg bid with meals or XR 500 mg with the evening meal	15 mg qd	4 mg daily either single or divided dose Better results with divided dose	Varies with each agent Glyburide 2.5 mg qd Glucotrol XL 5 mg qd Glynase 3 mg qd Amaryl 2 mg qd

TABLE 20.5. Oral Medications Commonly Used to Treat Type 2 DM (*Continued*)

Parameter	Metformin	Pioglitazone	Rosiglitazone	Sulfonylurea
Maximum dose	850 mg tid with meals or XR 2000 mg with the evening meal	45 mg qd	8 mg daily as either single or divided dose Better results with divided dose	Varies with each agent Glyburide 10 mg bid Glucotrol XL 20 mg qd Glynase 6 mg bid Amaryl 8 mg qd
Contraindications	Type 1 diabetes Renal dysfunction Hepatic dysfunction History of EtOH abuse Chronic conditions associated with hypoxia (asthma, COPD, CHF) Acute conditions associated with potential for hypoxia (CHF, acute MI, surgery) Situations associated with potential renal failure	Type 1 diabetes Liver disease Class III and IV CHF	Type 1 diabetes Liver disease Class III and IV CHF	Type 1 diabetes Hepatic dysfunction

Parameter	Repaglinide	Nateglinide	Acarbose	Miglitol
Mode of action	↑ Insulin secretion	↑ Insulin secretion	α-Glucosidase inhibition ↓ carbohydrate digestion and absorption from GI tract	α-Glucosidase inhibition ↓ carbohydrate digestion and absorption from GI tract

Glucose effects	Postprandial and fasting	Postprandial	Postprandial	Postprandial
Hypoglycemia as monotherapy	Yes; less than that seen with sulfonylureas	No	No	No
Weight gain	No	No	No	No
Insulin levels	↑	↑	↓ or ↔	↓ or ↔
Side effects	Rare hypoglycemia	Very rare hypoglyemia, as effects are glucose-dependent	GI (flatulence, abdominal distention, diarrhea)	GI (flatulence, abdominal distention, diarrhea)
Lipid effects	No change	No change	↓ or ↔	↓ or ↔
Starting dose for a 70-kg man	0.5 mg prior to meals	120 mg tid prior to meals	25 mg tid with first bite of each meal	25 mg tid with first bite of each meal
Maximum dose	16 mg daily in divided doses at meals/snacks	120 mg tid prior to meals	100 mg tid with first bite of each meal	100 mg tid with first bite of each meal
Contraindications	Type 1 diabetes	Type 1 diabetes	Type 1 diabetes Inflammatory bowel disease Bowel obstruction Cirrhosis Chronic conditions with maldigestion or malabsorption	Type 1 diabetes Inflammatory bowel disease Bowel obstruction Cirrhosis Chronic conditions with maldigestion and malabsorption

DECREASING INSULIN RESISTANCE/INCREASING INSULIN SENSITIVITY

Metformin hydrochloride and the thiazolidinediones work via different mechanisms. Metformin mainly inhibits the uncontrolled hepatic glucose production, while the thiazolidinediones mainly enhance skeletal muscle glucose uptake—the earliest defect in evolving type 2 DM.

Metformin (Glucophage), a true insulin sensitizer, decreases hepatic glucose production and enhances peripheral glucose utilization. It is an antihyperglycemic agent and does not stimulate insulin secretion; hence, when used as monotherapy it cannot induce hypoglycemia. Ideal candidates for treatment are overweight or obese type 2 DM patients. The potentially fatal side effect of lactic acidosis generally occurs only when metformin is used in contraindicated patients: those with renal insufficiency, liver disease, alcohol excess, or underlying hypoxic states (congestive heart failure, chronic obstructive pulmonary disease, significant asthma, acute myocardial infarction). Metformin should be discontinued the morning of (1) elective surgery that may require general anesthesia and (2) elective procedures using contrast materials (e.g., intravenous pyelogram, cardiac catheterization), and should not be restarted for 48 to 72 hours after the surgery/procedure, pending documentation of a normal serum creatinine. Adjustments in the individual's diabetes regimen will have to be made for this time period to maintain glycemic control. In the UKPDS, despite similar levels of glycemic control, the subset of obese type 2 DM patients treated with metformin had a statistically significantly lower cardiovascular event and death rate than the other groups.[41] Thus, metformin must be modulating other aspects of the cardiodysmetabolic syndrome.

Thiazolidinediones [pioglitazone (ACTOS) and rosiglitazone (Avandia)] are antihyperglycemic insulin-sensitizing agents that bind to the peroxisome proliferator-activated receptor (PPAR) and amplify the insulin signal. In addition to glucose lowering properties, they have purported beneficial effects on the other components of the cardiodysmetabolic syndrome. These agents may also assist in preservation of β-cell function via reduction in lipid deposition within the islets of Langerhans—a concept called lipotoxicity, a finding documented in animals. These agents can be safely used in patients with renal insufficiency without the need for dosage adjustment. A contraindication to their use is liver disease or elevations in hepatic transaminases. Edema is the commonest clinical adverse effect. Although the risk of transaminase elevation is rare, monitoring should be done every 2 months for the first year, and periodically thereafter. These agents are contraindicated in patients with New York grade III or grade IV congestive heart failure. Clinically, glucose lowering is very gradual with these agents, such that individualized downward titration in insulin dosage in insulin-treated type 2 DM patients may not be needed for at least 2 weeks, and the maximum effect may not be seen for up to 12 weeks.

α-GLUCOSIDASE INHIBITION

α-Glucosidase inhibition by acarbose (Precose) and miglitol (Glyset) has a primary mode of action of decreasing postprandial blood glucoses via direct interference with the digestion and absorption of dietary carbohydrate. These agents are most commonly used as adjunctive therapy rather than monotherapy. Both of these agents need to be dosed with the first bite of the meal. Increased intestinal gas formation, the most common side effect, is minimized with slow dose titration and does improve with continued administration.

Augmentation of Insulin Secretion

Sulfonylureas enhance insulin secretion and action. First-generation sulfonylureas (chlorpropamide, tolazamide, tolbutamide), although efficacious, have a higher risk of side effects, such as sustained hypoglycemia, the chlorpropamide flush (an Antabuse-like reaction), protein binding interference with certain medications, and syndrome of inappropriate diuretic hormone (SIADH) secretion. The second- and third-generation sulfonylureas are preferred owing to their increased milligram potency, shorter duration of action, and better side-effect profile.

Prior concerns about possible cardiotoxicity of sulfonylureas related to the University Group Diabetes Program (UGDP) Study have generally disappeared, given the emergence of data to support the safety of these agents from the cardiovascular prospective in the UKPDS. Glimepiride, a third-generation sulfonylurea, has theoretical benefits in terms of reduced risk of hypoglycemia, potentially lower risk of adverse cardiovascular effects, and perhaps reduced potential for secondary failure.

The insulin secretagogue in the meglitinide class, repaglinide (Prandin), is dosed prior to meals, producing an abrupt spurt of insulin secretion, designed to assist in the control of postprandial glucose levels. There is a potential, although unproven, for a reduction in weight gain so frequently seen with sulfonylureas. Theoretical potential to reduce secondary failure rates is also a purported benefit.

Nateglinide (Starlix), a phenylalanine derivative, is an insulin secretagogue, the effects of which are glucose-dependent. Nateglinide dosed prior to meals produces an abrupt spurt of insulin. However, in contrast to repaglinide, nateglinide restores early insulin secretion that is lost as β-cell function is declining prior to the development of type 2 DM. Early insulin secretion is important, shutting off hepatic glucose production in preparation for the prandial glucose rise. Weight gain is attenuated and hypoglycemia is very rare. Switching from a sulfonylurea to nateglinide can result in a slight rise in fasting glucoses; however, as postprandial glucoses are significantly improved, the HbA_{1c} may be maintained or lowered. This is due to the fact that postprandial glucose contributes more to the HbA_{1c} than fasting or preprandial glucoses do.

Insulin Therapy

To achieve the American Diabetes Association (ADA) goal HbA_{1c}, the vast majority of type 2 DM patients will require combination therapy. The concept of initiating pharmacotherapy with an insulin-sensitizing agent appears physiologically logical and, it is hoped, will assist in delaying or preventing sulfonylurea failure, frequently seen after 5 to 6 years of sulfonylurea monotherapy. Additionally, insulin sensitization will ameliorate many of the other components of the cardiodysmetabolic syndrome, thus, it is hoped, translating to reduced macrovascular disease. This hypothesis is currently being tested in several clinical trials.

Can type 2 DM be prevented? The Diabetes Prevention Program in type 2 DM is ongoing with metformin being used in the treatment group. In the HOPE trial, that nondiabetic patients at high risk to develop cardiovascular disease who were treated with ramipril 10 mg daily had a 34% risk reduction in the development of type 2 DM.[33] In the West of Scotland trial, the use of pravastatin reduced the risk of developing type 2 DM by 30%.[42] A recent Finnish lifestyle modification study demonstrated a 58% risk reduction in developing type 2 DM in patients with impaired glucose tolerance who were randomized to a program of intensive diet and exercise.[43]

Insulin therapy in type 2 DM patients is indicated in situations where patients are acutely decompensated and are more insulin-resistant due to intercurrent illnesses. Clearly, short-term insulin therapy can reestablish glycemic control acutely in many individuals. However, reevaluation of endogenous insulin production with C-peptide determinations is important. Most obese patients with type 2 DM have normal or fairly elevated C-peptide levels, assuming they are not glucotoxic from antecedent chronic hyperglycemia. The initiation of insulin therapy in a type 2 DM patient remains controversial in terms of indications and optimum insulin regimen. The dilemma revolves around the obese C-peptide–positive patient who was achieving good glycemic control in the short term with insulin. This individual often suffers progressive obesity and worsening glycemic control owing to worsening insulin resistance, thereby increasing requirements for exogenous insulin. Thus frequently insulin therapy in an obese C-peptide–positive patient fails to achieve its primary goal of sustained improved glycemic control. Additionally, perpetuation of the obese state, or indeed worsening thereof, in conjunction with progressive hyperinsulinemia raises concerns about the impact of this worsened metabolic milieu on hypertension, dyslipidemia, and the atherosclerotic process. Initiation of insulin therapy should therefore be undertaken cautiously in most patients and progress carefully monitored in terms not only of glycemic control but also of hypertension, dyslipidemia, and obesity.

Many insulin regimens have been used to treat type 2 DM, most being similar to those used in the type 1 setting. Trends have focused on the use of bedtime insulin therapy in these individuals on the grounds that it can maximally affect the dawn hepatic glucose output/disposal and peak insulin resistance, thereby achieving the best possible fasting blood glucose and minimizing glucotoxicity. Minimizing glucotoxicity facilitates daytime islet secretory function and minimizes the need for daytime insulin therapy.[44] Combination therapy with insulin-sensitizing agents and insulin seems theoretically sound, reducing the need for exogenous insulin. The data, however, support modest improvements in glycemic control and modest reduction in insulin requirements. It is the exceptional patient who is able to discontinue insulin therapy. One such regimen has been the use of a bedtime dose of intermediate-acting insulin at a dose of 0.2 units/kg of body weight coupled with daytime oral agents. An alternative to the bedtime intermediate-acting insulin is the use of insulin glargine starting at a dose of 10 units and titrating accordingly. Although hypoglycemia is relatively uncommon in type 2 DM patients owing to their fundamental insulin resistance, it can occur in those on insulin or sulfonylureas. Sulfonylureas should be used with caution in patients with hepatic or renal impairment and the elderly.

Gestational Diabetes Mellitus

Gestational DM (GDM) is an important entity in terms of maternal morbidity, fetal macrosomia, associated obstetric complications, and neonatal hypoglycemia. GDM should be sought in all patients using current screening and diagnostic guidelines (Table 20.1). Early, aggressive management can significantly improve outcome. The initial strategy for the patient with GDM is dietary control; when the goals of pregnancy are not being achieved (i.e., premeal and bedtime glucose <90 mg/dL and 1 hour postprandial glucose <120 mg/dL), insulin therapy is initiated. Given the data linking postprandial blood glucose levels to macrosomia, it is important that postprandial glucose levels are controlled adequately and that target glucose levels are achieved.[45,46] In our center the postprandial goal is most readily and predictably reached with premeal lispro insulin. To cover basal requirements we use a small dose of prebreakfast ultralente insulin and an overnight intermediate-acting insulin. As an alternative, premeal regular insulin and overnight intermediate-acting insulin can be used. Most women with GDM have reestablishment of euglycemia immediately postpartum. These individuals, however, should be counseled on the long-term risks of prior GDM for developing overt type 2 DM, which may occur in as many as 70% of these individuals.[47] Additionally, the hazards of persistent obesity, associated insulin resistance, dyslipidemia, hypertension, and potential for premature cardiovascular death must be addressed.[48]

Individuals with type 1 DM who are contemplating pregnancy should be in optimal glycemic control prior to conception to decrease the risk of congenital malformations and the incidence of maternal-fetal complications. The achievement of two consecutive HbA$_{1c}$ levels in the nondiabetic range is recommended before conception. Alternatively, CSII may be used to readily achieve these goals. Careful follow-up by a skilled management team is essential to an optimum outcome.[46] Insulin glargine has a category C rating for pregnancy and should not be used.

Contraception and DM

The use of oral contraceptives (OCs) in women with type 1 or type 2 DM has been an area of controversy,[46] with many believing that significant elevations occur in blood glucose along with an increased risk of vascular complications. In our experience the incidence of such problems is minimal given a woman who is normotensive and has an absence of vascular disease; therefore, we believe OCs can be safely used. Even for a woman in poor glycemic control, OCs are still the most effective form of contraception.

Diabetic Ketoacidosis

Diabetic ketoacidosis (DKA) is the ultimate expression of absolute insulin deficiency resulting in uncontrolled lipolysis, free fatty acid delivery to the liver, and ultimately accelerated ketone body production. Insulin deficiency at the level of the liver results in uncontrolled hepatic glucose output via gluconeogenesis and glycogenolysis. With insulin-mediated skeletal muscle glucose uptake being inhibited, hyperglycemia rapidly ensues. The attendant osmotic diuresis due to hyperglycemia results in progressive dehydration and a decreasing glomerular filtration rate. Dehydration may be compounded by gastrointestinal fluid losses (e.g., emesis from ketones or a primary gastrointestinal illness with concurrent diarrhea). Insensible fluid losses from febrile illness may further compound the dehydration.

Diagnosis of DKA is fairly characteristic in the newly presenting or established type 1 DM patient. The history of polydipsia, polyuria, weight loss, and Kussmaul's respirations are virtually pathognomonic. Physical examination is directed at assessing the level of hydration (e.g., orthostasis) and the underlying precipitating illness. Measurement of urine ketone, urine glucose, and blood glucose levels can rapidly confirm the clinical suspicion, with arterial pH, serum bicarbonate, and ketones validating the diagnosis. A thorough search for an underlying precipitating illness remains axiomatic (e.g., urosepsis, respiratory tract infection, or silent myocardial infarction). Treatment is directed at correcting (1) dehydration/hypotension; (2) ketonemia/acidosis; (3) uncontrolled hepatic glucose output/hyperglycemia; and (4) insulin resistance of the DKA/underlying illness. Of course specific treatment is directed to any defined underlying illnesses.

Dehydration and hypotension require urgent treatment with a 5- to 6-L deficit to be anticipated in most individuals. Initial treatment is 0.9% NaCl, with 1 to 2 L/hr being given for the first 2 hours and flow rates thereafter being titrated to the individual's clinical status. Use of a Swan-Ganz catheter is prudent in the individual with cardiac compromise. Potassium replacement at a concentration of 10 to 40 mEq/L is critical to replace the usual deficits of more than 5 mEq/kg once the patient's initial serum potassium level is known and urine output is documented. Giving 50% of the potassium as KCl and 50% as KPO_4 appears theoretically sound, but routine phosphate replacement has not been shown to alter the clinical outcome. Bicarbonate therapy is generally reserved for patients with a pH of less than 7.0, plasma bicarbonate less than 5.0 mEq/L, severe hyperkalemia, or a deep coma. Bicarbonate is administered by slow infusion 50 to 100 mEq over 1 to 2 hours with the therapeutic end point being a pH higher than 7.1

rather than normalization of the pH. Overzealous use of bicarbonate can result in severe hypokalemia with attendant cardiac arrhythmogenicity, paradoxical central nervous system acidosis, and possible lactic acidosis due to tissue hypoxia. Intravenous insulin therapy is initiated at a dose of 0.1 U/kg/hr with rapid titration every 1 to 2 hours should a 75 to 100 mg/dL/hr decrease in glucose not be achieved. Insulin therapy at this relatively high dose is needed to combat the insulin resistance of the hormonal milieu of DKA (i.e., high levels of glucagon, cortisol, growth hormone, and catecholamines). Given that hepatic glucose output is more rapidly controlled than ketogenesis, the insulin infusion rate can be maintained by switching the intravenous infusion to dextrose 5% to 10% when blood glucose is less than 250 mg/dL. The insulin infusion is continued until the patient is ketone-free, clinically well, and able to resume oral feeding. It is of paramount importance that subcutaneous insulin be instituted promptly at the time of refeeding.

Flow sheets should be generated documenting the following:

1. Patient admission weight relative to previous weights with serial weights every 6 to 12 hours, urine ketones, and fluid balance
2. Vital signs and mental status every 1 to 2 hours
3. Bedside glucose monitoring every 1 to 2 hours
4. Urine ketones every 1 to 2 hours
5. Fluid balance
6. Blood gases and arterial pH on admission, repeating until pH is over 7.1
7. Serum potassium on admission and then every 2 to 4 hours
8. Serum ketones on admission and then every 2 to 4 hours
9. Complete blood count, serum chemistries, chest roentgenogram, electrocardiogram, and appropriate cultures on admission
10. Abnormal chemistries other than potassium repeated every 4 hours until normal.[49,50]

References

1. Clinical practice recommendations: 2001. Diabetes Care 2001;24(suppl 1):S1–S133.
2. The European patient's charter. Diabetic Med 1991;8:782–3.
3. Landin-Olsson M, Nilsson KO, Lernmark A, Sunkvist G. Islet cell antibodies and fasting C-peptide predict insulin requirement at diagnosis of diabetes mellitus. Diabetalogia 1990;33:561–8.
4. Zeigler AG, Herskowitz RD, Jackson RA, Soeldner JS, Eisenbarth GS. Predicting type I diabetes. Diabetes Care 1990;13:762–75.
5. Keller RJ, Eisenbarth GS, Jackson RA. Insulin prophylaxis in individuals at high risk of type I diabetes. N Engl J Med 1993;341:927–8.
6. Shapiro AMJ, Lakey BS, Ryan EA, et al. Islet transplantation in seven patients with type 1 diabetes mellitus using a glucocorticoid-free immunosuppressive regimen. N Engl J Med 2000;343:230–8.
7. Helmrich SP, Ragland DR, Leung RW, Paffenbarger RS. Physical activity and reduced occurrence of non-insulin-dependent diabetes mellitus. N Engl J Med 1991;325:147–52.

8. UKPDS Group. UK prospective diabetes study XI: biochemical risk factors in type 2 diabetic patients at diagnosis compared with age-matched normal subjects. Diabetic Med 1994;11:533–44.

9. DeFronzo RA. The triumvirate: B-cell, muscle, and liver: a collusion responsible for NIDDM. Diabetes 1988;37:667–87.

10. Erikkson J, Franssila-Kallunki A, Ekstrand A. Early metabolic defects in persons at increased risk for non-insulin-dependent diabetes mellitus. N Engl J Med 1989;321:337–43.

11. DeFronzo RA, Bonadonna RC, Ferrannini E. Pathogenesis of NIDDM. Diabetes Care 1992;15:318–68.

12. Clark PM, Hales CN. Measurement of insulin secretion in type 2 diabetes: problems and pitfalls. Diabetic Med 1992;9:503–12.

13. Bjornstorp P. Metabolic implications of body fat distribution. Diabetes Care 1991;14:1132–43.

14. Ferrannini E, Buzzigoli G, Bonadonna B, et al. Insulin resistance in essential hypertension. N Engl J Med 1987;317:350–7.

15. Zavaroni I, Bonora E, Pagliara M, et al. Risk factors for coronary artery disease in healthy persons with hyperinsulinemia and normal glucose tolerance. N Engl J Med 1989;320:703–6.

16. Kern TS, Engerman RL. Arrest of glomerulonephropathy in diabetic dogs by improved glycemic control. Diabetologia 1990;33:522–5.

17. Diabetes Control and Complications Trial Research Group. The effect of intensive treatment of diabetes on the development and progression of long-term complications in insulin-dependent diabetes mellitus. N Engl J Med 1993;329:977–86.

18. UKPDS Group. Intensive blood-glucose control with sulfonylureas or insulin compared with conventional treatment and risk of complications in patients with type 2 diabetes (UKPDS 33). Lancet 1998;352:837–53.

19. UKPDS Group. Association of glycaemia with macrovascular and microvascular complications of type 2 diabetes (UKPDS 35): prospective observational study. BMJ 2000;321:405–11.

20. UKPDS Group. Association of systolic blood pressure with macrovascular and microvascular complications of type 2 diabetes (UKPDS 36): prospective observational study. BMJ 2000;321:412–9.

21. National committee for clinical laboratory standards. Development of designated comparison methods for analytes in the clinical laboratory, 2nd ed., proposed guideline. NCCLS publication NRSCL6-P2. Villanova, PA: NCCLS, 1993.

22. Viberti GC. Etiology and prognostic significance of albuminuria in diabetes. Diabetes Care 1988;11:840–8.

23. Deckert T, Feldt-Rasmussen B, Borch-Johnson K, Jensen T, Kofoed-Gnevoldsen A. Albuminuria reflects widespread vascular damage: the Steno hypothesis. Diabetologia 1989;32:219–26.

24. Marshall SM. Screening for microalbuminuria: which measurement? Diabetic Med 1991;8:706–11.

25. Hamwi GL. Changing dietary concepts in therapy. In: Danowski TS, ed. Diabetes mellitus: diagnosis and treatment. New York: American Diabetes Association, 1964;73–8.

26. Wood FC, Bierman EL. Is diet the cornerstone in management of diabetes? N Engl J Med 1986;1244–7.

27. Zehrer C, Hansen R, Bantl J. Reducing blood glucose variability by use of abdominal injection sites. Diabetes Educator 1990;16:474–7.
28. Skyler JS, Skyler DL, Seigler DE, O'Sullivan M. Algorithms for adjustment of insulin dosage by patients who monitor blood glucose. Diabetes Care 1981;4:311–8.
29. Frykberg RG. Management of diabetic foot problems (Joslin Clinic). Philadelphia: Saunders, 1984.
30. Singerman LJ. Early-treatment diabetic retinopathy study: good news for diabetic patients and health care professionals [editorial]. Diabetes Care 1986;9:426–9.
31. Lewis EJ, Hunsicker LG, Bain RE, Rohde RD. The effect of angiotensin-converting enzyme inhibition on diabetic nephropathy. N Engl J Med 1993;329:1456–62.
32. The Heart Outcomes Prevention Evaluation (HOPE) Study Investigators. Effects of an angiotensin-converting enzyme inhibitor, ramipril, on cardiovascular events in high risk patients. Lancet 2000;342:145–53.
33. The Heart Outcomes Prevention Evaluation (HOPE) Study Investigators. Effects of ramipril on cardiovascular and microvascular outcomes in people with diabetes mellitus: results of the HOPE study and MICRO-HOPE sub-study. Lancet 2000;345:253–9.
34. Tuttle KR, Bruton JL, Perusek MC, Lancaster JL, Kopp DT, DeFronzo RA. Effect of strict glycemic control on renal enlargement in insulin-dependent diabetes mellitus. N Engl J Med 1991;324:1626–32.
35. ALLHAT Collaborative Research Group. Major cardiovascular events in hypertensive patients randomized to doxazosin vs. chlorthalidone: the antihypertensive and lipid-lowering treatment to prevent heart attack trial (ALLHAT). JAMA 2000;283:1967–75.
36. Expert panel on detection, evaluation, and treatment of high blood cholesterol in adults. Executive summary of the third report of the national cholesterol education program (NCEP) expert panel on detection, evaluation, and treatment of high blood cholesterol in adults. JAMA 2001;285:2486–97.
37. Flynn MD, Tooke JE. Aetiology of diabetic foot ulceration: a role for the microcirculation? Diabetic Med 1992;9:320–9.
38. Skyler JS. Insulin treatment: therapy for diabetes mellitus and related disorders. Alexandria, VA: American Diabetes Association, 1991;127–37.
39. Chan NH, Baldeweg S, Tan TMM, Hurel SI. Inhaled insulin in type 1 diabetes. Lancet 2001;357:1979.
40. Bhatia V, Wolfsdorf JI. Severe hypoglycemia in youth with insulin-dependent diabetes mellitus: frequency and causative factors. Pediatrics 1991;88:1187–93.
41. UKPDS Group. Effect of intensive blood-glucose control with metformin on complications in overweight patients with type 2 diabetes (UKPDS 34). Lancet 1998;352(9131):854–65.
42. Freeman DJ, Norrie J, Sattar N, et al. Pravastatin and the development of diabetes mellitus: evidence for a protective treatment effect in the West of Scotland Coronary Prevention Study. Circulation 2001;103:346–7.
43. Tuomilehto J, Lindstorm J, Eirksson JG, et al. Prevention of type 2 diabetes mellitus by changes in lifestyle among subjects with impaired glucose tolerance. N Engl J Med 2001;344:1343–50.
44. Groop LC, Widèn E, Ekstrand A, et al. Morning or bedtime NPH insulin combined with sulfonylureas in treatment of NIDDM. Diabetes Care 1992;15:831–4.
45. Proceedings of the Third International Workshop-Conference on Gestational Diabetes Mellitus. Diabetes 1991;40(suppl 2):1–201.

46. Jovanovic-Peterson L, Peterson CM. Pregnancy in the diabetic woman: guidelines for a successful outcome. Endocrinol Metab Clin North Am 1992;33:433–56.
47. Kaufmann RC, Amankwah KS, Woodrum J. Development of diabetes in previous gestational diabetic [abstract]. Diabetes 1991;40:137A.
48. Kaufmann RC, Amankwah KS, Woodrum J. Serum lipids in former gestational diabetics [abstract]. Diabetes 1991;40:192A.
49. Kozak GP, Rolla AR. Diabetic comas. In: Kozak GP, ed. Clinical diabetes mellitus. Philadelphia: Saunders, 1982;109–45.
50. Siperstein MD. Diabetic ketoacidosis and hyperosmolar coma. Endocrinol Metab Clin North Am 1992;33:415–32.

Case Presentation

Subjective

Patient Profile

Harold Nelson is a 76-year-old married man.

Presenting Problem

"Blood sugar going up and down."

Present Illness

Mr. Nelson has been diabetic for 24 years. He was initially diet-controlled but has taken glyburide, 5 mg daily, in the morning for the past 3 years. For about 2 months, he has noted wide swings in his blood sugar levels from 60 to more than 300 mg/dl on home blood glucose monitoring. He has had no shakiness or sweating at times of low blood sugar, although sometimes he feels inappropriately weak and sleeps more than usual. His appetite is fair, and he has lost some weight in the past few weeks.

Past Medical History, Social History, and Family History

All are unchanged since his previous visits 2 and 9 months ago (see Chapters 5 and 18).

Habits

Unchanged except that he reports drinking alcoholic beverages "a little more than usual."

Review of Systems

Occasional constipation. Sometimes he has lower leg pain after walking.

- What additional medical history might be important? Why?
- What might you ask to clarify his alcohol use?
- What might you ask to further evaluate the leg pain?
- Have you listened carefully to what Mr. Nelson is trying to tell you?

Objective

Vital Signs

Height, 5 ft 7 in; weight, 160 lb (a decrease of 6 lb in 2 months); blood pressure, 162/84; pulse, 74; respirations, 20; temperature, 37.0°C.

Examination

The patient is ambulatory and alert. The eyes, ears, nose, and throat—including a funduscopic examination—are normal. The chest is clear to percussion and auscultation. The heart has a regular sinus rhythm, and no murmurs are present. On the abdominal examination, there is no mass or tenderness, and the liver is palpable about 1 cm below the right costal margin. There are Heberden's nodes of both hands and osteoarthritic swelling of other joints, especially the knees. The deep tendon reflexes are normal, and there is no decreased perception of pinprick in the lower extremities.

Laboratory

An office determination reveals a blood sugar of 270 mg/dl approximately 2 hours after breakfast.

- What more data would you obtain from the physical examination, and why?
- What might you do to help clarify the patient's lower leg pain?
- What—if any—laboratory tests would you order today? Explain.
- What—if any—diagnostic imaging would you order today? Why?

Assessment

- What are possible causes of Mr. Nelson's problems with blood sugar control? How would you explain this to the patient?
- Could the presenting complaint be related to problems in the family? How might you assess this possibility?
- What are possible causes of the weight loss? Of the leg pain?
- What might be the meaning of these problems to the patient? How might you address this issue?

Plan

- Describe your therapeutic recommendations for the patient. How would you explain this to Mr. Nelson?
- Describe your advice regarding diet, alcohol use, and exercise.
- How might you involve other family members in dealing with the problem?
- What continuing care would you advise?

21

Human Immunodeficiency Virus Infection and Acquired Immunodeficiency Syndrome

STEVEN P. BROMER AND RONALD H. GOLDSCHMIDT

Care for patients with human immunodeficiency virus (HIV) infection requires excellence in all aspects of family practice. The family physician's roles include providing patient education to prevent uninfected persons from becoming infected, identifying and counseling infected persons, delivering comprehensive medical care, initiating and monitoring antiretroviral (ARV) therapy, providing prophylaxis against opportunistic infections, managing the acquired immunodeficiency syndrome (AIDS), and providing support and care for the family. New manifestations of HIV disease, diagnostic protocols, and drug recommendations for HIV disease change on a regular basis, so familiarity with sources of updated information and guidelines on HIV care is essential[1] (Table 21.1).

The striking benefits of combination antiretroviral ther-apy, sometimes called highly active antiretroviral therapy (HAART), have changed the implications of HIV disease dramatically.[2] The demonstrated effectiveness of ARV therapy in reducing opportunistic infections and decreasing mortality has made the hope of a normal life span with a high quality of life a real possibility for HIV-positive persons.

Despite substantial progress in the medical management of HIV infection, the AIDS epidemic continues to exact a tremendous toll on families, communities, and society. The World Health Organization estimates that there are more than 40 million people infected with HIV worldwide and more than 3 million deaths annually. In North America as many as 45,000 new infections occur annually.[3] Minority communities in the United States are disproportionately affected and the proportion of women infected continues to increase.[4] Family-centered approaches to prevention and treatment are needed to address the new challenges created by the changing epidemic.

Risk Factors, Risk Reduction, and Patient Education

HIV is usually transmitted from person to person by the passage of blood or body fluids such as semen and vaginal secretions. Urine, sweat, and saliva are not gen-

TABLE 21.1. Internet Resources for HIV Management

www.hivatis.org	Up-to-date Public Health Service guidelines on use of antiretroviral medications, prophylaxis against opportunistic infections and other important management issues in HIV disease
www.cdc.gov	HIV/AIDS and other sexually transmitted disease guidelines from the Center for Disease Control and Prevention
www.hivinsite.ucsf.edu	Comprehensive site with information on treatment, prevention and policy from the University of California at San Francisco
www.hopkins-aids.edu	Comprehensive site with access to resources for treatment, prevention and policy from Johns Hopkins University AIDS Service
www.ucsf.edu/hivcntr	Web site of the National HIV Telephone Consultation Service (Warmline) and the National Clinicians' Post-Exposure Prophylaxis Hotline (PEPline); based in the National HIV/AIDS Clinicians' Consultation Center at San Francisco General Hospital, sponsored by the Health Resources and Services Administration
www.actis.org	A resource of federally and privately funded HIV/AIDS clinical trials; sponsored by the United States Department of Health and Human Services

erally considered to be infectious. Persons engaging in unprotected sexual activity and intravenous drug use with needle-sharing account for most cases of HIV infection. The risk of transfusion-related infection is very low and is estimated to be about 1 in every 677,000 units of donated blood.[5] Vertical transmission occurs in 25% of children of infected mothers who are not receiving ARV therapy. Effective ARV therapy decreases this transmission rate dramatically.[6] Casual transmission (in the absence of sexual contact or passage of blood) from person to person does not seem to occur. Transmission from infected patients to health care workers occurs at a rate of approximately 0.3% (one seroconversion for every 333 needlesticks or similar injury) and constitutes an uncommon but important transmission category. The use of timely postexposure prophylaxis with ARV medications can decrease the risk of transmission following a needlestick injury when the source patient is known to be HIV-positive.[7] Universal blood and body fluid precautions are essential for minimizing health care worker risk.

Physicians should assess their patients' risk for HIV infection by obtaining a sexual and drug history. Education about the use of condoms is essential for all persons who do not remain celibate or in a mutually monogamous relationship. Intravenous drug users can be encouraged to enter a drug treatment program. Those who do not abstain from intravenous drug use must be educated about safe needle use through a needle exchange program or by cleaning their injection equipment with bleach. Physicians' offices should have health education materials about HIV and sexually transmitted diseases openly available for patients and families to read and take with them. HIV-positive patients also need to be counseled about risk reduction both to protect themselves from other infections and to prevent transmission of HIV to their partners.

Counseling and Testing

Counseling and testing for HIV should be offered to all patients who have risk factors for HIV infection. Patients who have unexplained constitutional symptoms should also be offered HIV counseling and testing. Physicians should keep acute HIV infection in the differential diagnosis for patients presenting with a febrile illness who have a recent history of risk activities. Acute HIV infection usually causes a flu-like illness (Table 21.2) with symptoms of fever, myalgia, sore throat, and fatigue. On exam patients may have elevated temperatures, postural hypotension, mucous membrane ulcerations, maculopapular rash, adenopathy, and neurologic signs consistent with aseptic meningitis.[8] Patients with acute HIV infection may benefit from early ARV therapy and need to be counseled about risk reduction to prevent transmission of the virus to others.

Counseling about HIV is the beginning of a critical medical intervention.[9] During the pretest counseling sessions, the physician and patient need to discuss the patient's risk of being infected, ongoing activities that put the patient or others at risk, and methods of future risk reduction. Before offering testing, the physician should assess whether the patient appears psychologically and socially prepared for the results and if support from friends and family is available. A discussion of the complications of the HIV antibody testing including false-positive results, false-negative results, possible loss of confidentiality, and family and social disruption precedes obtaining informed consent for testing. The difference between confidential and anonymous testing needs to be discussed. Although confidential testing can be done in the physician's office, it results in charted documentation that can reveal HIV status to health care workers and others who process medical records. To avoid possible breaches of confidentiality and to ensure anonymity, the patient can be referred to an anonymous test site or obtain home testing.

Testing to establish the diagnosis of HIV infection usually requires an enzyme-linked immunosorbent assay (ELISA) screening test followed by either a West-

TABLE 21.2. Acute Retroviral Syndrome: Associated Signs and Symptoms

Common symptoms	Fever
	Myalgia
	Fatigue
	Sore throat
	Headache
	Rash
Common signs	Elevated temperature
	Maculopapular rash
	Mucous membrane ulcers (including oral and genital lesions)
	Adenopathy

ern blot (WB) or immunofluorescent antibody (IFA) confirmatory test. A "window period" of several weeks to 3 months exists between the time of infection and seroconversion with the development of specific antibodies against HIV. During this time patients can be viremic and infectious but not have sufficient levels of antibodies to result in positive serologic testing. For seronegative patients with recent at-risk activities, retesting at 3 to 6 months is advised. If there is strong clinical suspicion of recent HIV infection, antigen assays such as a plasma HIV RNA viral load or P24 antigen assay can be checked, but a positive antigen test needs to be interpreted with care because of concerns for false-positive results in these assays. A positive result needs to be confirmed with standard antibody tests in the future. In a few patients, serologic evidence of HIV infection may be delayed beyond 6 months.

All patients should receive their test results during a face-to-face posttest counseling session. For patients testing HIV positive, this session likely marks a turning point in their life. Patients should be told clearly that the test is positive, and that they are infected with HIV. It is important to reassure patients that HIV positivity does not mean they are at risk of becoming ill in the near future. Because HIV infection has a long asymptomatic phase and because of continuing advances in the treatment of HIV, there may be many years before problems arise. Upon hearing an HIV-positive result, however, patients may be in some degree of psychological shock and might not be able to assimilate much information. A commitment to ongoing care should be the focus of the first posttest counseling session. Perhaps the most important intervention that family physicians can make is to provide reassurance that they will remain the patient's personal physician while assembling a multidisciplinary team to help the patient address the challenges of the new diagnosis. At future visits, the family physician can offer to meet with the family and members of the patient's social network to help the patient combat isolation and identify particular challenges faced in coping with the diagnosis. The posttest counseling session is also important for patients who test negative for HIV. These patients need to be counseled about risk reduction and helped to develop specific plans to prevent future exposures.

Medical Management of HIV Disease

Health Care Maintenance

The seropositive patient requires routine health care maintenance and special attention to specific signs, symptoms, and laboratory markers for HIV disease progression. Routine health care maintenance includes a comprehensive history and physical examination with special attention to a history of sexually transmitted diseases and physical findings of skin and oral conditions. Laboratory evaluation includes a routine complete blood count including platelet count, chemistry panel, hepatitis and syphilis serologies, and markers of HIV disease (see below). A chest roentgenogram is required for persons with a history of cardiopulmonary problems but is not required for all HIV-infected persons. Women should have Pap smears performed and repeated at 6 months. Annual influenza vaccination and one-time pneumococcal vaccination should be administered. Hepatitis A and B vaccination is recommended if patients do not have serologic evidence of immunity. Polio vaccination for HIV-infected persons and their family members should be with the inactivated (intramuscular) preparation.

Because HIV infection contributes to an increased risk of progression from latent to active tuberculosis (TB), it is essential to screen all HIV positive patients for TB. A purified protein derivative (PPD) skin test for TB in HIV-infected persons is considered positive for TB infection with a 5-mm (rather than the usual 10-mm) reaction. PPD-negative patients should be screened annually. For HIV-infected persons known to be at high risk for TB (injection drug users, homeless persons, and persons from countries with a high incidence of TB) even a negative tuberculin skin test cannot eliminate the possibility of co-infection with TB. Patients with positive tuberculin skin tests and those with a high risk of TB require a chest roentgenogram to exclude active TB. Once active disease has been ruled out, patients should be offered treatment for latent TB with either isoniazid 300 mg daily for 9 months or rifampin 600 mg daily with pyrazinamide 2 g daily for 2 months.[10]

Laboratory Markers of HIV Disease

$CD4^+$ lymphocyte counts and plasma HIV RNA viral load measurements are essential tools in monitoring HIV disease. Depletion of $CD4^+$ lymphocytes is the hallmark of HIV disease and is an important marker of the degree of immunosuppression and predictor of the risk for opportunistic infections. The normal range for $CD4^+$ lymphocyte counts is broad and variable, so multiple measurements are required to detect trends. Viral load testing provides an assessment of viral activity and the patient's ability to control viral replication as well as the effectiveness of antiretroviral medications. The viral load also helps to predict the rate of decline in $CD4^+$ counts, with high viral loads predicting more rapid depletion of $CD4^+$ cells. $CD4^+$ counts and viral loads should be measured three to four times per year, in patients both receiving and not receiving antiviral therapy. In addition, viral load and $CD4^+$ counts should be checked within 2 months of starting a new antiviral regimen and if any significant clinical events occur.

Antiretroviral Therapy

Effective combination ARV therapy is a powerful medical intervention that can control viral replication and preserve immune function for HIV-positive patients, but it does not cure HIV infection. ARV agents can have substantial short-term and long-term side effects and toxicities. In addition, a patient's virus can become resistant to all agents currently in use. Guidelines for antiretroviral therapy change frequently.[1,11]

Prior to prescribing ARV medications, the family physician must assess the patient's ability to adhere to complex treatment regimens. Unlike therapeutics in other chronic diseases, such as diabetes or hypertension, the consequence of non-adherence to HIV medications can be the rapid development of resistance and permanent loss of clinical benefit.[12] Therefore, if a patient is unlikely to adhere to a medication regimen, it is better to postpone starting treatment until more supports are in place to help the patient adhere or other areas of the patient's life are more organized. Involving family members as well as utilizing the resources of case managers, clinical pharmacists, social workers, and other members of the care team can help with adherence issues.

Controversy exists over the best time to begin ARV therapy. The most recent guidelines on the use of antiretroviral agents from the Department of Health and Human Services[12] recommend starting ARV therapy in all patients who are symptomatic from HIV disease regardless of CD4$^+$ count and in asymptomatic patients with CD4$^+$ counts below 200 cells/mm^3. There is controversy about starting antiretroviral therapy in asymptomatic patients with CD4$^+$ counts between 200 and 350, but most experts recommend offering therapy to these patients. The guidelines recommend considering therapy for patients with CD4$^+$ counts between 350 and 500 cells/mm^3 who have high viral loads [greater than 55,000 copies by polymerase chain reaction (PCR) RNA assay or 30,000 copies on branched DNA assay]. Many clinicians would not treat patients with CD4$^+$ counts greater than 350 cells/mm^3 who have viral loads less than 55,000 (PCR RNA) or 30,000 (branched DNA) copies. These patients need regular CD4$^+$ cell counts and viral load testing to monitor disease progression and to assess the need for beginning therapy.

Initial antiviral regimens include at least three drugs, often from several different classes of agents. Common regimens are two nucleoside analogues with either one or two protease inhibitors, two nucleoside analogues with a nonnucleoside analogue, or three nucleoside analogues (Table 21.3). The goal of an initial regimen in patients without prior treatment is suppression of the viral load to undetectable levels and preservation or improvement in CD4 counts. Patients need to have CD4$^+$ counts and viral load testing by 8 weeks after starting a regimen, with the expectation of a log reduction in the pretreatment viral load. Depending on the initial viral load, it may take up to 6 months to achieve undetectable viral loads, so regimens should not be changed in the first few months unless there is clear virologic failure.

Patients failing antiviral regimens or patients with extensive history of antiviral use need special consideration in devising regimens that have the best chance of success. It is essential to obtain a complete history of ARV use, including the chronology of ARV regimens, CD4$^+$ counts and viral loads, as well as the reasons for change or discontinuation of specific medications. Resistance tests that measure either genotypic or phenotypic resistance to antiviral medications may play an important role in helping guide treatment options.[13] Given the complexity of the decisions involved in choosing or changing ARV regimens, it is reasonable for physicians without extensive experience with these medications to

TABLE 21.3. Common Antiretroviral Medications

Medication	Dose	Comment and side effects
Nucleoside reverse transcriptase inhibitors (NRTIs)[a,b]		
Zidovudine (AZT, Retrovir)[a,b]	200 mg tid or 300 mg bid	Anemia, neutropenia, headaches, nausea, malaise
Didanosine, (DDI, Videx, Videx EC)	200 mg bid or 400 mg qd	Need to take on empty stomach; diarrhea, pancreatitis, peripheral neuropathy, lactic acidosis
Zalcitabine (DDC, Hivid)	0.75 mg tid	Peripheral neuropathy, oral ulcers
Stavudine (D4T, Zerit)	20–40 mg bid	Peripheral neuropathy, insomnia, lactic acidosis, lipoatrophy
Lamivudine (3TC, Epivir)[a,b]	150 mg bid	Headache, fatigue, peripheral neuropathy, lactic acidosis
Abacavir (Ziagen)[b]	300 mg bid	Nausea, headache, malaise, hypersensitivity reaction, lactic acidosis, lipoatrophy
Non-nucleoside reverse transcriptase inhibitors (nNRTIs)		
Efavirenz (Sustiva)	600 mg qhs	Dizziness, anxiety, headache, nightmares, hepatitis; avoid during pregnancy; mixed P-450 enzyme inducer and inhibitor
Nevirapine (Viramune)	200 mg qd × 14 days then 200 mg bid	Rash, hepatitis, nausea, vomiting, diarrhea, fatigue, headaches, rare hematologic toxicity; P-450 enzyme inducer.
Delavirdine (Rescriptor)	400 mg tid	Rash, nausea, headache, hepatitis; P-450 enzyme inducer
Protease inhibitors (PIs)		
Nelfinavir (Viracept)	750 mg tid or 1250 mg bid (see dual PI regimens below)	Take with food; diarrhea, hyperlipidemias, abnormal fat accumulation, insulin resistance, hepatitis
Indinavir (Crixivan)	800 mg tid (see dual PI regimens below)	Take on empty stomach; nephrolithiasis, hyperlipidemias, abnormal fat accumulation, insulin resistance, diarrhea and asymptomatic hyperbilirubinemia

436

Drug	Dosage	Notes
Ritonavir (Norvir)	600 mg bid (see dual PI regimens below)	Take with food; potent P-450 enzyme inhibitor; nausea, vomiting, diarrhea, anorexia, hepatitis, hyperlipidemias, abnormal fat accumulation, insulin resistance, circumoral paresthesias
Saquinavir soft gel (Fortovase)	1200 mg tid (see dual PI regimens below)	Take with food; headache, confusion, hyperlipidemias, abnormal fat accumulation, insulin resistance, nausea, diarrhea, hepatitis
Amprenavir (Agenerase)	1200 mg bid (see dual PI regimens below)	Take with food; nausea, vomiting, diarrhea, hyperlipidemias, abnormal fat accumulation, oral paresthesias, headache, rash and hepatitis
Dual PI combinations		
Lopinavir/ritonavir (Kaletra)	400 mg/100 mg bid (three capsules); increase to four capsules if also giving efavirenz or nevirapine	Take with food; nausea, diarrhea, rash, headache, hyperlipidemia, insulin resistance
Ritonavir/indinavir	200 mg/800 mg bid or 400 mg/400 mg bid	OK to take with food; see individual agents
Ritonavir/saquinavir soft gel	400 mg/400 mg bid	See individual agents
Ritonavir/amprenavir	200 mg/600 mg bid	See individual agents

Source: Adapted from Goldschmidt and Dong.[1]
[a]AZT/3TC available as Combivir 300 mg/150 mg.
[b]AZT/3TC/Abacavir available as Trizavir 300 mg/150 mg/300 mg.

consult with colleagues who have more experience or with telephone resources such as the National HIV Telephone Consultation Service (Warmline) at (800) 933-3413 of the Department of Family and Community Medicine at San Francisco General Hospital.

All patients taking ARV therapy need both laboratory and clinical monitoring for adverse medication effects. Complete blood count and a chemistry panel with liver function tests should be included. Because many antiviral medications alter lipid metabolism, fasting lipid levels should be monitored. If lipid abnormalities develop, alternative regimens can be considered or the patient can be treated with lipid-lowering agents. Patients taking protease inhibitors have a higher incidence of hyperglycemia, which can be treated with dietary counseling or antihyperglycemic medications if needed. Often the most troubling side effects for patients are changes in body habitus from loss of subcutaneous adipose tissue in the face and limbs and accumulation of visceral adipose tissue in the abdomen. A very serious toxicity from antiviral medications is the development of potentially fatal lactic acidosis with multisystem organ failure. Patients on antiviral medications with complaints of malaise, dyspnea, and nonspecific gastrointestinal complaints should be evaluated for hyperlactatemia and liver abnormalities.[14] Potentially fatal hypersensitivity reactions to ARV medications can occur and need to be considered especially in patients restarting ARV regimens.

Management of the Immunocompromised Patient

Not all patients are able to benefit from ARV therapy because of intolerance to ARV medications, an inability to adhere to complex regimens, or virologic failure secondary to viral resistance. These patients are at risk of progressive decline in immune function and in developing opportunistic infections and malignancies. In this setting, it is especially important to maintain a close doctor–patient relationship to optimize care and to help address the medical, psychological, and social consequences of illness and disability.

Prophylaxis Against Opportunistic Infections

Preventing *Pneumocystis carinii* pneumonia (PCP) and other opportunistic infections decreases morbidity and mortality in immunocompromised patients.[15,16] When CD4$^+$ lymphocyte counts fall to fewer than 200 cells/mm^3 or when patients develop symptoms of advanced HIV disease, prophylaxis against PCP should be initiated. Prophylaxis has been shown to delay or prevent the development of PCP and improve the survival and health of HIV-infected persons. Trimethoprim-sulfamethoxazole (TMP-SMX), one double-strength tablet daily, is the drug of choice. For patients unable to tolerate TMP-SMX, alternative regimens are available. Prophylaxis against toxoplasmosis is generally provided by standard TMP-SMX regimens for PCP prophylaxis.

Prophylaxis against *Mycobacterium avium* complex (MAC) disease has been recommended for all patients with fewer than 50 CD4$^+$ lymphocytes/mm^3. Azithromycin or clarithromycin are the drugs of choice. Primary prophylaxis against fungal, herpes simplex, herpes zoster, and cytomegalovirus infections is not routinely recommended. Primary and secondary prophylaxis against many opportunistic infections can be discontinued if patients are able to maintain CD4$^+$ counts above the high-risk levels for more than 6 months while on ARV therapy. Recommendations for prophylaxis and discontinuation of prophylaxis change as more data become available. The most recent recommendations can be accessed through the Internet resources listed in Table 21.1.

Clinical Manifestations of AIDS

Nonspecific Symptoms and Signs

Nearly all patients with progressive HIV disease develop weight loss,[17] weakness, malaise, and anorexia. Unexplained fevers are common with advanced HIV disease. Investigation for specific organ system disease and opportunistic infections and malignancies is the first step in evaluating these symptoms and signs. This investigation includes evaluations for pulmonary disease including PCP and disseminated MAC infection.[18] Sepsis caused by bacteria and fungi (including cryptococcal sepsis) can also be identified. When no specific pathogenic process can be found, constitutional symptoms and signs are usually attributed to the HIV infection itself. Fevers can be treated with nonsteroidal antiinflammatory drugs (NSAIDs), but these drugs can be especially nephrotoxic in AIDS patients. Weight loss, especially from loss of muscle mass, needs to be aggressively worked up and treated.[19]

Skin and Oral Cavity

Skin and oral cavity lesions are the most frequent first manifestations of AIDS.[20] A form of seborrheic dermatitis is the most common skin condition found in HIV-infected persons. This condition is readily treated with a combination of low-strength hydrocortisone cream plus ketoconazole cream. Drug rashes can be bothersome and serious. Careful investigation to identify and discontinue the offending drug (including nonprescription drugs the patient may be taking without the physician's knowledge) is essential.

Kaposi's sarcoma (KS) is an AIDS-defining condition. The violaceous to brown lesions can occur anywhere on the body. A biopsy can be required, especially to distinguish KS from bacillary angiomatosis, a bacterial condition that can produce similar lesions. KS does not require treatment unless the lesions are cosmetically bothersome, bulky, or painful, or the patient wishes the lesions to be treated. Other skin conditions include bacterial folliculitis, fungal rashes, and molluscum contagiosum. Herpes zoster infections (shingles) can occur early in HIV disease. Herpes simplex infections of the perioral and perirectal areas can be extensive and persistent. Treatment with oral acyclovir is usually effective, but extensive lesions require intravenous acyclovir. Disseminated herpes simplex and zoster infections usually require intravenous acyclovir treatment.

Oral candidiasis (thrush) is not an AIDS-defining condition. Thrush takes the form of white plaques that can be scraped from the tongue or other areas of the oral mucosa. Oral candidiasis can also present in an inflammatory form with erythema and atrophy but without white plaques. Treatment with topical or systemic antifungal agents is effective. Oral hairy leukoplakia is a viral lesion that appears on the lateral borders of the tongue. Because this condition is asymptomatic and recedes spontaneously, no treatment is required. Other oral conditions include KS, angular cheilitis secondary to candidal infection, and periodontal disease.

EYES

Cytomegalovirus (CMV) retinitis usually occurs when $CD4^+$ lymphocyte counts are lower than 50 cells/mm^3. Hemorrhages, perivascular exudates, and white, gray, or yellow discoloration of the peripheral retina are characteristic. When CMV retinitis is identified, treatment with ganciclovir (Cytovene) or foscarnet (Foscavir) should be instituted, as progression to blindness can occur rapidly and without warning.[21] Cotton-wool spots are nonspecific signs of ischemia that are frequently noted on funduscopic examination of many AIDS patients. These small white lesions with indistinct margins can come and go and do not threaten vision.

LYMPH NODES AND HEMATOPOIETIC SYSTEM

Generalized lymphadenopathy caused by HIV-induced nodal hyperplasia is common and does not require biopsy or specific treatment. Treatable causes of lymphadenopathy, including lymphoma, tuberculosis, fungal infections, and KS, should be considered when suspicious clinical syndromes are present, lymphadenopathy is asymmetric, or prominent hard lymph nodes are present. Biopsy may be required in these instances.

All blood cell lines can be affected by HIV infection. Neutropenia is common, with reductions in the absolute neutrophil count to fewer than 300 to 500 neutrophils/mm^3 frequently occurring in the patient with AIDS. Careful observation, blood cultures, and consideration of empiric antibiotic treatment are required for severe neutropenia. Granulocyte/macrophage-stimulating factors can help raise the neutrophil count to noncritical levels in the presence of drug-induced granulocytopenia. Anemia caused by HIV disease can require transfusions or erythropoietin therapy. Macrocytosis is a normal hematologic response to zidovudine therapy and does not require or respond to treatment. Some patients receiving zidovudine develop anemia with or without macrocytosis, requiring discontinuation of the drug or blood transfusion. Thrombocytopenia can occur early in the course of HIV infection and does not appear to predict disease progression, nor is it a condition that requires treatment. Thrombocytopenia late in the course of HIV disease does not require treatment unless bleeding is present.[22]

LUNGS

Pulmonary disease is a significant cause of morbidity and mortality in HIV-infected persons.[23] The symptoms and signs can vary from only minimal shortness of breath or nonproductive cough to severe respiratory distress. The physical examination usually reveals tachypnea. Rales and cough with purulent sputum are not usually present unless bacterial pneumonia or pulmonary tuberculosis is present. Evaluation is based on the findings of the chest radiograph and arterial blood gas measurements. X-ray findings of PCP and other pulmonary processes in AIDS typically show diffuse interstitial infiltrates or alveolar infiltrates. Thoracic and mediastinal lymphadenopathy and pleural effusions, when present, may indicate fungal disease, *Mycobacterium tuberculosis* infection, lymphoma, or pulmonary KS. Pleural effusions do not occur with PCP alone. The chest film is normal in 10% of patients with PCP. A negative high-resolution computed tomography (CT) scan of the chest in these patients can rule out PCP but a positive study is not specific for PCP. Arterial blood gas measurements usually show substantial hypoxemia with hypocarbia. Lactic dehydrogenase levels are frequently elevated in patients with AIDS pulmonary disease but do not provide sufficient information on which to base differential diagnostic decisions. Abnormalities of chest radiographs or arterial blood gases require further diagnostic investigation to establish the pathologic diagnosis.

PCP is one of the most common pulmonary disease in immunocompromised patients with HIV. Examination of pulmonary specimens for *P. carinii* requires sputum induction or bronchoscopy; patients with PCP do not spontaneously expectorate sputum containing *P. carinii* organisms. *P. carinii* cysts can be detected for at least 3 weeks after initiation of therapy. Therefore, patients seriously ill with presumptive PCP should be treated empirically, with diagnostic procedures performed later.

First-line treatment of PCP is with intravenous or oral TMP-SMX. The duration of PCP therapy is 3 weeks. TMP-SMX has the added advantage of treating possible concurrent bacterial pneumonia. Patients with PaO$_2$ less than 70 mm Hg should receive concurrent corticosteroids.[24] Patients with moderate to severe PCP are usually hospitalized to provide monitoring and ensure proper medication administration. Marked clinical worsening after 1 week or failure to respond after 2 weeks of therapy is a reasonable indication for changing to an alternative agent. Patients with mild PCP who have adequate home support services can be treated as outpatients with oral medications. Oral treatment of PCP is with TMP-SMX or with dapsone plus trimethoprim. PCP recurrences can be treated with the same agent that was successful on previous episodes.

Other pulmonary pathogenic processes to be considered include pneumonia (most commonly caused by *Haemophilus influenzae*, *Streptococcus pneumoniae*, *Legionella pneumophila*, and *Mycoplasma pneumoniae*), tuberculosis, MAC, and KS.

GASTROINTESTINAL TRACT

Esophagitis with dysphagia, odynophagia, and retrosternal pain can be caused by *Candida albicans*, CMV, or herpes simplex virus. Candidal esophagitis, which is an AIDS-defining disease, is most common. In patients with coexisting oral candidiasis, systemic treatment with fluconazole or ketoconazole should be initiated as an empiric trial. If the patient does not have oral candidiasis or a previous case diagnosis of AIDS, esophagoscopy with biopsies and cultures is advised to establish the diagnosis and direct therapy. Treatment of CMV esophagitis with ganciclovir or foscarnet and of herpes esophagitis with acyclovir is usually effective.

Chronic diarrhea with weight loss can occur in immunocompromised patients. Bacterial cultures and parasite determination should be performed to identify treatable causes such as *Shigella*, *Salmonella*, and *Campylobacter* infections or *Cryptosporidium* or other parasitic infestations. *Clostridium difficile* titers should be determined.

Perianal disease, most commonly caused by herpes simplex virus infections, requires prolonged therapy with oral acyclovir. Extensive perianal disease requires intravenous therapy.

Liver disease can be the result of drug toxicity, hepatitis, or other infections and malignancies. Patients with laboratory findings suggesting a predominantly obstructive pattern (elevated alkaline phosphatase) should undergo ultrasound examination to rule out hepatic masses or biliary tract obstruction. An AIDS-associated cholangiopathy with strictures and papillary stenosis can be identified by upper endoscopy with retrograde cholangiography. Sphincterotomy can effectively palliate symptoms of a biliary tract obstruction. When the ultrasound examination is negative, MAC disease, tuberculosis, fungal diseases, or other infiltrative hepatic processes should be considered.

GYNECOLOGIC PROBLEMS

Women with HIV infection can have severe, persistent vaginal candidiasis (see Chapter 16). Prolonged or repeated antifungal treatment is often necessary. Cervical dysplasia and cancer are also more frequent and more aggressive than in women not infected with HIV. Papanicolaou smears should be examined every 6 months; dysplasia should be evaluated by colposcopy.[25]

RENAL AND ADRENAL DISEASE

The most common renal problem is drug toxicity. Special attention is required when patients are taking TMP-SMX, NSAIDs, or other drugs known to cause nephrotoxicity. HIV-associated nephropathy with renal failure can occur, most commonly among patients who have been intravenous drug users, hypertensive patients, or those who have coexisting intrinsic renal disease. Adrenal insufficiency, characterized by hypotension and blunted stress response, can occur.

Neurologic Problems

Neurologic problems[26,27] occurring in immunocompromised patients include peripheral neuropathies, myelopathies, and central nervous system (CNS) disorders. The most common CNS disorder is the AIDS dementia complex and is usually a late manifestation of HIV disease. Dementia can present with cognitive impairment, motor disturbances, or behavioral dysfunction. The most typical presentation is confusion, forgetfulness, and lethargy. Predominant features can also include ataxia and clumsiness. Behavioral changes are dominated by apathy, listlessness, and withdrawal. The major cause of the AIDS–dementia complex is HIV infection of the brain. The diagnosis is one of exclusion of other treatable causes of CNS disease. Treatment with effective ARV regimens can improve dementia.

The differential diagnosis of CNS disorders includes cryptococcal meningitis, toxoplasmic encephalitis, CNS lymphoma, and progressive multifocal leukoencephalopathy. Cryptococcal meningitis can present with the AIDS–dementia complex, fever, photophobia, headache, or stiff neck. Serum and cerebrospinal fluid cryptococcal antigen tests are positive more than 90% of the time. Treatment with amphotericin B or fluconazole is usually effective.[28] Toxoplasmic encephalitis[29] can present as the AIDS–dementia complex but also can cause seizures and focal neurologic signs. Empiric treatment is usually given when suspicious lesions on CT or magnetic resonance imaging scans are noted. Failure to respond clinically or radiologically within 2 weeks can be an indication for a brain biopsy to rule out lymphoma and other CNS problems.

Lymphomas

Multisystem lymphomas, including non-Hodgkin's lymphoma,[30] can occur in the thoracic and abdominal lymph nodes, gastrointestinal tract, bone marrow, brain, and other organs. Systemic disease can be treated with combination chemotherapy and/or radiation therapy.

HIV Disease in Children

Infection with HIV can occur transplacentally, at the time of delivery, and with breast-feeding. Because treatment with ARV therapy can greatly reduce the rate of perinatal transmission, all pregnant women at risk for HIV infection should be offered counseling and testing. HIV-infected mothers should be counseled about the benefits of ARV therapy and offered treatment. They should be discouraged from breast-feeding when there are safe alternatives.

The diagnosis of HIV infection in infants is complicated by the presence of maternal antibodies for HIV until the age of 15 months. A definitive diagnosis can usually be made earlier with viral assays. HIV DNA PCR is the preferred assay for detecting infection. Infants born to HIV-positive mothers should be tested within 48 hours of birth. A positive test should be confirmed with a repeat test as soon as possible. If the initial test is negative, follow-up testing should occur at 1 to 2 months and again at 3 to 6 months of age. Infants at risk for HIV infection should be given PCP prophylaxis with TMP-SMX at age 4 to 6 weeks until HIV infection has been ruled in or out.[31]

HIV-infected children should have CD4$^+$ counts with CD4$^+$ percentages and viral load testing every 3 months. Because children have higher CD4$^+$ counts than adults, percentage of CD4$^+$ cells is a better marker of immunosuppression than absolute CD4$^+$ counts. HIV-infected children should receive PCP prophylaxis for the first year of life regardless of CD4$^+$ count, with subsequent prophylaxis based on immune status. HIV-positive children should receive routine diphtheria/pertussis/tetanus (DPT), *H. influenzae* type b (HiB), and inactivated (intramuscular) poliovirus vaccine at standard intervals. Mumps/measles/rubella (MMR) vaccination should be given on schedule unless the child is profoundly immunocompromised. Oral poliovirus vaccine should not be given to HIV-infected children or to household members living with immunocompromised persons. Influenza and pneumococcal vaccines are recommended for children with symptomatic HIV infection.

In children, immunosuppression from AIDS usually presents with constitutional symptoms (e.g., fever and failure to thrive), oral candidiasis, lymphadenopathy, hepato-splenomegaly, and persistent or recurrent bacterial infections. Viral infections can also be severe and persistent. Pulmonary manifestations include PCP and lymphocytic interstitial pneumonitis. Gastrointestinal complications include diarrhea and candidal esophagitis. Neurologic and developmental problems also occur and must be evaluated thoroughly.

ARV therapy in children has been shown to slow disease progression and lower mortality. Therapy should be considered in HIV-infected children with evidence of immunosuppression. As in adults, issues of adherence need to be addressed prior to starting therapy. Families with HIV-positive children need a family-centered approach from a multidisciplinary care team.

References

1. Goldschmidt RH, Dong BJ. Treatment of AIDS and HIV-related conditions: 2001. J Am Board Fam Pract 2001;14:283–309.
2. The Concerned Action on Seroconversion to AIDS and Death in Europe. Survival after introduction of HAART in people with known duration of HIV-1 infection. Lancet 2000;355:1158–9.
3. The World Health Organization. AIDS Epidemic Update: December 2000. Available at *www.who.int.*
4. Centers for Disease Control and Prevention. HIV/AIDS Surveillance Report, 2000. Available at *www.cdc.gov/hiv/stats/hasr1201.htm.*
5. Kleinman S, Busch MP, Korelitz JJ, Schreiber GB. The incidence/window period model and its use to assess the risk of transfusion-transmitted human immunodeficiency virus and hepatitis C virus infection. Transfusion Med Rev 1997;11(3):155–72.
6. Mandelbrot L, Landreau-Mascaro A, Rekacewicz C, et al. Lamivudine-zidovudine

combination for prevention of maternal–infant transmission of HIV-1. JAMA 2001;285:2083–93.

7. Centers for Disease Control and Prevention. Updated Public Health Service guidelines for the management of health-care worker exposures to HIV and recommendations for postexposure prophylaxis. MMWR 2001;50:1–52.

8. Schacker T, Collier A, Hughes J, Shea T, Corey L. Clinical and epidemiologic features of primary HIV infection. Ann Intern Med 1996;125:257–64.

9. Goldschmidt RH, Legg JJ. Counseling patients about HIV test results. J Am Board Fam Pract 1991;4:361–3.

10. Havlir DV, Barnes PF. Tuberculosis in patients with human immunodeficiency virus infection. N Engl J Med 1999;340:367–73.

11. Panel on Clinical Practices for Treatment of HIV Infection. Guidelines for the use of antiretroviral agents in HIV-infected adults and adolescents. 2001. Available at *www.hivatis.org*.

12. Chesney MA, Ickovics J, Hecht FM, Sidipa G, Rabkin J. Adherence: a necessity for successful HIV combination therapy. AIDS 1999;13(suppl A):S271–8.

13. Hirsch MS, Brun-Vezinet F, D'Aquila RT, et al. Antiretroviral drug resistance testing in adult HIV-1 infection. JAMA 2000;283:2417–26.

14. Carr A, Cooper DA. Adverse effects of antiretroviral therapy. Lancet 2000;356:1423–30.

15. Kovacs JA, Masur H. Prophylaxis against opportunistic infections in patients with human immunodeficiency virus infection. N Engl J Med 2000;342:1416–29.

16. Center for Disease Control and Prevention. 1999 USPHA/IDSA guidelines for the prevention of opportunistic infections in persons infected with human immunodeficiency virus. MMWR 1999;43(RR-10):1–67.

17. Grunfeld C, Feingold KR. Metabolic disturbances and wasting in the acquired immunodeficiency syndrome. N Engl J Med 1992;327:329–37.

18. Horsburgh CR Jr. *Mycobacterium avium* complex infection in the acquired immunodeficiency syndrome. N Engl J Med 1991;324:1332–8.

19. Nemechek PM, Polsky B, Gottlieg MS. Treatment guidelines for HIV-associated wasting. Mayo Clin Proc 2000;75(4):386–94.

20. Berger TG, Obuch ML, Goldschmidt RH. Dermatologic manifestations of HIV infection. Am Fam Physician 1990;41:1729–42.

21. Holland GN, Tufail A. New therapies for cytomegalovirus retinitis. N Engl J Med 1995;333:658–9.

22. Glatt AE, Anand A. Thrombocytopenia in patients infected with human immunodeficiency virus: treatment update. Clin Infect Dis 1995;21:415–23.

23. Miller R. HIV-associated respiratory disease. Lancet 1996;348:307–12.

24. Consensus statement on the use of corticosteroids as adjunctive therapy for *Pneumocystis carinii* pneumonia in the acquired immunodeficiency syndrome: the National Institutes of Health–University of California Expert Panel for Corticosteroids as Adjunctive Therapy for *Pneumocystis carinii* pneumonia. N Engl J Med 1990;323:1500–4.

25. Legg JJ. Women and HIV. J Am Board Fam Pract 1993;6:367–77.

26. Simpson DM, Tagliati M. Neurologic manifestations of HIV infection. Ann Intern Med 1994;121:769–85.

27. Newton HB. Common neurologic complications of HIV-1 infection and AIDS. Am Fam Physician 1995;51:387–98.

28. Saag MS, Powderly WG, Cloud GA, et al. Comparison of amphotericin B with flu-

conazole in the treatment of acute AIDS-associated cryptococcal meningitis. N Engl J Med 1992;326:83–9.
29. Luft BJ, Hafner R, Korzun AH, et al. Toxoplasmic encephalitis in patients with the acquired immunodeficiency syndrome. N Engl J Med 1993;329:995–1000.
30. Little RF, Gutierrez M, Jaffe ES, Pau A, Horne M, Wilson W. HIV-associated non-Hodgkin lymphoma: incidence, presentation and prognosis. JAMA 2001;285:1880–5.
31. The Working Group on Antiretroviral Therapy and Medical Management of HIV-Infected Children. Guidelines for the use of antiretroviral agents in pediatric HIV infection. 2000. Available at *www.hivatis.org*.

CASE PRESENTATION

Subjective

PATIENT PROFILE

Mark McCarthy is a 28-year-old single male restaurant waiter.

PRESENTING PROBLEM

"Cough and HIV-positive."

PRESENT ILLNESS

Mark has had a cough for 3 weeks with a recurrent low-grade fever. His cough has been productive of gray-yellow sputum with an occasional fleck of blood. He was found 10 months ago to be HIV-positive when he requested the test after several worrisome sexual contacts.

PAST MEDICAL HISTORY

Unremarkable since tonsillectomy, age 5.

SOCIAL HISTORY

The patient dropped out of college to organize a rock group that disbanded 2 years ago. He now works as a waiter in his parents' restaurant.

HABITS

Smokes one and a half packs of cigarettes daily. He uses no alcohol. He drinks four cups of coffee a day and occasionally smokes marijuana.

FAMILY HISTORY

His father, aged 54, is diabetic and has coronary artery disease. His mother, aged 51, and sister are living and in good health.

REVIEW OF SYSTEMS

Over the past month, he has had a poor appetite and believes that he has lost 3 to 5 pounds.

- What additional information about the history of present illness would be pertinent?
- What additional information about his HIV history might be pertinent? How would you elicit this information?
- What information about his current life style and work might be important? How would you frame this inquiry?
- What might be Mr. McCarthy's unstated reasons for the visit today? Why might this be important?

Objective

VITAL SIGNS

Height, 5 ft 9 in; weight, 145 lb; blood pressure, 110/72; pulse, 78; respirations, 24; temperature, 38.2°C.

EXAMINATION

The patient is a thin white man who does not appear acutely ill but coughs from time to time while speaking. The eyes, ears, nose, and throat are unremarkable except for mild pharyngeal injection. There are a few enlarged cervical nodes bilaterally. The chest has scattered rhonchi at both bases. The heart has a normal sinus rhythm with no murmurs. The skin has a few dark, slightly elevated areas of pigmentation on the dorsum of the hands.

- What other information obtained from the physical examination might be important? Why?
- Are there other areas of the body that you might examine? Why?
- What—if any—laboratory tests should be ordered today?
- What—if any—diagnostic imaging should be ordered today?

Assessment

- Pending the outcome of the tests you have ordered, what is your diagnostic assessment? How would you explain this to the patient?
- How would you assess Mr. McCarthy's knowledge of his health status and prognosis?

- What might be the meaning of the current illness to the patient? How would you address this issue?
- Describe the family implications of the illness.

Plan

- What are your specific recommendations for this patient? How would you explain this to the patient?
- What—if any—changes would you advise in his future work responsibilities?
- Mr. McCarthy's parents ask for an explanation of their son's illness. How would you respond?
- What are your recommendations for continuing care?

22
Anxiety Disorders

DEBORAH S. McPHERSON

Anxiety disorders are among the most frequently occurring mental disorders in the general population. They encompass a group of conditions that share pathologic anxiety as a principal disturbance of mood with resultant effects on thought, behavior, and physiologic activity. This category of disorders includes panic disorder with agoraphobia, generalized anxiety disorder, social anxiety disorder, obsessive-compulsive disorder, and posttraumatic stress disorder.

Panic Disorder with Agoraphobia

Panic disorder is a common, chronic, and potentially disabling psychiatric condition that frequently presents in the primary care setting. The disorder is characterized by the experience of two or more unexpected panic attacks followed by persistent concern about future attacks or change in behavior to avoid panic attacks. Panic attacks are characterized as discrete episodes of intense fear or discomfort associated with numerous somatic and cognitive symptoms (Table 22.1). Symptoms occur abruptly and reach their maximum intensity within 10 to 15 minutes. Episodes rarely persist longer than 30 minutes.[1] By definition, panic attacks are not caused by any underlying medical condition, due to the effects of a drug or substance, or attributable to another psychiatric disorder (Table 22.2).

Panic attacks are common, with 15% of respondents in the National Comorbidity Survey reporting at least one in their lifetime; 3% of respondents reported a panic attack in the month preceding the survey.[2] Panic disorder has a lifetime prevalence of 2% to 4% in adults and occurs twice as often in women as in men. In half of the patients, agoraphobia is also present. In these cases, patients avoid situations or places where help may be unavailable or escape difficult if a panic attack occurs. Symptoms can become so severe that patients are almost totally disabled. Patients are unable to predict when attacks will occur, although certain situations may be associated with the attacks, such as driving a car or using public transportation. The disorder usually begins in late adolescence to middle adulthood and is infrequent after age 50. Early onset carries a greater risk of comorbidity, chronicity, and impairment. Between 50% and 65% of patients with panic disorder have had at least one episode of depression, and 20% to 30% suffer from

TABLE 22.1. Common Symptoms of Panic Attacks

Autonomic	Neurologic
Sweating	Dizziness
Chills	Paresthesias
Hot flushes	Trembling
Cardiopulmonary	Psychiatric
Chest pain	Depersonalization
Palpitations	Derealization
Shortness of breath	Intense fear
Tachycardia	
Gastrointestinal	
Choking	
Nausea	

alcoholism or substance abuse.[3] About 20% of patients have attempted suicide at least once.[4]

Differential Diagnosis

Because of the associated somatic symptoms, patients with panic disorder frequently present to the family physician's office. Unfortunately, the diagnosis can be missed because the symptoms mimic cardiopulmonary, gastrointestinal, and neurologic illnesses. Medical conditions that should be excluded are coronary artery disease, mitral valve prolapse, hypoglycemia, thyroid dysfunction, asthma, and partial complex seizures. In addition, many over-the-counter medications, herbal therapies, caffeine, and alcohol may precipitate or exacerbate symptoms of panic disorder. A careful history and physical examination and appropriate laboratory studies, when indicated, are sufficient to identify an underlying medical disorder.[5]

TABLE 22.2. Diagnostic Criteria for Panic Disorder with Agoraphobia

A. Both 1 and 2
  1. Recurrent unexpected panic attacks
  2. At least one of the attacks has been followed by 1 month (or more) of one (or more) of the following:
    a. Persistent concern about having additional attacks
    b. Worry about the implications of the attack or its consequences (e.g., losing control, having a heart attack, "going crazy")
    c. Significant change in behavior related to the attacks
B. Presence of agoraphobia
C. Panic attacks are not due to the direct physiologic effects of a substance (e.g., drug abuse, medication) or a general medical condition (e.g., hyperthyroidism)
D. Panic attacks are not better accounted for by another mental disorder, such as social phobia (e.g., occurring on exposure to feared social situations), specific phobia (e.g., on exposure to a specific phobic situation), obsessive-compulsive disorder (e.g., on exposure to dirt in someone with an obsession about contamination), posttraumatic stress disorder (e.g., in response to stimuli associated with a severe stressor), or separation anxiety disorder (e.g., in response to being away from home or close relatives)

Source: American Psychiatric Association,[1] with permission.

Management

Treatment of panic disorder consists of counseling and pharmacotherapy in conjunction with cognitive behavioral therapy (CBT). Because of the chronic nature of this disorder, patients should recognize that sustained improvement requires long-term adherence to the prescribed regimen.

BEHAVIORAL THERAPY

Cognitive-behavior therapy treatment may be used alone or in conjunction with pharmacotherapy. In CBT, exposure exercises are used to desensitize the patient to situations that provoke panic attacks and to assist patients in learning symptom management skills. Systematic desensitization is especially effective when coupled with family and physician support. Exposure to phobic situations should be encouraged. Family members frequently adapt to the agoraphobic's fears, so successful treatment often changes family dynamics. Cognitive restructuring is also emphasized to change the patient's thought process during panic attacks. Response rates of up to 60% have been demonstrated using CBT alone.[6]

PHARMACOLOGIC THERAPY

Four classes of medication may be used in the treatment of panic disorder. All four are effective, but they differ in terms of safety and tolerability as well as their activity in treating comorbid conditions. Overall, pharmacotherapy is effective in the majority of patients with panic disorder, but should be maintained for at least 12 months to minimize the risk of recurrence.

Selective serotonin reuptake inhibitors (SSRIs) are considered first-line therapy for panic disorder because of their efficacy and low side-effect profile, especially among patients with comorbid depression or suicidal risk factors. Reduction of frequency and severity of panic attacks is appreciated as early as the second week of therapy. In all agents in this class, up to 80% improvement in frequency has been reported. SSRIs have been shown to be equally effective in both men and women and in patients with or without agoraphobia in clinical trials. Currently, only sertraline (Zoloft) and paroxetine (Paxil) are approved by the Food and Drug Administration (FDA) for the treatment of panic disorder. Because pharmacokinetic properties vary within the class, patients who fail to respond to one agent should be given a trial of another. Side effects include nausea, diarrhea, insomnia, and sexual dysfunction. Initial agitation may also occur during titration, especially with fluoxetine.[7] Recommended starting and therapeutic doses of medications used in the treatment of panic disorder are given in Table 22.3.[8]

If treatment is effective and panic attacks have been eliminated after 12 to 18 months, dose reduction can begin over the next 4 to 6 months. Treatment with SSRIs may continue indefinitely as tolerated if any symptoms persist, the patient retains comorbid psychiatric conditions, has a history of prior relapse, or is experiencing significant stress and is concerned about relapse.

Table 22.3. Medications Used in Panic Disorder

Class	Starting dose	Recommended dose
Selective serotonin reuptake inhibitors (SSRIs)		
Citalopram (Celexa)	10 mg	20–60 mg/day
Fluoxetine (Prozac)	5–10 mg qd	20–80 mg/day
Fluvoxamine (Luvox)	25–50 mg qd	50–300 mg/day
Paroxetine (Paxil)	10 mg qd	40–60 mg/day
Sertraline (Zoloft)	25 mg qd	50–200 mg/day
Benzodiazepines		
Alprazolam (Xanax)	0.25–0.5 mg tid	2–10 mg/day
Clonazepam (Klonopin)	0.25 mg bid	1–4 mg/day
Monoamine oxidase inhibitors (MAOIs)		
Phenelzine (Nardil)	15 mg tid	60–90 mg/day
Tricyclic antidepressants (TCAs)		
Desipramine (Norpramin)	10 mg qd	25–300 mg/day
Imipramine (Tofranil)	10 mg qd	50–300 mg/day
Nortriptyline (Pamelor)	10 mg qd	25–150 mg/day

Until recently, the tricyclic antidepressants (TCAs) were considered first-line therapy in panic disorder. Within this class, imipramine (Tofranil) at 50 to 300 mg/day, nortriptyline (Pamelor) at 25 to 150 mg/day, and desipramine (Norpramin) at 25 to 300 mg/day have demonstrated effectiveness.[9] Important disadvantages of TCAs include the potential for orthostatic hypotension and direct cardiac effects that can lead to potentially fatal arrhythmias in overdosage. TCAs have a relatively slow onset of action and initial worsening of anxiety may occur during dose titration.[10]

Monoamine oxidase inhibitors (MAOIs) have been successfully used in the treatment of panic disorder for many years. The most commonly used agent is phenelzine (Nardil), although tranylcypromine (Parnate) is also effective. In recent years, these medications have given way to more effective and safer products as first-line treatment. The MAOIs require a strict adherence to a tyrosine free diet to prevent hypertensive crisis and have the potential for serious drug–drug interactions with many over-the-counter preparations. Side effects include orthostatic hypotension, insomnia, weight gain, and sexual dysfunction. The recommended starting dose of phenelzine (Nardil) is 15 mg tid with a gradual increase to the lowest effective total dose between 60 and 90 mg/day.

Benzodiazepines are effective in the treatment of panic disorder, are generally well tolerated, and have a rapid onset of action. Because of their ability to potentiate the effects of alcohol and their potential for physical dependence, however, their utility is limited to treating acutely distressed patients until a more appropriate agent reaches maximal effectiveness. Both alprazolam (Xanax) given at 0.25 to 0.5 mg tid to a maximum dose of 10 mg/day and clonazepam (Klonopin) given at 0.25 mg bid to a maximum dose of 4 mg/day are approved by the FDA in the treatment of panic disorder. Benzodiazepines may cause sedation, poor coordination, and memory impairment. Withdrawal symptoms may become evident between doses in the form of rebound anxiety. While these medications are considered short acting in younger adults, they should be used judiciously in elderly patients.

Patients with panic disorder are frequently seen by family physicians and present no immediate need for referral. Family physicians may consider home visits for the treatment of agoraphobic patients until they are able to return to a more active lifestyle. Referral is appropriate when first- or second-line pharmacotherapy is ineffective or for patients who are suffering from comorbid substance abuse or who are actively suicidal.

Generalized Anxiety Disorder

Generalized anxiety disorder (GAD) is characterized by unrealistic and excessive worry about life circumstances in disproportion to actual problems. Patients with GAD may have extended periods of time when they're not consumed by their worries, but report feeling anxious most of the time. Symptoms are typically associated with three different categories: excessive physiologic arousal such as muscle tension, irritability, and insomnia; distorted cognitive processes including poor concentration and unrealistic assessment of problems; and poor coping strategies such as avoidance, procrastination, and poor problem-solving skills. Symptoms must be present for at least 6 months and must adversely impact the patient's life (Table 22.4).[1]

TABLE 22.4. Diagnostic Criteria for Generalized Anxiety Disorder

A. Excessive anxiety and worry (apprehensive expectation), occurring more days than not for at least 6 months, about a number of events or activities (such as work or school performance).
B. The person finds it difficult to control the worry.
C. The anxiety and worry are associated with three (or more) of the following six symptoms (with at least some symptoms present for more days than not for the past 7 months). Note: Only one item is required in children.
    1. Restlessness or feeling keyed up or on edge
    2. Being easily fatigued
    3. Difficulty concentrating or mind going blank
    4. Irritability
    5. Muscle tension
    6. Sleep disturbance (difficulty falling or staying asleep, or restless unsatisfying sleep)
D. The focus of the anxiety and worry is not confined to features of an axis I disorder, e.g., the anxiety or worry is not about having a panic attack (as in panic disorder), being embarrassed in public (as in social phobia), being contaminated (as in obsessive-compulsive disorder), being away from home or close relatives (as in separation anxiety disorder), gaining weight (as in anorexia nervosa), having multiple physical complaints (as in somatization disorder), or having a serious illness (as in hypochondriasis); and the anxiety and worry do not occur exclusively during posttraumatic stress disorder.
E. The anxiety, worry, or physical symptoms cause clinically significant distress or impairment in social, occupational, or other important areas of functioning.
F. The disturbance is not due to the direct physiologic effects of a substance (e.g., drug of abuse, medication), or a general medical condition (e.g., hyperthyroidism) and does not occur exclusively during a mood disorder, a psychotic disorder, or a pervasive developmental disorder.

Source: American Psychiatric Association,[1] with permission.

Lifetime prevalence of GAD is 4.1% to 6.6%, but in patients presenting to physicians' offices the prevalence is twice the rate found in the general community.[11] As with panic disorder, GAD is more common in women, with an onset typically in the early 20s. The condition tends to be chronic, with periods of exacerbation and remission, although symptoms can be intensified by stressful life events. Patients rarely seek psychiatric help, but often present to their family physician with multiple nonspecific complaints.

Diagnosis

Because the difference between normal anxiety and GAD is sometimes unclear and GAD frequently presents with comorbid psychiatric disorders, the diagnosis can be challenging. More than 70% of GAD patients have had at least one panic attack. Depression is very common, with a 67% lifetime prevalence of major depressive episodes.[12] Patients with persistent anxiety, worry, or multiple nonspecific complaints should first be evaluated for an underlying medical condition. Medical disorders frequently associated with anxiety include hyperthyroidism, Cushing's disease, mitral valve prolapse, carcinoid syndrome and pheochromocytoma. Additionally, medications such as corticosteroids, digoxin, thyroxine, and theophylline may cause anxiety. Patients should also be asked about any herbal products or over-the-counter medications they might be using as well as their use of alcohol, nicotine, caffeine, or illicit drugs.[13] Because of the significant overlap of symptoms and comorbidity with other psychiatric illness, GAD should be considered a diagnosis of exclusion. Unlike panic disorder, the anxiety experienced in GAD is usually specific and chronic. GAD may be contrasted with major depression on the basis of the neurovegetative symptoms frequently seen in depression. Restlessness and motor tension are more commonly found in cases of GAD. Somatization disorder should also be considered in the differential diagnosis. In this disorder, multiple chronic physical complaints occur, which involve several organ systems. While GAD patients often present with mainly somatic complaints, they are usually much more limited in scope than in somatization disorder.[14]

Management

BEHAVIORAL THERAPY

Mild anxiety should be treated initially with counseling. Patients should be advised to discontinue all stimulants including caffeine and nicotine as well as to participate in a regular exercise program most days of the week.[15] Biofeedback, progressive relaxation, and stress management may be used in individual and group settings and may include family participation. Family members should be included as much as possible to help the patient develop problem-solving skills and to provide an alternative perspective on the patient's problems.[16] Cognitive-behavior therapy may also be helpful in identifying and redirecting anxious thoughts.[17]

PHARMACOLOGIC THERAPY

In patients with significant impairment of daily function, use of benzodiazepines should be considered. A favorable response is likely if significant depression is lacking, the patient is aware of the psychological basis for their anxiety, and there has been a prior favorable response to benzodiazepines. Results are usually seen within 1 week with development of tolerance to the sedation, impaired concentration, and amnesic effects of these medications within several weeks.[18] Benzodiazepines act primarily by decreasing vigilance and eliminating somatic symptoms such as muscle tension rather than by decreasing anxiety. These agents should be used cautiously in elderly patients, beginning with the lowest therapeutic dose available of lorazepam (Ativan), oxazepam (Serax) or temazepam (Restoril), because of their favorable method of metabolism by conjugation.[19] Several alternatives are available as listed in Table 22.3. All benzodiazepine therapy can lead to physical dependence. Withdrawal symptoms include irritability, anxiety, and insomnia, and tend to be more severe at higher doses or in patients with a prior history of substance abuse. After 6 to 8 weeks of therapy, medication may be gradually discontinued. Reduction of the dose by 25% or less per week minimizes withdrawal symptoms. Rebound anxiety may occur at the end of the tapering process, but typically persists for less than 72 hours.

Buspirone (BuSpar) may also be considered as first-line therapy for chronic anxiety. Unlike benzodiazepines, symptomatic relief of anxiety with buspirone may require 2 to 3 weeks of treatment. The initial dosage of buspirone is 5 mg tid with titration to symptom relief or to a maximum dose of 20 mg tid. Dosage should be increased by 5 mg per day every 2 to 3 days to avoid symptoms of headache or dizziness.[20] In patients taking benzodiazepines during the initial period, tapering of the benzodiazepine should not begin until the patient reaches a daily dose of 20 to 40 mg of buspirone. Side effects associated with buspirone include dizziness, nausea, headache, nervousness, and light-headedness.

Venlafaxine extended release (Effexor XR) is a serotonin-norepinephrine reuptake inhibitor (SNRI) that has been studied specifically in the treatment of GAD. In randomized, double-blind, placebo-controlled trials, venlafaxine was shown to significantly reduce symptoms of anxious mood, tension, irritability, restlessness, and startle response in patients with anxiety. Currently, venlafaxine extended-release is the only FDA approved treatment for GAD. The recommended starting dosage is 75 mg/day with an increase of 75 mg/day at 4-day intervals to a maximum of 225 mg/day. Reduced dosages should be used in patients with renal impairment.[21] The most common side effects include asthenia, sweating, nausea, constipation, anorexia, dry mouth, and blurred vision. Modest yet sustained elevations in blood pressure have also been reported.

Point of Referral

Indications for referral include difficulty establishing a psychiatric diagnosis in patients with comorbid psychiatric illnesses, and the patient's failure to respond to standard treatment. Referral to a mental health professional should occur for CBT either as primary therapy or in addition to pharmacologic therapy prescribed by the family physician.

Social Anxiety Disorder

Social anxiety disorder, or social phobia, is described as an intense, irrational, and persistent fear of being scrutinized or negatively evaluated by others (Table 22.5).[1] Most commonly, patients report fear of public speaking or performance, but the disorder can encompass any social interaction and may be generalized as well as specific. Exposure to the feared situation almost always induces anxiety, and anticipation of the event or situation interferes significantly with the patient's normal routine or relationships. The patient is usually aware that the fear is irrational and excessive, but this awareness does not reduce the physical and psychological symptoms associated with the disorder. These symptoms may include diaphoresis, blushing, tachycardia, trembling, and halting or rapid speech. Fears of fainting and loss of bowel or bladder function are also common.

TABLE 22.5. Diagnostic Criteria for Social Phobia

A. A marked and persistent fear of one or more social or performance situations in which the person is exposed to unfamiliar people or to possible scrutiny by others. The individual fears that he or she will act in a way (or show anxiety symptoms) that will be humiliating or embarrassing. Note: In children, there must be evidence of the capacity for age-appropriate social relationships with familiar people and the anxiety must occur in peer settings, not just in interactions with adults.
B. Exposure to the feared social situation almost invariably provokes anxiety, which may take the form of a situationally bound or situationally predisposed panic attack. Note: In children, the anxiety may be expressed by crying, tantrums, freezing, or shrinking away from social situations with unfamiliar people.
C. The person recognizes that the fear is excessive or unreasonable. Note: In children, this feature may be absent.
D. The feared social or performance situations are avoided or else are endured with intense anxiety or distress.
E. The avoidance, anxious anticipation, or distress in the feared social or performance situation(s) interferes significantly with the person's normal routine, occupation (academic) functioning or social activities or relationships, or there is marked distress about having the phobia.
F. In individuals under 18 years of age, the duration is at least 6 months.
G. The fear or avoidance is not due to the direct physiologic effects of a substance (e.g., a drug of abuse, a medication) or a general medical condition and is not better accounted for by another mental disorder (e.g., panic disorder with or without agoraphobia, separation anxiety disorder, body dysmorphic disorder, a pervasive developmental disorder or schizoid personality disorder).
H. If a general medical condition or another mental disorder is present, the fear in criterion A is unrelated to it (e.g., the fear is not of stuttering, trembling in Parkinson's disease, or exhibiting abnormal eating behavior in anorexia nervosa or bulimia nervosa.)

Specify if:
  Generalized: If the fears include most social situations (also consider the additional diagnosis of avoidant personality disorder).

Source: American Psychiatric Association,[1] with permission.

Left untreated, social anxiety disorder is chronic and may result in severe disability. Avoidance of social situations may reduce symptoms but has no impact on the underlying psychological distress. Significant academic and occupational limitations can occur as a result of the disorder. Patients are frequently unable to complete their education and may remain in less rewarding careers as a result of their persistent fears and anxiety.[22]

The lifetime prevalence of social anxiety disorder has been estimated at about 13%. Social phobia is slightly more common in women and usually begins in childhood or adolescence. Rarely does onset occur after age 25; however, symptoms may become more apparent as new social and occupational situations arise throughout adulthood.[23] About half of the patients report an association of the onset of their phobia with a specific experience, with the remainder reporting social anxiety for most of their lives.[24–26] Because patients are typically unwilling to acknowledge their fears in an interview format, brief screening questions can be used to improve the detection of social anxiety disorder. In a recent study of 9375 patients, the following yes-or-no statements were found to be 89% sensitive in detecting social phobia: (1) "Being embarrassed or looking stupid is among my worst fears"; (2) "Fear of embarrassment causes me to avoid doing things or speaking to people"; (3) "I avoid activities in which I am the center of attention."[27]

Complications and Comorbidity

Depression, addiction, and suicide are frequently associated with social anxiety disorder. The lifetime risk of depression is increased by four times, and nearly one fifth of patients presenting with social phobia also abuse alcohol.[25] Longitudinal data suggest that social anxiety disorder preexists in 70% of cases of substance abuse, emphasizing the importance of early detection and treatment of this disorder.[26]

Management

BEHAVIORAL THERAPY

The most effective therapy in treating social phobia is focused on reducing anxiety by reducing avoidance behavior. Components of CBT include anxiety management techniques, improvement in social coping skills, cognitive restructuring, and finally gradual exposure. Treatment may require up to 24 sessions and can be conducted individually or in groups. Up to 75% of patients have demonstrated benefit from CBT, even after discontinuing sessions. Relapse rates are significantly higher following discontinuation of effective pharmacotherapy, supporting the consideration of CBT as initial treatment in appropriate patients.[28]

Pharmacologic Therapy

Selective serotonin reuptake inhibitors (SSRIs) are considered an appropriate first-line therapy for generalized social anxiety disorder. Controlled trials of paroxetine (Paxil), fluvoxamine (Luvox), and sertraline (Zoloft) have demonstrated acute treatment improvement rates in 50% to 75% of patients.[29] A recent open trial of citalopram (Celexa) has shown effectiveness as well.[30] As a class, these agents provide the benefit of an antidepressant, are non–habit-forming, and have a relatively low side-effect profile. Because of their delayed onset of action, the SSRIs are not appropriate for acute anxiety episodes. Common adverse reactions include nausea, dry mouth, headache, and sexual dysfunction. SSRIs should not be used within 2 weeks of MAOIs because of the potential for serious or fatal interactions.

Benzodiazepines have long been effectively used in the treatment of acute social phobia because of their rapid onset and tolerability. Improvement rates of 40% to 80% have been demonstrated in controlled studies of alprazolam (Xanax) and clonazepam (Klonopin).[31] Benzodiazepines should be used cautiously in patients with a history of substance abuse because of their ability to produce physical dependence. With the introduction of effective long-term treatments, benzodiazepines are frequently used in low doses for initial symptom relief in combination with SSRIs and CBT.

Controlled clinical trials demonstrate that approximately two third of patients with generalized social anxiety disorder will achieve improvement with MAOIs. The typical recommendation for treatment is phenelzine (Nardil), 45 to 90 mg per day.[32] Careful consideration should be given to dietary restrictions and risks associated with the use of MAOIs. Strict adherence to a low tyramine diet is required to prevent potentially fatal hypertensive reactions. Many over-the-counter medications are contraindicated in patients using MAOIs, including several antihistamines and decongestants. Common adverse effects include weight gain, sedation, postural hypotension, and sexual dysfunction.

While controlled trials using beta-blockers for generalized social phobia have shown little effectiveness, these agents are clinically effective in low doses episodically for performance anxiety.[33] Typically, propranolol (Inderal) 10 to 40 mg is used. These agents are contraindicated in patients with asthma, sinus bradycardia, second- or third-degree heart block, congestive heart failure, and cardiogenic shock.

Obsessive-Compulsive Disorder

Obsessions are recurrent, intrusive thoughts, impulses, or images that are perceived as inappropriate, grotesque, or forbidden (Table 22.6).[1] Obsessions are uncontrollable, and patients often feel they will unwillingly act upon these impulses. Common themes include contamination, self-doubt, need for order or symmetry, or loss of control of violent or sexual impulses.

Compulsions are repetitive behaviors or thoughts that reduce the anxiety accompanying the obsessions. They may include physical behaviors such as checking locks or hand washing or mental acts such as counting or praying. Patients are frequently aware that their behavior is excessive and irrational.

TABLE 22.6. Diagnostic Criteria for Obsessive-Compulsive Disorder

A. Obsessions or compulsions
    Obsessions as defined by 1, 2, 3, and 4:
    1. Recurrent and persistent thoughts, impulses, or images that are experienced, at some time during the disturbance, as intrusive and inappropriate and that cause marked anxiety or distress.
    2. The thoughts, impulses, or images are not simply excessive worries about real-life problems.
    3. The person attempts to ignore or suppress such thoughts, impulses, or images or to neutralize them with some other thought or action.
    4. The person recognizes that the obsessional thoughts, impulses, or images are a product of his or her own mind (not imposed from without, as in thought insertion).
    Compulsions as defined by 1 and 2:
    1. Repetitive behaviors (e.g., hand-washing, ordering, checking) or mental acts (e.g., praying, counting, repeating words silently) that the person feels driven to perform in response to an obsession, or according to rules that must be applied rigidly.
    2. The behaviors or mental acts are aimed at preventing or reducing distress or preventing some dreaded event or situation; however, these behaviors or mental acts either are not connected in a realistic way with what they are designed to neutralize or prevent or are clearly excessive.
B. At some point during the course of the disorder, the person has recognized that the obsessions or compulsions are excessive or unreasonable. Note: This does not apply to children.
C. The obsessions or compulsions cause marked distress, are time-consuming (take more than 1 hour a day), or significantly interfere with the person's normal routine, occupational (or academic) functioning, or usual social activities or relationships.
D. If another axis I disorder is present, the content of the obsessions or compulsions is not restricted to it (e.g., preoccupation with food in the presence of an eating disorder; hair pulling in the presence of trichotillomania; concern with appearance in the presence of body dysmorphic disorder; preoccupation with having a serious illness in the presence of hypochondriasis; preoccupation with sexual urges or fantasies in the presence of paraphilia; or guilty ruminations in the presence of major depressive disorder).
E. The disturbance is not due to the direct physiologic effects of a substance (e.g., a drug of abuse, a medication) or a general medical condition.

Specify if:
With poor insight: If, for most of the time during the current episode, the person does not recognize that the obsessions and compulsions are excessive or unreasonable.

Source: American Psychiatric Association,[1] with permission.

Obsessive-compulsive disorder (OCD) occurs equally in men and women, although the onset is frequently earlier in men. While once considered rare, OCD is now recognized as relatively common with a lifetime prevalence of 2.5%.[34] Age of onset is usually during late adolescence or early adulthood, although some childhood presentations have been reported. Presentation in late adulthood is rare and should prompt an investigation for an organic cause. The onset may be insidious or acute; however, the disorder is usually chronic. Even in patients receiving appropriate treatment, elimination of symptoms is uncommon. Prognosis is most favorable when the onset is mild, the disorder begins in adulthood, obsessions are more prominent than compulsions, and treatment is sought promptly.

Because of the nature of the disorder, patients may present as a result of a secondary physical symptoms such as extremely dry skin from repeated hand washings. A supportive, nonthreatening approach is recommended because the patient's embarrassment and fears concerning the compulsive behavior cause reluctance to disclose the source of symptoms. Useful screening questions include: "Do you ever find that certain thoughts and images keep coming into your head even though you try to keep them out? Do these thoughts make sense or do they seem absurd or silly? Do you sometimes feel that you must do certain things over and over even though you don't want to? Does this seem reasonable or does this seem excessive?" Affirmative answers to these questions may prompt further evaluation for OCD.

Differential Diagnosis

Depressive disorders, GAD, and hypochondriasis should be considered when symptoms resembling OCD occur. Of significance in diagnosing OCD is the patient's perception of the obsessive thinking. In patients with depression or GAD, excessive worries may resemble obsessive thinking, but the patient considers these ruminations to be realistic and appropriate. In OCD, the patient usually recognizes the obsessions as absurd. Hypochondriasis is more similar to OCD because of the unrealistic nature of the obsessions with disease; however, the patient rarely experiences compulsions. Physical disorders that may present with symptoms similar to OCD include encephalitis, diabetes insipidus, head trauma, Huntington's chorea, and some brain tumors.

Management

BEHAVIORAL THERAPY

The basis of behavioral therapy for OCD involves increasing exposure to the feared object or obsession while preventing patients from performing their usual rituals. Therapy is usually continued for 8 to 10 weeks and may involve family members, especially if the family is supporting the patient's disorder by assisting in the compulsive behavior. Although the exposure technique can be difficult for both the patient and the family, 80% to 90% of patients with OCD are improved after behavior therapy.[35]

PHARMACOLOGIC THERAPY

Patients with a purely obsessional disorder, comorbid depression, or an inability to comply with behavioral therapy often have improvement with pharmacologic therapy. SSRIs have demonstrated effectiveness in treating OCD with significantly fewer side effects than TCAs. Their ease of use and relative safety have improved the opportunity for treatment of OCD by family physicians. In general, higher doses of SSRIs must be used to treat OCD than in the treatment of depression. Fluoxetine (Prozac) at 40 to 80 mg/day, paroxetine (Paxil) at 20 to 60 mg/day, sertraline (Zoloft) at 50 to 200 mg/day, and fluvoxamine (Luvox) up to 300 mg/day, have all been demonstrated to be effective to some extent in OCD patients.[36] Because fluvoxamine is dosed twice daily, this agent presents an increased risk of serotonin withdrawal due to incorrect dosing over that of the remaining agents in this class. Side effects associated with SSRIs include nausea, diarrhea, insomnia, and sexual dysfunction.

Clomipramine (Anafranil), a TCA, has been shown to be effective in OCD in doses from 150 to 250 mg/day. While therapy must often continue for at least a year, the dose may be reduced once improvement in the obsessive symptoms is established. TCA side effects are dose dependent and include seizures, weight gain, sedation, anticholinergic effects, impotence, and cardiac conduction delays. Regardless of the choice of therapy, termination of pharmacotherapy will usually result in the return of symptoms.

Posttraumatic Stress Disorder

Posttraumatic stress disorder (PTSD) is characterized by a cluster of symptoms that occur following experience of a profound trauma such as rape, combat, natural disaster, or sudden violent death of a friend or family member (Table 22.7).[1] Four categories of criteria are required to accurately diagnose PTSD. A traumatic event occurred in which the patient witnessed or experienced actual or threatened death or serious injury and responded with intense fear, helplessness or horror. Upon exposure to memory cues, the event is reexperienced through intrusive flashbacks, recollections, or nightmares. The patient avoids trauma-related stimuli and feels emotionally numb or disassociated. The patient has increased arousal indicated by irritability, difficulty sleeping, hypervigilance, difficulty concentrating, or increased startle response. In addition, these symptoms must persist for more than 1 month and significantly interfere with the patient's occupation and/or social life.[1]

PTSD is the fifth most prevalent psychiatric disorder, with a lifetime prevalence of 8% to 12%. Although often associated with war, it is estimated that more than 50% of people will experience a traumatic event severe enough to cause PTSD at some time in their lives. Of those exposed to such an event, 20% will develop PTSD.[37] Symptoms usually begin within 3 months of the traumatic event. Having had a psychiatric disorder prior to the trauma or a family history of psychiatric disorders increases the risk of developing PTSD. Developing PTSD also increases the risk of subsequent psychiatric problems. Up to 80% of patients with PTSD have a comorbid psychiatric disorder. The most common comorbidities include depression, dysthymia, GAD, substance abuse, panic disorder, bipolar disorder, phobias, and dissociative disorders.[38] In a recent study, the risk for a major depressive episode increased by 5.7-fold in men and 3.4-fold in women compared to individuals without this disorder. Risk for mania increased by 15.5-fold in men and 4.1-fold in women. Additionally, patients with PTSD were six

TABLE 22.7. Diagnostic Criteria for Posttraumatic Stress Disorder

A. The person has been exposed to a traumatic event in which both of the following were present:
  1. The person experienced, witnessed, or was confronted with an event or events that involved actual or threatened death or serious injury, or a threat to the physical integrity of self or others.
  2. The person's response involved intense fear, helplessness, or horror. Note: In children, this may be expressed instead by disorganized or agitated behavior.

B. The traumatic event is persistently reexperienced in one (or more) of the following ways:
  1. Recurrent and intrusive distressing recollections of the event, including images, thoughts, or perceptions. Note: In young children repetitive play may occur in which themes or aspects of the trauma are expressed.
  2. Recurrent distressing dreams of the event. Note: In children there may be frightening dreams without recognizable content.
  3. Acting or feeling as if the traumatic event were recurring (includes a sense of reliving the event that occurs on awaking or when intoxicated). Note: In young children trauma-specific reenactment may occur.
  4. Intense psychological distress at exposure to internal or external cues that symbolize or resemble an aspect of the traumatic event.
  5. Physiologic reactivity on exposure to internal or external cues that symbolize or resemble an aspect of the traumatic event.

C. Persistent avoidance of stimuli associated with the trauma and numbing of general responsiveness (not present before the trauma), as indicated by three (or more) of the following:
  1. Efforts to avoid thought, feelings, or conversations associated with the trauma
  2. Efforts to avoid activities, place, or people that arouse recollections of the trauma
  3. Inability to recall an important aspect of the trauma
  4. Markedly diminished interest or participation in significant activities.
  5. Feeling of detachment or estrangement from others
  6. Restricted range of affect (e.g., unable to have loving feelings)
  7. Sense of foreshortened future (e.g., does not expect to have a career, marriage, children, or a normal life span)

D. Persistent symptoms of increased arousal (not present before the trauma), as indicated by two (or more) of the following:
  1. Difficulty falling or staying asleep
  2. Irritability or outbursts of anger
  3. Difficulty concentrating
  4. Hypervigilance
  5. Exaggerated startle response

E. Duration of the disturbance (symptoms in criteria B, C, and D) is more than 1 month.

F. The disturbance causes clinically significant distress or impairment in social, occupational, or other important area of functioning.

Specify if:
  Acute: if duration of symptoms is less than 3 months
  Chronic: if duration of symptoms is 3 months or more

Specify if: *With delayed onset* if onset of symptoms is at least 6 months after the stressor

Source: American Psychiatric Association,[1] with permission.

times more likely to attempt suicide. Notably, these risks return to normal levels when patients achieve remission of their PTSD symptoms.[39]

Diagnosis

The diagnosis of PTSD during an office visit can be challenging. Patients frequently do not offer information about traumatic events or typical PTSD symptoms. In addition, depression and substance abuse may obscure the underlying disorder. It is essential to approach the patient with an empathetic and nonjudgmental attitude to elicit a history of trauma. In the case of adult trauma, questions may be asked directly, such as, "Have you ever been physically attacked or threatened? Have you ever been in a severe accident or disaster?" Childhood trauma often requires an approach that established normality. "Many persons are troubled by frightening events from their childhood. Have you ever had thoughts like this?"[40]

Management

The treatment of PTSD is complicated because of the wide range of symptoms and likelihood of predisposing factors and comorbid conditions. In general, the goals of treatment are to reduce symptoms, improve coping mechanisms, reduce disability, and lower comorbidity. These goals can be achieved through patient education, pharmacotherapy and psychotherapy.

Behavioral Therapy

Individual or group therapy plays an important role in the treatment plan of PTSD. CBT or exposure therapy, which uses repeated, detailed imagining of the trauma in a controlled environment, can help patients learn to cope with their anxiety through desensitization. Other effective skills gained through behavioral therapy include cognitive restructuring, anger management, and relapse prevention. Group therapy often enables patients to benefit from empathy provided by other survivors while directly confronting their grief and anxiety. PTSD can have devastating effects on family members as well, so family therapy is often warranted.[41]

Pharmacologic Therapy

While behavioral therapy is indicated for all patients with PTSD, appropriate pharmacologic therapy can reduce symptoms associated with reexperiencing, avoidance, and hypervigilance. In addition, effective treatment of coexisting conditions improves the success of behavioral therapy. SSRIs have demonstrated the broadest range of efficacy and lowest side effect profile in the treatment of PTSD. Sertraline (Zoloft) is the only SSRI approved by the FDA specifically for the treatment of PTSD.[42] Fluvoxamine (Luvox) has effectiveness in reducing obsessional thoughts and eliminating insomnia.[43] TCAs and MAOIs have historically been used in the treatment of PTSD, but have essentially been replaced by the use of SSRIs. Because of the frequent use of alcohol and other contraindicated substances by patients with PTSD, MAOI and benzodiazepine use is discouraged. Trazodone (Desyrel) at doses of 50 to 200 mg has a unique role in promoting sleep through sedative properties and suppression of rapid eye movement sleep, thereby reducing the nightmares associated with PTSD.[44] Antiadrenergic agents are often effective in reducing nightmares, hypervigilance, startle reactions, and outbursts of rage. Clonidine (Catapres), 0.2 mg tid, titrated from 0.1 mg at bedtime is typically used. Propranolol (Inderal) in doses of 60 to 640 mg/day and guanfacine (Tenex) 1 to 2 mg/day at bedtime may also be considered. Blood pressure should be checked periodically with long-term use of these agents because of the potential for hypotension.[45]

Referral

Family physicians are trained to initiate counseling and begin first-line pharmacotherapy. If symptoms persist despite use of a combination of an SSRI, trazodone, and clonidine, psychiatric consultation should be obtained before sedative or hypnotic agents are used. In most cases, PTSD patients require referral to a mental health professional for psychotherapy.

References

1. American Psychiatric Association. Diagnostic and statistical manual of mental disorders, 4th ed. Washington, DC: American Psychiatric Association, 1994;411–7.
2. Eaton WW, Kessler RC, Wittchen HU, Magee WJ. Panic and panic disorder in the United States. Am J Psychiatry 1994;151:413–20.
3. Marshall JR. Alcohol and substance abuse in panic disorder. J Clin Psychiatry 1997;58(suppl 2):46–9.
4. Gorman J. Recent developments in understanding panic disorder leading to improved treatment strategies. Primary Psychiatry 1996;3:31–8.
5. Roy-Byrne PP, Stein MB, Russo J. Panic disorder in the primary care setting: comorbidity, disability, service utilization, and treatment. J Clin Psychiatry 1999;60: 492–9.
6. Liebowitz MR. Panic disorder as a chronic illness. J Clin Psychiatry 1997;58(suppl 13):5–8.
7. Nutt DJ. Antidepressants in panic disorder: clinical and preclinical mechanisms. J Clin Psychiatry 1998;59(suppl 8):24–8.
8. Vanin JR, Vanin SK. Blocking the cycle of panic disorder: ways to gain control of the fear of fear. Postgrad Med 1999;105:141–6.
9. Saeed SA, Bruce TJ. Panic disorder: effective treatment options. Am Fam Physician 1998;57:2405–12.
10. Mavissakalian MR, Perel JM. Imipramine treatment of panic disorder with agoraphobia. J Psychiatry 1995;152:673–82.
11. Schweizer E, Rickels K. Strategies for treatment of generalized anxiety in the primary care setting. J Clin Psychiatry 1997;58(suppl 3):76–80.

12. Rickels K, Schweizer E. The clinical course and long-term management of generalized anxiety disorder. J Clin Psychopharmacol 1990;10:101–8.
13. Wise MG, Griffies WS. A combined treatment approach to anxiety in the medically ill. J Clin Psychiatry 1995;56(suppl 2):14–19.
14. Noyes R, Woodman C, Garvey MJ, et al. Generalized anxiety disorder vs. panic disorder. Distinguishing characteristics and patterns of comorbidity. J Nerv Ment Dis 1992;180:369–79.
15. Taylor CB, Sallis JF, Needle R. Relation of physical activity and exercise to mental health. Public Health Rep 1985;100:195–202.
16. Mathews A. Why worry? The cognitive function of anxiety. Behav Res Ther 1990;28:455–68.
17. Butler G, Fennell M, Robson P, Gelder M. Comparison of behavior therapy and cognitive behavior therapy in the treatment of generalized anxiety disorder. J Consult Clin Psychol 1991;59:167–75.
18. Schweizer E. Generalized anxiety disorder. Longitudinal course and pharmacologic treatment. Psychiatr Clin North Am 1995;18:843–57.
19. Shorr RI, Robin DW. Rational use of benzodiazepines in the elderly. Drugs Aging 1994;4:9–20.
20. Davidson JR, DuPont RL, Hedges D, Haskins JT. Efficacy, safety and tolerability of venlafaxine extended release and buspirone in outpatients with generalized anxiety disorder. J Clin Psychiatry 1999;60(8):528–35.
21. Silverstone PH, Ravindran A. Once-daily venlafaxine extended release (XR) compared with fluoxetine in outpatients with depression and anxiety: Venlafaxine XR 360 Study Group. J Clin Psychiatry 1999;60(1):22–8.
22. Schneier FR, Johnson J, Hornig CD, Liebowitz MR, Weissman MM. Social phobia: comorbidity and morbidity in an epidemiological sample. Arch Gen Psychiatry 1992;49:282–8.
23. Kessler RC, McGonagle DK, Zhao S, et al. Lifetime and 12-month prevalence of DSM-III-R psychiatric disorders in the United States. Results from the National Comorbidity Survey. Arch Gen Psychiatry 1994;51:8–19.
24. Ost LG, Hugdahl K. Acquisition of phobias and anxiety response patterns in clinical patients. Behav Res Ther 1981;19:439–47.
25. Schneier FR, Martin LY, Liebowitz MR, Gorman JM, Fyer AJ. Alcohol abuse in social phobia. J Anx Disord 1989;3:15–23.
26. Kushner MG, Sher KJ, Beitman BD. The relation between alcohol problems and the anxiety disorders. Am J Psychiatry 1990; 147:685–95.
27. Bruce TJ, Saeed SA. Social anxiety disorder: a common, underrecognized mental disorder. Am Fam Physician 1999;60:2311–22.
28. Juster HR, Heimberg RG. Social phobia: longitudinal course and long-term outcome of cognitive-behavioral treatment. Psychiatr Clin North Am 1995;18:821–42.
29. Stein MB, Liebowitz MR, Lydiard RB, Pitts CD, Bushnell W, Gergel I. Paroxetine treatment of generalized social phobia (social anxiety disorder): a randomized controlled trial. JAMA 1998;280:708–13.
30. Bouwer C, Stein DJ. Use of the selective serotonin reuptake inhibitor citalopram in the treatment of generalized social phobia. J Affect Disord 1998;49:79–82.
31. Davidson JR, Potts N, Richichi E, Krishnan R, Ford SM, Smith R. Treatment of social phobia with clonazepam and placebo. J Clin Psychopharmacol 1993;13:423–8.
32. Versiani M, Nardi AE, Mundim FD, Alves AB, Liebowitz MR, Amrein R. Pharma-

cotherapy of social phobia. A controlled study with moclobemide and phenelzine. Br J Psychiatry 1992;161:353–60.

33. Turner SM, Beidel DC, Jacob RD. Social phobia: a comparison of behavior therapy and atenolol. J Consult Clin Psychol 1994;62:350–8.

34. Karno M, Golding JM, Sorenson SB, Burnam MA. The epidemiology of obsessive-compulsive disorder in five US communities. Arch Gen Psychiartry 1988;45:1094–9.

35. Abramowitz JS. Effectiveness of psychological and pharmacological treatments for obsessive-compulsive disorder: a quantitative review. J Consult Clin Psychol 1997;65:44–52.

36. Greist JH, Jefferson JW, Kobak KA, Katzelnick DJ, Serlin RC. Efficacy and tolerability of serotonin transport inhibitors in obsessive-compulsive disorder. A meta-analysis. Arch Gen Psychiatry 1995;52:53–60.

37. Kessler RC, Sonnega A, Bromet E. Posttraumatic stress disorder in the National Comorbidity Study. Arch Gen Psychiatry 195;52:1048–60.

38. Brady KT. Posttraumatic stress disorder and comorbidity: recognizing the many faces of PTSD. J Clin Psychiatry 1997;58(suppl 9):12–5.

39. Kessler RC. Posttraumatic stress disorder: the burden to the individual and to society. J Clin Psychiatry 2000;61(suppl 5):4–12.

40. Blank AS Jr. Clinical detection, diagnosis, and differential diagnosis of post-traumatic stress disorder. Psychiatr Clin North Am 1994;17:351–83.

41. Foa EB, Heast-Ikeda D, Perry KJ. Evaluation of a brief cognitive behavioral program for the prevention of chronic PTSD in recent assault victims. J Consult Clin Psychol 1995;63:948–55.

42. Brady KT, Sonne SC, Roberts JM. Sertraline treatment of comorbid posttraumatic stress disorder and alcohol dependence. J Clin Psychiatry 1995;56:502–5.

43. Marmar CR, Schoenfeld F, Weiss DS, et al. Open trial of fluvoxamine treatment for combat-related posttraumatic stress disorder. J Clin Psychiatry 1996;57(suppl 8):66–72.

44. Friedman MJ. Current and future drug treatment for posttraumatic stress disorder patients. Psychiatr Ann 1998;28:461–8.

45. Silver JM, Sandberg DP, Hales RE. New approaches in the pharmacotherapy of PTSD. J Clin Psychiatry 1990;51(suppl 10):33–8.

CASE PRESENTATION

Subjective

PATIENT PROFILE

Nancy Nelson is a 40-year-old female accountant.

PRESENTING PROBLEM

"Feeling nervous."

PRESENT ILLNESS

Mrs. Nelson reports a long history of recurrent anxiety, becoming worse over the last 3 years. Her hands are often moist and tremulous, and she has trouble falling asleep at night. Her symptoms are worse with new people and when with clients at work. She is fearful of making mistakes on the job, especially on clients' tax returns. She has trouble relaxing even on weekends and vacations. She feels some relief when she takes a drink of alcohol.

PAST MEDICAL HISTORY

She has had three urinary tract infections over the past year; the last was treated 4 months ago.

SOCIAL HISTORY, HABITS, AND FAMILY HISTORY

Are unchanged since her last visit 4 months ago (see Chapter 15).

REVIEW OF SYSTEMS

She reports occasional urinary frequency and one- to two-time nocturia.

- What additional medical history would you like to know? Why?
- What is a likely reason for today's visit?
- What more would you like to know about her symptoms at work?
- What might Mrs. Nelson be trying to tell you today?

Objective

GENERAL

The patient appears tense and fidgets with her hair and fingers during the interview.

VITAL SIGNS

Blood pressure, 118/60; pulse, 74 and regular; respirations, 18.

EXAMINATION

The eyes, ears, nose, and throat are normal; the neck and thyroid are unremarkable; the hands are cool with slightly moist palms. No tremor is present.

- What additional information—if any—might you include in the physical examination, and why?
- Are there other areas of the body that should be examined today? Why?
- What physical diseases might cause Mrs. Nelson's symptoms? How might you eliminate these as diagnostic possibilities?
- What laboratory tests or diagnostic imaging—if any—would you obtain today? Why?

Assessment

- What is your diagnostic assessment? How would you explain this to Mrs. Nelson?
- Might today's complaint be a "ticket of admission" to discuss other problems? Explain.
- Might her symptoms be related to life events that have not yet been discussed, and how would you elicit this information?
- What might be the impact of this illness on the family? On coworkers?

Plan

- Describe your therapeutic recommendation. How would you explain this to Mrs. Nelson?
- What—if any—life-style changes would you advise?
- Would you recommend consultation or referral? Explain.
- What continuing care would you recommend?

23
Depression

RUPERT R. GOETZ, SCOTT A. FIELDS,
AND WILLIAM L. TOFFLER

Depression in primary care settings has been a particular focus of recent attention.[1,2] To effectively treat patients with the many common presentations of depression, family physicians need a systematic understanding of the types of depressive disorders. We first explore diagnostic and therapeutic concepts, highlighting the structure behind the current understanding of these disorders. Then we discuss the application of these concepts to the process of evaluation and treatment of patients, including special populations.

Epidemiology

Almost half of all office visits resulting in a mental disorder diagnosis are to nonpsychiatrists, mostly physicians in primary care. Patients seen in this setting may be in an earlier, less organized stage of illness. Table 23.1 summarizes the prevalence of depressive disorders. Generally, women are at higher risk than men, as are patients with other medical or psychiatric conditions.

Etiology

Mechanisms of depression in three main areas have been investigated: biologic abnormalities, psychological causes, and social factors. These areas are summarized in the biopsychosocial model of Engel.[3] The ultimate causes of these disorders remain unclear. Clinically, etiologic differentiation and specific biologic tests remain limited in their usefulness. Genetic factors may play a role in increased susceptibility. First-degree relatives of a patient with depressive disorder have about a 25% to 30% likelihood of major depression or bipolar disorder. Twin studies have shown concordance for major depression of 50% for monozygotic twins and 25% for dizygotic twins.[4] The variation in risk makes unlikely a single depressive disorder gene with predictable penetrance for specific disorders.

Psychological factors have long been considered important in depression. Cog-

TABLE 23.1. Epidemiology of Depressive Disorders in the General Population

Disorder	Current prevalence (%)	Lifetime prevalence (%)
Major depression	3–6	10–20
Dysthymia	1	2–3
Bipolar disorder	<0.5	0.5–1.0

nitive-behavioral theory holds that cognitive distortions, activated by a stressor, lead some individuals to unrealistically negative and demeaning views of themselves, the world, and the future. Some theories of depression place a high value on the patient's function within society. That is, patients cannot be understood outside their social context.

Diagnosis

The *Diagnostic and Statistical Manual of Mental Disorders*, 4th edition, revised (DSM-IV) divides mood disorders into 10 categories: major depression; bipolar I; bipolar II; dysthymic; cyclothymic; those due to general medical conditions; those due to substance abuse; and depressive, bipolar, and mood disorders not otherwise specified.[5]

Diagnostic Criteria

A *major depressive disorder* requires the patient to have a major depressive episode (Table 23.2), and there should never have been a manic, hypomanic, or mixed episode. Symptoms should cause significant impairment and not be due

TABLE 23.2. DSM-IV Diagnostic Criteria for a Major Depressive Episode

A. Five of the following nine symptoms are present for at least 2 weeks
   1. Depressed mood
   2. Diminished interest or pleasure
   3. Significant appetite or weight change
   4. Sleep disturbance (insomnia or hypersomnia)
   5. Psychomotor agitation or retardation
   6. Fatigue or loss of energy
   7. Feelings of worthlessness or inappropriate guilt
   8. Diminished ability to think or concentrate
   9. Recurrent thoughts of death or suicide
B. Not a mixed episode
C. Causes significant distress or impairs function
D. Not attributable to medical condition or substance abuse
E. Not attributable to bereavement

Note: A mnemonic may be useful to recall these criteria: Depression is worth seriously memorizing extremely gruesome criteria, sorry (DIWSMEGCS). These initials stand for: Depressed mood, Interest, Weight, Sleep, Motor activity, Energy, Guilt, Concentration, and Suicide.[6]
Source: Adapted from American Psychiatric Association,[5] with permission.

TABLE 23.3. DSM-IV Diagnostic Criteria for Dysthymic Disorder

A. Depressed mood for at least 2 years
B. Two of the following six symptoms
    1. Poor appetite or overeating
    2. Insomnia or hypersomnia
    3. Low energy or fatigue
    4. Low self-esteem
    5. Poor concentration or difficulty making decisions
    6. Feelings of hopelessness
C. Never interrupted for more than 2 months at a time
D. No major depression during the first 2 years
E. Never had a manic episode
F. Not superimposed on a psychotic disorder
G. Not attributable to medical conditions or substance abuse
H. Causes significant distress or impairment

Source: Adapted from American Psychiatric Association,[5] with permission.

to substances or bereavement. Either depressed mood or loss of interest or pleasure is required. Once the diagnosis is made, the severity (mild, moderate, severe), result of treatment (partial or full remission), and presence or absence of psychotic features are noted.

Dysthymia is used to describe a specific disorder rather than a "mild depression." It is diagnosed when two of six criteria (Table 23.3) are met over a period of 2 years, uninterrupted by more than a 2-month period and not initiated by a major depression.

Bipolar disorders are divided into types I and II, the former characterized by at least one manic (Table 23.4) or mixed episode, the latter by at least one hypomanic episode and major depressive episodes. Mania is distinguished from hypomania by the longer duration and presence of marked impairment in social or occupational functioning or the need for admission to a hospital because of danger to self or others. A mixed episode is defined as fitting criteria for major depressive and manic episodes together for 1 week.

Analogous to dysthymia, *cyclothymia* is a disorder characterized by hypomanic

TABLE 23.4. DSM-IV Diagnostic Criteria for Manic Episode

A. Distinct period of elevated, expansive or irritable mood for 1 week
B. Three of the following seven symptoms (four if the mood is only irritable)
    1. Inflated self-esteem or grandiosity
    2. Decreased need for sleep
    3. More talkative than usual or pressure to keep talking
    4. Flight of ideas or experience of racing thoughts
    5. Distractibility
    6. Increased goal directed activity or psychomotor agitation
    7. Excessive involvement with pleasurable activities with potential painful consequences
C. Not a mixed episode
D. Disturbance causes marked impairment
E. Not based on medical conditions or substance abuse

Source: Adapted from American Psychiatric Association,[5] with permission.

and depressed episodes over 2 years, never without depressive symptoms for longer than 2 months. Mood disorders caused by general medical conditions and substance-induced mood disorders are now included within the group of depressive disorders, and atypical disorders are divided into three "not otherwise specified" categories.

In family practice and other primary care settings, depressed patients usually present with physical complaints. Depression may co-occur with medical problems such as chronic pain or human immunodeficiency syndrome (HIV), or with substance abuse. Thus, an organic basis for the disturbance must first be ruled out. The condition should also not be attributable to a primary psychotic disorder. Depressive disorders can be linked in a diagnostic algorithm (Fig. 23.1). The important role of early detection of medical disorders and a possible manic episode is emphasized by its placement near the top of the sequence. There is a spectrum of disease that should be considered. While the criteria for diagnosing major depression are well defined by DSM-IV, subthreshold depressive symptoms have a significant impact on patients' ability to function and quality of life. Depression has also been associated with other adverse outcomes such as increased medical morbidity and mortality.

Related Diagnoses

Several other disorders present with dysphoria as the chief complaint or prominent feature. They should be considered as part of a differential diagnosis (Fig. 23.2).

Cognitive Disorders

Cognitive mood disorders may include both depressed and manic presentations together with indications of an underlying medical disorder in the physical, mental status, or laboratory examination. In particular, abnormalities in cognitive testing, such as disorientation, memory deficits, and attention and concentration difficulties should raise the concern of a cognitive disorder.

Delirium and dementia may have prominent depressive symptoms. Delirium, characterized by inability to sustain attention, is more likely in elderly or medically ill patients. It is often acute in onset and shows fluctuation. Dementia begins insidiously. Affective lability, periods of apathy, and concentration and memory problems are prominent. Differentiation from the "pseudodementia of depression" may be difficult, and treatment may have to be directed at a depressive disorder to clarify the diagnosis. Alcohol and drug abuse and dependence disorders fall into the category of substance-related mental disorders. The classification of the psychiatric disorders induced by substances into each category emphasizes the importance of distinguishing them as a first priority.

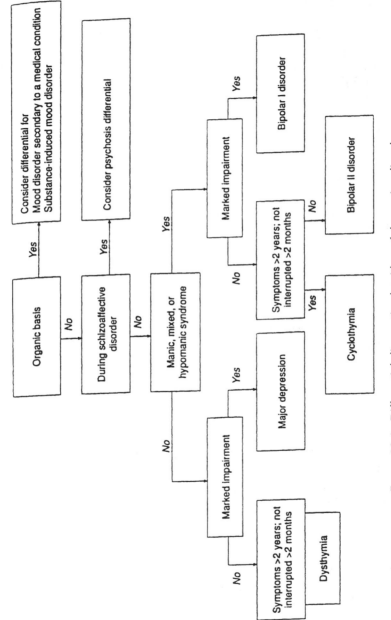

FIGURE 23.1. Differential diagnostic algorithm of depressive disorders.

474

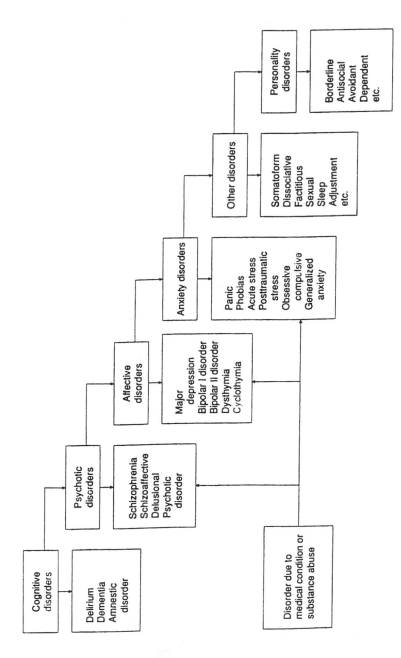

FIGURE 23.2. Implied differential diagnostic cascade of psychiatric disorders.

475

PSYCHOTIC DISORDERS

Psychotic disorders are characterized by loss of reality contact. When the depressive symptoms meeting criteria for a major depressive episode or for mania are present as well, a diagnosis of a schizoaffective disorder is made. Differentiation from the depressive disorders with psychotic features is possible when there is a 2-week history of psychosis in the absence of depressive symptoms. Occasionally, treatment for both disorders over time is required to clarify the underlying diagnosis.

ANXIETY DISORDERS

Anxiety disorders, in particular panic and posttraumatic stress disorder, may have severe dysphoria as the presenting complaint. The prominence of anxiety and vegetative signs characteristic of depression may help define the diagnosis (see Chapter 22).

SOMATOFORM DISORDERS

With somatoform disorders, such as chronic pain (somatoform pain disorder) and hypochondriasis, a patient who meets criteria for the depressive disorder should be assigned this diagnosis in addition to the somatoform diagnosis.

PERSONALITY DISORDERS

Personality disorders are characterized by long-standing, pervasive, maladaptive personality traits; they therefore also often include significant dysphoria. The presence of a personality disorder should not obviate the diagnosis of a major depressive disorder. However, a patient who has suffered from intense constant distress since adolescence is much less likely to respond to biologic treatments than a patient with major depression alone.

BEREAVEMENT

Grief, though intense, must be seen within its cultural context. The duration may be variable, though morbid preoccupation with worthlessness, prolonged and marked functional impairment, and marked psychomotor retardation may raise the concern that the patient is suffering from a major depression (see Chapter 26).

Evaluation

A clear series of diagnostic and therapeutic steps allows differentiation of disorders and logical treatment choice. Formal screening tools, such as the Beck Depression Inventory[7] or simple screening questions about loss of interest or pleasure may be helpful in identifying whom to evaluate.

1. History: A thorough evaluation should include safety, current history and review of systems, prior episodes of depression (including psychosis, suicide ideation and attempts), treatments, prior medical problems, childhood and developmental difficulties, and family and social histories. The question of suicidal risk is the initial overriding concern. Together with this consideration the degree of the patient's competence to participate in treatment planning must be assessed.[8] History of previous manic episodes must be investigated. Vegetative signs, including changes in sleep, appetite, weight, and sexual functioning, should be explored because of their relevance for medication choice.
2. Mental status examination: The general appearance of the patient must be noted. Abnormalities in the patient's cognitive function should raise the suspicion of an organic etiology. Loose associations, flight of ideas, or loss of reality contact point toward psychosis. Abnormal emotional states are the hallmark of depressive disorders. Irritability and euphoria may speak for mania. Rating scales such as the Mini-Mental Status Examination or the Beck Depression Inventory may be helpful for objectifying this examination.
3. Laboratory evaluation: Laboratory workup of depression should include basic chemistries, complete blood count, and thyroid studies. Patients evaluated for depression are at increased risk for physical disorders.
4. Consultation: Each family physician must define when to refer a patient. Physician variables regarding consultation include experience with particular drugs, comfort with psychotherapeutic modalities, and availability of reliable consultants. Patient variables include trust in the physician, openness to referral, specific diagnostic characteristics such as psychosis, or treatment failure. Admission of a suicidal patient or treatment with electroconvulsive therapy (ECT) generally requires psychiatric consultation.

Treatment Principles

The patient's safety must be established. Voluntary or involuntary hospitalization must be offered when such safety is in doubt. No-harm contracts may be useful for assessing the risk to the patient; they cannot replace a comprehensive plan. Biologic, psychological, and social interventions must be prioritized. A return visit for more extended evaluation and treatment planning may be necessary.

In the context of depression, several rules based on diagnostic considerations or documented clinical confidence have been formulated to guide treatment[9]:

1. Treat medical disorders that underlie the depression first.
2. Address alcohol and drug abuse before attempting other interventions.
3. When a patient meets criteria for major depression, make the diagnosis and provide medical treatment.
4. When a patient does not fully meet these criteria, psychotherapy alone or a treatment trial with antidepressants may be reasonable.

5. A 6-week treatment period at full, recommended strength may be considered an adequate medication treatment trial.
6. In the presence of psychosocial issues, psychotherapy should be provided in addition to biologic treatments.
7. The effect of treatment should be monitored, and patients who fail follow-up appointments should be actively reengaged in treatment.

When a patient does not respond to the initial treatment strategy, the history is reviewed for hidden alcohol or drug abuse, unrecognized underlying medical problems, or subtle psychotic symptoms. Patient compliance and determination of antidepressant blood levels are considered. The treatment plan is reviewed and revised as appropriate. Strategies used when there has been no response include changing to another antidepressant, such as tricyclics, or augmentation with lithium or thyroid.

Treatment

Biologic Therapies

Differentiation of unipolar from bipolar depressive disorders is crucial because the basic treatment strategies differ. The mainstay of therapy for major depression is the antidepressant, although mood stabilizers and neuroleptics are used adjunctively. Conversely, the main treatment for bipolar disorders is a mood stabilizer, and adjunctive use of neuroleptics and antidepressants may be required.

When major depression is present, treatment with antidepressants should (and in some cases of dysthymia may) be offered. The compounds differ little in their antidepressant efficacy, but their side-effect profiles are diverse (Table 23.5). Choice is dictated by the desire to achieve or avoid certain side effects. Obviously, cost is also an important consideration, highlighted by managed care. Use of antidepressants in patients with bipolar disorders may increase the number of cycles per year and may provoke a manic episode.

SELECTIVE SEROTONIN REUPTAKE INHIBITORS (SSRIs)

The SSRI antidepressants (e.g., citalopram, fluoxetine, fluvoxamine, paroxetine, and sertraline) with almost exclusive serotonin activity have favorable side-effect profiles. Due to ease of use (often once-a-day dosing), they have become a frequent first choice, despite their cost. They have low sedative and anticholinergic properties. There is also a very low risk of death from overdose. They are activating and should be given during the day. This activation may trigger agitation, anxiety, and restlessness (akathisia), which can be disconcerting to the patient. Resulting or primary sleep difficulties may require addition of a medication such as diphenhydramine or a sedating antidepressant, such as trazodone.

Interactions with other medications can lead to dangerous side effects. These are most often mediated through effects on the cytochrome P-450 hepatic isoen-

TABLE 23.5. Effects and Side Effects of Common Antidepressants

Generic and trade names	Chemical type	Mean $t_{1/2}$ (hours)	Sedation	Anticho-linergic	Orthostasis	Usual dosage[a] (mg/day)	Cost[b] ($/month)	Watch for
Amitriptyline Elavil Endep	Tricyclic tertiary amine	35	+++	+++	+++	75–300	5.30 47.99 44.36	
Amoxapine Asendin	Dibenzoxapine	8	++	+++	+	100–300	180.81	EPS
Bupropion Wellbutrin	Aminoketone	15	+	+	+	75–450	67.60	Seizures, agitation
Citalopram Celexa	SSRI	35	+/–	0	0	20–60	69.99	Baseline liver function and thyroid tests
Clomipramine Anafranil	Tricyclic tertiary amine	25	+++	+++	++	75–200	98.10	
Desipramine Norpramin Pertofrane	Tricyclic secondary amine	20	+	+	+	75–200	53.36 105.62	
Doxepin Sinequan Adapin	Tricyclic tertiary amine	15	+++	++	++	75–200	16.94 57.27 48.20	
Fluoxetine Prozac	SSRI	100	0	0	0	20–60	64.75	Insomnia, anxiety
Fluvoxamine Luvox	SSRI	15	+	0	0	50–300	69.99	Avoid with cisapride, diazepam, pimozide, and MAOIs
Imipramine Tofranil Janimine	Tricyclic tertiary amine	20	++	++	+++	75–200	5.40 88.94	
Maprotiline Ludiomil	Tetracyclic	25	++	++	++	75–225[c]	64.37 81.15	Seizures, rash
Nefazodone Serzone	SSRI	5	+/–	+/–	0	200–600	49.68	Headache, nausea

TABLE 23.5. Effects and Side Effects of Common Antidepressants

Generic and trade names	Chemical type	Mean $t_{1/2}$ (hours)	Sedation	Anticho-linergic	Orthostasis	Usual dosage[a] (mg/day)	Cost[b] ($/month)	Watch for
Mirtazapine Remeron	Piperazino-azepine	30	+	+	+	15–45	69.99	Agranulocytosis
Nortriptyline Pamelor Aventyl	Tricyclic secondary amine	35	+	+	+	50–150	60.51 78.43 74.92	
Paroxetine Paxil	SSRI	20	+/–	+/–	0	20–50	54.60	Headache, nausea
Protriptyline Vivactil	Tricyclic secondary amine	80	+	+++	++	15–40	83.82	
Sertraline Zoloft	SSRI	25	+/–	0	0	50–200	58.23	
Trazodone Desyrel	Triazolo-pyridine	7	+++	+/–	++	100–400	34.37 99.02	Priapism
Trimipramine Surmontil	Tricyclic tertiary amine	20	+++	++	++	75–200	67.74	
Venlafaxine Effexor	Phenethylamine	7	0	0	0	75–300	59.96	Headache, nausea

Treat the elderly with approximately half the recommended dosage of each of these medications.
+++ = marked; ++ = moderate; + = mild; +/– = equivocal; 0 = none.
SSRI = selective serotonin reuptake inhibitor; EPS = extrapyramidal symptoms; MAOI = monoamine oxidase inhibitor.
[a]Dosage: usual daily maintenance dose.
[b]Based on wholesale price listings, 1995.
[c]Maprotiline: ceiling dose due to possible seizures.

zymes. Different antidepressants affect differing subsystems, thus current drug interaction tables should be used when prescribing them with other medications.

Tricyclic and Related Antidepressants

These classic antidepressants include, for example, amitriptyline, imipramine, nortriptyline, and desipramine (from most sedating to least). They are well studied, effective, and generally the least inexpensive. These drugs are also known as serotonin-norepinephrine reuptake inhibitors. Newer preparations include clomipramine and venlafaxine. These preparations may be especially helpful if the SSRIs are ineffective.

Once a medication is chosen, a low starting dose is generally initiated. Incremental increases are made until the expected target range is reached, a clinical response is noted, or unacceptable side effects occur. Such dosage increases are often tolerated every 3 or 4 days. Full therapeutic effects on their mood and energy can be expected after approximately 4 weeks, yet sleep may improve within a few days. The patient may experience increased energy before mood and depressive thought patterns are reversed. Thus the early treatment phase is potentially more dangerous for a patient with suicidal thoughts. Because beneficial effects and side effects vary greatly in individual patients, frequent visits, initially weekly or even more often, are required until the depression has been alleviated.

When the patient has achieved remission of the depression, the medication should be continued for a minimum of 4 to 5 months. In cases of recurring or severe depression, continued medication for a longer period, possibly years, may be best. Once the decision to stop treatment has been made, dosage should be reduced slowly over several weeks while observing for any signs of relapse for several months.

Other Antidepressants

Newer medications include bupropion, mirtazapine, nefazodone, trazodone, and venlafaxine. Bupropion may cause fewer sexual side effects, yet it must be taken in several daily doses. Mirtazapine may be useful in depression with anxiety or insomnia. Nefazodone and venlafaxine may combine the usefulness of the two prior drugs, and trazodone's sedation may make it particularly useful when sleep is impaired. Monoamine oxidase inhibitors are rarely used and have largely been supplanted by SSRIs. The risk of a hypertensive crisis can be avoided by excluding foods high in tyramine.

Mood Stabilizers

Lithium is one of the most effective mood stabilizers also used to augment antidepressants. It has antidepressant properties for the bipolar patient with depression as well as antimanic properties for the patient with elevated mood; it works best when used prophylactically. It is excreted renally, so changes in fluid balance or dietary salt intake can dramatically affect the lithium level and produce toxicity. Side effects include gastrointestinal disturbances, hypothyroidism, and nephrogenic diabetes insipidus. Carbamazepine, gabapentin, topiramate, and valproate represent alternatives to lithium in bipolar disorders.

Psychological Therapies

When asked, significant numbers of patients requiring treatment for depression prefer psychotherapy to medications. For mild cases of major depression, interpersonal and cognitive-behavioral treatments should be used first. Combination of psychotherapy with antidepressants may be particularly indicated in patients maintained on medications, patients with severe neurotic character problems, and in the context of marital conflict.[10] There may be significant differences in the usefulness of these therapies for the short-term versus the long-term treatment of depression. Particularly when both biologic and psychological treatments are suggested, clear agreements, possibly contractual, are necessary between collaborating providers specifying who is responsible for care.

Electroconvulsive Therapy

Psychiatric referral for ECT remains a useful, effective option for treatment of severe depression and mania. Studies have shown it to be as effective or superior to other antidepressant treatments. It is contraindicated in a patient with recent stroke, space-occupying intracranial lesions, or recent myocardial infarction. There are no scientifically valid studies showing longer-term memory loss or disturbances in the ability to learn new information. Maintenance antidepressant treatment should follow to prevent relapse.

Social Treatments

Implications of the depression for marital, family, job, and social functioning must be considered and addressed. The patient's support network must be explored. Expectations regarding length of complete or partial disability should be discussed early. Social work interventions can hasten full recovery, which may otherwise be delayed or even made impossible.

Special Populations

Children

Social withdrawal, poor school performance, a phobia, aggression, self-deprecation, and somatic complaints may herald depression, in which case standardized testing of children may be helpful. Biologic treatments are generally considered to be effective for major depression in children and adolescents. The dosage of medications must take into consideration the lower fat/muscle ratio, which leads to a decreased volume for distribution of the drug. The relatively larger liver in children leads to more rapid metabolism of the tricyclic agents than in adults. Prepubertal children can have more dramatic swings in blood levels; therefore, doses should be divided three times daily, a practice that can likely be discontinued in the adolescent. Psychotherapy is frequently necessary, at times with inclusion of the whole family in treatment.

Elderly Population

Distinction between somatic (vegetative) symptoms of depression and physical problems is a common problem in the elderly (see Chapter 5). Vague somatic discomforts may herald depression. Psychotic symptoms may be subtle and focus on somatic complaints. When symptoms of cognitive impairment accompany depression, three main disorders must be distinguished: delirium, pseudodementia of depression, and depression in dementia. Delirium is characterized by its course, but the latter two diagnoses may be more difficult to delineate. A family history of depressive disorder, concern about the deficits, and an inability to try hard at cognitive tasks all speak for depression.

A treatment trial with antidepressants to influence the reversible portion of the patient's dysfunction may be helpful. Side effects require particular attention. Of most concern are excess sedation, cardiac arrhythmias, orthostatic hypotension, and anticholinergic syndromes. Medications are usually begun at half the normal dosages for the average adult patient, and changes are made less frequently. Side effects should be monitored carefully and levels determined when questions arise. ECT may be useful in elderly patients with refractory depression, psychotic symptoms, medication intolerance, or medical compromise, as rapid progression to severe nutritional depletion is not uncommon.

References

1. Cole S, Raju M, Barrett J. The MacArthur Foundation depression education program for primary care physicians (section 9: participant's monograph). Gen Hosp Psychiatry 2000;22:334–46.
2. Webb MR, Dietrich AJ, Katon W, Schwenk TL. Diagnosis and management of depression. Am Fam Physician 2000; (monograph no. 2):1–19.
3. Engel G. The need for a new medical model: a challenge for biomedicine. Science 1977;196:129–36.
4. Torgersen S. Genetic factors in moderately severe and mild affective disorders. Arch Gen Psychiatry 1986;43:222–6.
5. American Psychiatric Association. Diagnostic and statistical manual of mental disorders, 4th ed., rev. Washington, DC: APA, 2000.
6. Andreasen NC, Black DW. Introductory textbook of psychiatry. Washington, DC: American Psychiatric Press, 1990;191.
7. Beck AT, Ward CH, Mendelson M, Mock J, Erbaugh J. An inventory for measuring depression. Arch Gen Psychiatry 1961;4:561–71.
8. Gutheil TG, Bursztajn H, Brodsky A. The multidimensional assessment of danger-

ousness: confidence assessment in patient care and liability prevention. Bull Am Acad Psychiatr Law 1986;14:123–9.

9. American Psychiatric Association. Practice guidelines for the treatment of patients with major depressive disorders (revised). Am J Psychiatry 2000;157(suppl):1–45.

10. Scott WC. Treatment of depression by primary care physicians: psychotherapeutic treatments for depression. In: Informational report of the Council on Scientific Affairs, American Medical Association. Chicago: AMA, 1991.

CASE PRESENTATION

Subjective

PATIENT PROFILE

Mary Nelson is a 71-year-old married female retired teacher.

PRESENTING PROBLEM

"No energy and sleeping poorly."

PRESENT ILLNESS

For the past 2 months, Mrs. Nelson has noted tiredness and disturbed sleep. She lacks energy all day, yet sleeps for only short periods at night and wakes each morning about 4 a.m. unable to fall asleep again. Her appetite is poor, and she sometimes cries inappropriately. She has had several similar episodes in the past treated with antidepressants. Her last visit, about 8 months ago, focused on management of her hypertension (see Chapter 8).

PAST MEDICAL HISTORY

She is hypertensive on hydrochlorothiazide for 10 years, with an ACE-inhibitor added 8 months ago.

SOCIAL HISTORY, HABITS, AND FAMILY HISTORY

All are unchanged since her previous visit.

REVIEW OF SYSTEMS

She occasionally notes daytime somnulence, especially during the afternoon. She believes she has lost some weight recently.

- What additional medical history might help clarify the problem?
- How might you inquire about life events that could be contributing to Mrs. Nelson's problem?
- What might have prompted the visit today? How would you elicit this information?
- What more might you like to know about the daytime sleepiness?

Objective

Vital Signs

Weight, 119 lb (decrease of 3 lb since her previous visit 8 months ago); blood pressure, 142/76; pulse, 70.

Examination

The patient has a flat affect, speaks slowly, and becomes tearful several times during the interview. The eyes, ears, nose, and throat are normal. There are no abnormalities of the neck and thyroid. The hands are warm, and there is no tremor.

- What additional data—if any—might you obtain from the physical examination? Why?
- What physical diseases—if any—might account for today's symptoms? How would you examine for these possibilities?
- What—if any—laboratory tests would you obtain today?
- What physical findings—if present—would suggest that the problem is other than a primary affective disorder? Explain.

Assessment

- What is your diagnostic assessment? How would you explain this to the patient?
- How might the family be contributing to the illness?
- How might you assess the possibility of suicidal intent? Describe how you would frame this inquiry.
- What is likely to be the meaning of this illness to the patient? To the family?

Plan

- Describe your specific recommendations. How would you present these to Mrs. Nelson?
- What community resources—if any—might be useful in caring for this patient's problem? How would you gain involvement of these other professionals?
- If Mrs. Nelson indicated that she had thoughts of suicide, what would you do?
- What continuing care would you advise?

24
Care of Acute Lacerations

BRYAN J. CAMPBELL AND DOUGLAS J. CAMPBELL

The optimum management of lacerations requires knowledge of skin anatomy and the physiology of wound healing. Such knowledge facilitates proper management of wounds of varying depth and complexity. By understanding the healing process, the family physician can maximize the options for repair and minimize the dangers of dehiscence and infection. The goals of primary closure are to stop bleeding, prevent infection, preserve function, and restore appearance. The patient always benefits from a physician who treats the patient gently, handles the tissue carefully, understands anatomy, and appreciates the healing process.[1,2]

Skin Anatomy

Figure 24.1 represents a model of the skin and the underlying tissue down to structures such as bone or muscle. Two additional features of skin anatomy that affect the repair of injuries are cleavage lines and wrinkles. Lines of cleavage are also known as Langer's lines. These lines are formed by the collagen bundles that lie parallel in the dermis. An incision or repair along these lines lessens disruption of collagen bundles and decreases new collagen formation and therefore causes less scarring. Wrinkle lines are not always consistent with Langer's lines. If a laceration is not in an area of apparent wrinkling, following the basic outline of Langer's lines results in the best repair.

Wound Healing

Phase One: Inflammatory Phase

The substrate, or inflammatory, phase occurs during the first 5 to 6 days after injury. Leukocytes, histamines, prostaglandins, and fibrinogen, delivered to the injury site via blood and lymphatic channels, attempt to neutralize bacteria and foreign material. The amount of inflammation present in a wound is related to the presence of necrotic tissue, which is increased by dead space and impaired

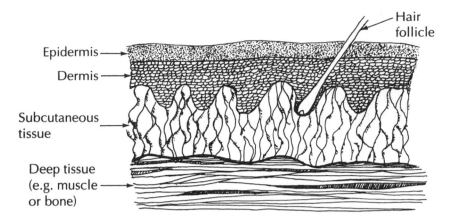

FIGURE 24.1. Model of skin and subcutaneous tissue.

circulation. Specific measures that reduce the inflammatory response include debridement, removal of foreign material, cleaning, control of bleeding, and precise tissue coaptation.

Phase Two: Fibroblastic Phase

The fibroblastic, or collagen, phase occupies days 6 though 20 after injury. Fibroblasts enter the wound rapidly and begin collagen synthesis, which binds the wound together. As the collagen content rises, the wound strength increases until the supporting ligature can be removed. Compromise of the vascular supply can inhibit the development of collagen synthesis and interfere with healing.

Phase Three: Maturation (Remodeling) Phase

The wound continues to undergo remodeling for 18 to 24 months, during which time collagen synthesis continues and retraction occurs. Normally during this time the scar becomes softer and less conspicuous. The prominent color of the scar gradually fades, resulting in a hue consistent with the surrounding skin. Aberrations of the maturation process can result in an unsightly scar such as a keloid. Such scars are due to a combination of inherited tendencies and extrinsic factors of the wound. Proper technique in wound care and repair minimizes the extrinsic contribution to keloid formation. If it is necessary to revise an unsightly scar, the ideal delay is 18 months or more after the initial repair.

Anesthesia

Under most circumstances it is preferable to anesthetize the wound prior to preparation for closure. Before applying anesthesia, the wound is inspected using a slow, gentle, aseptic technique to ascertain the extent of injury including an assessment of the neurovascular supply. At this time a decision is made to refer the patient if the complexity of the wound warrants consultation.

Topical Agents

When appropriate, topical anesthesia is ideal, as pain can be relieved without causing more discomfort or anxiety. Small lacerations may be closed without additional medications.

PAC (Pontocaine/Adrenaline/Cocaine) and TAC (Tetracaine/Adrenaline/Cocaine)

Pontocaine or tetracaine 2%/aqueous epinephrine (adrenaline) 1:1000/cocaine (PAC) is the most commonly used topical agent.[3,4] It may be prepared in a 100-mL volume by mixing 25 mL of 2% tetracaine, 50 mL of 1:1000 aqueous epinephrine, 11.8 g of cocaine, and sterile normal saline to a volume of 100 mL.

Placing a saturated pledget over the wound for 5 to 15 minutes often provides adequate local anesthesia. Blanching of the skin beyond the margin of the wound allows an estimation of adequate anesthesia. Further anesthesia may be applied by injection if necessary.

Emla

Emla is a commercially available preparation of 2.5% lidocaine/2.5% prilocaine in a buffered vehicle. It is squeezed onto the skin surface and covered with an occlusive dressing. Its efficacy is similar to that of TAC, but it takes nearly twice as long to anesthetize the skin (30 minutes). The same guideline of skin blanching applies to the use of Emla.

Ethyl Chloride

A highly volatile fluid, ethyl chloride comes in commercially prepared glass bottles with a sprayer lid. This fluid can be sprayed onto the skin surface by inverting the bottle and pressing the lid. The flammable fluid chills the skin rapidly. The agent may be applied until skin frosting occurs. It provides brief anesthesia, allowing immediate placement of a needle without causing additional pain.

Injectable Agents

Lidocaine

Lidocaine produces moderate duration of anesthesia (about 1–2 hours) when used in a 1% or 2% solution. When mixed with 1:100,000 aqueous epinephrine, the anesthetic effect is prolonged (2–6 hours), and there is a local vasoconstrictive effect. Any anesthetic mixed with epinephrine should be used with caution on fingers, toes, ears, nose, or the penis to avoid risk of ischemia and subsequent necrosis. Occasional toxicity occurs with lidocaine, but most reactions are due to inadvertent intravascular injection. Manifestations of toxicity include tinnitus, numbness, confusion, and rarely progression to coma. True allergic reactions are unusual.

It is possible to reduce the discomfort of lidocaine injection by buffering the solution with the addition of sterile sodium bicarbonate.[5-8] A solution of 9 mL of lidocaine plus 1 mL of sodium bicarbonate (44 mEq/50 mL) is less painful to inject but provides the same level of anesthesia as the unbuffered solution. It is also possible to buffer other injectable agents including those with epinephrine. However, epinephrine is unstable at a pH above 5.5 and is commercially prepared in solutions below that pH. Therefore, any buffered local anesthetic with epinephrine must be used within a short time of preparation.[9] Warming a buffered solution to body temperature provides additional reduction of the pain of injection. Buffering also appears to increase the antibacterial properties of anesthetic solutions.[10]

ADDITIONAL AGENTS

Mepivacaine (Carbocaine) produces longer anesthesia than lidocaine (about 45–90 minutes). It is not used with epinephrine. Reactions are similar to those seen with lidocaine. Procaine (Novocain) works quickly but has a short duration (usually less than 30–45 minutes). It has a wide safety margin and may be used with epinephrine. Bupivacaine (Marcaine) is the longest-acting local anesthetic (approximately 6–8 hours). It is often used for nerve blocks or may be mixed with lidocaine for problems that take longer to repair. It is also useful for injecting into a wound to provide postprocedural pain relief. It may be mixed with epinephrine and is available in 0.25%, 0.50%, and 0.75% solutions.

DIPHENHYDRAMINE

Diphenhydramine (Benadryl) may also be used as an injectable anesthetic.[11] It is somewhat more painful to inject than lidocaine but has an efficacy similar to that of lidocaine. Diphenhydramine may be prepared in a 0.5% solution by mixing a 1-mL vial of 50 mg diphenhydramine with 9 mL of saline. This solution is useful when a patient claims an allergy to all injectable anesthetics.

Anesthetic Methods

INFILTRATION BLOCKS

Infiltration blocks are useful for most laceration repairs. The wound is infiltrated by multiple injections into the skin and subcutaneous tissue. Using a long needle and a fan technique decreases the number of injection sites and therefore decreases the pain to the patient. Using a 27-gauge or smaller needle to inject through the open wound margin also minimizes the patient's discomfort, as does moving from an anesthetized area slowly toward the unanesthetized tissue.

FIELD BLOCKS

Field blocks result in similar pain control but may distort the wound margin less and are useful where accurate wound approximation is necessary (e.g., the vermillion border). The area around the wound is injected in a series of wheals completely around the wound, thereby blocking the cutaneous nerve supply to the laceration. This technique is more time-consuming but produces longer-lasting anesthesia. Another option to reduce the initial pain of the injection is to produce a small wheal using buffered sterile water and then injecting the anesthetic through the wheal. The buffered water has a brief anesthetic action.

NERVE BLOCKS

Nerve blocks are most commonly effected by injecting a nerve proximal to the injury site. The most frequent use of this technique is the digital block performed by injecting anesthetic into the webbing between the digits at the metacarpophalangeal joint on each side of the digit (Fig. 24.2). Mouth and tongue lacerations are repairable using dental blocks. It is useful to receive practical instruction in such blocks from a dental colleague.

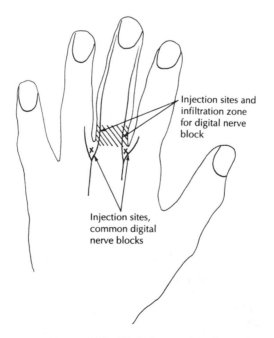

FIGURE 24.2. Digital nerve block.

Sedation

The Task Force on Sedation and Analgesia by Non-Anesthesiologists[12] provides excellent protocols for sedative use by family physicians. Under adequate observation sedative agents can help the doctor deal with difficult patients. For all agents described herein, it is imperative that there be appropriate monitoring and that adequate resuscitation equipment be readily available. The welfare of the patient is of prime concern, and such medications should not be used solely for the provider's convenience.

Ketamine

Ketamine is a phencyclidine derivative. It provides a dissociative state resulting in a trance-like condition and may provide amnesia for the procedure. Ketamine can be administered by many routes, but the most practical for laceration repair is the oral method. It usually results in significant analgesia without hypotension, decreased heart rate, or decreased respiratory drive. The use of proper monitoring and the availability of resuscitation equipment is mandatory. Oral ketamine can be prepared by adding 2.5 mL of ketamine hydrochloride injection (100 mg/mL) to 7.5 mL of flavored syrup. It is then given at a dose of 10 mg/kg. Sedation occurs over 20 to 45 minutes after ingestion. The most common side effects include nystagmus, random extremity movements, and vomiting during the recovery stage.[13]

Midazolam (Versed)

Midazolam is a benzodiazepine with typical class effects of hypnosis, amnesia, and anxiety reduction. It is readily absorbed and has a short elimination half-life. It may be given as a single dose via the nasal, oral, rectal, or parenteral route. The rectal route is useful when the patient is combative. A cooperative patient prefers oral or nasal administration (oral dose 0.5 mg/kg; nasal dose 0.25 mg/kg, by nasal drops). Injectable midazolam is used to make a solution that may be given orally or nasally. The drug should be made into a 5 mg/mL solution. For oral use it may be added to punch or apple juice to improve the taste. The maximum dose for children by any route is 8 mg.

For rectal administration, a 6-French (F) feeding tube is attached to an angiocath connected to a 5-mL syringe. The lubricated catheter is then inserted into the rectum and the drug injected followed by a syringe full of air to propel the medication into the rectum. The tube is then withdrawn and the patient's buttocks are held together for approximately 1 minute. The dose is 0.45 mg/kg by this route. The medication may begin to work as soon as 10 minutes after administration. Side effects may be delayed, so the patient should be observed for at least an hour as the duration of a single dose lasts about an hour. Some burning can occur when the nasal route is used. Inconsolable agitation may appear regardless of the route of administration. This side effect of agitated crying resolves after several hours. Vomiting may also occur.[12,14,15]

Fentanyl

Fentanyl is a powerful synthetic opioid that produces rapid, short-lasting sedation and analgesia. Like other opioids, its effects are reversible, and it has limited cardiovascular effects. Although it can be given in many forms, oral transmucosal fentanyl citrate (OTFC) is available commercially in a lollipop (Fentanyl Oralet). This drug, commonly used as an preanesthetic medication, is available in three dosage forms (200, 300, and 400 mg). The dose for adults is 5 mg/kg to a maximum of 400 mg regardless of weight. Pediatric dosages begin at 5 mg/kg to a maximum of 15 mg/kg or 400 mg (whichever is less). Children weighing less than 15 kg should not receive fentanyl. OTFC effects are apparent 5 to 10 minutes after sucking the Oralet. The maximum effect is usually achieved about 30 minutes after use, but effects may persist for several hours. Side effects are common but usually minor. About half of patients develop transient pruritus, 15% notice dizziness, and at least one third develop vomiting. The most dangerous effect is hypoventilation, which can be fatal.[12,16,17] Oversedation or respiratory depression responds to naloxone.

Nitrous Oxide

Nitrous oxide is a rapid-acting anesthetic that works within 3 to 5 minutes with a similar duration after cessation of administration.[18] Commercial equipment is available to deliver a mixture of nitrous oxide and oxygen at various ratios (usually 30–50% N_2O/50–70% O_2). Side effects include nausea in about 10% to 15% of patients with occasional emesis. The efficacy of nitrous oxide is known to be variable. Although some patients object to the use of the mask, many patients prefer using a specially designed self-administration mask. Nitrous oxide can cause expansion of gas-filled body pockets, and for that reason it should not be used in patients with head injuries, pneumothoraces, bowel obstructions, or middle ear effusions.

Wound Preparation

Proper preparation of a wound can improve the success of aesthetically acceptable healing. The wound should be closed as soon as possible, although most lacerations heal well if closed within 24 hours after the injury. After anesthesia, proper cleansing should be accomplished by wiping, scrubbing, and irrigating with normal saline using a large syringe with or without a 22-gauge needle, which produces enough velocity to clean most wounds. Antiseptic soaps such as hexachlorophene (pHisoHex), chlorhexidine gluconate (Hibiclens), or povidone-iodine (Betadine) can also be used, but one should be aware that all of these cleansing agents with the exception of normal saline will delay wound healing to some extent by destroying fibroblasts and leukocytes as well as bacteria. Sterile scrub brushes may be useful for cleaning grossly contaminated lesions.

After washing and irrigation, the area is draped with sterile towels to create a clean field. The wound is then explored using sterile technique to confirm the depth of injury, ascertain whether injury to underlying tissue has occurred, rule out the presence of any foreign body, and determine the adequacy of anesthesia. After examination, debridement is performed if necessary.

Debridement is the process of converting an irregular dirty wound to a clean one with smooth edges. Wound margins that are crushed, mangled, or devitalized are excised unless it is unwise to do so. Tissue in areas such as the lip or eyelid should be removed with extreme caution. It is pointless to increase the deformity when a somewhat imperfect scar can provide a more functional result. If a considerable amount of tissue has been crushed, initial removal of all the damaged tissue may result in undesirable function (such as would occur if the skin over a joint was removed). Such injuries should be closed loosely using subcutaneous absorbable sutures. The scar can be revised later if necessary.

The initial incision is made with a scalpel followed by excision with a pair of sharp tissue scissors. The edges should be perpendicular to the skin surface or even slightly undercut to facilitate eversion of the skin margins (Fig. 24.3). In hairy areas incisions should parallel the hair shafts to minimize the likelihood of hairless areas around the healed wound (Fig. 24.4).

After debridement the skin edges are held together to see if it is possible to approximate them with minimal tension. Generally, it is necessary to undermine the skin to achieve greater mobility of the surface by releasing some of the subcutaneous skin attachments that prevent the skin from sliding (Fig. 24.5). This step takes place in the subcutaneous layer and can be done with a scalpel or scis-

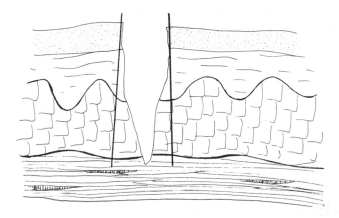

FIGURE 24.3. Slight undercutting of the wound edges facilitates slight eversion of the wound edge.

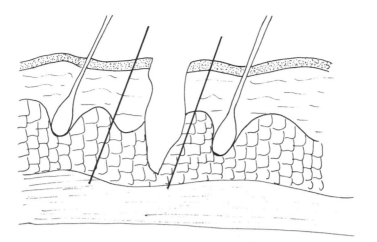

FIGURE 24.4. Parallel debridement in a hairy area avoids damaging hair follicles.

sors. The wound is then undermined circumferentially about 4 to 5 mm from the edge of the margin. The undermining should be equal across the wound and widest where the skin needs to move the most, usually the center of the cut.

Hemostasis can be accomplished most easily by simple pressure on the wound site for 5 to 10 minutes. If pressure is unsuccessful, bleeders may be carefully cauterized or ligated. Cautery or ligation can hinder healing if large amounts of tissue are damaged. Small vessels can be controlled with absorbable suture if necessary, but large arterial bleeders may need to be controlled with permanent ligature if it is possible to do so without compromising the distal circulation. If

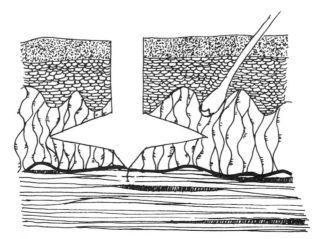

FIGURE 24.5. Undermining the subdermal layer facilitates closure.

oozing persists, the wound is closed with a drain (e.g., a sterile rubber band or Penrose drain) left in the wound several days. An overlying pressure dressing minimizes bleeding. Advancing the drain every other day permits healing with minimal hematoma formation.

Wound Closure

Suture options are listed in Table 24.1. Absorbable materials are gradually broken down and absorbed by tissue; nonabsorbable sutures are made from chemicals that are encapsulated by the body and thus isolated from tissue. Monofilament sutures are less irritating to tissue but are more difficult to handle and require more knots than braided sutures. Stitches placed through the epidermis are done with nonabsorbable materials to minimize the tissue reactivity that occurs with absorbable stitches. Reverse cutting needles in a three-eighths or one-half circle design are available in various sizes for each type of suture.

A well-closed wound has three characteristics: the margins are approximated without tension, the tissue layers are accurately aligned, and dead space is eliminated. Deep stitches are placed in layers that hold the suture, such as the fat–

TABLE 24.1. Common Suture Materials

Suture	Advantages	Disadvantages
Absorbable		
Catgut	Inexpensive	Low tensile strength
		Strength lasts 4–5 days
		High tissue reactivity
Chromic catgut	Inexpensive	Moderate tensile strength and reactivity
Polyglycolic acid (Dexon)	Low tissue reactivity	Moderately difficult to handle
Polyglactic acid (Vicryl)	Easy handling	Occasional "spitting" of suture
	Good tensile strength	due to absorption delay
Polyglyconate (Maxon)	Easy handling	Expensive
	Good tensile strength	
Nonabsorbable		
Silk	Handles well	Low tensile strength
	Moderately inexpensive	High tissue reactivity
		Increased infection rate
Nylon (Ethilon, Dermilon)	High tensile strength	Difficult to handle; slippery, so many knots needed
	Minimal tissue reactivity	
	Inexpensive	
Polypropylene	No tissue reaction	Expensive
(Proline SurgiPro)	Stretches, accommodates swelling	
Braided polyester	Handles well	Tissue drag if uncoated
(Mersilene, Ethiflex)	Knots secure	Expensive
Polybutester (Novofil)	Elastic, accommodates swelling and retraction	Expensive

fascial junction or the derma–fat junction. A buried knot technique is the preferred method for placing deep sutures. Deep sutures provide most of the strength of the repair, and skin sutures approximate the skin margins and improve the cosmetic result (Fig. 24.6).

Suture Techniques[19–21]

Simple Interrupted Stitch

A simple interrupted stitch is placed by passing the needle through the skin surface at right angles, placing the suture as wide as it is deep. The goal is to place sutures that slightly evert the edge of the wound (Fig. 24.7). This maneuver produces a slightly raised scar that recedes during the remodeling stage of healing and leaves a smooth scar. The opposite margin is approximated using a mirror image of the first placement. Following the natural radius of the curved needle places the suture in such a way as to evert the wound margin. It can be modified to correctly approximate the margins when the wound edges are asymmetric[1] (Fig. 24.8). Occasionally a wound exhibits excessively everted margins. By reversing the usual approach and taking a stitch that is wider at the top than at the base, the wound can be inverted, improving the cosmetic appearance (Fig. 24.9). A useful general rule is that the entrance and exit points should be 2 mm from the margin for facial wounds but may be farther apart on other surfaces.[1,2]

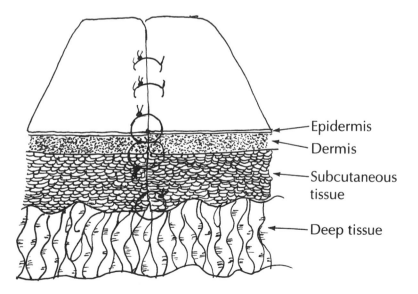

FIGURE 24.6. Layer closure showing sutures in the epidermis, at the dermal–epidermal junction, and at the dermal–fat junction.

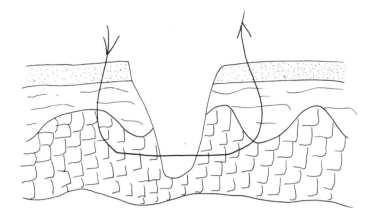

FIGURE 24.7. Simple interrupted suture with placement to facilitate wound eversion.

The open-loop knot (Fig. 24.10) avoids placing the suture under excessive tension and facilitates removal of the stitch. The first throw of the knot with two loops ("surgeon's knot") is placed with just enough tension to approximate the wound margin. The second throw, a single loop, is tied, leaving a little space so no additional tension is place on the first loop. Subsequent throws can be tightened snugly without increasing tension on the wound edge. Pulling all the knots to the same side of the wound makes suture removal easier and improves the aesthetics of the repair. As a rule of thumb one should put at least the same num-

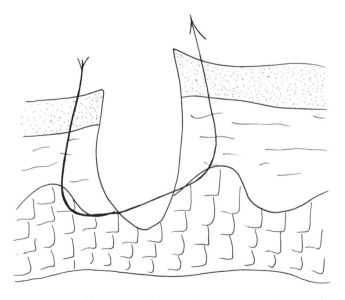

FIGURE 24.8. Placement of suture in an asymmetric wound.

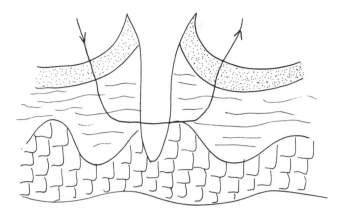

FIGURE 24.9. Suture placement in a wound with everted edges.

ber of knots of a monofilament suture as the size of the ligature (e.g., five knots with 5-0 suture).

Vertical or Horizontal Mattress Suture

The vertical mattress suture promotes eversion and is useful where thick layers are encountered or tension exists. Two techniques may be used. The classic method first places the deep stitch and closes with the superficial stitch (Fig. 24.11). The short-hand method[22] is performed by placing the shallow stitch first,

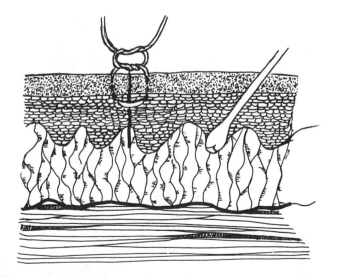

FIGURE 24.10. Model of skin showing surgeon's knot.

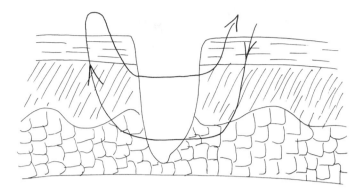

FIGURE 24.11. Vertical mattress suture.

pulling up on the suture (tenting the skin), and then placing the deeper stitch. Horizontal mattress sutures also have the advantage of needing fewer knots to cover the same area.

Intracuticular Running Suture

The intracuticular running suture, utilizing a nonabsorbable suture, can be used where there is minimal skin tension. It results in minimal scarring without suture marks. Controlled tissue apposition is difficult with this method, but it is a popular technique because of the cosmetic result. The suture ends do not need to be tied but can be taped in place under slight tension (Fig. 24.12).

Three-Point Mattress Suture

The three-point or corner stitch is used to minimize the possibility of vascular necrosis of the tip of a V-shaped wound. The needle is inserted into the skin of the wound edge on one side of the wound opposite the flap near the apex of the wound (Fig. 24.13A,B). The suture is placed at the mid-dermis level, brought across the wound, and placed transversely at the same level through the apex of the flap. It is then brought across the wound and returned at the same level on the opposite side of the V parallel to the point of entry. The suture is then tied, drawing the tip of the wound into position without compromising the blood supply (Fig. 24.13C). This method can also be used for stellate injuries where multiple tips can be approximated in purse-string fashion.

Running or Continuous Stitch

The running stitch is useful in situations where speed is important (e.g., a field emergency) because individual knots do not have to be tied. It is appropriate for

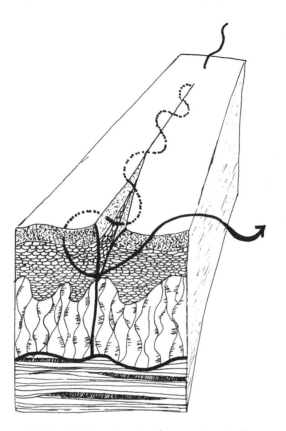

FIGURE 24.12. Intracuticular running stitch.

use on scalp lacerations especially, because it is good for hemostasis. The continuous method does not allow fine control of wound margins (Fig. 24.14).

Specific Circumstances

Lacerations Across a Landmark

Lacerations that involve prominent anatomic features or landmarks, such as the vermilion border of the lip or the eyebrow, require special consideration. Commonly a laceration is closed from one end to the other, but in special situations it is advisable to place a retention stitch (a simple or vertical mattress stitch) to reapproximate the landmark border accurately. The remainder of the wound can then be closed by an appropriate method. If the retention stitch is under significant tension when the repair seems complete, it should be removed and replaced.

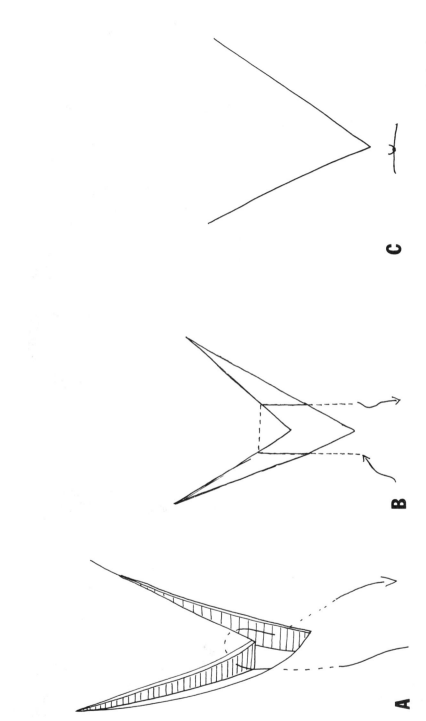

FIGURE 24.13. Three-point stitch. (A) Three-dimensional view showing suture placement. (B) Schematic view. (C) Finished stitch.

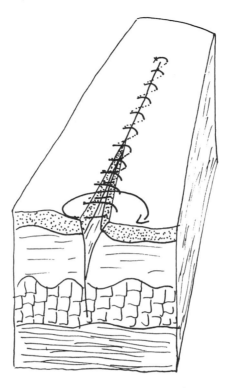

FIGURE 24.14. Running stitch.

Beveled Lacerations

A frequently seen injury, the beveled laceration, tempts the physician to close it as it is; but the undercut flap may not heal well owing to disruption of the blood supply. The margins of the wound should be modified, as shown in Figure 24.15. The edges are squared, undermined, and closed in layers.

Dog Ears

Dog ears, a common problem, results from wound closure where the sides of the laceration are unequal. One side bunches up, and a mound of skin occurs. It also occurs when an elliptical wound is closed in the center, leaving excess tissue at each end. To correct the problem, the dog ear is tented up with a skin hook, and a linear incision is made along one side. The excess triangle is then grasped at the tip and a second linear incision is made (Fig. 24.16). This maneuver allows closure in a single line.

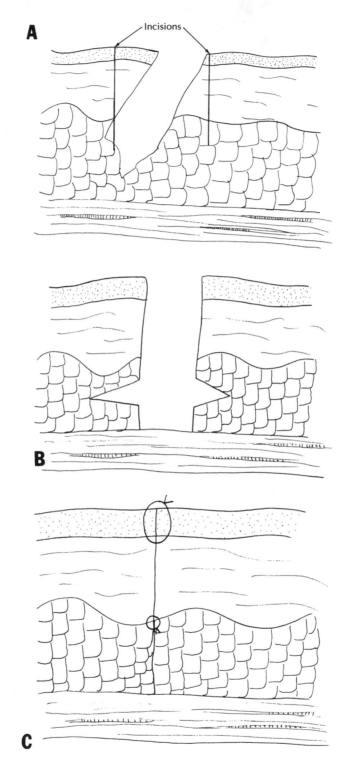

FIGURE 24.15. Closure of beveled wound. (A) Squaring beveled edges. (B) Undermining the fat layer. (C) Layered closure.

504

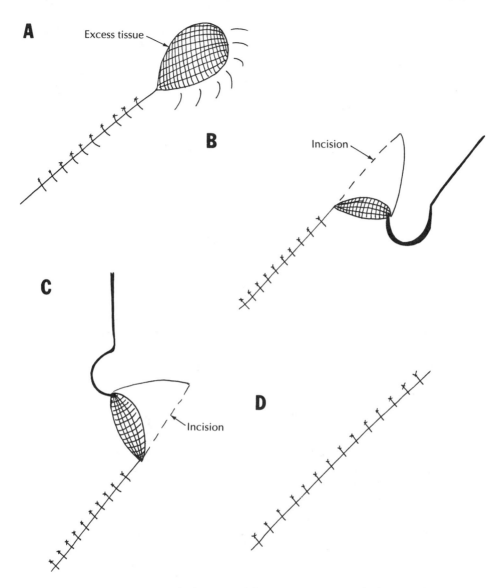

FIGURE 24.16. Correction of "dog ear." (A) Excess tissue at end of repair. (B) Tenting the dog ear and first incision. (C) Pulling flap across initial incision and position of second incision. (D) Appearance of final closure.

Complex Lacerations

A wound may occur with unequal sides with a hump of tissue on one side. This lump of tissue may be excised using the technique described above for removal of dog ears. The triangular defect is then closed using a modification of the three-point mattress suture, the four-point technique shown in Figure 24.17. The resulting closure forms a T-shaped repair.

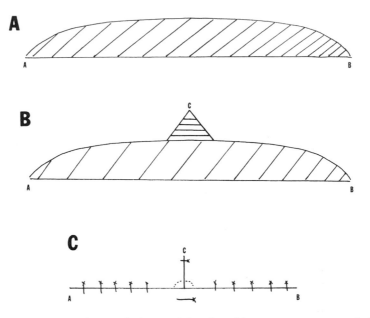

FIGURE 24.17. Unequal wound closure. (A) Sides of laceration are unequal. (B) Excise triangle of tissue on longer side. (C) T-closure showing four-point suture.

Finger Injuries

AMPUTATED FINGERTIP

If the area of the fingertip amputation is less than 1 cm^2, the wound can be handled by careful cleansing, proper dressings, and subsequent healing by secondary intention. If the wound is larger, the complexity of treatment increases. If the amputation is beveled dorsally and distally, a conservative approach without suturing or grafting usually results in good healing. An unfavorable angle requires more extensive repair.[23] Referral to a plastic or hand surgeon may be warranted.

NAIL BED INJURIES

Nail bed injuries can be managed by saving the nail and reapproximating nail matrix lacerations with fine absorbable sutures. It may be necessary to remove the nail to repair an underlying nail bed tear. The nail may then be replaced and held in position with several sutures, allowing the nail to act as a splint.

Alternatives to Suturing

Suturing has been an effective method for closing wounds for centuries, but options for skin suturing are now available. They may even represent more cost-effective methods of wound closure.

Staples

One option is the use of skin staples, which have been used for years in the operating room as the final closure for a variety of incisions. Typically, staples are used on the skin in wounds that would be closed in a straight line. The skin is closed with staples after other layers are closed by suturing. The most significant advantage to the use of staples is the decreased time necessary to close the skin. An assistant may be required to position the skin properly.[24]

Adhesives

The most commonly used tissue glues are related to cyanoacrylate ester known as Super Glue. Tissue glues for superficial wounds have the advantage of rapid closure, minimal physical and emotional trauma to the patient, and absence of a foreign body in the wound.[25,26] They may also be less expensive to use than traditional methods of closure.

Histoacryl Blue, a.k.a. Dermabond, has been commercially available in Canada since 1975, and in the United States since 1998. It is a safe alternative to suturing.[27–29] Hemostasis must be achieved before applying the glue. Because some chemicals used for hemostasis such as Monsel's solution will prevent the adhesive from bonding to the skin, care must be taken to avoid skin edges. Layered closure may be accomplished using deep, absorbable sutures combined with surface adhesive. Surface sutures combined with adhesive should be avoided because the adhesive will bond to the suture material and may make removing the suture difficult. Only wounds that are under no tension are appropriate for adhesive, such as those on the face and the forearm. Even wounds such as on the foot are generally inappropriate because as soon as the patient steps on the foot, pressure is generated across the wound edges. After hemostasis and cleansing have been achieved, the wound must be approximated using gloved fingers (vinyl is preferred to latex because it also not bond as well to the adhesive), metal instruments (preferred because metal also does not bond as tightly to the adhesive as plastic), Steri-strips, or specially manufactured closure devices for use with the adhesive. With the wound edges approximated, a layer of adhesive is applied to the top of the wound and allowed to polymerize. Two more subsequent layers should be applied and allowed to polymerize over the top of the first layer. Some other precautions: Because the adhesive is a very thin, runny liquid, gravity should be utilized to keep the liquid from running into eyes, the wound itself, or other undesirable areas. If adhesive does get on the cornea in spite of appropriate precautions, it does not cause damage and may be left to come off within a few days. Other methods to control the spread of the adhesive include sponges lightly moistened with saline or use of Vaseline around the area. The patient should be instructed to keep the wound dry for 7 to 10 days because moisture weakens the bonding strength. The wound can either be left open to air, or covered with a clean bandage. Petroleum-based products should also be avoided on the adhesive because of a weakening effect.

Postrepair Management

Most wounds should be protected during the first 1 to 2 days after repair. Frequently a commercial bandage may be used; but when the wound is still oozing, a pressure dressing is applied. The initial layer is a nonstick gauze dressing available in sterile packages, such as Adaptic, Telfa, or Xeroderm. A gauze pad is then placed and held in place by roller gauze, elastic wrap, or elastic tape. Dressings are removed and the wound reexamined at 48 to 72 hours. If a drain has been placed, it should be advanced every 24 to 48 hours. If the wound is under significant tension, additional support can be achieved by using Steri-Strips or bulky supportive dressings, including splints that are commercially available or custom-made from plaster or fiberglass.

Most wounds can be left open after the first 24 to 48 hours. It is important to remove wet dressings from a repair because the skin maceration that results from them may prolong healing and increase the risk of infection. Initial epithelialization takes place during the first 24 hours, and thereafter it is permissible to wash the wound briefly. Lacerations on the scalp and face may be impractical to bandage.

Wounds should be reexamined for infection or hematoma formation after 2 to 3 days if there is any concern at the time of repair. Contaminated wounds and wounds that have been open longer than 24 hours have a greater likelihood of infection.

Timing of suture removal should be individualized, based on wound location, the mechanical stress placed on the repair, and the tension of the closure. Facial sutures should be removed within 3 to 5 days to minimize the possibility of suture tracks. Supporting the repair with Steri-Strips may decrease the likelihood of dehiscence. In skin areas that are not highly mobile (e.g., the back or extremities) sutures are left in place for 7 to 10 days. On fingers, palms, soles, and over joints, the sutures remain in place at least 10 to 14 days and sometimes longer. Table 24.2 is a sample instruction sheet for patients.

TABLE 24.2. Instructions for Patients

1. Keep wound dressings clean and dry. Protect dressings from moisture when bathing.
2. If the dressing gets wet, remove it and reapply a clean, dry dressing.
3. Remove the dressing after 2 days and reapply every 2 days unless instructed otherwise.
4. If any of the following signs appears, contact your physician or clinic immediately:
    A.   Wound becomes red, warm, swollen, or tender.
    B.   Wound begins to drain.
    C.   Red streaks appear near the wound or up the arm or leg.
    D.   Tender lumps appear in the armpit or groin.
    E.   Chills or fever occur.
5. Because of your particular injury the doctor would like your wound check in _____ days.
6. Please return for removal of your stitches in _____ days.
7. You received the following vaccinations:
    A.   Tetanus toxoid _____
    B.   DT (diphtheria/tetanus) _____
    C.   DPT (diphtheria/pertussis/tetanus) _____

Concurrent Therapy

Preventing infection is an important aspect of laceration treatment. Puncture wounds and bites usually should not be closed because the risk of infection negates the advantage of closure. Dog bites can usually be safely closed, however. Sometimes a gaping puncture wound on the face requires closure for cosmetic reasons despite the risk of infection.

Antibiotic Usage

Antibiotic prophylaxis is probably not helpful in most circumstances unless given in sufficient quantity to obtain good tissue levels while the wound is still open. If extensive repair is necessary, intravenous antibiotics should be started during wound closure. Animal and human bite wounds are often treated by post-closure antibiotics. The efficacy of this practice remains controversial, but antibiotics are often given because of the extensive contamination that occurs with bite wounds, especially those from cats. Amoxicillin-clavulanate covers the typical bacteria of bite wounds. Doxycycline and ceftriaxone are alternative medications.[29]

Tetanus Prophylaxis

Tetanus prophylaxis is a crucial part of the care of the lacerated patient; it is imperative that the immunization status of the patient be documented. Patients most likely to be inadequately immunized are the elderly, who may have never received a primary series. Table 24.3 is a summary of the guide published by the Centers for Disease Control and Prevention. Whenever passive immunity is required, human tetanus immune globulin (TIg) is preferred. The usual dose of TIg

TABLE 24.3. Guide to Tetanus Prophylaxis During Routine Wound Management

History of adsorbed tetanus toxoid (doses)	Clean, minor wounds		All other wounds[a]	
	Td[b]	TIg	Td[b]	TIg
Unknown or <3	Yes	No	Yes	Yes
≥Three[c]	No[d]	No	No[e]	No

[a]Such as, but not limited to, wounds contaminated with dirt, feces, soil, and saliva; puncture wounds; avulsions; and wounds resulting from missiles, crushing, burns, and frostbite.
[b]For children <7 years old; DPT (DT if pertussis vaccine is contraindicated) is preferred to tetanus toxoid alone. For persons ≥7 years of age Td is preferred to tetanus toxoid alone.
[c]If only three doses of *fluid* toxoid have been received, a fourth dose of toxoid, preferably an adsorbed toxoid, is given.
[d]Yes, if >10 years since last dose.
[e]Yes, if >5 years since last dose. (More frequent boosters are not needed and can accentuate side effects.)
Td = tetanus-diphtheria toxoid; TIg = tetanus immune globulin; DPT = diphtheria/pertussis/tetanus.

is 500 units IM. Tetanus toxoid and TIg should be given through separate needles at separate sites.[30,31]

References

1. Brietenbach KL, Bergera JJ. Principles and techniques of primary wound closure. Prim Care 1986;13:411–31.
2. Snell G. Laceration repair. In: Pfenninger JL, Fowler GC, eds. Procedures for primary care physicians. St. Louis: Mosby, 1994;12–19.
3. Bonadio WA, Wagner V. Efficacy of TAC topical anesthetic for repair of pediatric lacerations. Am J Dis Child 1988;142:203–5.
4. Hegenbarth MA, Altieri MF, Hawk WH, Green A, Ochsenschlager DW, O'Donnell R. Comparison of topical tetracaine, adrenaline, and cocaine anesthesia with lidocaine infiltration for repair of lacerations in children. Ann Emerg Med 1990;19:63–7.
5. Matsumoto AH, Reifsnyder AC, Hartwell GD, Angle JF, Selby JB, Tegtmeyer CJ. Reducing the discomfort of lidocaine administration through pH buffering. J Vasc Interv Radiol 1994;5:171–5.
6. Bartfield JM, Ford DT, Homer PJ. Buffered versus plain lidocaine for digital nerve blocks. Ann Emerg Med 1993;22:216–19.
7. Mader TJ, Playe SJ, Garb JL. Reducing the pain of local anesthetic infiltration: warming and buffering have a synergistic effect. Ann Emerg Med 1994;23:550–4.
8. Brogan BX Jr, Giarrusso E, Hollander JE, Cassara G, Mararnga MC, Thode HC. Comparison of plain, warmed, and buffered lidocaine for anesthesia of traumatic wounds. Ann Emerg Med 1995;26:121–5.
9. Murakami CS, Odland PB, Ross BK. Buffered local anesthetics and epinephrine degradation. J Dermatol Surg Oncol 1994;20:192–5.
10. Thompson KD, Welykyj S, Massa MC. Antibacterial activity of lidocaine in combination with a bicarbonate buffer. J Dermatol Surg Oncol 1993;19:216–20.
11. Ernst AA, Marvez-Valls E, Mall G, Patterson J, Xie X, Weiss SJ. 1% lidocaine versus 0.5% diphenhydramine for local anesthesia in minor laceration repair. Ann Emerg Med 1994;23:1328–32.
12. Task Force on Sedation and Analgesia by Non-Anesthesiologists. Practical guidelines for sedation and analgesia by non-anesthesiologists. Anesthesiology 1996;84:459–71.
13. Qureshi FA, Mellis PT, McFadden MA. Efficacy of oral ketamine for providing sedation and analgesia to children requiring laceration repair. Pediatr Emerg Care 1995;11:93–7.
14. Connors K, Terndrup TE. Nasal versus oral midazolam for sedation of anxious children undergoing laceration repair. Ann Emerg Med 1994;24:1074–9.
15. Shane SA, Fuchs SM, Khine H. Efficacy of rectal midazolam for the sedation of preschool children undergoing laceration repair. Ann Emerg Med 1994;24:1065–73.
16. Schutzman SA, Burg J, Liebelt E, et al. Oral transmucosal fentanyl citrate for the premedication of children undergoing laceration repair. Ann Emerg Med 1994; 24:1059–64.
17. Clinical considerations in the use of fentanyl Oralet. North Chicago, IL: Abbott Laboratories, 1995;1–16.
18. Gamis AS, Knapp JF, Glenski JA. Nitrous oxide analgesia in a pediatric emergency department. Ann Emerg Med 1989;18:177–81.
19. Moy RL, Lee A, Zolka A. Commonly used suture materials in skin surgery. Am Fam Physician 1991;44:2123–8.

20. Epperson WJ. Suture selection. In: Pfenninger JL, Fowler GC, eds. Procedures for primary care physicians. St. Louis: Mosby, 1994;3–6.
21. Moy RL, Waldman B, Hein DW. A review of sutures and suturing techniques. J Dermatol Surg Oncol 1992;18:785–95.
22. Jones JS, Gartner M, Drew G, Pack S. The shorthand vertical mattress stitch: evaluation of a new suture technique. Am J Emerg Med 1993;11:483–5.
23. Ditmars DM Jr. Finger tip and nail bed injuries. Occup Med 1989;4:449–61.
24. Edlich RF, Thacker JG, Silloway RF, Morgan RF, Rodeheaver GT. Scientific basis of skin staple closure. In: Haval Mutaz B, ed. Advances in plastic and reconstructive surgery. Chicago: Year Book, 1986;233–71.
25. Osmond MH, Klassen TP, Quinn JV. Economic comparison of a tissue adhesive and suturing in the repair of pediatric facial lacerations. J Pediatr 1995;126(6):892–5.
26. Quinn JV, Drzewiecki A, Li MM, et al. A randomized, controlled trial comparing tissue adhesive with suturing in the repair of pediatric facial lacerations. Ann Emerg Med 1993;22:1130–5.
27. Applebaum JS, Zalut T, Applebaum D. The use of tissue adhesive for traumatic laceration repair in the emergency department. Ann Emerg Med 1993;22:1190–2.
28. Fisher AA. Reactions to cyanoacrylate adhesives: "instant glue." Cutis 1995:18–22, 46,58.
29. Lewis KT, Stiles M. Management of cat and dog bites. Am Fam Physician 1995; 52:479–85.
30. Centers for Disease Control. Tetanus prophylaxis during routine wound management. MMWR 1991;40(RR-10):1–28.
31. Richardson JP, Knight AL. The management and prevention of tetanus. J Emerg Med 1993;11:737–42.

CASE PRESENTATION

You are called by the hospital emergency department staff at 6 p.m. One of your patients is there with a hand laceration. You go there to meet him.

Subjective

PATIENT PROFILE

Ken Nelson is a 47-year-old married male home builder.

PRESENTING PROBLEM

"I cut my hand today."

PRESENT ILLNESS

Five hours ago, the patient cut his right hand on sheet metal at work. He finished his work shift and now presents at the end of the day for treatment.

PAST MEDICAL HISTORY

No serious illness or hospitalization.

SOCIAL HISTORY

Ken Nelson is a self-employed building contractor who lives with his wife and 16-year-old daughter.

HABITS

He does not use tobacco or alcohol. He drinks one thermos of coffee per day.

FAMILY HISTORY

Not recorded because of the limited nature of today's problem.

- What more would you like to know about the injury? Why might this information be important?
- What do you need to know about his tetanus immunizations status?

- What are pertinent safety issues that should be elicited?
- What might be the significance of the 5-hour delay in seeking care? How would you inquire about this?

Objective

VITAL SIGNS

Blood pressure, 132/86; pulse, 66.

EXAMINATION

There is a 4-cm-long linear laceration of the lateral right hand; the wound extends into the subcutaneous tissues. The patient has full active and passive motion of the hand and fingers. There is no loss of neurologic function.

- What further information—if any—regarding the physical examination might be important?
- What are some concerns regarding hand injuries, and how would you examine to address these possibilities?
- How can you determine that neurologic function is intact?
- In what circumstances would you obtain laboratory testing or diagnostic imaging?

Assessment

- What are some concerns regarding this injury? How would you describe these concerns to the patient?
- If the patient had lost sensory perception to one of his fingers, what would you do?
- Is this a teachable moment for accident prevention? How would you approach this issue with the patient?
- What are pertinent insurance issues in regard to this injury?

Plan

- How would you prepare the wound for suturing, and what suture material would you use? Describe special considerations in suture technique for hand lacerations.
- What would be your recommendation regarding tetanus prophylaxis?
- Mr. Nelson asks about returning to work. How would you respond?
- What aftercare would you recommend for this injury?

25
Athletic Injuries

MICHAEL L. TUGGY AND CORA COLLETTE BREUNER

Family physicians routinely treat many athletic injuries in their clinical practice. The benefits of long-term exercise in the prevention of common illnesses such as cardiovascular disease, osteoporosis, and falls in the elderly are well established. With the increased interest in fitness in the general population, the number of people resuming more active exercise as they age is increasing. Injuries sustained in childhood or adolescence may have long-term effects that can hamper later attempts at physical activity.[1] For all ages of patients, proper training and prevention can lead to lifelong participation in athletic activities.

Most sports injuries are related to overuse injuries and often are not brought to the attention of the family physician until the symptoms are advanced. Traumatic injuries are more readily diagnosed, but may have more serious long-term sequelae for the life of the athlete. Sport selection has a great impact on risk of injury. The adolescent athlete is probably at highest risk for injury due to sport selection, presence of immature growth cartilage at the growth plates and joint surfaces, and lack of experience.[2] High-risk sports selected by young adults also have higher degrees of risk, which can be modified to lessen injury rates by training and education. Table 25.1 lists common sports activities and their relative injury rates.

Mechanisms of Injury

Direct trauma is a common mechanism that leads to injury. Deceleration injuries are the most common form of serious injury, resulting in significant blunt trauma or joint injury. The athlete's momentum, enhanced by self-generated speed, gravity, and equipment, is translated into energy when impact occurs. This energy is then absorbed by the body in the form of blunt trauma, torsion of joints, or transfer of stress within the skeleton.

Collision sports, such as football or rugby, and high-velocity sports, such as alpine skiing, have much higher rates of significant musculoskeletal injury due to the combination of speed and mass effect on impact. Factors that affect the extent of injury include tensile strength of the ligaments and tendons of affected joints, bony strength, flexibility, and ability of the athlete to reduce the impact.

TABLE 25.1. Common Sports Injuries and Injury Rates

Sports activity	Common injuries	Injury rate (per 1000 exposures)
Running	Tibial periostitis, stress fracture Metatarsal stress fractures	14
Football	ACL/MCL tears Shoulder dislocation/separation Ankle sprain	13
Wrestling	Shoulder dislocation MCL, LCL tears	12
Gymnastics	Spondylolysis/spondylolisthesis Ankle sprains	10
Alpine/telemark skiing	ACL/MCL tears Skier's thumb Shoulder dislocation	9
Basketball	Ankle sprains Shoulder dislocation/separation	4
Baseball	Lateral epicondylitis Rotator cuff tear	4
Cross-country skiing	Ankle sprains Lateral epicondylitis	3

ACL = anterior cruciate ligament; LCL = lateral collateral ligament; MCL = medial collateral ligament.

This is where appropriate conditioning for a sport reduces injury risk. Not only are endurance and strength training important, but also practicing falls or recovery from falls can help the athlete diffuse the energy of the fall or impact. Athletes should be encouraged to use the appropriate safety equipment and to train comprehensively for their sport.

Overuse injuries comprise the most common form of sports injuries seen by the family physician. These injuries are induced by repetitive motion leading to microscopic disruption of a bone–tendon or bone–synovium interface. This microtrauma initiates an inflammatory response. If the inflammatory response is not modulated by a rest phase or is excessive due to mechanical factors, then degradation of the tendon or bone may occur. Predisposing factors that lead to overuse injuries include poor flexibility, imbalance of strength of opposing muscle groups, mechanical deformity (e.g., pes planus), inadequate rest between exercise periods, and faulty equipment.[3] Adolescent athletes are especially vulnerable to such injuries, especially in areas where growth cartilage is present in the epiphyseal or apophyseal attachments of major muscle groups. Elderly athletes also are at higher risk because of preexisting degenerative joint disease (DJD) and poor flexibility.

Overuse injuries can be classified in four stages. Stage 1 injuries are symptomatic only during vigorous exercise and stage 2 during moderate exercise. Stage 3 injuries are symptomatic during minimal exercise, and the symptoms usually last up to 24 hours after exercise has ceased. Stage 4 injuries are painful at rest with no exercise to exacerbate the symptoms. Most overuse injuries are seen at later stages by physicians (stage 3 or 4) and require significant alteration in training schedules to allow healing of the injury. Progressive inflammation from overuse can eventually lead to tendon disruption, periostitis (stress reaction), true stress fractures, or cartilaginous degeneration. Early periostitis may only appear as a "fluffiness" of the cortical margin with compensatory cortical thickening underlying it (Fig. 25.1). In more advanced cases, the margin is clearly blurred and the cortex significantly thickened. If symptoms suggest a significant stress reaction but x-rays are negative, then a bone scan is indicated. True stress fractures can be visualized on plain film while stress reactions (periostitis) are best seen on bone scan. Because stress fractures are inflammatory in nature, the complication rates due to delayed or nonunion are higher than those with traumatic fractures.[4] The results of improper treatment of these injuries can be severe, resulting in permanent degenerative changes or deformity. The primary care provider plays an important role not only in diagnosing the injury early (and thus shortening the rehabilitation period) but also in stressing prevention with proper training guidance and timely intervention.

Traumatic Injuries

Physicians providing coverage for athletic events must recognize high-risk situations for serious injuries and evaluate the safety of the sports environment. Asking the following questions when first evaluating a patient with a traumatic injury helps suggest the correct diagnosis and focus the physical examination: During what sport did the injury occur? How did the injury occur? Where does it hurt? What aggravates the pain? Did other symptoms accompany the injury? Did swelling occur and if so, how soon? How old is the athlete? Has the athlete been injured before? Once these questions are answered, the physician should then perform a focused musculoskeletal and neurovascular exam.

Ankle Injuries

Ankle injuries are ubiquitous and constitute the most common acute musculoskeletal injury, affecting the entire spectrum of grade school to professional athletes. It is estimated that 1 million people present with ankle injuries each year, with an average cost of $300 to $900 for diagnosis and rehabilitation requiring 36 to 72 days for complete rehabilitation. Basketball players have the highest rate of ankle injuries, followed by football players and cross-country runners.[5] Eighty-five percent of athletes with ankle sprains have inversion injuries. The most common structures injured with inversion are the three lateral ligaments that support the ankle joint: the anterior and posterior talofibular ligaments, and the calcaneofibular ligament (Fig. 25.2). The other primary mechanism of ankle sprains is eversion, accounting for 15% of ankle injuries. In general, these

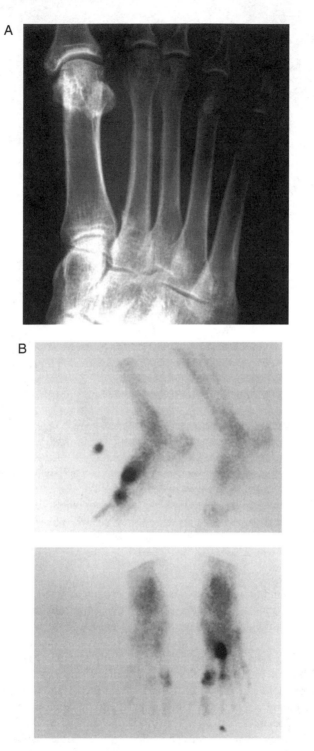

FIGURE 25.1. (A) Periostitis of the proximal second metatarsal characterized by thickening of the cortex and "fluffy" appearance of the medial margin of the cortex. (B) The confirmatory bone scan identified two areas of significant inflammation of the second metatarsal.

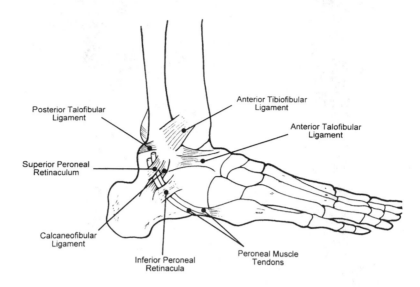

FIGURE 25.2. Lateral view of major ankle ligaments and structures.

are more severe than inversion injuries because of a higher rate of fractures and disruptions of the ankle mortise, leading to instability. The deltoid ligament is the most common ligament to be injured in eversion injuries. Fifteen percent of all complete ligament tears are associated with avulsion fractures of the tibia, fibula, talus, or the base of the fifth metatarsal. Epiphyseal growth plate injuries may be present in the young athlete who sustains an ankle injury. Clinical evidence for an epiphyseal injury of the distal fibula or tibia is bony tenderness about two finger breadths proximal to the tip of the malleolus.[6]

DIAGNOSIS

The examination in the immediate postinjury period may be limited by swelling, pain, and muscle spasm. Inspection should focus on an obvious deformity and vascular integrity. Ankle x-rays are necessary only if there is inability to bear weight for four steps both immediately and in the emergency department, or if there is bony tenderness at the posterior edge or tip of either malleoli.[7] The patient should be reexamined after the swelling has subsided, as the second examination may be more useful in pinpointing areas of tenderness. A pain-free passive and active range of motion of the ankle should be determined in all aspects of movement. The anterior drawer test should be used to assess for joint instability. A positive test, which entails the palpable and visible displacement of the foot more than 4 mm out of the mortise, is consistent with a tear of the anterior talofibular ligament and the anterior joint capsule.[8] Injuries to the lateral ligament complex are assigned grades 1, 2, or 3 depending on the amount of effusion and functional disability.

MANAGEMENT

Immediate treatment is applied according to the RICE (rest, ice, compression, and elevation) protocol.

Rest. The athlete can exercise as long as the swelling and pain are not worse within 24 hours. Exercise should include simple weight bearing. If there is pain with walking, crutches are required with appropriate instructions on use until the athlete is able to walk without pain.

Ice. Ice should be applied directly to the ankle for 20 minutes at a time every 2 hours, if possible, during the first 1 to 2 days. Icing should continue until the swelling has stopped.

Compression. Compression can be applied in the form of a horseshoe felt adhesive (0.625 cm). An elastic wrap will do but is not optimal. The compression dressing is worn for 2 to 3 days. Air stirrup braces are recommended to allow dorsiflexion and plantar flexion and effectively eliminate inversion and eversion. For grade 3 sprains, casting for 10 to 14 days may be an option.

Elevation. The leg should be elevated as much as possible until the swelling has stabilized.

ORTHOPEDIC REFERRAL

Indications for orthopedic referral include the following factors: fracture–dislocation, evidence of neurovascular compromise, penetrating wound into the joint space, and grade 3 sprain with tendon rupture. All patients with ankle injuries should begin early rehabilitation exercises, including passive range of motion and graduated strength training immediately after the injury.

Overview of Knee Injuries

It has been estimated that during each week of the fall football season at least 6000 high school and college players injure their knees, 10% of whom require surgery.[9] Even more discouraging are the results of a 20-year follow-up study of men who had sustained a knee injury in high school. The investigators found that 39% of the men continued to have significant symptoms, 50% of whom had radiographic abnormalities.[9] Knee braces, while popular, have not been proven to be effective in preventing knee ligament injuries. The best time to evaluate the knee is immediately after the injury. Within an hour of a knee injury, protective muscle spasm can prevent a reliable assessment of the joint instability. The following day there may be enough joint effusion to preclude a satisfactory examination. When evaluating knee injuries, compare the injured knee to the uninjured knee. The Pittsburgh Decision Rules delineate evidence-based guidelines for when radiographs should be obtained. In general, any sports injury that involves a fall or torsional stress to the knee resulting in an effusion would mandate a knee radiograph. Knee radiographs are necessary to rule out tibial eminence fractures, epiphyseal fractures, and osteochondral fractures. Finally, an evaluation of the neurovascular status of the leg and foot is mandatory.

Meniscus Injuries

Meniscus injuries can occur from twisting or rotation of the knee along with deep flexion and hyperextension. Symptoms include pain, recurrent effusions, clicking, and with associated limited range of motion. Meniscus flaps may become entrapped within the joint space, resulting in locking or the knee "giving out."

DIAGNOSIS

Classically, meniscus tears are characterized by tenderness or pain over the medial or lateral joint line either in hyperflexion or hyperextension. This should be differentiated from tenderness along the entire medial collateral ligament elicited when that ligament is sprained. When the lower leg is rotated with the knee flexed about 90 degrees, pain during external rotation indicates a medial meniscus injury (McMurray's test).

MANAGEMENT

After a meniscus injury, the athlete should follow the RICE protocol. Crutch usage should be insisted upon to avoid weight bearing until the pain and edema have diminished. In most athletes, an orthopedic referral should be considered for arthroscopy in order to repair the damaged meniscus. Plan for follow-up to initiate a rehabilitative program and return to sports.

Medial Collateral Ligament (MCL) Sprain

The MCL ligament is the medial stabilizer of the knee and it is usually injured by an excessive valgus stress of the knee. The resulting stress can result in a first-, second-, or third-degree sprain. MCL tears are often associated with medial meniscus injury. Lateral collateral ligament tears are unusual and are caused by an inwardly directed blow (varus force) to the inside of the knee.

DIAGNOSIS

The player is usually able to bear some weight on the leg immediately after the injury. Medial knee pain is usually felt at the time of the injury and the knee may feel "wobbly" while the player walks afterward. The examination will reveal acute tenderness somewhere over the course of the MCL, usually at or above the joint line. The integrity of the MCL is assessed by applying a valgus stress to the knee while holding the tibia about a third of the way down and forcing it gently laterally while holding the distal femur in place. A patient with a partial (grade 1 or 2) tear of a collateral ligament will have marked discomfort with valgus and varus testing. The athlete with a complete (grade 3) tear of a collateral ligament may have surprisingly little pain on testing but remarkably increased laxity of the ligament. Swelling, ecchymosis over the ligament or a joint effusion, usually develops within several hours of the injury.

MANAGEMENT

A grade 1 sprain is treated with the RICE protocol. Running should be restricted until the athlete is pain free in knee flexion. Generally in 5 to 10 days there will be complete recovery, and with physician clearance, the player can resume full activity. The management of more serious sprains should be directed by an orthopedist.

Anterior Cruciate Ligament (ACL) Injury

This is the most frequent and most severe ligament injury to the knee. It usually occurs not with a direct blow to the knee, but rather from torsional stress coupled with a deceleration injury. These injuries are seen when an athlete changes direction while running and the knee suddenly "gives out."

DIAGNOSIS

A "pop" is often felt during the injury. The player falls on the field in extreme pain and is unable to continue participating. A bloody effusion will develop in 60% to 70% of athletes within the next 24 hours. One of three tests can be employed to test for ACL insufficiency: the anterior drawer, the Lachman maneuver, or the pivot shift test. The *anterior drawer test* should be performed with the knee in 30 degrees of flexion. The injured leg is externally rotated slightly to relax the hamstrings and adductor muscles. The examiner kneels lateral to the injured leg, stabilizes the femur with one hand, and directs a gentle but firm upward force with the other hand on the proximal tibia. If the tibia moves anteriorly, then the ACL has been torn. The *Lachman test* is performed with the hamstrings relaxed and the knee placed in 15 to 20 degrees of flexion. With one hand on the femur just above the knee to stabilize it, the tibia is pulled forward with the opposite hand placed over the tibial tuberosity. If the ACL is intact, the tibia comes to a firm stop. If the ligament is torn the tibia continues forward sluggishly. A *pivot shift test* is performed with the ankle and leg held under the examiner's arm. The leg is abducted and the knee extended. Place the knee in internal rotation with gentle valgus stress to the knee. The hands are placed under the proximal tibia while the knee is flexed to about 25 degrees. If the lateral tibial condyle rotates anteriorly (subluxes forward) during the flexion maneuver, then the test is positive.

Posterior cruciate ligament injuries are usually caused by a direct blow to the upper anterior tibia or posterior forces applied to the tibia while the knee is in flexion. This might apply to a karate player who is kicked in the area of the tibial tuberosity while the foot is firmly on the ground, or to someone who falls forward onto a flexed knee. Posterior cruciate ligament tears are detected by posterior displacement of the tibial tuberosity (the *sag sign*) when the leg is held by the heel with the hip and knee flexed.

MANAGEMENT

Initial management of ACL tears follows the RICE protocol along with immobilization and crutches, with instructions on their use. The rehabilitation requires the early initiation of quadriceps contractions to prevent atrophy and promote strengthening. Protective bracing with a hinged knee brace may be appropriate for certain athletes. Referral to an orthopedist should be made acutely if there is evidence on x-ray of an avulsion fracture of the ACL attachments or subacutely for possible arthroscopic repair if there is joint laxity.

Patellar Dislocation

This injury can result from a blow to the patella or when an athlete changes direction and then straightens the leg. It is most common in athletes with significant valgus deformity of the knee joint and in adolescents.

DIAGNOSIS

The dislocation usually occurs laterally, but the medial joint capsule and retinaculum may also be torn, sometimes simulating or actually associated with a medial collateral ligament sprain. The dislocation usually reduces spontaneously and the athlete will have a painful swollen knee due to hemarthrosis and tenderness at the medial capsule. Lateral pressure on the patella while gently extending the knee will be met with obvious anxiety and resistance.

MANAGEMENT

If there is no obvious evidence of fracture, an attempted reduction of the dislocation can be made by first extending the knee. It can be helpful to massage the hamstring muscle and ask the athlete to relax it. As the patient allows more knee extension, exert gentle midline pressure directed to the lateral aspect of the patella. The patella should relocate in seconds to minutes. Difficulty with this maneuver suggests a fracture or displaced chondral fragment; the next step would be to splint the knee and refer to an emergency room for radiographs and reduction. Postreduction management follows the RICE protocol, with crutch use for those who can't bear weight. The leg should be elevated while the edema persists, with immediate quadriceps strengthening exercises to prevent atrophy.

Neck Injuries

Injuries to the head and neck are the most frequent catastrophic sports injury. The four common school sports with the highest risk of head and spine injury are football, gymnastics, ice hockey, and wrestling. Nonschool sports risks far outweigh those from organized sports. Common causes of head injuries in this group are trampoline use, cycling, and snow sports.[10] Fortunately, many neck injuries are minimal strains, diagnosed after a quick history and physical examination. Axial loading is the most common mechanism for serious neck injury. Classic examples include the football player "spearing" or tackling head first, and the hockey player sliding head first into the boards. Axial loading can produce spinal fracture, dislocation, and quadriplegia at very low impact velocities— lower than for skull fractures. Extension spinal injuries are more serious than flexion injuries. With extension spine injury (whiplash), the anterior elements are disrupted and the posterior elements are compressed. In flexion injury, the anterior elements are compressed, causing anterior vertebral body fracture, chip fracture, and occasionally anterior dislocation.

DIAGNOSIS

When an athlete is unconscious and motionless, an initial assessment is mandatory. Athletes with focal neurologic deficits or marked neck pain should be suspected of having cervical spine injury until cleared by x-ray examination.

MANAGEMENT

The ABC (airway, breathing, and circulation) of emergency care apply, along with neck stabilization and initiation of emergency transport. Cervical spine injury is assumed until proven otherwise. Proper stabilization precautions must be carried out while the athlete is removed from the playing field or injury site. If the athlete is wearing a helmet, it should not be removed until arrival in the emergency room.

Closed Head Injuries

The definition of concussion by the Neurosurgical Committee on Head Injuries is "a clinical syndrome characterized by immediate and transient posttraumatic impairment of neural function, such as the alteration of consciousness, disturbance of vision, equilibrium, etc., due to brainstem involvement."[11] There is also a complication of concussion called a " second-impact syndrome" in which fatal intracerebral edema is precipitated by a second blow to the head of an athlete who has persisting symptoms from an earlier concussion.[12] Fortunately, this syndrome is rare. If athletes have any persisting symptoms from any degree of concussion, they should not be allowed to play. Postconcussion syndrome consists of headache (especially with exertion), labyrinthine disturbance, fatigue, irritability, and impaired memory and concentration. These symptoms can persist for weeks or even months. Both football and snowboarding are common sports associated with closed head injuries.

Epidural hematoma results when the middle meningeal artery, which is embedded in a bony groove in the skull, tears as a result of a skull fracture, crossing this groove. Because the bleeding in this instance is arterial, accumulation of clot continues under high pressure and, as a result, serious brain injury can occur. Subdural hematomas are caused by the shearing forces applied to the bridging arachnoid veins that surround the brain.

Diagnosis

Reviewing the recognition and classification of concussion can simplify its management (Table 25.2). The classic description of an epidural hematoma is that of loss of consciousness in a variable period, followed by recovery of consciousness after which the patient is lucid. This is followed by the onset of increasingly severe headache; decreased level of consciousness; dilation of one pupil, usually on the same side as the clot; and decerebrate posturing and weakness, usually on the side opposite the hematoma. Patients with acute subdural hematoma are more likely to have a prolonged lucid interval following their injury and are less likely to be unconscious at admission than patients with epidural hematomas.

Management

Patients with closed head injuries need a thorough neurologic evaluation, usually including a computed axial tomography (CAT) scan or magnetic resonance

TABLE 25.2. Grading of Head Injuries and Management

Grade of concussion	Symptoms	Management
1	Brief confusion, <30 min, no LOC	No head imaging required unless focal deficit appears or LOC develops; may return to activity with head protection in 7 days
2	Prolonged amnesia or confusion, >30 min, no LOC	No head imaging required unless focal deficit appears or LOC develops; may return to activity with head protection in 21 days
3a	LOC <5 min; amnesia, confusion common	Computed tomography or magnetic resonance imaging recommended to rule out hemorrhage; no further sports activity with risk of head injury for remainder of season; helmet use in the future is strongly recommended
3b	LOC ≥5 min	

LOC = loss of consciousness.

imaging (MRI). Return to competition should be deferred until all symptoms have abated and the guidelines described in Table 25.2 have been followed. Adequate head protection in skiers, snowboarders, and football players is an appropriate prevention measure and should be mandatory if the patient has a history of a previous concussion.

Shoulder Dislocation

Shoulder dislocation may occur when sufficient impact tears the anterior joint capsule of the glenohumeral joint, resulting in a slippage of the humeral head out of the glenoid fossa. In anterior glenohumeral dislocation there are two mechanisms of injury: a fall onto an outstretched hand, or a collision with a player or object with the shoulder abducted to 90 degrees and externally rotated. While the shoulder may dislocate posteriorly, an anterior-inferior dislocation is the most common. Careful examination to rule out humeral neck fracture is important before reduction of the shoulder in the field. Small avulsion fractures can occur at the attachment of the supraspinatus tendon (Fig. 25.3), but this injury will not preclude immediate reduction of the shoulder.

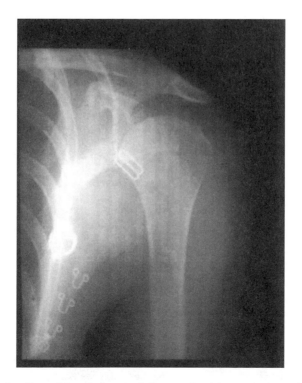

FIGURE 25.3. Small avulsion fracture of the proximal humerus in a skier who sustained a shoulder dislocation.

DIAGNOSIS

Athletes who have anterior shoulder dislocation will often state that the shoulder has "popped out" and complain of excruciating pain. The athlete is unable to rotate the arm and has a hollow region just inferior to the acromion with an anterior bulge caused by the forward displacement of the humeral head. Subluxation of the shoulder may occur when the humerus slips out of the glenohumeral socket and then spontaneously relocates. Posterior subluxations are seen more commonly in athletes who use repetitive overhand motion such as swimmers and baseball and tennis players.

MANAGEMENT

Anterior dislocation is the only shoulder injury that requires prompt manipulation. The Rockwood technique involves an assistant who applies a long, folded towel around the ipsilateral axilla, crossing the upper anterior/posterior chest. Gentle traction is applied while the physician applies in-line traction at 45 degrees abduction on the injured extremity. Traction is gradually increased over several minutes. Successful reduction will manifest as a "thunk" when the humerus relocates in the glenoid cavity. If started immediately, the dislocation should be reducible in 2 to 3 minutes. Postreduction radiographs are required. With the Stimson technique, the patient lies prone on a flat surface with the arm hanging down. A 5-pound weight is tied to the distal forearm. The reduction will usually take place within 20 minutes.[13] Scapular manipulation in a similar position has also been described as another method to relocate the shoulder with minimal traction.[13] If these attempts at early reduction are unsuccessful, reduction using analgesia or anesthesia can be attempted in the emergency room. In the patient who dislocates for the first time, the shoulder should be immobilized for 2 to 3 weeks. Rehabilitation may reduce the rate of recurrence with goals being the restoration of full shoulder abduction and strengthening of the rotator cuff muscles.[14]

Acromioclavicular (AC) Separation

Acromioclavicular separation may be caused by a direct blow to the lateral aspect of the shoulder or a fall on an outstretched arm. AC separations are classified as grades 1, 2, or 3 as determined by the involvement of the AC and/or the coracoclavicular ligaments.

DIAGNOSIS

There will be discrete tenderness at the AC joint. In grade 1 AC separation, there is tenderness to palpation at the AC joint but no visible defect. Grade 2 or grade 3 AC separation will cause a visible gap between the acromion and the clavicle. A grade 2 separation involves a partial tear of the AC ligaments; a grade 3 separation is due to a complete tear of the AC ligaments. When a grade 2 or 3 separation is suspected, a radiograph should be obtained of both shoulders to rule out fracture and to delineate the grade of separation. With grade 2 injuries, the clavicle is elevated by one half the width of the AC joint due to the disruption of the AC joint. With grade 3 injuries both the AC and coracoclavicular ligaments are disrupted with resultant dislocation of the AC joint and superior migration of the clavicle.

MANAGEMENT

Initial management of AC separations requires the shoulder to be immobilized in a sling. The extent of medical intervention is determined by the grade of the injury. Those with grade 1 and 2 injuries may be treated conservatively with sling immobilization for 7 to 14 days. When symptoms subside, controlled remobilization and strengthening of the shoulder should begin. There is ongoing controversy regarding conservative versus operative management of the grade 3 injury. An orthopedic referral should be made for these athletes.

Brachial Plexus Injury

A brachial plexus injury, or "burner" or "stinger," is a temporary dysfunction of the neural structures in the brachial plexus after a blow to the head, neck, or shoulder. Burners are reported in football, wrestling, ice hockey, skiing, motocross, soccer, hiking and equestrian sports.[15] Several mechanisms probably contribute to injuries to the brachial plexus, usually involving lateral flexion of the cervical spine with concomitant depression of one of the shoulders. Lateral flexion with rotation and extension of the cervical spine toward the symptomatic side causes a direct compression of the nerve roots, while lateral flexion with shoulder depression causes a traction injury to the nerves.[16]

DIAGNOSIS

Typically the player experiences a sharp burning pain in the shoulder with paresthesia or dysesthesia radiating into the arm and hand. The patient may have associated sensory deficits, decreased reflexes, and weakness of the deltoid, biceps, supraspinatus, or infraspinatus muscles.

MANAGEMENT

If the neurologic findings return to normal within a few minutes, the athlete may return to play. In 5% to 10% of patients, signs and symptoms will persist requiring referral to either a neurologist or a physiatrist.

Thumb and Finger Injuries

Extensor injuries of the distal phalangeal joints occur when there is avulsion of the extensor tendon from the distal phalanx with and without a fracture. This results in a "mallet "or "drop" finger. Proximal phalangeal joint injuries occur when there is avulsion of the central slip of the distal phalanx, resulting in a flexion "boutonniere" deformity. Metacarpophalangeal (MCP) joint sprain of the thumb ("gamekeeper's" thumb) is caused by a fall on an outstretched hand, causing forced abduction to the thumb.

DIAGNOSIS

The distal or proximal phalanx is flexed and lacks active extension in extensor tendon ruptures. It is imperative that any distal interphalangeal (DIP) injury be evaluated for full extension to avoid missing a extensor tendon rupture. Gamekeeper's thumb causes pain and swelling over the ulnar aspect of the MCP joint and is made worse by abducting or extending the thumb. Complete tears of the ulnar collateral ligament are demonstrated by marked laxity in full extension.

MANAGEMENT

An x-ray should be obtained in all of the above injuries to rule out intraarticular fractures or avulsions that require orthopedic referral. In extensor tendon injuries, continued splinting of the distal finger joint in extension for at least 6 weeks is necessary. The treatment for a gamekeeper's thumb requires a thumb spica cast or splint protection for 4 to 6 weeks. During activity, the thumb can be protected by taping it to the index finger to prevent excessive abduction. A complete tear of the ulnar collateral ligament requires orthopedic referral for surgical repair.[17] Minor sprains can be rehabilitated in 3 to 4 weeks.

Specific Overuse Injuries

Shoulder Impingement Syndromes

Overuse injuries of the shoulder are most commonly seen in swimming, throwing, or racquet sports. Swimmers almost uniformly develop symptoms of this injury to varying degrees, especially those swimmers who regularly perform the butterfly stroke. Repetitive motions that abduct and retract the arm followed by antegrade (overhand) rotation of the glenohumeral joint can lead to impingement of the subacromial bursa and the supraspinatus tendon. Early in the course, only the subacromial bursa may be inflamed, but with progressive injury supraspinatus tendonitis develops and may become calcified. Other muscles that make up the rotator cuff can also be strained with this motion and eventually can lead to rotator cuff tears.

DIAGNOSIS

Patients with impingement will complain of pain with abduction to varying degrees and especially with attempts to raise the arm above the level of the shoulder. The pain radiates deep from the subacromial space to the deltoid region and may be vague and not well localized. Palpation of the subacromial bursa under the coracoacromial ligament will often elicit pain deep to the acromion, as will internal rotation of the arm when abducted at 90 degrees with the elbow also flexed at 90 degrees. A second maneuver to detect impingement is to extend the arm forward so it is parallel to the ground and then internally rotate and abduct the arm across the chest while stabilizing the shoulder with the examiner's hand. Both maneuvers narrow the subacromial space to elicit symptoms. The "painful arc"—pain only within a limited range of abduction—may indicate an advanced calcific tendonitis of the supraspinatus tendon. Radiographic imaging may be useful if this finding is present, as calcific tendonitis may require more invasive treatment.

Management

Modification of shoulder activity and antiinflammatory measures [the RICE protocol, nonsteroidal antiinflammatory drugs (NSAIDs)] are instituted early. Swimmers will need to alter the strokes during their training periods and reduce the distance that they swim to the point that the pain is decreasing daily. Rehabilitation exercises should consist of both aggressive shoulder stretching to lengthen the coracoacromial ligament and improve range of motion. The use of an upper arm counterforce brace will alter the fulcrum of the biceps in such a way as to depress the humeral head further. Strength training of the supraspinatus and biceps internal and external rotator muscles should be performed to aid in depressing the humeral head when stressed, thus increasing the subacromial space. In advanced calcific tendonitis, steroid injection into the subacromial bursa or surgical removal of the calcific tendon may be required.[18]

Tennis Elbow (Lateral Epicondylitis)

Lateral epicondylitis is characterized by point tenderness of the lateral epicondyle at the attachment of the extensor carpi radialis brevis. The most common sports that cause this syndrome are tennis, racquetball, and cross-country skiing.[19] The mechanism of injury in all of the sports is the repetitive extension of the wrist against resistance. Adolescent or preadolescent athletes are at highest risk of significant injury if the growth plate that underlies the lateral epicondyle is not yet closed. If the inflammation of the epicondyle is not arrested, the soft growth cartilage can fracture and rotate the bony attachment of the extensor ligaments, requiring surgical reimplantation of the epicondyle. Without surgery, a permanent deformity of the elbow will result.

Diagnosis

Patients will complain of pain with active extension of the wrist localized to the upper forearm and lateral epicondyle. There is usually marked tenderness of the epicondyle itself. Pain with grasping a weighted cup (Canard's test) or with resisted dorsiflexion is also diagnostic. X-ray studies are not necessary but may show calcific changes to the extensor aponeurosis in chronic cases. Comparison views of the unaffected elbow may be helpful in the adolescent in whom a stress fracture is suspected and the growth plate is not yet closed. Stress fractures of the lateral epicondyle are best diagnosed with a technetium-99 (Te-99) bone scan.

MANAGEMENT

Rest, NSAIDs, and ice to the area are the initial treatment modalities. Modification of the gripped object (racquet or ski pole) with a thicker grip will reduce the stress on the extensors. A counterforce brace worn over the belly of the forearm extensors or a volar cock-up splint can be used to relieve symptoms and alter the dynamic fulcrum of the muscles. Steroid injections superficial to the aponeurosis can be used in more refractory cases but should be limited to three injections.[20] Steroids should not be used in patients who may have a stress fracture or if the growth plates have not yet closed. Gradual return to the sport may begin immediately in grade 1 or 2 injuries, or as soon as the tenderness has resolved in higher grade injuries.

Lumbar Spondylolysis/Spondylolisthesis

Spondylolysis (fracture of the pars interarticularis) of the vertebrae results from repeated forced hyperextension of the spine. Spondylolisthesis (slippage of one vertebrae over another) may result from the facet joint degeneration induced by spondylolysis. Young preadolescent gymnasts are at highest risk for developing spondylolysis but it can also be seen in weight lifters, runners, swimmers who perform the butterfly stroke, divers, and football players.[21] In one large study, up to 10% of adolescent female gymnasts had spondylolysis.[22] Spondylolisthesis usually occurs in older teens and develops primarily at the L5-S1 joint. Their prognosis is worse than those with isolated spondylolysis.

DIAGNOSIS

The athlete usually complains of unilateral back pain that worsens with rotation of the trunk. There is usually regional spasm of the paraspinous musculature and the hamstrings. Pain from spondylolisthesis may cause radicular symptoms in the L5-S1 distribution. Lateral and anteroposterior (AP) x-rays of the spine may not reveal pars interarticularis pathology so oblique films should be added. Even if the x-rays are normal, if the diagnosis is suspected, restriction of the activity is necessary until repeat films are done in 4 to 6 weeks. A Te-99 bone scan is a sensitive test for detecting pars interarticularis fractures or stress reactions.

MANAGEMENT

Rest is essential in both of these conditions. Bone scans can be used to follow the healing process but costs may be prohibitive. Resolution of symptoms is an adequate indicator of healing. The athlete may continue to train in sports that do not result in hyperextension or rotation of the spine (e.g., cycling, stair-climbing) as long as the back symptoms are improving. Referral to a physical therapist for neutral spine stability exercises is warranted.

Low-grade spondylolisthesis can be managed conservatively by restriction of activity until the pain has resolved. Serial x-rays every 4 to 6 months can monitor progression in athletes who returned to their sport after the symptoms resolved. High-grade spondylolisthesis (>25% displacement of the vertebral body) can also be managed conservatively, but the patient must be permanently restricted from contact or collision sports. Bracing or surgical repair of spondylolisthesis may be required if pain is severe or persistent nerve root irritation is present.[23]

Retropatellar (Patellofemoral) Pain Syndrome

Retropatellar pain syndrome (RPPS) is most commonly found in patients participating in running, hiking, or cycling. The symptoms probably represent the majority of knee pain complaints in athletes. Retropatellar pain is caused by the repetitive glide of the patella over the femoral condyles, which can lead to inflammation of the retropatellar synovium or the cartilage itself. The glide of the patella is usually laterally displaced in athletes who have recurrent symptoms. Factors that increase this friction are instability of the knee from previous injury, valgus deformity of the knee, deficient vastus medialis obliquus muscle strength, patella alta, or recent increase in running program. Relative valgus stress on the knee is created in patients with abnormal Q angles, pes planus, femoral anteversion, or external tibial torsion causing lateral displacement of the patella. If progressive, RPPS can progress to chondromalacia patellae with destruction of the retropatellar cartilage.

DIAGNOSIS

Patients with RPPS present with vague retropatellar or peripatellar pain, which is usually most significant several hours after exercise. Walking downhill or downstairs, bending at the knees, and kneeling exacerbates pain symptoms. In more advanced cases, pain can be constant, occur during and after exercise. Oddly, patients often experience pain if the knee is not moved enough; i.e., if left flexed for several minutes, pain will develop. The examination of the knee should first include inspection of the patient's entire leg, feet, and hips to assess for a significant Q angle, torsional deformities, leg length discrepancy, or pes planus. On palpation of the knee, the lateral posterior margins of the patella should be palpated with the patella deviated laterally to detect tenderness of the retropatellar surface. This should also be repeated on the medial aspect of the patella with medial deviation. Effusions are usually absent in RPPS. A compression test of the patella is performed with the patient relaxing and then flexing the quadriceps group while the patella is displaced distally by the examiner. Fine crepitus with this test may indicate synovial inflammation but it is not specific. Coarse crepitus or popping with significant pain is indicative of chondromalacia. Sunrise views of the knees may reveal radiographic evidence of retropatellar degeneration, but usually these findings are present only in advanced cases and are not necessary for diagnosis.[24]

MANAGEMENT

For athletes with symptoms only at higher training levels, reduction of the exacerbating activity and NSAID use are the first steps. If the patient has a grade 3 or 4 injury, then cessation of the exacerbating activity for 2 to 4 weeks until the pain is no longer present at rest is necessary. Selective strengthening of the vastus medialis obliquus (VMO), orthotics, and alteration of mechanical forces when pedaling (for cyclists) can also relieve symptoms. Lateral deviation of the foot while extending the knee allows more medial tracking of the patella during exercise and forces the VMO to perform more of the quadriceps function. Stretching to reduce both hamstring and quadriceps tension is an important component of the rehabilitation of RPPS. As with all overuse injuries, a graduated increase in exercise duration at a rate of 10% per week, with relative rest periods every 3 to 4 weeks, may prevent recurrence of the symptoms.

Tibial Periostitis ("Shin Splints")

Tibial periostitis is the most common overuse injury in recreational runners and is often confused with other lower leg pain syndromes.[25] Any pain in the tibial area is often labeled "shin splints" but must be differentiated from anterior compartment syndrome, patellar tendonitis, or a simple muscular strain. The primary cause of tibial periostitis is mechanical; the attachment of a calf muscle is strained due to the pounding of running on a mechanically deficient foot. A recent increase in duration of running often triggers shin splints if the increase is too rapid and there is no rest phase. Over 4 to 8 weeks after such increases in training, this condition progresses to involve the bone by disrupting the periosteum and cortex.

DIAGNOSIS

Most patients with this syndrome have pes planus, which results in tibialis posterior tendonitis initially. Their pain is localized to the lower third of the medial aspect of the tibia. Patients with pes cavus have anterior tibialis tendonitis with pain localized laterally on the middle or upper tibia. If other calf flexors are involved, the pain may be deep in the calf, resembling a deep vein thrombosis (DVT). Homans' sign may be positive in these patients because the posterior aspect of the tibia is inflamed. If point tenderness is present, x-ray studies are indicated, with careful attention being paid to subtle changes in the cortical margin in the area of pain.

MANAGEMENT

Table 25.3 delineates rehabilitation strategies for this injury. The importance of adequate rest and graduated resumption of exercise with cycled rest phases cannot be overemphasized.[26] Aggressive stretching of the calf muscles, twice daily icing the affected area, and NSAIDs are essential adjuncts to adjustments in the training program. Corrective arch supports for either pes planus or pes cavus are necessary if these conditions are present. Combining strength training with resumption of running will enhance tendon healing and adaptive cortical thickening.

Jones' Fractures (Proximal Fifth Metatarsal Fractures)

Overuse injuries of the foot can occur in multiple sites including the metatarsal, tarsal, and sesamoid bones. Jones' and sesamoid bone fractures have very high rates of nonunion (50–90%).[27] These stress fractures must be detected and treated early to prevent this complication. Jones' fractures are primarily seen in distance runners, especially in those with a recent increase in activity. There is usually a history of antecedent pain for several weeks at the attachment of the peroneus brevis tendon to the proximal fifth metatarsal.

TABLE 25.3. Overuse Injuries: Staging and Rehabilitation

Stage	Symptoms	Rehabilitation
1	Pain with maximal exertion, resolves after event; nonfocal exam	Decrease activity to 50–70%, ice, NSAIDs for 7 days; every other day training
2	Pain with minimal exertion, resolves in <24 hours; minimal tenderness	Decrease activity to 50%, ice, NSAIDs for 10-14 days; every other day training
3	Pain despite rest, not resolved within 48 hours; tender on exam, mild swelling of tendon	Stop activity 2–4 weeks or until pain free; ice, NSAIDs; resume training at 50%, increase by 10% per week; every 4 weeks reduce to 50%
4	Continual pain, stress fracture, point tenderness and swelling	Immobilize if indicated; rest 4–6 weeks until pain free; ice, NSAIDs; resume training at 50%, increase by 10% per week; every 4 weeks reduce to 50%

NSAID = nonsteroidal antiinflammatory drug.

DIAGNOSIS

Pain and tenderness at the site are universal. Inversion of the ankle, causing stress of the peroneus brevis tendon, or attempts to evert the foot against stress also localize pain to the proximal head of the fifth metatarsal. Radiographs may show evidence of cortical thickening, sclerotic changes within the medullary bone, or a true fracture line. The more proximal the fracture, the higher the risk of delayed union. If the radiographs are negative, but if there is significant tenderness, then a bone scan should be performed because of the high rate of false-negative radiographs for this fracture.

MANAGEMENT

All athletes with evidence of stress fracture on bone scan or sclerotic changes on x-ray should be referred for possible screw placement.[28] If there is evidence only of a periosteal reaction, without visible fracture or medullary sclerosis, the foot should be placed in a non–weight-bearing short leg cast for 4 to 6 weeks and follow-up films obtained when pain-free to ensure that healing has been complete. Despite appropriate care, avascular necrosis may occur, requiring grafting of the bone. After the fracture is healed, the athlete may gradually return to the activity, with close follow-up to prevent recurrence of symptoms.[29]

Prevention of Injuries

The primary focus of injury prevention stems from understanding the mechanisms of injury. In contact or collision sports, appropriate protective equipment is essential in reducing the severity of injuries sustained by the participants. Wearing protective helmets substantially reduces risk of head injuries in many collision sports. In sports where the risk of falls is prominent, use of wrist guards and knee pads can reduce injuries to these joints. Alpine skiers must use releasable bindings that are adjusted appropriately for their weight and skill level to reduce the risk of ligamentous knee injuries. Overuse injuries can be prevented by developing graded training programs that allow time for compensatory changes in tendons and bones to prevent inflammation. Orthotics and focused training of muscle groups can correct mechanical problems that could lead to overuse injuries.

The second aspect of injury prevention is maximizing the strength, proprioceptive skills, and the flexibility of the athlete. Appropriate off-season and preseason training of athletes, coaches, and trainers can substantially reduce injuries during the regular season.

References

1. Cook PC, Leit ME. Issues in the pediatric athlete. Orthop Clin North Am 1995; 26:453–64.
2. Patel DR. Sports injuries in adolescents. Med Clin North Am 2000;84:983–1007.

3. Brody DM. Running injuries. Clin Sym 1987;39:23–5.
4. Hulkko A, Orava S. Stress fractures in athletes. Int J Sports Med 1987;8:221–6.
5. Clanton TO, Porter DA Primary care of foot and ankle injuries in the athlete. Clin Sports Med 1997;16:435–66.
6. Brostrom L. Sprained ankles, I. Anatomic lesions in recent sprains. Acta Chir Scand 1964;128:483–95.
7. Stiell IG. Decision rules for the use of radiography in acute ankle injuries. JAMA 1993;269:1127–32.
8. Perlman M, Leveille D, DeLeonibus J, et al. Inversion lateral ankle trauma: differential diagnosis, review of the literature and prospective study. J Foot Surg 1987;26:95–135.
9. Dyment PG. Athletic injuries. Pediatr Rev 1989;10(10):1–13.
10. Proctor MR, Cantu RC. Head and spine injuries in young athletes. Clin Sports Med 2000;19:693–715.
11. Committee on Head Injury Nomenclature of the Congress of Neurological Surgeons. Glossary of head injury including some definitions of injury to the cervical spine. Clin Neurosurg 1966;12:386.
12. Cantu RC. Second impact syndrome. Physician Sports Med 1992;20:55–66.
13. Hergengroeder AC. Acute shoulder, knee and ankle injuries. Part 1: diagnosis and management. Adolesc Health Update 1996;8(2):1–8.
14. Blake R, Hoffman J. Emergency department evaluation and treatment of the shoulder and humerus. Emerg Med Clin North Am 1999;17:859–76.
15. Aronen JC, Regan K. Decreasing the incidence of recurrence of first time anterior shoulder dislocations with rehabilitation. Am J Sports Med 1984;12:283–91.
16. Archambault JL. Brachial plexus stretch injury. J Am Coll. Health 1983;31(6):256–60.
17. Vereschagin KS, Weins JJ, Fanton GS, Dillingham MF. Burners, don't overlook or underestimate them. Phys Sportsmed 1991;19(9):96–106.
18. Kahler DM, McLue FC. Metacarpophalangeal and proximal interphalangeal joint injuries of the hand, including the thumb. Clin Sports Med 1992;11:5–76.
19. Smith DL, Campbell SM. Painful shoulder syndromes: diagnosis and management. J Gen Intern Med 1992;7:328–39.
20. Safran MR. Elbow injuries in athletes: a review. Clin Orthop 1995;310:257–77.
21. Mehlhoff TL, Bennett B. The elbow. In: Mellion MB, Walsh WM, Shelton GL, eds. The team physician handbook. Philadelphia: Hanley & Belfus, 1990. p. 334–45.
22. Wilhite J, Huurman WW. The thoracic and lumbar spine. In: Mellion MB, Walsh WM, Shelton GL, eds. The team physician handbook. Philadelphia: Hanley & Belfus, 1990. p. 374–400.
23. Jackson DW, Wiltse LL. Low back pain in young athletes. Phys Sportsmed 1974;2:53–60.
24. Smith JA, Hu SS. Disorders of the pediatric and adolescent spine. Orthop Clin North Am 1999;30:487–99.
25. Davidson K. Patellofemoral pain syndrome. Am Fam Physician 1993;48:1254–62.
26. Batt ME. Shin splints—a review of terminology. Clin J Sports Med 1995;5:53–7.
27. Stanitski CL. Common injuries in preadolescent and adolescent athletes. Sports Med 1989;7:32–41.
28. Orava S, Hulkko A. Delayed unions and nonunions of stress fractures in athletes. Am J Sports Med 1988;16:378–82.
29. Lawrence SJ, Bolte MJ. Jones fractures and related fractures of the fifth metatarsal. Foot Ankle 1993;14:358–65.

CASE PRESENTATION

Subjective

PATIENT PROFILE

Kendra Nelson is a 16-year-old female high school sophomore.

PRESENTING PROBLEM

"Ankle injury."

PRESENT ILLNESS

Three hours ago, Kendra twisted her left ankle while playing basketball in the high school gym. She noted immediate pain and swelling, and she can bear almost no weight on the ankle. However, she states that "the pain is not really bad."

PAST MEDICAL HISTORY

Kendra had a similar ankle sprain about 4 months ago.

SOCIAL HISTORY, HABITS, AND FAMILY HISTORY

These are unchanged since her last office visit for viral influenza 7 months ago (see Chapter 10).

- What additional history regarding the injury might be helpful?
- How might today's problem relate to the injury 4 months ago?
- What might be significant regarding Kendra's assessment of the pain?
- What might be the meaning of this injury to Kendra? How would you inquire about this?

Objective

GENERAL

The patient hops, rather than walks, to the examination room using the left lower extremity only for balance.

VITAL SIGNS

Blood pressure, 102/64; pulse, 74.

EXAMINATION

The left ankle is swollen and ecchymotic. It is tender laterally, and there is limited range of motion. The dorsalis pedis pulse is normal.

LABORATORY

An office x-ray with routine views of the ankle reveals soft tissue injury with swelling most prominent laterally. There are no bony abnormalities, and the ankle mortise is intact.

- What more would you include in the physical examination?
- What would be evidence on physical examination to help differentiate between soft tissue injury and fracture?
- Have you seen other patients with similar findings? If so, what was the diagnostic assessment and outcome of therapy?
- What are possible complications of this injury, and how would you examine for these?

Assessment

- Based on the findings described above, what is your diagnosis? How would you explain this to Kendra?
- Describe the tissue and pathologic changes involved in this injury.
- What are the implications of this injury for the family and the school?
- If the ankle mortise seemed unstable, what would you do differently?

Plan

- What would be your therapy of this injury? How would you explain your plan to Kendra and her parents?
- Kendra asks about weight-bearing, return to school, and participation in sports. What would you advise?
- What should you tell the school about the injury? How will you communicate this information?
- What follow-up would you advise?

26
Care of the Dying Patient

FRANK S. CELESTINO

Family physicians have traditionally prided themselves on comprehensive and continuous provision of care throughout the human life cycle. When managing the terminal phases of illness, however, most clinicians have had little formal education directed at the experience of human suffering and dying.[1,2] For many physicians the task and challenge of caring for a dying patient can seem overwhelming. The aging of the United States population, the development and widespread use of life-prolonging technologies, the ascendence of managed care emphasizing the central role of the primary care physician, media attention, the growing discomfort with futile treatment, the public's interest in physician-assisted suicide and the demand for better palliation have all fueled a growing need for physicians to master the art and science of helping patients achieve death with dignity.[3–5] This need has led to a series of major initiatives to improve palliative care education for both clinicians and the public, including the Education for Physicians in End-of-Life Care Project of the American Medical Association, the Faculty Scholars in End-of-Life Care Program of the Department of Veteran Affairs, the Improving Residency Training in End-of-Life Care Program of the American Board of Internal Medicine, the Project on Death in America of the Soros Foundation, and the Last Acts Program of the Robert Wood Johnson Foundation.[3,6]

This chapter reviews the key components of a comprehensive care program for terminally ill patients (Table 26.1).[7–9] The focus is on optimum care of patients who experience prolonged but predictable dying. Classically, these individuals have had disseminated cancer. It is now recognized that a much broader array of dying patients—those with acquired immunodeficiency syndrome, end-stage renal or cardiac disease, emphysema, and degenerative neurologic diseases—deserve such comprehensive palliative care. For a more detailed discussion of the topics covered in this chapter, the reader can consult two recent theme issues that exhaustively review the cultural, spiritual, political, ethical, economic, social, and medical aspects of terminal care.[10,11]

TABLE 26.1. Components of a Comprehensive Care Plan for Dying Patients

Compassionate and professional communication of diagnosis, treatment options, and prognosis

Psychosocial support of the patient and family
    Includes developing an understanding of the cultural and religious (spiritual) meaning of suffering and death for the patient and family
    Emphasizes continuity to allay fears of abandonment

Implementation of a comprehensive, evidence-based palliative care program
    Multidisciplinary in nature (physicians, nurses, clergy, social workers, pharmacists, nutritionists, lawyers, patient advocates)
    Hospice involvement
    Establishment and clarification of advance care directives (living wills, durable power of attorney for health care, autopsy and organ donation wishes, dying in hospital versus at home), and attitudes toward physician-assisted suicide
    Pain management (WHO and ACS guidelines)
    Nonpain symptom treatment (including behavioral/psychiatric issues)
    Nutritional support

Acknowledgment and management of financial and reimbursement issues

Bereavement management

WHO = World Health Organization; ACS = American Cancer Society.

Cultural Context of Dying and Suffering

The last 50 years have witnessed the increasing medicalization of death in the United States, with most patients now dying in hospitals instead of at home.[3,9–12] The Council on Scientific Affairs of the American Medical Association (AMA)[9] has emphasized that "in the current system of care, many dying patients suffer needlessly, burden their families, and die isolated from families and community." The AMA council and others[3,6] have cited the advance directives movement, the rising public enthusiasm for euthanasia and physician-assisted suicide, the popularity of the hospice, sensationalized court cases, and the establishment of organizations such as Americans for Better Care of the Dying and the Hemlock Society as evidence of increasing uneasiness with medicine's response to dying. They call for acceptance of dying as a normal part of the human life cycle, expanded research into terminal care, educational programs for all health professionals, and better reimbursement for terminal care.[5,6]

Communication of Diagnosis, Therapy Plans, and Prognosis

Several recent reviews have highlighted a number of sources of communication difficulties with dying patients, including social factors, patient and family barriers, and issues specific to physicians.[13–17] Buckman[13] addressed two specific tasks of communication in terminal care: breaking bad news and engaging in therapeutic dialogue. His six-step protocol is a useful paradigm for all health care practitioners: (1) getting started, which includes such issues as location, eye contact, personal touch, timing, and participants; (2) finding out how much the patient already knows and understands; (3) learning how much the patient wants to know; (4) sharing appropriate amounts of information, with attention to aligning and educating; (5) responding to the patient's and family's feelings; and (6) planning ongoing care and follow-through.

There is usually no reason to provide detailed answers to questions the patient has not yet asked. The concept of gradualism—revealing the total truth in small doses as the illness unfolds—allows the patient the opportunity to develop appropriate coping strategies. However, it is important not to use euphemisms (such as swelling or lump), but to acknowledge the presence of cancer when confirmation is in hand. One must also realize that many patients do not hear the bad news accurately when it is first presented, and reexplanation is often needed.

Not only has the primacy of patient autonomy in modern medicine encouraged truth telling, but studies reveal that patients greatly prefer open, honest communication.[13-17] Overall, the drive for disclosure must be counterbalanced by the realization that the terminally ill patient struggles to maintain a sense of hope in the face of an increasingly ominous medical situation. Clinicians must continue to nurture hope in their dying patients through appropriate optimism around aspects of treatment, achievable goals, and prognosis, combined with timely praise for the patient and family's efforts to achieve spiritual healing and death with dignity. When physicians apply good communication skills (including attending to both verbal and nonverbal signals, exploring incongruent affect, and empathically eliciting patients' perspectives) and actively work to reduce barriers to mutual understanding, patients experience a reduction in both physical and psychological aspects of suffering.

One of the most difficult tasks is predicting how long the patient will live. With improved computing and statistical tools, more accurate objective estimates of survival are often available.[18] Despite these advances prognostication for many patients remains an imperfect science. One approach is to provide a conservative estimate that allows the patient and family to feel proud about "beating the odds" and exceeding expectations.

Psychosocial Support of the Patient and Family

One of the greatest challenges facing clinicians is to adequately address the multitude of psychosocial needs of dying patients and their families.[19] Kubler-Ross was one of the first to study and popularize the notion that terminally ill individuals often experience predictable stages of emotional adaptation and response to the dying process.[20] The five stages were characterized as shock and denial, anger, bargaining, depression, and acceptance. Although duration of these stages and the intensity and sequencing with which they are experienced are highly variable from one individual to the next, accurate recognition of the patient's psychological stage allows the clinician to optimize communication, support, and empathy to meet new needs as they arise.

In addition to the needs delineated in Table 26.1, and the desire for truth telling and a sense of hopefulness, dying patients above almost all else want assurance that the physician (and others) will not abandon them.[21] There is often great fear of dying alone in an environment separated from loved ones and worry about being repulsive to others because of loss of control over bodily functions. Terminally ill patients often seek physical expressions of caring, such as touching, hugging, and kissing. Regardless of their formal involvement with organized religion, they also often seek closure on the spiritual issues of their lives. Many individuals find great solace in life review: the pleasures, pains, accomplishments, and regrets. Most desire some input into making decisions about their care. The above list of concerns applies as much to the family as to the patient. Although in many circumstances family members are critical to the success of terminal care, one must recognize not only caregiver depression and burnout but also dysfunctional family relationships that impede successful physician management.

An often underappreciated aspect of successful supportive care is developing understanding of the symbolic meaning of suffering and dying for the individual patient. Experiences of illness and death and beliefs about the appropriate role of healers are profoundly influenced by a patient's cultural[22] and religious[19,22,23] background. Efforts to use racial or ethnic background alone as predictors of beliefs or behaviors may lead to stereotyping of patients and culturally insensitive care for the dying. Koenig and Gates-Williams[24] provide a protocol to assess the impact of culture. They recommend assessing, in addition to ethnicity, (1) the vocabulary most appropriate for discussing the illness and death; (2) who has decision-making power—the patient or the larger family unit; (3) the relevance of religious beliefs (death, afterlife, miracles, sin); (4) the attitude toward dead bodies; (5) issues of age, gender, and power relationships within both the family and the health care team; and (6) the patient's political and historical context (e.g., poverty, immigrant status, past discrimination).

Comprehensive Palliative Care

At some point in the course of a chronic illness, it becomes clear that further therapeutic efforts directed at cure or stabilization are futile. Emphasis then shifts from curative to palliative care with an enhanced focus on optimal function and quality of life. According to the World Health Organization (WHO), palliative care "affirms life, regards dying as a normal process, neither hastens nor postpones death, provides relief from pain and other distressing symptoms, integrates the psychological and spiritual aspects of care, offers a support system to help patients live as actively as possible until death and provides support to help the family cope during the patient's illness and in their own bereavement."[25]

Hospice

In the United States, palliative care is most effectively provided by the now more than 2000 hospice organizations that coordinate the provision of high-quality interdisciplinary care to patients and families much more effectively and efficiently than most physicians could do on their own.[26] The first hospice was opened in South London by Dr. Cicely Saunders in 1967, with the concept first appearing in America by 1974. Philosophically, the objectives of hospice and palliative care are the same. Hospice care, which is provided regardless of ability to pay, has grown from an alternative health care movement to an accepted part of the American health care system, with Medicare reimbursement beginning in 1982. Hospice organizations provide a highly qualified, specially trained interdisciplinary team of professionals (nurses, pharmacists, counselors, pastoral care, patient care coordinators, volunteers) who work together to meet the physiologic, psychological, social, spiritual, and economic needs of patients and families facing terminal illness.[26] Classically, more than 80% of hospice patients have had disseminated cancer, but in recent years patients with chronic diseases that are deemed inevitably terminal within 6 months have become eligible as well. The hospice team collaborates continuously with the patient's attending physician (who must certify the terminal condition), to develop and maintain a patient-centered, individualized plan of care. Hospice medical services and consultation are available 24 hours a day, 7 days a week, though minute-to-minute personal care of the patient by the hospice team is not feasible and must be provided by family or volunteers. Hospice care, though aimed at allowing the patient to remain at home if desired, continues uninterrupted should the patient need acute hospital care or a hospice inpatient unit.

Advance Directives

Because it is now possible to keep sick patients alive longer at greater cost with lesser quality of life, patients and physicians have welcomed the emphasis on advance directives planning. *Advance directive* is an "umbrella" term that refers to any directive for health care made in advance of serious, cognition-impairing illness that robs the patient of decision-making capability.

Two general types of directive are widely recognized.[27] With the instructional type the patient specifies in writing certain circumstances and, in advance, declines or accepts specific treatments. The second type involves appointment of a health care agent, a person to whom is delegated all authority about medical decisions. Each type of directive has its strengths and drawbacks, and they should be seen as complementary, not competitive.

The advance directives movement seems to fit well with an emphasis on patient autonomy and the economic reality of needing to conserve health costs. Unfortunately, studies have revealed that advance directives may make little difference in the way patients are treated at the end of life and reduce costs only modestly.[28,29] Similar drawbacks have applied to the Patient Self-Determination

Act, which when implemented in 1991 was designed to encourage competent adults to complete advance directives and to help identify those patients who previously had executed such documents on admission to acute or long-term facilities. Nonetheless, in practice the discussions among physician, patient, and family leading up to establishment of a formal directive are often of greater importance than the documents themselves. When a terminally ill patient calmly discusses foreseeable events and choices leading up to death, the effect on anxious family members can be dramatic and salutary. Such discussions ideally occur relatively early after a terminal illness is diagnosed so as to avoid a crisis situation in which the patient becomes incapacitated and the family must assume responsibility for clinical decisions in the absence of knowledge about their loved one's preferences. State statutes vary widely regarding living wills and health care proxies as well as the authority granted to close friends or family members in the common situation where an incapacitated person has left no advance directives.

Physicians must realize that most dying patients at some point contemplate suicide and that a small but significant number, in one way or another, will ask their physicians to help hasten death.[30,31] With the publicity surrounding doctor-aided suicides in Michigan and the onslaught of state and federal judicial and legislative activity concerning physician-assisted suicide (PAS), clinicians caring for dying patients must explore their own moral stance in this challenging area so as to deal more effectively with patient suffering. Fortunately, approval of PAS in Oregon (and the Netherlands) has greatly stimulated clinicians' interest in palliative care, especially when abuses of the PAS process are uncovered.[31]

Inherent in any discussion of advance directives is the concept of the loss of "decision-making capacity." This catch-phrase obscures the fact that in common practice decisional capacity is difficult to assess. The elements of capacity seem straightforward: Can the person indicate a choice and do so free of coercion? Can the person manipulate relevant information meaningfully and understand the consequences of choosing each of the options? Searight[32] published a helpful, clinically relevant interview framework for assessing patient medical decision-making capacity. Such approaches verify that early dementia does not by itself usually prevent patients from participating in advance directives discussions.

Pain Management

Symptom management, especially achieving pain relief (see Chapter 5), remains the first priority for the attending physician and palliative care team.[3,7–9,25,33–35] Without effective control of pain and other sources of physical distress, quality of life for the dying patient is unacceptable, and progress on the psychological work of dying is aborted. The very prospect of pain induces fear in the patient, and frustration, anxiety, fatigue, insomnia, boredom, and anger contribute to a lowered threshold for pain. Thus treatment of the entire patient contributes to pain control.

Despite decades of evidence that physicians can and should be successful in controlling cancer pain, studies continue to reveal undertreatment and multiple barriers to effective cancer pain management.[6,33-35] Physicians have been guilty of inadequate knowledge of pain therapies, poor pain assessment, overconcern about controlled substances' regulations, and fear of patient addiction and tolerance. On the other hand, patients may be reluctant to report pain accurately. The health care system also presents impediments by giving cancer pain treatment low priority and inadequate reimbursement, along with restrictive regulation of controlled substances.

Pain during terminal illness and with cancer may be of two types: (1) nociceptive (somatic/visceral) and (2) neuropathic.[25,33-35] Somatic/visceral pain arises from direct stimulation of afferent nerves due to tumor infiltration of skin, soft tissue, or viscera. Somatic pain is often described as dull or aching and is well localized. Bone and soft tissue metastases are examples of somatic pain. Visceral pain tends to be poorly localized and is often referred to dermatomal sites distant from the source of the pain.

Neuropathic pain results from injury to some element of the nervous system because of the direct effect of the tumor or as a result of cancer therapy (surgery, irradiation, or chemotherapy). Examples include brachial or lumbosacral plexus invasion, spinal nerve root compression, or neuropathic complications of drugs such as vincristine. Neuropathic pain is described as sharp, shooting, shocklike, or burning and is often associated with dysesthesias. Unlike somatic/visceral pain, neuropathic pain may be relatively less responsive to opioids, whereas antidepressants, anticonvulsants, or local anesthetics may have good efficacy.

An optimum pain management program includes assessing the pathophysiology of the patient's pain, taking a pain history, noting response to prior therapies, discussing the patient's goals for pain control, assessing psychosocial contributors to pain, and frequently reevaluating the patient after changes in treatment. Use of visual analogue or other pain scales is particularly useful for initial assessment and follow-up. This technique is in keeping with the new Joint Commission on Accreditation of Healthcare Organizations (JCAHO) standards of pain assessment, which encourage viewing pain as a vital sign.

Classically, the management of pain in terminally ill patients has involved multiple modalities: analgesic drugs, psychosocial and emotional support, palliative irradiation and surgery, and anesthesia-related techniques, such as nerve blocks, which can be both diagnostic and therapeutic.[33-35] Sometimes chemotherapy, radiopharmaceuticals, or hormonal therapies are of some help with cancer pain.

Analgesics are the mainstay for management of cancer and terminal illness pain. Traditionally, they have been classified into three broad categories: nonopioids (aspirin, acetaminophen, nonsteroidal antiinflammatory agents), opioids (with morphine the prototype), and adjuvant analgesics (antidepressants, anticonvulsants, local anesthetics, capsaicin, corticosteroids, and neuroleptics).

Because patients with advanced disease often have mixed types of pain, drugs from different classes are often combined to achieve optimal pain relief. This concept, together with the principle of using the simplest dosing schedule and the least-invasive modalities first, form the basis for WHO's "analgesic ladder" approach to pain management.[25] This approach, which has been validated in clinical trials worldwide and championed by other agencies,[25] recommends nonopioids for mild to moderate pain (step 1), adding opioids (including tramadol) for persistent or increasing pain (step 2), and finally increasing the opioid potency or dose as the pain escalates (step 3). At each step, adjuvant medications are considered based on the underlying causes of the pain. The ladder-based protocol should not be seen as rigid, as therapy must always be individualized, with doses and intervals carefully adjusted to provide optimal relief of pain with minimal side effects.

Although many opioid analgesics exist, morphine remains the gold standard. Morphine has a simple metabolic route with no accumulation of clinically significant active metabolites. There are a wide variety of preparations, making it easy to titrate or change routes of administration. When switching narcotics or routes of administration, physicians must be familiar with the well-publicized charts of equianalgesic dosing equivalents.[33–35]

Regardless of the choice of specific drug, doses should be given on a regular schedule, by the clock, to maintain steady blood levels. Additional rescue doses can be superimposed as needed on the baseline regimen. Transdermal fentanyl has been another option for achieving steady-state blood levels.

There is no ceiling effect for morphine dosing. The hallmark of tolerance development is shortening of the duration of analgesic action. Physical dependence is expected, and addiction is rare. Sharp increases in dosage requirements usually imply worsening of the underlying disease. Opioid side effects—constipation, nausea, vomiting, mental clouding, sedation, respiratory depression—are watched for vigilantly, anticipated, and prevented if possible. Constipation is so pervasive an issue that all patients on opioids should be started on a bowel management regimen that may include fluid, fiber, stool softeners, laxatives, enemas, or lactulose.

Regarding adjuvants, corticosteroids provide a range of effects, including mood elevation, antiinflammatory activity, antiemetic effects, appetite stimulation (helpful with cachexia), and reduction of cerebral and spinal cord edema. They may be helpful for bone and nerve pain. Megestrol may also stimulate appetite. Antidepressants in lower doses (e.g., 10–100 mg of the prototype amitriptyline) and anticonvulsants (especially gabapentin) help alleviate neuropathic pain and provide innate analgesia as well as potentiation of opioids. In standard doses the antidepressants are mood elevating, with particularly promising results achieved with the newer selective serotonin reuptake inhibitors. Psychostimulants (e.g., methylphenidate) may be useful for reducing opioid-induced respiratory depression and sedation when dosage adjustment is not feasible. Bisphosphonates and radiopharmaceuticals can be helpful with bone pain.

Physical and psychosocial modalities can be used with drugs to manage pain during all phases of treatment. Physical modalities include cutaneous stimulation, heat, cold, massage, pressure, gentle exercise, repositioning, biofeedback, transcutaneous electrical nerve stimulation, aroma therapy, acupuncture, and even immobilization (casting). A variety of cognitive-behavioral interventions can also be employed: relaxation, guided imagery, distraction, reframing, psychotherapy, and support groups.

Nonpain Symptom Management

Dying patients struggle with numerous losses and fears that are exacerbated by debilitating and often demeaning nonpain symptoms, including nausea, vomiting, anorexia, diarrhea, bowel impaction, depression, anxiety, delirium, cough, dyspnea, visceral or bladder spasms, hiccups, decubiti, and xerostomia. To preclude unnecessary suffering, clinicians must utilize diverse methods to optimize palliative care and provide a relatively symptom-free death.[3,7–9,36] Morphine is of particular help with dyspnea.[33] The key is to search for reversible causes of these diverse symptom complexes before resorting to medication management, which in extreme cases of unrelieved suffering can include legally and morally sanctioned "terminal" sedation (the so-called double-effect phenomenon).[7–9,36]

Anorexia with decreased intake is distressing to families. In addition, concerns about providing adequate nutrition and hydration have arisen on both a moral and symptom relief basis. Studies have revealed that hunger is a rare symptom, and that thirst and dry mouth are usually easily managed with local mouth care and sips.[10,11,37] Thus food and fluid administration are now thought not to play a significant role in providing comfort to terminally ill patients, nor is such provision thought to be morally mandated (though the symbolic meaning of feeding efforts should not be overlooked). Interestingly, force feeding and total parenteral nutrition tend to shorten survival, and tube feedings do not decrease aspiration risk.[37]

Bereavement and Grief

Most family members suffer psychologically during the dying of a loved one and then go through an expected process of bereavement. A multitude of feelings—shock, disbelief, a general numbing of all affect, protest, relief, guilt, anguish, emotional lability, tearfulness—accompany the first days to weeks of grieving, eventually giving way to less intense feelings that in normal circumstances are largely resolved within 1 year. The mourning period is a time of physical vulnerability, with bereaved persons likely to suffer impaired immune status and behavioral problems.[38]

The family physician is often best situated to provide ongoing bereavement services. The 13-month bereavement support offered by hospice agencies and community grief support groups can be utilized. Key tasks for the physician providing care to the bereaved include validating and normalizing feelings, not medicating emotions simply because they are intense, assessing the progress of the family's grief work, identifying and intervening in abnormal grief, and using age-appropriate models and interactional styles.[38] Short-acting benzodiazepines can be helpful during the first 1 to 2 weeks if family members need relief from sleeplessness and extreme tearfulness.

Special Needs of Dying Children

Although most of the previously mentioned principles of comprehensive terminal care apply equally well to dying children, several additional considerations should be emphasized.[39,40] Communication must include age and developmentally appropriate vocabulary. Although most children do not develop an accurate understanding of dying until age 7 to 8, those as young as 4 to 5 recognize that they are gravely ill. Physicians should openly discuss with parents what role they wish to play in discussions of diagnosis, prognosis, and death.

Multidisciplinary hospice involvement may be even more important for children than adults. Likewise, studies have verified that most terminally ill children, as well as their families, fare better when the caring and dying occur at home.[39,40] Clinicians must remain cognizant of sibling issues such as feelings of neglect or jealousy. Siblings may need reassurance that they are not in some way responsible for the child's dying. In general, siblings should be encouraged to participate in the care of their dying loved one.

Conclusion

The challenge in providing terminal care is to form an accurate understanding of the needs and preferences of the dying patient and to fit the delivery of care to those needs. The fundamental rule is that good care involves giving patients options and some sense of control. Physicians must realize that patients' needs are shaped in unusual ways by factors (cultural and religious) that fall outside the comfortable biomedical domain.

References

1. Billings JA, Block S. Palliative care in undergraduate medical education. JAMA 1997;278:733–8.
2. Rabow MW, Hardie GE, Fair JM, McPhee SJ. End-of-life care content in 50 textbooks from multiple specialties. JAMA 2000;283:771–8.
3. Cassell CK, Field MJ, eds. Approaching death: improving care at the end of life. Washington, DC: National Academy Press, 1997.
4. Block SD, Bernier GM, Crawley LM, for the National Consensus Conference on Medical Education for Care Near the End of Life. Incorporating palliative care into primary care education. J Gen Intern Med 1998;13:768–73.
5. Mularski RA. Educational agenda for interdisciplinary end of life curricula. Crit Care Med 2001;29(2 suppl):N16–23.
6. Emmanuel LL, von Gunten CF, Ferris FD. Gaps in end-of-life care. Arch Fam Med 2000;9:1176–80.
7. Task Force on Palliative Care. Precepts of palliative care. J Palliat Med 1998;1: 109–12.
8. Cassell CK, Foley KM, eds. Principles for care of patients at the end of life: an emerging consensus among the specialties of medicine. New York: Millbank Memorial Fund, 1999.

9. Council on Scientific Affairs, American Medical Association. Good care of the dying patient. JAMA 1996;275:474–8.
10. Winker MA, Flanagin A, eds. Theme issue: end-of-life care. JAMA 2000;284:2413–528.
11. Matzo ML, Lynn J, eds. Death and dying. Clin Geriatr Med 2000;16:211–398.
12. Fox EJ. Predominance of the curative model of medical care. JAMA 1999;278:761–3.
13. Buckman R. How to break bad news: a guide for health care professionals. Baltimore: Johns Hopkins University Press, 1992.
14. Siegler EL, Levin BW. Physician–older patient communication at the end of life. Clin Geriatr Med 2000;16:175–204.
15. von Gunten CF, Ferris FD, Emanuell LL. Ensuring competency in end of life care—communication and relational skills. JAMA 2000;284:3051–7.
16. Balaban RB. A physician's guide to talking about end of life care. J Gen Intern Med 2000;15:195–200.
17. Quill TE. Initiating end of life discussions with seriously ill patients: addressing the "elephant in the room." JAMA 2000;284:2502–7.
18. Christakis NA. Death foretold: prophecy and prognosis in medical care. Chicago: University of Chicago Press, 2000.
19. Block SD. Psychological considerations, growth, and transcendence at the end of life—the art of the possible. JAMA 2001;285:2898–905.
20. Kubler-Ross E. On death and dying. New York: Macmillan, 1969.
21. Singer PA, Martin DK, Kelner M. Quality end of life care: patient perspectives. JAMA 1999;281:163–8.
22. Vincent JL. Cultural differences in end of life care. Crit Care Med 2001;29(2 suppl):N52–5.
23. Daaleman TP, VandeCreek L. Placing religion and spirituality in end of life care. JAMA 2000;284:2514–7.
24. Koenig BA, Gates-Williams J. Understanding cultural differences in caring for dying patients. West J Med 1995;163:244–9.
25. Jadad AR, Bowman GP. The WHO analgesic ladder for cancer pain management. JAMA 1995;274:1870–3.
26. Lynn J. Serving patients who may die soon—the role of hospice and other services. JAMA 2001;285:925–32.
27. Fischer GS, Arnold RM, Tulsky JA. Talking to the older adult about advance directives. Clin Geriatr Med 2000;16:239–54.
28. Lynn J. Rethinking fundamental assumptions: SUPPORT's implications for future reform. J Am Geriatr Soc 2000;48:S214–21.
29. Emanuel EJ. Cost savings at the end of life: what do the data show? JAMA 1996;275:1907–14.
30. Emanuell LL. Facing requests for physician-assisted suicide—toward a practical and principled clinical skill set. JAMA 1998;280:643–7.
31. Nuland SB. Physician-assisted suicide and euthanasia in practice. N Engl J Med 2000;342:583–4.
32. Searight HR. Assessing patient competence for medical decision making. Am Fam Physician 1992;45:751–9.
33. Cherny NI. The management of cancer pain. CA 2000;50:70–116.
34. Abrahm JL. Advances in pain management for older adult patients. Clin Geriatr Med 2000;16:269–311.
35. Chang HM. Cancer pain management. Med Clin North Am 1999;83:711–36.

36. Bruera E, Neumann CM. Management of specific symptom complexes in patients receiving palliative care. Can Med Assoc J 1998;158:1717–26.
37. Huang Z, Ahronheim C. Nutrition and hydration in terminally ill patients: an update. Clin Geriatr Med 2000;16:313–25.
38. Casarett D, Kutner JS, Abrahm J, for the ACP-ASIM End of Life Consensus Panel. Life after death—a practical approach to grief and bereavement. Ann Intern Med 2001;134:208–15.
39. Masri C, Farrell CA, Lacroix J, Rocker G, Shesnie SD. Decision-making and end of life care in critically-ill children. J Palliat Care 2000;16(suppl):S45–52.
40. American Academy of Pediatrics Committee on Bioethics and Committee on Hospital Care. Palliative care for children. Pediatrics 2000;106:351–7.

Case Presentation

Subjective

Patient Profile

Samuel Nelson is a 48 year old single male farm worker.

Presenting Problem

"Weight loss and shortness of breath"

Present Illness

Samuel Nelson is brought to the office by his mother, who has been concerned about her son's recent loss of some 25 pounds in weight. He has also been coughing more than usual, and the cough has been productive of blood-streaked sputum over the past few weeks. For the past 10 days, he has been unable to work because of weakness.

Past Medical History

Mr. Nelson is a heavy smoker and has had chronic obstructive pulmonary disease for more than 5 years. He had pneumonia treated as an outpatient 3 years ago.

Social History, Habits, and Family History

These were recorded at his last visit about 7 months ago (See Chapter 13) and there has been no change since that time.

- What are the diagnostic possibilities at this stage of the visit?
- What additional data might help clarify what is wrong with this patient?
- What might be the significance of the patient being unable to work?
- What might be the relevance of the mother accompanying her adult son to this office visit?

Objective

Vital Signs

Height, 5 ft, 10 in; weight, 154 lb; blood pressure, 110/62; pulse, 92; respirations, 36; temperature, 37.2°C.

EXAMINATION

The patient is sitting on the edge of the examination table, pale and short of breath. He appears chronically ill, with evidence of recent weight loss. The eyes appear sunken and the oral cavity is slightly dry. There is a palpable left supraclavicular lymph node with a diameter of approximately 3 cm. Breathing is labored; on examination of the chest, there are decreased breath sounds and dullness to percussion at the apex posteriorly and at the left lung base. The heart rate is 90-94 beats per minute with a regular sinus rhythm and no murmur audible. The liver is enlarged 2 to 3 centimeters below the right costal margin.

LABORATORY AND DIAGNOSTIC IMAGING

A chest roentgenogram performed in the office reveals a 6 by 8 centimeter mass in the left lung apex, with prominent hilar adenopathy and a pleural effusion at the left costophrenic sulcus. An office hemoglobin level is 9.4 grams/dl.

- What more—if anything—should be recorded in the physical examination? Why?
- What further diagnostic tests should be performed?
- What are the likely implications of these findings and what would you tell the patient and his mother today?
- What would you do next?

CONTINUING CARE

Upon your referral, Mr. Nelson was examined and treated at the regional medical center. Extensive testing, including needle biopsy of the lung lesion, revealed adenocarcinoma of the left lung with pleural effusion and widespread metastasis including bone, liver and brain. Following a course of palliative therapy, the patient has been returned to you for terminal care.

Assessment

- The patient and his family ask about the outlook for the weeks and months ahead. How would you respond?
- Mr. Nelson's sister, a paralegal employed by a local legal firm, asks about the relationship between the patient's lung cancer and his exposure to pesticides and other chemicals in his work. How would you respond?
- What are some of the implications of this disease for the family?

- What are some symptoms or physical findings—if they develop—that you would consider especially worrisome? Explain.

Plan

- You sense that the patient and family are concerned that they will be somehow left on their own to deal with the illness and eventual death. How can you reassure them?
- Mr. Nelson reports that he has pain in the mid-back that has awakened him from sleep the past few nights. How would you deal with this problem?
- How would you address the issue of advance directives with this patient and family?
- What might be the role of hospice in the care of this patient? When and how would you discuss this with the family?
- When this patient eventually dies, how do you believe you will feel and how will you deal with your feelings?

27

The Family Physician's Role in Responding to Biological and Chemical Terrorism

Alan L. Melnick

The September 11, 2001 events in New York City and Washington D.C. abruptly changed our perspectives about the likelihood that terrorists could direct weapons of mass destruction against civilian communities in the United States. On October 4, 2001, the Centers for Disease Control and Prevention (CDC) and their state and local partners reported a case of inhalational anthrax in Florida.[1] Over the following several weeks, public health authorities reported additional cases from Florida and New York City. Investigations revealed that the intentional release of *Bacillus anthracis* was responsible for these cases.[2] By November 9, 22 cases (17 confirmed and 5 suspected) of bioterrorism-related anthrax were reported from Washington D.C., Florida, New Jersey and New York City.[3] Ten of these cases were the inhalational form, resulting in 4 deaths; the other 12 cases were cutaneous anthrax. Of the 10 inhalation cases, most were people who had processed, handled, or received letters containing *B. anthracis* spores.

The association of anthrax with mail increased the level of public alarm. State and territorial public health officials responding to a CDC survey from September 11 through October 17 estimated their health departments had received 7000 reports of potential bioterrorist threats. Potential threats included suspicious packages, letters containing powder, and potential dispersal devices. Nearly 5,000 of these reports required telephone follow-up and about 1,000 of the reports led to testing of suspicious materials at a public health laboratory.[4] Public health officials were not alone. Patients deluged physicians' offices with concerns about suspicious envelopes and packages and concerns about anthrax symptoms. Although only four areas of the United States had identified bioterrorism-associated anthrax infections, physicians and public health officials across the nation were obliged to respond to bioterrorist hoaxes and threats, as well as anxious patients.

These events illustrate how family physicians and other primary care physicians have been and will be on the front line in detecting and responding to terrorist threats and events. This chapter will provide information useful for understanding the role of family physicians in responding to biologic and chemical terrorism including:

- The features of terrorist attacks distinguishing them from other forms of disasters

- The type of biologic or chemical agent terrorists are likely to use
- The clinical manifestations of these agents, including the routes of exposure
- How to identify patients at risk of exposure
- How to prevent disease in those exposed
- How to treat terrorist-caused illness
- How to work with local and state public health authorities in detecting and responding to terrorist caused illness
- Resources available for families traumatized by terrorism

Features of Terrorist Biologic Attacks

Historically, most planning for an emergency response to terrorism has focused on overt attacks with immediate effects, such as bombings and attacks using chemicals. In comparison to chemicals and explosives, the impact of biologic agents is more likely to be covert and delayed. As the recent anthrax events demonstrated, biologic agents do not have an immediate impact due to the interval between exposure and the onset of illness (the incubation period).[5] Because of ongoing disease transmission, biologic agents can result in continuing onset of new cases at multiple locations. Consequently, the most likely first responders to future biologic attacks will be family physicians and other health care providers.

Family physicians must be vigilant for indications that terrorists have released a biologic agent. These indications include:[6]

1. An unusual temporal or geographic cluster of illness. For example, the occurrence of similar symptoms in people who attended the same public event or gathering or patients presenting with clinical signs and symptoms suggestive of an infectious disease outbreak should raise suspicion. One indication may be two or more patients presenting with an unexplained febrile illness associated with sepsis, pneumonia, respiratory failure, rash, or a botulism-like syndrome with flaccid muscle paralysis. Suspicion should be heightened if these symptoms occurred in previously healthy persons.
2. An unusual age distribution for common diseases. For example, an increase in what looks like chicken pox in adult patients, but may be smallpox.
3. A large number of cases of acute flaccid paralysis with prominent bulbar palsies, suggestive of a release of botulinum toxin.

Biologic Agents Terrorists are Likely to Use

Terrorists can choose from countless biological agents, and the list can seem overwhelming. However, to best protect our patients and their families, family physicians should focus their attention on the agents that terrorists are most likely to use and that have the greatest potential for mass casualties. The CDC has defined three categories of biologic agents, "A," "B," and "C" with potential as weapons, based on several criteria:[5]

- Ease of dissemination or transmission
- Potential for major public health impact such as high mortality
- Potential for public panic and social disruption
- Requirements for public health preparedness

Based on these criteria, Category A contains seven agents of highest concern for the CDC:

- *Bacillus anthracis* (Anthrax)
- *Yersinia pestis* (Plague)
- *Variola major* (Smallpox)
- *Clostridium botulinum* toxin (Botulism)
- *Francisella tularensis* (Tularemia)
- Filoviruses (Ebola hemorrhagic fever, Marburg hemorrhagic fever)
- Arenaviruses (Lassa [Lassa fever], Junin [Argentine hemorrhagic fever], and related viruses).

This Chapter will focus on these biologic agents. Those interested in additional information on agents not covered in this chapter, including those in Categories B and C, should visit the CDC web site at http://www.bt.cdc.gov (last accessed 6/22/02).

Anthrax

Exposure Evaluation

An adequate history is the most essential step in the clinical evaluation for anthrax. When taking a history, family physicians should ask questions regarding the patient's concern about exposure with two goals in mind:

- First, assess the probability of exposure. By doing so, physicians can determine whether the patient is at risk for anthrax disease, whether to notify public health officials and law enforcement agencies and whether to begin preventive or curative treatment. Given the volume of patient telephone calls, physicians should consider training their nursing staff to triage the calls to reduce the number of patients requiring evaluation that is more extensive.
- Second, review with the patient his/her level of risk. If patients come to the office for further evaluation, the visit provides opportunities to educate patients and the public on how to evaluate their risk and how to take reasonable measures to protect themselves and their families.

Over a telephone call or during an office visit, questions physicians and their staff should ask their patients include:

- Have you been exposed to a situation where anthrax transmission has been confirmed or under investigation?
- Have you had any contact with a substance believed to be contaminated with anthrax?
- When, where and under what circumstances did the contact occur?
- What was the nature of the contact (skin, inhalation, ingestion)?
- Was any powder suspended in the air?
- Did other people come into contact with the substance?
- Were you exposed to a suspicious package/mail item? If so, why was it suspicious?
- Were you exposed to something else, why do you believe it was contaminated?
- Where is the substance/package? Is it contained safely (e.g., in a plastic zip-lock bag)?

Law enforcement authorities have released guidelines on identification of packages/envelopes potentially contaminated with anthrax. Characteristics of suspicious packages include:

- Inappropriate or unusual labeling
- Excessive postage
- Handwritten or poorly typed addresses
- Misspellings of common words
- Strange return address or no return address
- Incorrect titles or title without a name
- Not addressed to a specific person
- Marked with restrictions, such as "Personal," "Confidential," or "Do not x-ray"
- Marked with any threatening language
- Postmarked from a city or state that does not match the return address
- Powdery substance felt through or appearing on the package or envelope
- Oily stains, discoloration, or odor
- Lopsided or uneven envelope
- Excessive packaging material such as masking tape, string, etc.
- Excessive weight
- Ticking sound
- Protruding wires or aluminum foil

Anthrax: Clinical Presentation

Anthrax can present as one of three types of infection in humans: inhalational, cutaneous and gastrointestinal. Cutaneous anthrax is the most common naturally occurring form, with about 224 cases reported between 1944 and 1994 in the United Sates. Until the recent terrorist attacks, inhalational anthrax had not been reported since 1978. Gastrointestinal anthrax, which follows ingestion of insufficiently cooked contaminated meat, is relatively uncommon. This chapter will focus on inhalational and cutaneous forms of the disease.

Inhalational Anthrax

Inhalational anthrax results from the deposition of spores into the alveolar spaces. Inhalational anthrax does not cause a typical bronchopneumonia, so the term anthrax pneumonia is misleading. Postmortem study of those who died following the 1979 accidental release of anthrax spores in Sverdlovsk (in the former Soviet Union) revealed hemorrhagic thoracic lymphadenitis and hemorrhagic mediastinitis in all patients. About half of the patients had hemorrhagic meningitis as well. The clinical presentation of inhalational anthrax is in two stages. Patients first develop nonspecific symptoms, including fever, dyspnea, cough, headache, vomiting, chills, weakness, abdominal pain and chest pain. Signs of illness and laboratory studies are nonspecific during the first stage, which could last from hours to a few days. The second stage develops abruptly, with sudden fever, dyspnea, diaphoresis (often drenching) and shock. Stridor may result from massive lymphadenopathy and expansion of the mediastinum. A chest radiograph most often shows a widened mediastinum consistent with lymphadenopathy.[7]

The mortality rate of occupationally acquired inhalational anthrax cases in the United States is 89%, but most of these cases occurred before the development of critical care units, and in some cases, before the advent of antibiotics. During the October 2001 terrorist-caused outbreak, 6 out of 10 of the early inhalational anthrax cases survived, signifying that early diagnosis and treatment is critical to improving survival.

Many patients with a low risk of exposure but concerned about anthrax will have symptoms of an influenza-like illness. Influenza-like illness (ILI) is a non-specific respiratory illness characterized by fever, fatigue, cough and other symptoms.[8] Besides influenza, ILI has many other causes including other viruses, such as rhinoviruses, respiratory syncytial virus (RSV), adenoviruses, and parainfluenza virus. Other, less common causes of ILI are bacterial, such as *Legionella* spp, *Chlamydia pneumoniae*, *Mycoplasma pneumoniae*, and *Streptococcus pneumoniae*.

The 10 cases of inhalational anthrax following the October 2001 terrorist event provide epidemiologic clues helping physicians differentiate inhalational anthrax from ILI. Nine of the 10 cases occurred among postal workers, persons exposed to letters or areas known contaminated with anthrax spores, and media employees. Inhalational anthrax is not transmissible from person to person. Consequently, nine of the ten cases were located in only a few communities. In comparison, viral causes of ILI are spread person-to-person, causing millions of cases each year across all communities. In addition, non-anthrax causes of ILI have a typical seasonal pattern. Pneumococcal disease, influenza and RSV infection generally peak in the winter, mycoplasma and legionellosis are more common in the summer and fall, rhinoviruses and parainfluenza virus infections usually peak during the fall and spring, and adenoviruses circulate throughout the year.

Table 27.1 shows how clinical signs and symptoms identified in the October 2001 cases can help physicians distinguish other causes of ILI from inhalational anthrax. Most cases of non-anthrax ILI are associated with nasal congestion and

TABLE 27.1. Clinical Findings of Inhalational Anthrax, Laboratory Confirmed Influenza, and Other Causes of Influenza-Like Illness[8]

Symptom/Sign	Inhalational anthrax (n=10)	Laboratory-confirmed influenza	ILI from other causes
Elevated temperature	70%	68%–77%	40%–73%
Fever or chills	100%	83%–90%	75%–89%
Fatigue/malaise	100%	75%–94%	62%–94%
Cough (minimal or nonproductive)	90%	84%–93%	72%–80%
Shortness of breath	80%	6%	6%
Chest discomfort or pleuritic chest pain	60%	35%	23%
Headache	50%	84%–91%	74%–89%
Myalgias	50%	67%–94%	73%–94%
Sore throat	20%	64%–84%	64%–84%
Rhinorrhea	10%	78%	68%
Nausea or vomiting	80%	12%	12%
Abdominal pain	30%	22%	22%

rhinorrhea. In comparison, only one of the 10 patients in the October 2001 outbreak complained of rhinorrhea. A history of influenza vaccination does not help differentiate inhalational anthrax from other causes of ILI. The vaccine does not prevent ILI caused by infectious agents other than influenza, and many persons vaccinated against influenza will still get ILI. Therefore, receipt of vaccine does not increase the probability of inhalational anthrax as a cause of ILI, especially among persons who have no probable exposure to anthrax.

Chest radiograph findings can help differentiate non-anthrax ILI from inhalational anthrax. In the October 2001 outbreak, all ten inhalational anthrax patients presented with abnormal chest radiographs, seven with mediastinal widening, seven with infiltrates and eight with pleural effusion. In comparison, most cases of ILI are not associated with radiographic findings of pneumonia.[8] A chest radiograph showing a widened mediastinum in a previously healthy person with evidence of severe flu-like symptoms is essentially pathognomonic of advanced inhalational anthrax.

The most useful microbiologic test for anthrax is a standard blood culture, which should show growth within 6 to 24 hours. Physicians should order blood cultures only for patients in situations where they suspect bacteremia and not routinely on all patients with ILI symptoms who have no probable exposure to anthrax. When ordering blood cultures, physicians must alert the laboratory to the possibility of anthrax, so that the lab performs appropriate biochemical testing and species identification.

Cutaneous Anthrax[7]

Cutaneous anthrax follows the deposition of the organism into the skin, especially areas with previous cuts or abrasions. Exposed areas, such as the arms, hands, face and neck are the most frequently affected. After the spore begins germinating in the skin, toxin production causes local edema. The initial pruritic macule or papule enlarges into an ulcer by day two. Next, 1–3 mm vesicles may appear, discharging clear or serosanguinous fluid containing numerous organisms on Gram stain. A painless, depressed, black eschar follows, frequently associated with extensive local edema. Over the next 1–2 weeks, the eschar dries, loosens, and falls off, most often leaving no permanent scar. Lymphangitis and painful lymphadenopathy can occur with associated systemic symptoms. Antibiotic therapy does not change the course of the skin manifestations, but it does reduce the likelihood of systemic disease, reducing the mortality rate from 20% to near zero.[4]

Anthrax: Treatment

A high index of suspicion, prompt diagnosis and immediate initiation of effective antimicrobial treatment are critical for treating inhalational anthrax. Physicians must report suspected or confirmed cases of anthrax to local and state public health authorities immediately. Because of the high associated mortality, the CDC recommends two or more known effective antibiotics. The recommendations could change as we gather more experience with treating anthrax. Ciprofloxacin or doxycycline is recommended for initial intravenous therapy until susceptibility results are available. Other antibiotics suggested for use in combination with ciprofloxacin or with doxycycline include rifampin, vancomycin, imipenem, chloramphenicol, penicillin and ampicillin, clindamycin and clarithromycin.[9] The toxin produced by *B. anthracis* is a major cause of the morbidity associated with the disease. One study suggested corticosteroids as adjunct therapy for inhalational anthrax associated with extensive edema, respiratory failure and meningitis.[9,10]

Ciprofloxacin and doxycycline are also the drugs of choice for cutaneous anthrax. For patients with signs of systemic involvement, such as extensive edema or head and neck lesions, the CDC recommends intravenous therapy with multiple antibiotics. Corticosteroids may be helpful for toxin mediated morbidity associated with extensive edema or swelling of the head and neck areas. A 7–10 day course of antibiotics is typically effective for cutaneous anthrax. However, the CDC recommends 60 days of treatment for patients with bioterrorist induced cutaneous anthrax, because many of these patients are also at risk for aerosol exposure.[9]

Anthrax: Preventive Therapy

To protect the public, the highest priority is to identify people at risk of exposure and respond appropriately to protect them. The circumstances of any potential exposure rather than laboratory test results should be the main factor in decisions regarding antibiotic prophylaxis. After taking a history, physicians should offer antibiotic prophylaxis to patients with an exposure or contact with an item or environment known or suspected to be contaminated with *B. anthracis*, regardless of laboratory tests.[9] Although nasal swabs for anthrax culture can detect anthrax spores, negative cultures DO NOT rule out exposure. Therefore, nasal cultures are useful for epidemiologic purposes, but not for determining whether individual patients should receive antibiotic prophylaxis.

The latest recommendations from the CDC[11] recommend initiating antimicrobial prophylaxis pending additional information when:

- A patient is exposed to an air space where a suspicious material may have been aerosolized (e.g., near a suspicious powder-containing letter during opening)
- A patient has shared the air space likely to be the source of an inhalational anthrax case

After initial prophylaxis, physicians should continue antimicrobial prophylaxis for 60 days for:

- Patients exposed to an air space known to be contaminated with aerosolized *B. anthracis*
- Patients exposed to an air space known to be the source of an inhalational anthrax case
- Patients along the transit path of an envelope or other vehicle containing *B. anthracis* that may have been aerosolized (e.g., a postal sorting facility in which an envelope containing *B. anthracis* was processed)
- Unvaccinated laboratory workers exposed to confirmed *B. anthracis* cultures

Physicians should not provide antimicrobial prophylaxis:

- For prevention of cutaneous anthrax
- For autopsy personnel examining bodies infected with anthrax when appropriate isolation precautions and procedures are followed
- For hospital personnel caring for patients with anthrax
- For persons who routinely open or handle mail in the absence of a suspicious letter or credible threat

Table 27.2 summarizes the CDC recommendations for initial and continued post exposure prophylaxis. The antibiotic of choice for preventing inhalational anthrax in exposed pregnant women is ciprofloxacin 500 mg twice a day for 60 days. Physicians may consider prophylactic therapy with amoxicillin, 500 mg three times daily for 60 days for instances in which the specific *B. anthracis* strain has been proven penicillin sensitive (MMWR 11/2/01, notice to readers)

Physicians must be careful in prescribing prophylactic antibiotics because they have been associated with adverse health effects among patients taking them for short-term treatment of bacterial infections. In addition, few data exist regarding the use of these antimicrobials for longer periods, such as the 60 days recommended for anthrax prophylaxis. Anthrax vaccination requires an initial six dose series and an annual booster. Current supplies are limited and the production capacity is modest. Given the costs and logistics of a large-scale vaccination pro-

TABLE 27.2. CDC Recommendations for Post-Exposure Prophylaxis For Prevention of Inhalational Anthrax After Intentional Exposure to *Bacillus Anthracis*[4]

Category	Initial therapy	Duration
Adults (including immunocompromised persons)	Ciprofloxacin 500 mg po BID Or Doxycycline 100 mg po BID	60 days
Pregnant women	Ciprofloxacin 500 mg po BID	60 days
Children	Ciprofloxacin 10–15 mg/kg po Q 12 hrs (maximum 1 gm per day) Or Doxycycline: >8 yrs and 45 kg: 100 mg po BID >8 yrs and ≤ 45 kg: 2.2 mg/kg po BID ≤8 yrs: 2.2 mg/kg po BID	60 days

gram, the low likelihood of an attack in any given community, and the effectiveness of prophylactic antibiotics for those exposed, the CDC does not recommend vaccination of the population.

Plague

Pneumonic plague, the most likely clinical presentation of *Yersinia pestis* infection associated with a terrorist attack, is different from that of naturally occurring plague, which is associated with the presence of painful infected lymph nodes, or buboes. Another difference from the naturally acquired infection is that pneumonic plague is transmissible from person to person through respiratory droplets. A pneumonic plague outbreak would result with symptoms initially resembling those of other serious respiratory illnesses.[12] After an incubation period of 1–6 days, patients would present with an acute and often fulminant course of malaise, fever, headache, myalgia, and cough with mucopurulent sputum, hemoptysis, chest pain and clinical sepsis. Prominent gastrointestinal symptoms, including nausea, vomiting, abdominal pain and diarrhea might be present. The pneumonia rapidly progresses to dyspnea, stridor and cyanosis. Gram-negative rods may be seen on gram stain of the sputum and the chest radiograph will show evidence of bronchopneumonia.[12] Patients rapidly progress to respiratory failure, shock and a bleeding diathesis.[13] Without appropriate therapy, the mortality rate is 100%

As with anthrax, early diagnosis is critical and requires a high index of suspicion. The sudden appearance of previously healthy patients with fever, cough, chest pain and a fulminant course should suggest the possibility of inhalational anthrax or pneumonic plague. There are no readily available rapid diagnostic tests for plague, and microbiologic studies are important in the diagnosis. Cultures of sputum, blood or lymph node aspirates should demonstrate growth within 24–48 hours after inoculation.

During a pneumonic plague epidemic, all persons developing a fever of 38.5 degrees C or above or a new cough should begin parenteral antibiotics. Infants with tachypnea should also receive treatment. Aminoglycosides are the most efficacious treatment for pneumonic plague. In a limited, contained outbreak, parenteral streptomycin or gentamicin is the drug(s) of choice. In a mass outbreak, in which parenteral therapy may not be available, the Working Group for Civil Biodefense recommends oral therapy with doxycycline (or tetracycline) or ciprofloxacin. In addition, patients with pneumonic plague will require supportive care to treat complications of gram-negative sepsis, including adult respiratory distress syndrome, disseminated intravascular coagulation, shock, and multiorgan failure.[12] Because the potential benefits outweigh the risks, in limited or contained situations, streptomycin or gentamicin are the drugs of choice for children; in mass outbreaks, children should receive doxycycline. Due to its association with irreversible deafness in children following fetal exposure, physicians should avoid using streptomycin in pregnant women and instead give gentamicin. If gentamicin is not available, doxycycline is the drug of choice for pregnant women, because the benefits outweigh the risk of fetal toxicity.

Although the plague vaccine was effective in preventing or ameliorating bubonic disease, it was not effective in preventing pneumonic plague or reducing its morbidity. Production of the vaccine ceased in 1999. Asymptomatic persons having household, hospital or other close contact (within 2 meters) with untreated patients should receive prophylactic therapy for 7 days. Physicians should watch case contacts closely, and begin treating for disease at the first sign of a fever or cough within 7 days of exposure. Contacts refusing antibiotic prophylaxis do not require isolation but should also receive treatment at the first sign of infection. Doxycycline is the drug of choice for post exposure prophylaxis for adults, children and pregnant women. Pregnant women unable to take doxycycline should receive ciprofloxacin or another fluoroquinolone.[12]

Wearing masks was effective in preventing person-to-person transmission of pneumonic plague in outbreaks early in the 20th century. Therefore, current guidelines recommend the use of surgical masks to prevent transmission in future outbreaks. Close contacts of confirmed cases that have received less than 48 hours of antibiotic therapy should wear masks and follow droplet precautions (gowns, gloves and eye protection). In addition, people should avoid unnecessary close contact until cases receive at least 48 hours of antibiotic therapy and exhibit some clinical improvement.

Smallpox (Variola)

Acute smallpox symptoms resemble those of other acute viral infections such as influenza. After an incubation period of 12–14 days (range 7–17 days), smallpox begins with a 2–4 day nonspecific prodrome of fever, myalgias, headache and backache before rash onset. Severe abdominal pain and delirium may be present. Physicians who have never seen the characteristic smallpox rash might confuse smallpox with chickenpox, but the rashes have distinct features. The typical varicella rash has a centripetal distribution, with lesions most prominent on the trunk and rarely seen on the palms and soles. The varicella rash develops in successive groups of lesions over several days, resulting in lesions of various stages of development and resolution. Varicella lesions are superficial. In contrast, the vesicular/pustular variola rash has a centrifugal distribution, most prominent on the face and extremities. Variola lesions develop at one time, and the pustules are characteristically round, tense and deeply embedded in the dermis. Secondary bacterial infection is uncommon. Death usually results from the toxemia associated with circulating immune complexes and soluble variola antigens. The case fatality rate in the unvaccinated population is 30%.[14]

Smallpox spreads from person-to-person by droplet nuclei or aerosols from the oropharynx of infected people and by direct contact. Contaminated clothing or bed linens can spread the virus. Patients are most infectious from rash onset through the first 7–10 days of rash.

The United States discontinued routine smallpox vaccinations in 1972. The susceptibility of people who received the vaccine 29 or more years ago is uncertain, because clinical studies have never measured the duration of immunity following vaccination. Therefore, we must assume that the U.S. population is highly susceptible to infection. Given the high case fatality rate, physicians suspecting a single case must treat it as an international health emergency and immediately contact local and state public health authorities.

Public health authorities do not recommend mass vaccination for smallpox at this time for several reasons:

- Current supplies are inadequate to vaccinate the entire population
- After an aerosol release of smallpox, public health authorities will make vaccine supplies available to affected communities. Post exposure vaccination is effective in preventing infection or lowering mortality up to 4 days after exposure.
- The risks of vaccine complications outweigh the likelihood of a smallpox attack. Potential complications include, but are not limited to post-vaccinial encephalitis, progressive vaccinia infection, eczema vaccinatum, generalized vaccinia, and inadvertent inoculation (transmission of vaccinia infection to close contacts or auto-inoculation from the vaccine site to other areas, including the eyes). Certain populations are at greater risk of complications, including patients with eczema, immune deficiency and pregnant women.
- Vaccinia immune globulin (VIG) is useful in treating some of the vaccine complications. However, like the vaccine itself, VIG is in short supply, and not enough is available to treat all the complications that could occur.

Currently, the only available treatments for patients with smallpox infection are supportive therapy and antibiotics for occasional superimposed bacterial infections. Given the incubation period and the lag time before physicians recognized the rash as smallpox, two weeks or more could pass between the release of the virus and the diagnosis of the first cases. With each generation of trans-

mission, the number of cases could expand by a factor of 10–20.[14] The best way
to interrupt disease transmission is to identify, vaccinate and observe those at
greatest risk of infection. Clearly, as soon as physicians make the first diagnosis, they should isolate their patients and vaccinate their household and other
face-to-face contacts. Physicians should give the vaccine to suspected cases to
ensure that a mistaken diagnosis does not place patients at risk for smallpox. An
emergency vaccination program should also include:

- Health care workers at clinics or hospitals that could receive patients
- Other essential disaster response personnel, such as police, firefighters, transit
  workers, public health staff, emergency management staff and mortuary staff
  that may have to handle bodies
- Because of the risk of dissemination, in an outbreak situation, all hospital employees and patients should receive vaccination. Immunocompromised patients
  or patients with other contraindications for vaccination should receive Vaccinia
  Immune Globulin (VIG)

Whenever possible, physicians should isolate patients in their home or other
non-hospital facility to avoid further disseminating of the disease. In addition,
hospitals and health care facilities treating patients with smallpox should take
special precautions to ensure that all bedding and clothing of smallpox patients
is autoclaved or laundered in hot water with bleach. Standard disinfectants, such
as hypochlorite or quaternary ammonia, are effective for cleaning viral-contam-
inated surfaces.

Botulism

Patients with botulism classically present with difficulty seeing, speaking and
swallowing.[15] Physicians can recognize botulism by its classic triad:[15]

- Symmetric, descending flaccid paralysis with prominent bulbar palsies (the "4
  Ds"—diplopia, dysarthria, dysphonia and dysphagia)
- Afebrile patient
- Clear sensorium

As the paralysis extends, patients lose head control, become hypotonic and
develop generalized weakness. Dysphagia and loss of the gag reflect may necessitate intubation and usually mechanical ventilation. Deep tendon reflexes,
present initially, gradually diminish, and patients may develop constipation.
The case fatality rate is 60% without respiratory support. Death results from
upper airway obstruction (due to pharyngeal and upper airway muscle paralysis) and inadequate tidal volume (diaphragmatic and accessory respiratory
muscle paralysis).[15] Because botulinum toxin does not penetrate the brain, severely ill patients are not confused or obtunded. However, the associated bulbar palsies create communication difficulties and can make patients appear
lethargic.

Early recognition of an intentional airborne release of botulinum toxin requires heightened clinical suspicion. Certain features are particularly suggestive:[15]

- Outbreak of a large number of cases of acute flaccid paralysis with prominent bulbar palsies
- Outbreak with an unusual botulinum toxin type
- Outbreak with a common geographic factor among cases (for example, airport, or work location) but without a common dietary exposure
- Multiple simultaneous outbreaks with no common source

Physicians seeing patients with findings suggestive of botulism should take a careful travel history, activity history, and a dietary history. They should ask patients if they know of anyone with similar symptoms. A single case of suspected botulism is a potential public health emergency because it reflects the possibility of contaminated food, available to others, or a release of aerosolized toxin. Therefore, physicians must immediately report suspect cases to their hospital epidemiologist and to their local and state public health departments. Laboratory testing is only available at the Centers for Disease Control and Prevention and some state public health laboratories.

Treatment includes supportive care and passive immunization with equine antitoxin. Patients must receive antitoxin at the first suspicion of botulism to minimize neurologic damage. The antitoxin will not reverse already existing paralysis. Physicians can obtain antitoxin from the CDC through their state and local health departments. Potential side effects include anaphylaxis, serum sickness, urticaria and other reactions suggestive of hypersensitivity, necessitating a small challenge dose before giving the full dose. Supportive care may include enteral tube or parenteral nutrition, intensive care, mechanical ventilation, treatment of secondary infections and monitoring for impending respiratory failure. Pregnant patients and children should receive the standard treatment, including antitoxin. The potential adverse effects of antitoxin and its limited availability outweigh its use as a prophylaxis for exposed patients without symptoms. In an outbreak situation, physicians should closely observe potentially exposed asymptomatic patients.

Tularemia

After inhalation of contaminated aerosol, *F. tularensis* causes an abrupt onset of an acute, nonspecific febrile illness beginning 3–5 days after exposure. Nearly half the patients have a dissociation of pulse and temperature. Symptoms include headaches, chills, and rigors, generalized body aches (often prominent in the low back), coryza and sore throat. Patients frequently develop a dry or slightly productive cough, with or without objective signs of pneumonia, such as purulent sputum, dyspnea, tachypnea, pleuritic pain or hemoptysis. Gastrointestinal symptoms, including nausea, vomiting and diarrhea may occur. Symptoms of untreated, continuing illness include sweats, fever, chills, progressive weakness, malaise, anorexia and weight loss. Many cases develop pleuropneumonitis over the ensuing days and weeks. The earliest chest radiograph findings may be peribronchial infiltrates, typically advancing to bronchopneumonia in one or more lobes, often accompanied by pleural effusions and hilar adenopathy.[16]

However, clinical signs may be minimal or absent, and some patients will show only one or several small, discrete infiltrates or scattered granulomatous lesions of the lung parenchyma or pleura. In other patients, however, the pneumonia can progress rapidly to respiratory failure and death. The case fatality rate with treatment is about 2%. Person-to-person transmission has not been documented.

Inhalation can occasionally cause the oropharyngeal form of tularemia, associated with stomatitis and exudative pharyngitis, sometimes with ulceration. Patients may develop pronounced cervical or retropharyngeal lymphadenopathy.

Because of the nonspecific symptoms, physicians and public health authorities would have difficulty distinguishing between a terrorist attack and a natural outbreak of community acquired infection, especially influenza and some atypical pneumonias. Several clues that would indicate an intentional cause would include:

- Abrupt onset of large numbers of acutely ill people
- Rapid progression of many cases from upper respiratory symptoms and bronchitis to life threatening pleuropneumonitis and systemic infection
- An unusual number of cases with findings of atypical pneumonia, pleuritis and hilar adenopathy
- Cases among young, previously healthy adults and children

Physicians who suspect inhalational tularemia should

- Promptly collect specimens of respiratory secretions and blood and alert the laboratory to the need for special diagnostic and safety procedures
- Immediately notify the hospital epidemiologist or infection control practitioner
- Immediately notify their state and local health departments

In a contained casualty situation, where resources are adequate for individual case management, the Working Group for Civil Biodefense recommends streptomycin as the drug of choice, with gentamicin as an alternative in children and adults. Gentamicin is the drug of choice for pregnant women.[16] In a mass casualty situation, oral doxycycline or ciprofloxacin is the treatment of choice for adults and children, with oral ciprofloxacin as the best choice for pregnant women.[16]

Due to the short incubation period and incomplete protection by available vaccines, the Working Group on Civilian Biodefense does not recommend Tularemia vaccination for post exposure prophylaxis. Treatment begun with streptomycin, gentamicin, doxycycline or ciprofloxacin during the incubation period is protective against symptomatic infection. Once public health officials become aware that terrorists have released a *F. tularensis* aerosol, they will attempt to identify people at risk of exposure. Those exposed patients who are still asymptomatic should receive prophylactic treatment with 14 days of doxycycline or ciprofloxacin. If health officials fail to detect the release until people start becoming ill, physicians should instruct their patients to begin a fever watch. Those who develop an unexplained fever or flu-like illness within 14 days of exposure should begin antibiotic treatment. Close contacts of cases do not require pro-phylaxis because person-to-person transmission does not occur.[16]

Hemorrhagic Viruses

The Centers for Disease Control and prevention has focused its efforts on four viral hemorrhagic fever (VHF) pathogens that are potential bioterrorist agents: Ebola, Marburg, Lassa and South American VHF viruses. None of these is na-tive to the United States, so an outbreak that epidemiologists cannot link to travel must raise suspicion of bioterrorism. Although person-to-person spread is not common through the inhalational route in a typical outbreak situation, a bioter-rorist-released aerosol could cause an outbreak through inhalational exposure.

The Filoviruses (Ebola and Marburg) can be transmitted person-to-person through contact with blood or body secretions of infected persons. The incuba-tion period for Ebola and Marburg viruses ranges from several days to 3 weeks following exposure. Clinical signs of Ebola and Marburg VHFs include the abrupt onset of fever, fatigue, stomach pain, headache and myalgias. Other signs and symptoms include nausea, vomiting abdominal pain, diarrhea, chest pain, cough and pharyngitis. Most patients develop a maculopapular rash, prominent on the trunk approximately five days after onset of illness. As the disease progresses, bleeding manifestations, such as petechiae, ecchymoses and hemorrhages ap-pear.[6] Severe cases may have chest pain and show signs of bleeding under the skin, in internal organs, and from body openings. The case-fatality rate for Ebola hemorrhagic fever is 36–88% and may be strain dependent. Marburg hemorrhagic fever has a reported case-fatality rate around 25%.

In nature, direct contact with infected rodents or their urine and droppings causes infection with arenaviruses (Lassa and South American VHFs). Infection can also result from inhalation of particles contaminated with rodent excretions. Direct contact with blood or body secretions from infected patients can also cause person-to-person transmission. The incubation period for the Lassa and Junin viruses is typically 1–3 weeks. In addition to the symptoms typical of Ebola and Marburg VHFs, Lassa fever frequently causes neurological symptoms, including hearing loss, tremors, and encephalitis as well as signs of respiratory distress. South American VHFs can cause severe hemorrhagic fever, and a spotted rash may be a prominent feature. Lassa virus infections cause mild or undetectable illness in most infected people, but about 20% of people develop severe disease. Overall case-fatality rates are about 1%, but 15–20% of persons requiring hos-pitalization for Lassa fever may die. Pregnant women are more at risk for severe Lassa infection. The South American VHFs such as Junin (the cause of Argen-tine hemorrhagic fever) have case-fatality rates of 15–30%.

Immediate notification of a suspected case of VHF to local or state health de-partments and CDC is essential for rapid diagnosis, investigation, and control activities. Other than supportive therapy, there is no effective treatment for Ebola or Marburg infections. Specifically, patients will require appropriate maintenance of fluids and electrolytes and careful monitoring of blood pressure. Physicians and other health care staff must avoid contact with body fluids from infected patients, including blood, saliva, urine, and feces). Strict barrier procedures are required for suspected VHF patients. Health care staff should wear gowns and gloves when attending patients, and they should consider using face-masks to prevent small-droplet exposure. Hospitals must separate VHF patients from other patients. Close personal contacts or medical personnel exposed to blood or body secretions from VHF patients require monitoring for fever or other symptoms during the established incubation period. According to the World Health Organization, ribavirin may be effective for treating some patients with Lassa Fever. Additional information about viral hemorrhagic fever viruses is available online at http://www.bt.cdc.gov/bioagents.asp.[17]

Chemical Agents Terrorists are Likely to Use

Chemical agents that terrorists might use range from warfare agents to toxic chemicals commonly used in industry.[5] The CDC Strategic Planning Workgroup criteria for determining priority chemical agents include

- Chemical agents already known to be used as weaponry;
- Availability of chemical agents to potential terrorists;
- Chemical agents likely to cause major morbidity or mortality;
- Potential of agents for causing public panic and social disruption; and
- Agents that require special action for public health preparedness

Industry introduces hundreds of new chemicals internationally each month, making it impossible for family physicians to prepare for each of them. Instead, physicians should concentrate on treating exposed persons by clinical syndrome rather than by specific agent. As with biologic attacks, physicians must be vigilant in recognizing an unusual temporal or geographic cluster of chemically induced illness. Because of the public health risk, physicians must notify their local and state health departments if they suspect a nerve agent release. In addition, when evaluating and treating potentially exposed patients, physicians should coordinate their activities with authorities responsible for sampling and decontaminating the environment. This chapter will discuss two of the chemical agents that terrorists might use, nerve agents and blister agents. Further information on these and other potential chemical agents is available on the CDC web site at http://www.bt.cdc.gov/Agent/AgentlistChem.asp. (Last accessed 6-23-02)

Nerve Agents

Regardless of the route of exposure, nerve agents cause symptoms due to potent inhibition of anticholinesterase.[18] Symptoms and signs include:

- Rhinorrhea
- Chest tightness
- Pinpoint pupils
- Shortness of breath
- Excessive salivation and sweating
- Nausea, vomiting, abdominal cramps
- Involuntary defecation and urination
- Muscle twitching
- Confusion
- Seizures
- Flaccid paralysis
- Coma
- Respiratory failure and death

The initial effects of nerve agents depend on the dose and route of exposure. For example, inhalation causes respiratory effects within seconds to minutes, including rhinorrhea, chest tightness and shortness of breath. Therefore, asymptomatic patients arriving at the hospital do not require admission or treatment if the only possible exposure was through inhalation. In addition, patients with inhalation exposure exhibiting only miosis or mild rhinorrhea do not require admission. On the other hand, a large exposure due to absorption through skin exposure may first present an hour later with abdominal pain, nausea and vomiting.[18]

Exposed patients with contaminated skin or clothing can contaminate rescuers and health care providers through direct contact or through off-gassing vapor. Therefore, all patients should undergo decontamination of eyes, clothing and skin before entering the hospital or emergency room treatment area. Health care providers, especially first responders at risk of exposure should wear the appropriate personal protective equipment. In addition, atropine administered repeatedly as necessary and pralidoxime (2-PAMCI) are antidotes for nerve agent toxicity. Pralidoxime is only effective if patients receive it within minutes to a few hours following exposure. Additional treatment consists of supportive measures, including airway support and mechanical ventilation. Some patients will exhibit resistance to ventilation due to bronchial constriction and spasm. This resistance lessons after atropine administration. Additional information on decontamination, first aid, personal protective equipment and treatment is available from the ATSDR (Agency for Toxic Substances and Disease Registry) web site at http://www.bt.cdc.gov/agent/nerve/Nervesfnl.pdf (last accessed 11-10-01)

Blister Agents: Nitrogen and Sulfur Mustards, Lewisite and Mustard-Lewisite Mixture

Nitrogen and sulfur mustards are vesicants that injure the skin, eye and respiratory tract. Within several minutes after exposure, they can cause cellular changes, although the clinical effects occur 1 to 24 hours later. Table 27.3 summarizes the clinical effects of nitrogen and sulfur mustards.[19] Because of the delayed effects, most patients with severe exposures to nitrogen or sulfur mustards will go home or elsewhere after their exposure and may only present later at emergency rooms or physicians' offices when they begin developing symptoms. Like other chemical agents, patients with nitrogen or sulfur mustard-contaminated skin or clothing can contaminate rescuers and health care providers by direct contact or through off-gassing vapor. Therefore, once health care providers are aware of an exposure, they should require all patients to undergo decontamination of eyes, clothing and skin before allowing them to enter the treatment area. Decontamination can also reduce tissue damage. Health care providers, especially first responders at risk of exposure, should wear the appropriate personal protective equipment.

There are no antidotes for nitrogen mustard or sulfur mustard toxicity. The medical management is only supportive for skin, ocular and respiratory exposure. One guideline physicians can follow is to keep skin, eye and airway lesions free from infection. Severe skin burns may require care in a burn unit. Patients with airway damage below the pharynx require oxygen and assisted ventilation as necessary with positive end expiratory pressure (PEEP). At the first sign of damage at or below the larynx, patients will require intubation and transfer to the critical care unit. Bronchodilators may be helpful for bronchoconstriction. Steroids are not of proven value, but they can be used if bronchodilators are ineffective. Due to the risk of bleeding and perforation, emesis induction is contraindicated. Further information regarding decontamination, first aid, personal protective equipment and treatment is available from the ATSDR at http://www.bt.cdc.gov/Agent/Blister/NMUSTARDfnl.pdf (Nitrogen mustard, last accessed 11-10-01) and http://www.bt.cdc.gov/Agent/Blister/SMUSTARDfnl.pdf (Sulfur mustard, last accessed 11-10-01).

Unlike the other blister agents, sulfur and nitrogen mustards, Lewisite and the Mustard-Lewisite Mixture cause symptoms immediately. Lewisite, a systemic poison, and Mustard-Lewisite Mixture are irritating to the skin, eyes and airways. Contact with the liquid or vapor forms can cause skin erythema and blistering, corneal damage and iritis, damage to the airway mucosa, pulmonary edema, diarrhea, capillary leakage and subsequent hypotension.[20] Patients with Lewisite or Mustard-Lewisite-contaminated skin or clothing can contaminate rescuers and health care providers by direct contact or through off-gassing vapor. Management of Lewisite or Mustard-Lewisite exposure is similar to that of nitrogen and sulfur mustard exposures with two exceptions. First, patients exposed to Lewisite or the mixture will have an abrupt onset of symptoms and will likely present to emergency rooms immediately after exposure. As with the other blister agents, patients will require supportive care for eye, skin, ingestion and airway exposures. The second exception is that an antidote is available for Lewisite exposure. British Anti-Lewisite (BAL), also known as dimercaprol, is a chelating agent than can reduce systemic effects from Lewisite. However, because of toxic side effects, only patients who have signs of shock or significant pulmonary in-

TABLE 27.3. Health Effects of Exposure to Nitrogen and Sulfur Mustards.[19]

	Nitrogen mustard	Sulfur mustard
Dermal	Erythema and blistering. Rash develops in several hours, followed by blistering in 6–12 hours. Severe exposure can cause second and third degree burns.	Erythema and blistering. Pruritic rash develops in 4–8 hours, followed by blistering in 2–18 hours. Severe exposure can cause second and third degree burns.
Ocular	Intense conjunctival and scleral inflammation, pain, swelling, lacrimation, photophobia and corneal damage	Most sensitive tissue to sulfur. Intense conjunctival and scleral pain, swelling, lacrimation, blepharospasm, and photophobia. Miosis may occur. Severe exposure can cause corneal edema, perforation, scarring and blindness.
Respiratory	Mucosal damage within hours that may progress over days. Nasal and sinus pain or discomfort, pharyngitis, laryngitis, cough and dyspnea. Pulmonary edema is uncommon.	Upper and lower airway inflammation within hours of exposure and progressing over several days. Burning nasal pain, epistaxis, sinus pain, laryngitis, loss of taste and smell, cough, wheezing and dyspnea. Pseudomembrane formation and local airway obstruction
Gastrointestinal	Ingestion can cause chemical burns and hemorrhagic diarrhea. Nausea and vomiting may occur after ingestion, dermal or inhalation exposure.	Ingestion can cause chemical burns and cholinergic stimulation. Nausea and vomiting may occur after ingestion or inhalation. Early nausea and vomiting is usually transient and not severe. Nausea, vomiting and diarrhea occurring several days after exposure indicates GI tract damage and is a poor prognostic sign.
Central Nervous System	High doses have caused tremors, seizures, incoordination, ataxia and coma in laboratory animals.	High doses can cause hyperexcitability, convulsions and insomnia.
Hematopoietic	Bone marrow suppression and increased risk for infection, hemorrhage and anemia	Bone marrow suppression and increased risk for infection, hemorrhage and anemia
Delayed effects	Potential menstrual irregularities, alopecia, hearing loss, tinnitus, jaundice, impaired spermatogenesis, generalized swelling and hyperpigmentation	Years after apparent healing of severe eye lesions, relapsing keratitis or keratopathy may develop.
Potential sequelae	Chronic respiratory and eye conditions following large exposures	Persistent eye conditions, loss of taste and smell, and chronic respiratory illness, including asthmatic bronchitis, recurring respiratory infections, and pulmonary fibrosis

jury should receive BAL. Only trained personnel, in consultation with a regional poison control center, should provide chelation therapy. Additional information regarding decontamination, first aid, personal protective equipment and treatment is available from the ATSDR at http://www.bt.cdc.gov/Agent/Blister/Lewisitefnl. pdf (last accessed 11-10-01).

Approach to the "Worried Well" Patient

By answering questions and addressing concerns, physicians can easily reassure patients and reduce the trauma that many families experience following terrorist events. Table 27.4 contains a list of suggested answers for questions patients are likely to ask. Physicians should consider consulting with their local public health officials for updates and additional information useful for addressing patient concerns.

In addition to addressing patient concerns, family physicians play an essential role in addressing symptoms related to trauma from real or imagined events. Patients can suffer from posttraumatic stress disorder, even if their families and friends are not immediate victims of violent events. Because the diagnosis of PTSD may be challenging, family physicians will need to have a good understanding of its diagnostic features so they can provide the appropriate care or preventive interventions for people at risk. Fortunately, information is available from the American Academy of Family Physicians, including an excellent article on the Primary Care Treatment of Post-traumatic Stress Disorder[21] and a patient handout at http://www.aafp.org/afp/20000901/1035.html (last accessed 11/17/2001). The web site also includes additional resources for families traumatized by terrorism. (Also see Chapter 22.)

Summary

Clearly, family physicians are on the front lines of detecting and responding to biologic and chemical attacks. Their roles include:

- Addressing patient concerns about their risks of terrorist-caused illness
- Participation in surveillance to detect an attack. This includes reporting potential exposures and any unusual cases or clusters of cases to local and state public health officials and law enforcement
- Working with public health officials to identify patients at risk of exposure and provide preventive treatment
- Working with public health officials to identify patients with terrorist-caused disease and providing effective treatment
- Educating patients and the community on the risks of biologic and chemical terrorism, and how to protect themselves and their families
- Detecting symptoms of psychological trauma following terrorist events, and providing compassionate counseling and treatment to address these symptoms

TABLE 27.4. Common Patient Questions and Suggested Answers

Question	Answer
What is my risk of getting anthrax from the mail?	The current risk of anthrax from exposure to an envelope or other object containing anthrax is low, because transmission from secondary aerosolization of anthrax spores is unlikely. Primary aerosolization results from the initial release of anthrax, whereas secondary aerosolization is due to the agitation (from wind or human activities) of particles that have settled after the primary release. The particles that have settled tend to be large and require large amounts of energy to be re-suspended in air. Therefore, residue on mail or packages is unlikely to cause any additional infections
How do I know if an item of mail is suspicious?	Share the FBI criteria with patients (see page 556)
How should I handle a suspicious envelope or package?	<ul><li>Do not shake or empty the contents of a suspicious package or envelope.</li><li>Do not carry the package or envelope, show it to others, or allow others to examine it.</li><li>Put the package or envelope on a stable surface; do not sniff, touch, taste, or look closely at it or any contents that may have spilled.</li><li>Alert others in the area about the suspicious package or envelope.</li><li>Leave the area, close any doors, and take actions to prevent others from entering the area.</li><li>If possible, shut off the ventilation system.</li><li>Wash hands with soap and water to prevent spreading potentially infectious material to face or skin. Seek additional instructions for exposed or potentially exposed persons.</li><li>If at work, notify a supervisor, a security officer, or a law enforcement official.</li><li>If at home, contact your local law enforcement agency.</li><li>If possible, create a list of persons who were in the room or area when this suspicious letter or package was recognized and a list of persons who also may have handled this package or letter. Give the list to both the local public health authorities and law enforcement officials.</li></ul>
Should my family purchase gas masks?	Gas masks are generally ineffective against communicable disease. In addition, they provide protection against chemicals only when properly fitted and tested. For complete protection, people would have to wear them 24 hours per day, 7 days per week, because we cannot predict the time and location of a terrorist attack. Therefore, we do not recommend purchasing gas masks.
Should my family be vaccinated for bioterrorist-used germs?	At this time, the risk of vaccine complications and the cost of vaccinating everyone in the United States. In addition, only the CDC and the military have the vaccines—they are not available in physicians' offices or at local health departments. In the case of a terrorist attack, public health authorities and physicians will quickly identify people at risk of exposure, and make vaccines and preventive antibiotics available to them.

573

TABLE 27.4. Common Patient Questions and Suggested Answers

Question	Answer
Should my family stockpile antibiotics just in case?	There are several reasons why public health authorities and most physicians recommend against stockpiling antibiotics. Specific antibiotics are effective only against specific infections, and we cannot predict which agents terrorists will use. People must take the antibiotics at the proper time after exposure for them to be effective, which means that they must know when they have been exposed. Antibiotics taken inappropriately can lead to resistant bacteria, which can put the entire community at risk. The CDC has stockpiled large amounts of antibiotics, and we will make these available immediately to exposed people within 12 hours of the recognition of an attack.
Should I get a laboratory test for anthrax?	No, and here is why: Nasal swabs and blood tests are inaccurate. • You can be exposed and still have a negative test. • On the other hand, a positive test DOES NOT mean you have inhaled enough germs to get sick. Therefore, decisions on whether to give preventive antibiotics must be based upon risk assessment rather than testing results. Testing is done only as part of the public health investigation into a confirmed or highly probable exposure. • The decision to test is a public health and law enforcement decision. • The public health lab will do the testing only in case of a credible threat.
Is our water supply safe from terrorism?	Yes. In general, routine water treatment (chlorine, filtering) in our public water systems would take care of biological agents terrorists might place in the system, just as they handle natural germs. If terrorists were to add chemical agents, the water would so dilute the chemicals that they would pose little threat.
What can my family do to protect itself?	The best thing for families to do: develop a disaster plan just as they would for natural disasters. The disaster plan should include an emergency communications plan, a meeting place, and a disaster supplies kit. Parents should check with their children's school to get a copy of the emergency plan of the school. More information is obtainable at the at the local Red Cross chapter or at the Red Cross web-site: http://www.redcross.org/services/disaster/keepsafe/unexpected.html.

In several ways, family physicians are particularly well suited to respond to terrorism. First, family physicians are widely dispersed, in rural and urban areas, making them accessible for patients wherever terrorist events might occur. Second, family physicians provide continuity care, essential for the appropriate care of patients and families with ongoing physical and emotional outcomes from violent events. Third, family physicians provide comprehensive care, and can take care of most of the health problems, including emotional issues, facing victims of terrorism. Fourth, family physicians understand how to coordinate care for patients, and can refer victims of terrorist attacks to other appropriate services as necessary. Most importantly, family physicians understand how to provide care in the context of family and community.[22] As the events of September/October 2001 demonstrated, terrorism affects entire communities, whether or not individuals directly experience physical outcomes from the attacks. Family physicians, who understand how their patients and families interact with their community, can help identify and treat problems at the community level. Although horrible, past terrorist events illustrate the pivotal role that family physicians play, working in partnership with public health officials to protect and promote the health of families and communities.

References

1. Centers for Disease Control and Prevention. Ongoing investigation of anthrax—Florida, October 2001. Morbidity and Mortality Weekly Report 50. 2001;40:877.
2. Centers for Disease Control and Prevention. Update: Investigation of anthrax associated with intentional exposure and interim public health guidelines. Morbidity and Mortality Weekly Report 50, 2001;41:889–93.
3. Centers for Disease Control and Prevention. Update: Investigation of bioterrorism-related anthrax and adverse events from antimicrobial prophylaxis. Morbidity and Mortality Weekly Report 50.2001;44:973–6.
4. Centers for Disease Control and Prevention. Update: Investigation of bioterrorism-related anthrax and interim guidelines for clinical evaluation of persons with possible anthrax. Morbidity and Mortality Weekly Report 50. 2001;43:941–8.
5. Centers for Disease Control and Prevention. Biological and chemical terrorism: Strategic plan for preparedness and response. Recommendations of the CDC Strategic Planning Workgroup. Morbidity and Mortality Weekly Report 49, no. RR04 (April 21, 2000): 1–14
6. Centers for Disease Control and Prevention. Recognition of illness associated with the intentional release of a biologic agent. Morbidity and Mortality Weekly Report 50. 2001;41:893–7.
7. Inglesby TV, Henderson DA, Bartlett JG, et al. Anthrax as a biological weapon. Medical and public health management. JAMA 1999:281(18):1735–45. Also available at http://www.bt.cdc.gov (last accessed 11/3/2001).
8. Centers for Disease Control and Prevention. Notice to readers: Considerations for distinguishing influenza-like illness from inhalational anthrax. Morbidity and Mortality Weekly Report 50. 2001;44:984–6.
9. Centers for Disease Control and Prevention Update: Investigation of bioterrorism-re-

lated anthrax and interim guidelines for exposure management and antimicrobial therapy, October 2001. Morbidity and Mortality Weekly Report 50, 2001;42: 909–19.

10. Dixon TC, Meselson M, Guillemin J. Anthrax. N Engl J Med 1999;341:815–26.

11. Centers for Disease Control and Prevention. Notice to Readers: Interim guidelines for investigation of and response to Bacillus anthracis exposures. Morbidity and Mortality Weekly Report 50. 2001;44 987–90.

12. Inglesby TV, Dennis DT, Henderson DA, et al. Plague as a biological weapon: Medical and public health management. JAMA 2000;283:2281–90. Also available at http://www.bt.cdc.gov (last accessed 11/3/2001)

13. Henning KJ , Layton M. Bioterrorism. In APIC Text of Infection Control and Epidemiology. Association of Professionals in Infection Control and Epidemiology Inc. Washington, D.C. (2000):Chapter 24:1–11.

14. Henderson DA, Inglesby TV, Bartlett JG, et al. Smallpox as a biological weapon: Medical and public health management. JAMA 1999;281:2127–37. Also available at http://www.bt.cdc.gov (last accessed 11/3/2001)

15. Arnon SS, Schechter R, Inglesby TV, et al. Botulinum toxin as a biological weapon: Medical and public health management. JAMA 2001:285:1059–70. Also available at http://www.bt.cdc.gov (last accessed 11/3/2001)

16. Dennis DT, Inglesby TV, Henderson DA, et al. Tularemia as a biological weapon: Medical and public health management. JAMA 2001;285:2763–73. Also available at http://www.bt.cdc.gov (last accessed 11/3/2001

17. Centers for Disease Control and Prevention. Viral hemorrhagic fevers: Fact sheets. http://www.cdc.gov/ncidod/dvrd/spb/mnpages/factmenu.htm. Last accessed 11/14/01.

18. Nerve Agents. Agency for Toxic Substances and Disease Registry. http://www.bt.cdc.gov/agent/nerve/Nervesfnl.pdf. Last accessed 11-14-01.

19. Blister Agents. Agency for Toxic Substances and Disease Registry. Nitrogen Mustard (HN-1) (C6H13Cl2N) CAS 538-07-8, UN 2810; Nitrogen Mustard (HN-2) (C5H11Cl2N) CAS 51-75-2, UN 2927;andNitrogen Mustard (HN-3) (C6H12Cl3N) CAS 555-77-1, UN 2810. http://www.bt.cdc.gov/Agent/Blister/NMUSTARDfnl.pdf. Last accessed 11-14-01.

20. Blister Agents. Lewisite (L) (C2H2AsCl3) CAS 541-25-3, UN 1556; and Mustard-Lewisite Mixture (HL) CAS Number not available, UN 2810 Agency for Toxic Substances and Disease Registry. http://www.bt.cdc.gov:80/Agent/Blister/Lewisitefnl.pdf. Last accessed 11-14-01.

21. Lange JT, Lange CL , Cabaltica RBG. Primary care treatment of post-traumatic stress disorder. American Family Physician 2000;62(5):1035–1040.

22. Saultz, JW. Textbook of Family Medicine. New York: McGraw-Hill. 2000.

28
Information Mastery: Practical Evidence-Based Family Medicine

CHERYL A. FLYNN, ALLEN F. SHAUGHNESSY,
AND DAVID C. SLAWSON

Remember Marcus Welby? He symbolized the ideal family doctor—knowledgeable even about rare conditions, caring and compassionate, making multiple house calls with his little black bag, and devoting his complete attention and the best resources for the care of a single patient.

Fast forward to the new millennium, with health maintenance organizations (HMOs), schedules with 20 to 40 patients per day, and a huge information explosion, yet still having the responsibility of knowing the latest updates in medicine. As family doctors, we strive to maintain the characteristics embodied by that fictitious symbol—good history and physical examination skills, an understanding of the patient in the context of the family and community, and the ability to meld the two in diagnostic and therapeutic decision making. Yet with the exponential growth of information, and rapidly expanding medical technologies, it seems easy to blink an eye and miss some important new development. Lifelong learning skills and strategies to manage the jungle of medical information are the new survival tools for today's family doctors.

Enter evidence-based medicine (EBM), which is defined as "the conscientious, explicit, and judicious use of the current best evidence in making decisions about the care of an individual patient."[1] This practice encourages us to apply the highest quality information available at the time in the care of our patients. Critics argue that we have been using evidence all along; EBM is merely a new name for an old practice. But EBM is not simply the use of research in practice. Rather it is a systematic process to answer clinical questions with the best evidence. It requires lifelong learning skills not generally taught in medical school. A 1984 study found that physicians' knowledge of treating hypertension was inversely related to the year they graduated from medical school.[2] A later study demonstrated that those who attended a school where EBM was taught had no such knowledge decline.[3]

If EBM has been practiced all along, then why would an ophthalmologist from a well-respected institution advise journal readers to use an eye patch to treat corneal abrasions despite knowing that there were seven randomized controlled trials showing no benefit and possible harm ("We've always done it this way")?[4,5]

If our profession incorporates evidence into practice routinely, why were only two of 28 landmark trials implemented in practice in the 3 years following publication.[6] If you are a clinician who already is using the best evidence in practice, then we challenge you to train your colleagues and help train our future physicians, because clearly as a profession we do not routinely practice using the best evidence.

The newer definition of EBM is one that incorporates the best evidence, clinical experience, and patient perspective into medical management plans—a patient-centered evidence-based practice. This chapter outlines a new and more useful model of EBM, especially fitting for family physicians; offers practical strategies for using evidence in answering clinical questions; outlines a model for keeping up to date with the latest medical developments; and addresses some key concepts in the application of evidence in clinical practice.

Information Mastery

The traditional EBM model involves five steps to solve a clinical problem: developing answerable clinical questions, searching for and selecting the best evidence, evaluating the quality of that information, interpreting and applying it back at the patient level, and assessing one's practice. Although seemingly complete, this model has some limitations, especially for the busy family physician.

First is the lack of feasibility. It is estimated that the average physician generates about 15 clinical questions per day. Although some questions are simply "What is this drug?" or "What's the proper dose?" more than half are focused on identifying the best treatment or diagnosis strategies. Since it takes an average of 20 minutes to perform a Medline search, one would need several hours of uninterrupted time per week just to *find* the evidence for answering these questions. It is understandable, then, that the majority of the questions generated in practice remain unanswered. The unfortunate part is that half of the answers would have the potential to influence practice.[7]

A second, essential element of an evidence-based practice is the ability to keep up to date with the latest developments. To seek answers only to those questions we generate may leave us in the dark about new or previously unconsidered therapies. Worse still, it may result in medical gossip[8]—finding an answer to your question without the context of all the research of that area may result in the inappropriate application of the evidence.

Finally, the traditional EBM model presumes that the only source of medical information is the literature. Colleagues are the first source clinicians turn to for answers during practice.[9] The medical information system is expansive, and includes the World Wide Web beckoning from your personal computer, pharmaceutical representatives knocking at your door, and continuing medical education (CME) programs making broad-based medical recommendations. These sources are in addition to the estimated 6000 articles published each day in medical journals.[10] Family physicians need tools to help sort through this overwhelming quantity of medical information.

Information mastery (IM) was designed to be more user-friendly for busy clinicians. All sources of medical information are not equally useful, but depend on three factors:

$$Usefulness = \frac{Relevance \times Validity}{Work}$$

Here, *work* refers to any resources devoted to finding and using information. This conceptual model tells us that sources requiring little work are more useful. However, if an information source is either irrelevant or invalid, then regardless of the work, its usefulness will still be zero; all three factors must be balanced. The latter sections of this chapter offer practical tips and examples of ways to minimize work when answering clinical questions or attempting to stay current with medical information developments.

Determining Relevance: DOEs, POEs, and POEMs

One strategy to minimize work is to first assess relevance. Only if the source of information passes the relevance criteria do you need to follow through with a validity assessment. In medicine, we naturally create a hierarchy of relevance. It is uncommon that we'd apply data that were based solely on test tubes or animal models directly to our patients. Within clinical studies, there is also an additional hierarchy of data, that between disease-oriented and patient-oriented evidence. Disease-oriented evidence (DOE) refers to outcomes of pathophysiology, etiology, and pharmacology. Often these include test results and may also be called surrogate markers. We count them as important because we assume these intermediate outcomes are directly linked to the final outcomes. Consider guidelines that tell us to check for proteinuria in the diabetic patient. Why is the amount of protein in the urine important? Because it represents a marker for renal disease, we assume that less protein means that patients won't need dialysis or at least the need is delayed. Instead of assuming that an intervention that alters the quantity of proteinuria delays the need for dialysis or helps our diabetics live longer, why not study the final outcomes of morbidity and mortality? Insisting on evidence that is linked to final outcomes eliminates the assumption step and lets us know that what we are doing for our patients is more like to help than harm. These final outcomes are patient-oriented evidence (POEs) which are outcomes of mortality, quality of life, and disease prevention.

Why is this distinction so important? DOEs represent what ought to be based on our understanding of pathophysiology. What "ought to be," however, may not always turn out to be true. The medical literature is wrought with examples of medical decisions based on intermediate outcomes that were found not to withstand the longer term studies evaluating POEs: external fetal monitoring for low-risk pregnancies, calcium channel blockers for hypertension, antiarrhythmics for premature ventricular contractions after a myocardial infarction. These and other examples of POEs and DOEs are outlined in Table 28.1.

Table 28.1. Examples of Disease-Oriented Evidence (DOEs) and
Patient-Oriented Evidence that Matters (POEMs)

DOEs	POEMs
DOEs that were supported by POEMs	
Pap smears detect premalignant cervical lesions.	Routine screening with pap smears decreases the rate of cervical cancer mortality.
Statins lower cholesterol.	In hyperlipidemic patients with cardiac disease, statins lower the risk of recurrent cardiac events and improve survival.
Beta-blockers and diuretics lower blood pressure in hypertensive patients.	Beta-blocker and diuretic treatment of hypertension decreases MI and stroke and increases survival.
DOEs that were contradicted by POEMs	
Antiarrhythmics eliminate PVCs seen on telemetry in patients post-MI.	Routine use of some antiarrhythmics increases mortality in post-MI patients.
External fetal monitoring (EFM) detects concerning fetal heart tracing patterns.	In uncomplicated pregnancy, use of EFM increases cesarean rates and no improvement in neonatal outcomes is noted.
Calcium channel blockers (CCBs) lower blood pressure in hypertensive patients.	CCBs have been shown to increase rates of stroke, MI, and mortality.[23]

MI = myocardial infarction; PVC = premature ventricular contraction.

Two additional criteria must be considered when determining the relevance of medical information. First is the frequency with which the problem studied is encountered in your practice. Obviously, common problems are deserving of more attention. Second is deciding whether the information matters to you as a clinician. Would this evidence, if true, oblige you to change your current practice? If the perfect study were conducted demonstrating that penicillin treatment of strep pharyngitis prevented rheumatic heart disease, this should have little impact on our practices. However, a study demonstrating that estrogen replacement worsens urinary incontinence in postmenospausal women may offer motivation to not recommend this treatment to incontinent women. In this latter case, where our practice should be altered, the POE becomes a POEM, patient-oriented evidence that matters. The next step is validating the information to determine whether it should be applied.

Assessing the Validity of New Information

New research is believable only when it has been shown to be internally and externally valid. Internal validity is how well the evidence reflects the truth. To apply the results from a well-done study, the patient population needs to be similar enough to your patient or clinical population. This generalizability of the information to your own practice is external validity.

Determining validity is the hardest part of EBM for most people. Readers are often overwhelmed by statistical jargon and want to just accept that the editors have done that for them. Key validity considerations for different study types are outlined in Table 28.2. Readers can get a more detailed explanation from the "User's Guide" series (go to *http://www.cche.net/principles/content_all.asp*).[11] The IM worksheets offer a simplified version of validity assessment and can be obtained from the authors on request. One tip to lessen the work of evaluating study quality is to do this step as a group, for example in a resident journal club, or rotating responsibility among your clinical partners. Another option is to seek "prevalidated" sources, those where a known EBM/IM expert has done the quality evaluation for you.

The IM model tells us that focusing our attention on common, valid POEMs will maximize usefulness and help us offer the best care to our patients. When encountering any information source, first assess relevance (is it a common POEM that, if true, changes practice?), and, only if relevant, proceed to do the work of validating the evidence.

Practicing Information Mastery

The vast amount of medical information available to us can be a jungle of opportunities and traps. We choose to enter this jungle for one of four reasons: to refresh our memories of something forgotten (retracing), out of interest (sporting), to answer clinical questions (hunting), and to keep up to date (foraging). For medical problems with which we have less clinical experience, our questions tend to be simplified: What are the causes of excessive vomiting in a 2-month-old? How does Crohn's disease usually present? These are background questions[12] and fall more into the first category of learning (or relearning). Sporting refers to seeking information that is uniquely interesting to us, our own research interests, or exploring the details about Aunt Agnes's zebra illness. Sporting, therefore, should be delegated to personal or academic time. Hunting and foraging have a direct impact on how we practice medicine and care for our patients

TABLE 28.2. Key Validity Issues for Different Types of Articles

Therapy	Diagnosis	Prognosis	Systematic reviews
Randomized controlled trial?	Cohort design?	Prospective following of an inception cohort?	Comprehensive search for studies?
Double blinding?	Consecutive enrollment of patients?	>80% follow-up?	A priori inclusion criteria defined?
Concealed allocation?	Appropriate reference standard applied to all patients?	Generalizability?	Validity assessment included of studies?
Explanation of follow-up and withdrawals?	Independent, blinded application of the new test?	Blind assessment of outcomes?	Test for homogeneity?
Intention to treat analysis?			Appropriateness of combining results?
Generalizability?			

every day and require the use of the best current information. This section offers practical suggestions for beginning your evidence-based practice: how to hunt, how to forage, and how to approach nonliterature sources of medical information. Remember, the usefulness equation is our model for all three: minimizing work, maximizing relevance, and maximizing validity.

Hunting

If a patient asks a question or one arises during patient care, we must find the answer. Right? Not necessarily. Doing so is the equivalent of reading every article encountered, and is likely not feasible. Thus the first consideration in hunting is deciding whether we actually need to hunt! This parallels the common criteria for relevance outlined above. A general rule to follow here is asking, "Will this answer apply to another patient before it becomes out of date?" If not, then it may not be worthwhile to hunt for the answer yourself. Suppose a patient with hairy cell leukemia asks your advice about the best treatment for her cancer. It's not likely that you as the family doctor will be prescribing that, nor is it likely that today's answer will be tomorrow's (or next year's) answer when you next encounter someone with this cancer. This question could be deferred to the patient's oncologist. Another patient whose psoriasis calms in the summer sun wonders if buying a light box for home use in the winter will help. Relative to other skin conditions, psoriasis is less common in primary care, but you will likely soon encounter other patients with this problem and proceeding to find an evidence-based answer is appropriate.

The next step is deciding when to hunt. Those newly in practice or those new to EBM will likely find it challenging to do evidence searches during busy office hours. Questions need not always be answered while patients are there; set a follow-up appointment and commit yourself to finding an answer before then. Keep a list of questions that arise during practice, prioritize them for relevance, and hunt for evidence-based answers whenever you can—during lunch or before returning patient phone calls, or when on call. Faculty might find some time during resident precepting. The bottom line here is to just do it; whatever steps you take toward answering clinical questions with evidence are steps toward an evidence-based practice. As your skills and information technology advance, finding answers "on the fly" will be easier. Programs that search multiple Internet sites simultaneously (TRIP, *http://www.tripdatabase.com*; SumSearch, *http://www.sumsearch.uthscsa.edu*), and newer evidence-based information tools (Medical Inforetriever, *http://www.medicalinforetriever.com*) are available on personal and handheld computers to bring evidence answers to the point of care.

Finally, knowing how and where to hunt is critical. Because a good answer begins with a good question, learning to ask well-constructed questions is the first step. Foreground questions are those specific questions about the best treatment or testing strategy; they arise more frequently as our medical experience increases and thus are best answered by using current evidence.[13] The four components of a good question form the PICO acronym:

*P*atient and problem information (age, race, severity of illness, setting, comorbid illnesses)

*I*ntervention proposed (which may represent medications, or advice, or screening tests)

*C*omparison group (no intervention, or standard of care)

*O*utcomes of interest (which should be POEMs).

This PICO format helps convert your clinical question into a search strategy that maximizes your chance of finding relevant information.

Developing reasonable searching techniques will also help minimize the work of hunting, although many busy clinicians will not have the time do to this on their own. A medical librarian (*http://www.crmef.org/curriculum*) can help train you to a sufficient level of skill for independent searching, addressing such things as Boolean search terms, truncation of keywords, and linking terms to medical subject headings. Established search strategies have been developed that help maximize the return of valid studies. For example, searching in PubMed offers the advantage of the clinical queries feature. Selecting the search purpose (therapy, diagnosis, prognosis, or etiology) links your clinical search terms with study design terms to improve the retrieval of more valid study types.

The last part of efficient hunting is knowing where to start. The medical information system can be envisioned as a pyramid (Fig. 28.1), with the most useful information, the most relevant and valid or predigested sources, at the top. Many of us were trained to look for evidence by searching Medline; however,

Drilling for the Best Information

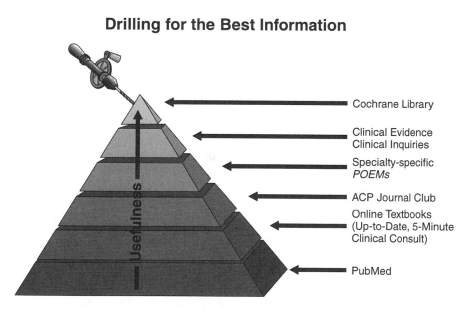

FIGURE 28.1. The medical information system depicted as a pyramid. The usefulness of the information increases as one climbs the pyramid.

this is the largest and least sorted database and therefore takes the most work to search. By starting at the top of the pyramid of sources and drilling down only as far as necessary to find a relevant and valid answer to the question, much time can be saved. The pyramid also shows us which databases are the most relevant and valid. Table 28.3 contains further information on each of these databases, as well as tools to search through the various databases.

It will likely take time and practice for the average clinician to develop efficient hunting skills. However, even asking questions and considering the quality of the evidence one finds are simple first steps in the continuum toward a more evidence-based practice.

Foraging

Doctors cite journal reading as one key method for keeping up to date; many of us have a bedside stack. In reality, though, we do a poor job of reading journals (or else there would be no stack!). Nor do we succeed at incorporating that information into practice. Instead of reading the stack, consider scanning the stack for relevant evidence. Read only the abstract conclusion and ask yourself the relevance question: Is this a common POEM that will change my practice? Read on to validate only those articles that pass the relevance criteria. In this way IM limits what we need to read, but also increases the responsibility of carefully assessing the information deemed relevant.

Even better strategies can be developed to forage the medical literature with less work and more likelihood of retrieving relevant and valid information. Four basic principles apply to a practical foraging strategy: (1) regularly casting a broad net, (2) being aware of the best sources of information, (3) using relevance criteria to screen information for usefulness, and (4) developing a retrieval system.

Since family physicians see a broad range of patients and problems, we especially have a need to be far-reaching in our attention to the medical literature. Scanning the most respected journals and all of our own specialty journals still leaves us at risk for missing a potentially relevant article. For example, a well-done trial was published in *Neurology* in 1998 demonstrating effective migraine prophylaxis from high-dose riboflavin.[13] Most family physicians do not read *Neurology* regularly and would have missed this potentially useful information. Since less than 4% of original research represents POEMs,[14] a lot of sieving is required to identify the few nuggets of gold. Even the journals with the highest POEM:DOE ratios—*JAMA, Lancet, British Medical Journal, Annals of Internal Medicine, Journal of Family Practice (JFP)*—have at most one or two articles per issue pertinent for family doctors.[14]

By perusing "POEM bulletin boards," we can let others do this filtering work for us. *JFP* POEMs is a site that can reduce the work of foraging. Editors scan more than 90 journals monthly, using the IM criteria to select articles of relevance specifically to family doctors. Eight of 25 to 30 relevant articles are selected each month and the summaries of the critical appraisal and key population and outcome information are published in the *JFP*. These reviews can be

TABLE 28.3. Explanation of the Databases in the Information Pyramid (see Fig. 28.1).

Database	Content/description	How to access
Cochrane Library	Database of SRs of therapeutics: high-quality MAs updated approximately every 2 years Database of abstracts of reviews of effectiveness DARE: validated summaries of published SRs/MAs Controlled Trials Registry	Cochrane SR abstracts available free online at *http://www.som.flinders.edu.au/fusa/cochrane/cochrane/revabstr/mainindex.htm* Full library available by subscription with quarterly updates
Clinical evidence	Text covering many clinical topics with full outline of evidence-supported treatments	In print; online version available from BMJ at *http://www.evidence.org*
Clinical inquiries	Database of evidence-based answers to a prioritized list of questions generated by FPs	2-4 are published each month in the JFP (available free online at *http://www.jfponline.com*) Soon will be housed in a searchable electronic database
JFP POEMs	Summaries of original research articles relevant to FPs with validity assessments	8 published each month in the JFP; search entire database of POEMs on the Web at *http://www.medicalinforetreiver.com*
ACP Journal Club	Critically appraised summaries of recent literature relevant to medical practice but not specifically for FPs	Available by subscription only
MD consult (5-minute consult)	Comprehensive collection of books, journals, news, and patient education sources	Available online for subscription fee (Accessed at *http://www.5mcc.com/*)
PubMed	National Library of Medicine's database with over 10 million citations Clinical queries feature links your search with built-in filters to better find validly designed studies for therapy, diagnosis, etiology, and prognosis	Accessed free at *http://www.ncbi.nlm.nih.gov.entrez/*

ACP = American College of Physicians; BMJ = *British Medical Journal*; EBM = evidence-based medicine; FP = family practitioner; JFP = *Journal of Family Practice*; MA = meta-analysis; SR = systematic review.

found and searched online at *www.medicalinforetriever.com*. The remaining studies are critically appraised and summarized in both the *Evidence-Based Practice* newsletter and the daily e-mail electronic newsletter (*InfoPointer*).

Other abstracting services do similar work. The American College of Physicians Journal Club (ACPJC) publishes validated summaries of original research. Although they cite relevance to medical practice as selection criteria, ACPJC does not target primary care specifically, nor does it use the IM relevance criteria.[15] Other services (Tips from Other Journals, Journal Watch) highlight potentially relevant research without a formal validity assessment. These may best be used by scanning the summaries and applying the relevance criteria to identify truly relevant information for your practice. Unfortunately, needing to personally perform a validity assessment greatly increases the work involved in applying the information into practice. Thus, secondary sources offering both relevant and valid information are preferred.

Newer electronic services are emerging that further lessen the work. Medical InfoPointer (*www.medicalinforetriever.com*) is an abstracting service that carefully evaluates research for relevance and validity and delivers a short synopsis with a "bottom line" recommendation of one article each day via e-mail. Bandolier on the Web (*bandolier@pru.ox.ac.uk*) is a British evidence-based medicine resource that will e-mail its monthly table of contents to interested readers.

Regardless of the strategies employed, the final and essential step of foraging is to create a retrieval system. The traditional version of this was cutting the article out from the journal and filing it your cabinet in some reasonable ordering system. Today's clinician needs to "file" the key information (population and intervention details, outcomes assessment and magnitude of results, and the original citation) in an electronic system on handheld or personal computer to make it available quickly during patient care. Web-based software (e.g., Avantgo) makes it possible to download Web pages to store in your electronic folders. Many of the foraging sites above also have searching capabilities—so if you remember that the riboflavin article for migraine prophylaxis was in *JFP* POEMs, you can quickly search that database to retrieve the answer in a matter of seconds. The paper version of foraging is still a great first step toward better information mastery. But ultimately, technology phobia or not, you'll likely need to develop some simple computer skills in searching and filing or you'll be left behind.

Other Medical Information Sources

As a general rule, when evaluating the usefulness of any source of information consider the work, the relevance, and the validity of the information. A sampling of information sources are highlighted below using the usefulness equation as the guide.

MEDICAL LITERATURE THAT IS NOT ORIGINAL RESEARCH

Summary reviews are those that paint a broad landscape of a clinical topic; they likely include the classic presentation, epidemiology, and diagnostic and therapeutic suggestions. We may be enticed by these reviews; they seem to be a low-work option, one stop shopping. Yet because the authors usually do not specify their methods for finding or evaluating the evidence, we are often not sure of the relevance and quality of information upon which recommendations are based. In fact, the quality of these reviews varies inversely with the level of expertise of the author,[16] suggesting that authors may begin with their conclusions and report only the data that support their recommendations, while ignoring contradictory reports! When reading summary reviews, if you stumble across advice that is contrary to your current practice, check whether the recommendation is based on a POEM, and if so (or if you can't tell), consider finding the original study yourself to evaluate the true usefulness. This added work makes this type of article less useful in the long run. Summary reviews may best be reserved for retracing, or when we have background rather than foreground questions.

Similar issues exist for clinical practice guidelines (CPGs). The intent of CPGs is to provide recommendations supported by available information that help clinicians make medical decisions. However, the quality of these seemingly low-work sources can vary greatly, from purely consensus-based opinion to a summary and synthesis of only quality evidence. Characteristics of quality CPGs include a brief summary statement for each recommendation, a long reference section pointing to original research, a methods section explaining how evidence was obtained and evaluated, and a detailed discussion of the evidence. Identifying an evidence table, a balance sheet, or some indication of the strength of the supporting evidence increases the likelihood of the CPG being evidence-linked. The relevance varies between and within CPGs; scanning for recommendations that are POEM-based can help identify those that are more relevant. Specific criteria for evaluating the validity of CPGs have been developed.[17]

CONTINUING MEDICAL EDUCATION (CME)

Doctors cite attendance at CME programs as the second most common strategy to keep up to date. Yet the passive, lecture-based CME rarely improves knowledge and almost never changes behavior. Since most CME talks are similar in structure to the summary type reviews, we may be falsely lulled into thinking we're learning a lot when in fact we're not. Interactive educational processes and those that incorporate an audit/feedback system are more likely to influence us. But to truly make CME useful requires your attention and participation as a member of the audience. Keep your ears open for any recommendation by the speaker that would change your current practice. Ask follow-up questions about the evidence on which the speaker based her suggestions. Was it POEM data? What was the quality of the data? Are the references available? Implement only those that are valid POEMs.

EXPERTS

In the context of medical information, an expert is anyone of whom we ask a clinical question. Most often we turn to "content experts," those with more expertise in the topic of inquiry. Yet the answers they give can often be quite subjective, based more on experience than valid data.[18,19] Clinical scientists are those with expertise in evaluating information for validity but may not necessarily be content experts. The best experts are YODAs (your own data analyzers),[20] who have and share the evidence basis for their recommendations, balancing it with their clinical experience. Our suggestion is to seek out the YODAs in your own community. When referring patients or asking questions of your consultants, include specific requests for the source of their recommendations. It may be solely experience based, but knowing this will help you keep your eyes and ears open for valid POEMs in the future.

PHARMACEUTICAL REPRESENTATIVES

Pharmaceutical representatives (PRs) are seemingly the source of medical information that requires the least amount of effort—they come to *you* often bringing lunch! Frequently the information they supply is not relevant (DOE based) or the methodology of the studies isn't sound. This serves to remind us that work must be balanced with relevance and validity to define usefulness. Ask for their sources to assess the usefulness of their information.

Even more helpful may be to ask PRs explicitly for the information needed to decide if their suggested therapy is better than what you currently prescribe. The STEPS mnemonic is a helpful way to remember these key questions. *S*afety refers to the long-term absence of harmful drug effects, whereas *t*olerability is the significance of more short-term side effects. Since we cannot judge whether a patient's headache is more significant than his stomach upset, the best measure of tolerability is pooled dropout rates from placebo-controlled trials. This information tells us who had side effects of any kind severe enough to warrant discontinuing the medication. *E*ffectiveness is not only whether the medication works— for POEM outcomes—but how well it works. We need to consider the clinical significance of the data presented (see application section). *P*rice refers to the cost not only of the medication but also of any associated monitoring required. *S*implicity is the ease of the medication regimen from the patient's perspective, and may influence compliance.

Application of Evidence

Clinical Significance

An important consideration in the application of evidence to individual patients is the clinical significance of the effect. It is not sufficient to ask whether one treatment is better than another; we need also to ask *how much* better. For example, one of the currently available antivirals is proven to shorten the duration of symptoms in adults with influenza (i.e., the statistical difference). But the amount of benefit is approximately a half day less of symptoms (i.e., the clinical difference). In the course of a 7-day illness, this may not seem worth the expense or risk of intestinal side effects to most patients. Yet to a busy stockbroker, taking the drug to possibly be able to return to work 4 hours sooner may be worthwhile. Clinical experience and patient perspective are the basis for deciding the clinical significance of such a finding.

The number needed to treat (NNT) is another measure of clinical significance. Calculated as the inverse of the rate difference, NNT tells us how many patients need to be treated for one to receive benefit. Consider two patients with elevated cholesterol: first is a 63-year-old male smoker with hypertension, total cholesterol of 250, and a high-density lipoprotein (HDL) of 35; the other is a 37-year-old woman with a total cholesterol of 328 and an HDL of 40. The statins have been shown to lessen the risk of a cardiac event by approximately 30%.[21] Intuitively we'd encourage the man to take lipid-lowering medication more so than the woman, because his cardiac risk is greater. NNT allows us to quantify the benefit for each. Using incidence data from the Framingham study[22] to calculate baseline risk, the man's 10-year risk of a cardiac event decreases from 30.4% to 20% and the woman's from 3.2% to 2.2% if treated with a statin. This yields NNTs of 9.6 and 100, respectively. Thus, the same medication yields a very different level of clinical benefit for each patient and should influence who receives treatment.

Clinical Jazz

If EBM were solely medical decision making based on evidence, it would become what critics call cookbook medicine, and could be done by computers. Either that, or we'd be paralyzed, unable to care for patients at all because there just aren't valid POEM data for much of what we do. Yet if we practiced only experience-based medicine, we may still be bloodletting our preeclamptic patients because some of them got better. Lest we consider this an unrealistic example, how many of us are victims of the latest bad experience bias? Objective evidence of this bias is seen in obstetricians whose cesarean section rates increase following an adverse event.[23] Clinical experience is important, but as the sole evidence source it is fraught with biases that would never be acceptable if presented in a research article: small sample sizes, lack of blinding or randomization, lack of standardized outcome measurements, and nonrandom loss to follow-up.

EBM is not really in competition with clinical experience. The newer definition of EBM integrates the use of evidence, balanced with clinical judgment and the patient's preferences. In the IM model, this is clinical jazz. And like fine jazz music, it requires structure—the evidence of valid POEMs—along with improvisation—our clinical experience. Following this structure can actually be liberating. Basing our decisions on well-done outcomes-based research helps us avoid being ping-ponged between conflicting recommendations and may increase our confidence with medical decision making. The simplicity of the structure allows us ample room for improvisation. We use our judgment every time we make a decision in the absence of ideal evidence: POEMs with study flaws, or valid

DOEs, or no existing evidence addressing our clinical questions. A key component of EBM in these situations is the awareness that our decisions are based on this lesser-than-ideal level of evidence and keeping our eyes open to replace that information when better quality data are available.[24]

Conditions with multiple valid POEMs, such as hypertension, provide opportunities to improvise as well. We rely on our clinical experience to apply most research data, since the patients we see in our offices are rarely as healthy, nor is our follow-up as rigorous, as those in randomized controlled trials.

Finally, our artistry and communication skills are needed to negotiate with patients whose preferences differ from the evidence. One patient may refuse colon cancer screening, despite high-quality relevant data in support of flexible sigmoid-oscopy; a mother may demand a computer tomography (CT) scan to evaluate her child, who has an acute headache but a normal exam and evidence demonstrating no need for a CT scan. A restricted view of EBM would suggest we only perform those services with evidence to support them; patient-centered medicine may seem like bowing to the patient's wishes regardless of the evidence. Clinical jazz is harmonizing the evidence, our experience, and our patients' views together to come to a reasonable decision. This is a true evidence-based medical practice!

References

1. Sackett DL, Rosenberg WMC, Gray JAM, Haynes RB, Richardson WS. Evidence based medicine: what it is and what it isn't. BMJ 1995;312:71–2.
2. Evans DE, Haynes RB, Gilbert JR, et al. Educational package on hypertension for primary care physicians. Can Med Assoc J 1984;130:719–22.
3. Shin JH, Haynes RB, Johnston ME. Effect of problem-based, self-directed undergraduate education on life-long learning. Can Med Assoc J 1993;148:969–76.
4. Slawson DC, Shaughnessy AF. Treatment of corneal abrasions. JAMA 1996; 275(11):837.
5. Flynn CA, D'Amico F, Smith G. Should we patch corneal abrasions? J Fam Pract 1998;47:264–70.
6. Fineburg HV. Clinical evaluation: how does it influence medical practice? Bull Cancer 1987;74:333–46.
7. Ely JW, Oheroff JA, Ebell MH, et al. Analysis of questions asked by family doctors regarding patient care. BMJ 1999;319:358–61.
8. Slawson DC, Shaughnessy AF, Bennett JH. Becoming a medical information master: feeling good about not knowing everything. J Fam Pract 1994;38:505–13.
9. Connelly DP, Rich EC, Curley SP, Kelly JT. Knowledge resource preferences of family physicians. J Fam Pract 1990;30:353–9.
10. Arndt KA. Information excess in medicine. Overview, relevance to dermatology, and strategies for coping. Arch Dermatol 1992;128:1249–56.
11. Oxman AD, Sacket DL, Guyatt GH. Users' guides to the medical literature. I. How to get started. JAMA 1993;270:2093–5.
12. Asking answerable clinical questions. In: Sackett DL, Straus SE, Richardson WS, Rosenberg W, Haynes RB, eds. Evidence-based medicine: How to practice and teach EBM, 2nd ed. Edinburgh: Churchill Livingstone, 2000;13–27.

13. Schoenen J, Jacquy J, Lenaerts M. Effectiveness of high-dose riboflavin in migraine prophylaxis: a randomized controlled trial. Neurology 1998;50:466–70.
14. Ebell MH, Barry HC, Slawson DC, Shaughnessy AF. Finding POEMs in the medical literature. J Fam Pract 1999;48:350–5.
15. Slawson DC, Shaughnessy AF. Becoming an information master. Using "medical poetry" to remove the inequities in health care delivery. J Fam Pract 2001;50:51–6.
16. Oxman AD, Guyatt GH. The science of reviewing research. Ann NY Acad Sci 1993;703:125–33.
17. Hayward RSA, Wilson MC, Tunis SR, Bass ER, Guyatt G. Users' guides to the medical literature. VIII. How to use clinical practice guidelines. A. Are the recommendations valid? JAMA 1995;274:570–4.
18. Slawson DC, Shaughnessy AF. Obtaining useful information from expert-based sources. BMJ 1997;314:947–9.
19. Chalmers TC. Informed consent, clinical research and the practice of medicine. Trans Am Clin Climatol Assoc 1982;94:204–12.
20. Shaughnessy AF, Slawson DC, Bennett JH. Becoming an information master: a guidebook to the medical information jungle. J Fam Pract 1994;39:489–99.
21. LaRosa JC, He J, Vupputuri S. Effect of statins on risk of coronary disease: a meta-analysis of randomized controlled trials. JAMA 1999;282:2340–6.
22. Anderson KM, Odell PM, Wilson PW, Kannel WB. Cardiovascular disease risk profiles. Am Heart J 1990;121:293–8.
23. Turretine MA, Ramirez MM. Adverse perinatal events and subsequent cesarean rates. Obstet Gynecol 1999;94:185–9.

INDEX